The
ABSITE REVIEW:
Practice Questions

2nd Edition

Steven M. Fiser MD

The ABSITE Review: Practice Questions
2nd Edition

Steven M. Fiser MD
Hancock Surgical Consultants, LLC
Richmond, Virginia

Contents:

Cell Biology

1. DNA polymerase is involved in:
   a. Transcription
   b. Translation
   c. Duplication
   d. Protein carboxylation

   Answer c. DNA polymerase is responsible for **duplication** of DNA. **DNA polymerase chain reaction** uses oligonucleotides to amplify specific DNA sequences (a tool used in research).

2. RNA polymerase is involved in:
   a. Transcription
   b. Translation
   c. Duplication
   d. Protein carboxylation

   Answer c. RNA polymerase is responsible for **transcription**, the process by which DNA is copied into mRNA.

3. Proteins are synthesized from:
   a. DNA
   b. rRNA
   c. tRNA
   d. mRNA

   Answer d. Ribosomes **translate** mRNA into specific proteins (amino acid sequences).

4. Anti-viral protease inhibitors used in patients with HIV work by:
   a. Preventing protein precursor cleavage
   b. Activating lysosomes
   c. Degrading ribosomes
   d. Inhibiting RNA polymerase

   Answer a. Protease inhibitors prevent viral replication by selectively binding viral proteases and preventing protein precursor cleavage, which is necessary for the production of infectious viral particles.

5. Steroid hormones:
   a. Bind a receptor on the plasma membrane and activate a plasma membrane enzyme
   b. Bind a cytoplasmic receptor, enter the nucleus, and affect transcription of mRNA
   c. Bind a receptor in the nucleus and affect transcription of RNA
   d. Do not enter the cell

   Answer b. Steroid hormones bind a receptor in the cell cytoplasm, enter the nucleus as a steroid-receptor complex, and then affect transcription of mRNA for protein synthesis. **Thyroid hormone** affects transcription after binding a receptor that resides in the nucleus. Steroid and thyroid hormones require 1-2 hours before having effects.

6. Cells divide during what phase of the cell cycle?
   a. G1
   b. S
   c. G2
   d. M

Answer d. Cells divide during the M phase (mitosis).

<u>Cell cycle - 4 phases</u>
   G1 - Most variable part, determines **cell cycle length**
      Growth factors affect cell during G1
   S (synthesis) - cell is preparing for division
      Protein synthesis, DNA replication (DNA polymerase)
   G2 (G2 checkpoint) – stops cell from proceeding into mitosis if there is **DNA damage** to allow **repair** (maintains DNA stability)
   M (mitosis) - cell divides

7.   Omeprazole acts by binding:
      a. H_2 Histamine receptor
      b.   H / K ATPase
      c.   Acetylcholine receptor
      d.   Gastrin receptor

      Answer b. Omeprazole blocks the proton pump (H / K ATPase) in parietal cells.

8.   Tyrosine kinase:
      a.   Phosphorylates tyrosine residues
      b.   Decarboxylates tyrosine residues
      c.   Carboxylates tyrosine residues
      d.   De-phosphorylates tyrosine residues

      Answer a. Tyrosine kinase phosphorylates tyrosine residues. **Imatinib** (Gleevec) is a receptor tyrosine kinase inhibitor used in patients with malignant GIST (gastro-intestinal stromal tumors).

9.   What receptor does erythromycin bind to increase gastro-intestinal motility?
      a.   Somatostatin receptor
      b.   Acetylcholine and dopaminergic receptors
      c.   GABA receptor
      d.   Motilin receptor

      Answer d. Erythromycin binds the motilin receptor and can be used to increase motility.

10.   What portion of the lipopolysaccharide complex accounts for its toxicity?
      a.   Lipid A
      b.   Lipid B
      c.   Lipid C
      d.   Lipid D

      Answer a. Lipid A is the toxic portion of the **lipopolysaccharide complex** found with gram negative sepsis. Lipid A is the most potent stimulant for **TNF-alpha** release.

11.   Of the following, which is the most critical component in the neovascularization of tumor metastases?
      a.   HER receptor
      b.   VEGF receptor
      c.   Neu receptor
      d.   FGF receptor

      Answer b. One of the most critical elements in the **neovascularization** of metastases is the **VEGF** (vascular endothelial growth factor) **receptor.** Many new chemotherapeutic strategies target the VEGF receptor (a tyrosine kinase) or VEGF itself.

12.   All of the following are true except:

a.   Desmosomes anchor cells to each other
b.   Hemidesmosomes anchor cells to platelets
c.   Gap junctions allow communication between cells
d.   Tight junctions are water impermeable

Answer b. Hemidesmosomes anchor cells to extra-cellular matrix.

Desmosomes and **hemidesmosomes** – anchor cells
(cell–cell and cell–extracellular matrix molecules, respectively)
Tight junctions – occluding junctions that occur between cells; form a water
impermeable barrier (eg skin epithelium, bladder epithelium)
Gap junctions – formed between cells to allow communication

13.   All of the following are true except:
a.   Keratin is found in hair and nails
b.   Desmin is found in muscle
c.   Vimentin is found in skin
d.   The above are intermediate filaments

Answer c. Vimentin is found in fibroblasts.

Intermediate filaments:
Keratin (hair and nails)
Desmin (muscle tissue)
Vimentin (fibroblasts)

14.   Protein kinase A is activated by
a.   Ca
b.   Diacylglycerol
c.   cAMP
d.   ADP

Answer c. Protein kinase A is activated by **cAMP** (a second messenger).
Adenylate cyclase forms cAMP from ATP.

15.   Protein kinase C is activated by:
a.   Ca
b.   ATP
c.   cAMP
d.   ADP

Answer a. Protein kinase C is activated by **Ca** or **diacylglycerol** (both second
messengers). Diacylglycerol (DAG) and inositol tri-phosphate (IP_3) and formed
from PIP_2 by phospholipase C. Ca is released from the mitochondria.

16.   All of the following are true except:
a.   Cholesterol increases plasma membrane fluidity
b.   Intra-cellular calcium level is very low compared to extra-cellular level
c.   G proteins are GTPases
d.   The Golgi apparatus is the major site of ATP production

Answer d. Mitochondria are the major site of ATP production.

Hematology

17. Which of the following is the correct order of responses following vascular injury:
    a. Vasoconstriction, thrombin generation, platelet adhesion
    b. Platelet adhesion, vasoconstriction, thrombin generation
    c. Thrombin generation, vasoconstriction, platelet adhesion
    d. Platelet adhesion, thrombin generation, vasoconstriction
    e. Vasoconstriction, platelet adhesion, thrombin generation

    Answer e. vasoconstriction, platelet adhesion, thrombin generation

18. Thromboxane:
    a. Decreases platelet aggregation by increasing release of calcium in platelets
    b. Decreases platelet aggregation by decreasing release of calcium in platelets
    c. Increases platelet aggregation by increasing release of calcium in platelets
    d. Increases platelet aggregation by decreasing release of calcium in platelets

    Answer c. Thromboxane causes platelet aggregation by **increasing Ca^{++}** in platelets. This results in exposure of the Gp IIb/IIIa receptor and platelet binding.

19. Prostacyclin:
    a. Decreases platelet aggregation and causes vasodilatation
    b. Decreases platelet aggregation and causes vasoconstriction
    c. Increases platelet aggregation and causes vasodilatation
    d. Increases platelet aggregation and causes vasoconstriction

    Answer a. Prostacyclin decreases platelet aggregation and causes vasodilatation (mediated through **increased cAMP** in platelets).

20. All of the following are true except:
    a. Prostacyclin is synthesized in endothelium
    b. Thromboxane is released from platelets
    c. ASA inhibits cyclooxygenase
    d. Thromboxane is regenerated in platelets within 24 hours after ASA Tx
    e. Bleeding risk is best assessed with history and physical exam

    Answer d. Thromboxane is <u>not</u> regenerated in platelets as cyclooxygenase is irreversibly inhibited and platelets do not have nuclear material to re-synthesize cyclooxygenase. Endothelium does contain DNA and can re-synthesize cyclooxygenase.

21. Which of the following is required in formation of the pro-thrombin complex:
    a. Magnesium
    b. Potassium
    c. Selenium
    d. Cobalamin
    e. Calcium

    Answer e. Calcium is required in formation of the prothrombin complex. The pro-thrombin complex (Xase complex) uses **X, V, calcium, platelet factor 3,** and **pro-thrombin** (Factor II).

22. Which of the following coagulation factors is not synthesized in the liver:
    a. Factor V
    b. Factor VI
    c. Factor VII
    d. Factor VIII
    e. Factor IX

Answer d. Factor VIII is synthesized in vascular endothelium. **vWF** (von Willebrand Factor) is also synthesized in vascular endothelium and is important in hemostasis (links GpIb receptor on platelets to collagen).

23. Which of the following deficiencies results in a normal PT (INR) and prolonged PTT:
    a. Factor VII
    b. Factor V
    c. Factor X
    d. Factor II
    e. Factor VIII

    Answer e. Factor VIII (8)

24. Which of the following deficiencies results in a prolonged PT (INR) and normal PTT:
    a. Factor VI
    b. Factor VII
    c. Factor VIII
    d. Factor IX
    e. Factor X

    Answer b. Factor VII (7)

25. Which of the following factors has the shortest half-life:
    a. Factor VI
    b. Factor VII
    c. Factor VIII
    d. Factor IX
    e. Factor X

    Answer b. Factor VII (7)

26. All of the following are Vit K dependent factors except:
    a. Factor II
    b. Factor V
    c. Factor VII
    d. Factor IX
    e. Factor X

    Answer b. Factor V

27. All of the following platelet problems are true except:
    a. Bernard-Soulier disease involves a GpIb receptor defect
    b. Glanzmann thrombasthenia involves a GpIIb/IIIa receptor defect
    c. Uremia involves down-regulation of vWF
    d. Vit K deficiency leads to decreased platelet production

    Answer d. Vit K deficiency leads to decreased Vit K dependent factor production (**II, VII, IX** and **X**; also **protein C** and **protein S**)

28. All of the following apply to von Willebrand disease except:
    a. Type III disease does not respond to DDAVP (desmopressin)
    b. Type I and III disease have reduced quantity of circulating vWF
    c. Type III is the MC type
    d. It is the MC congenital bleeding disorder
    e. The defect is in platelet adhesion

    Answer c. Type I is the most common type of von Willebrand disease.

29. All of the following are true for hemophilia A (Factor VIII deficiency) except:
    a. Factor VIII levels should be raised to 100% pre-op before major surgery
    b. 1st line therapy for hemarthrosis is aspiration of the joint

c. Factor VIII levels should be maintained at 80-100% for 14 days post-op after major surgery
d. Hemophilia A and hemophilia B have the same bleeding risk which is dependent on factor levels

Answer b. 1st line therapy for **hemarthrosis** is **recombinant factor VIII and ice.** Range of motion exercises are started well after the bleeding is controlled for hemarthrosis.

First line Tx (and often **definitive Tx**) for any bleeding issues (eg joint, intra-cerebral, contained GI bleed [eg duodenal hematoma]) associated with **hemophilia A** is **Factor VIII replacement** (for Hemophilia B – Factor IX).

30. All of the following are true of hemophilia A and B except:
    a. Patients with severe, life-threatening bleeds and high factor VIII or IX antibody titers should be treated with Factor VII concentrate
    b. DDAVP is not effective for Hemophilia B
    c. Both have prolonged PT
    d. Both are sex linked recessive

    Answer c. Both hemophilia A and B have **prolonged PTT**. DDAVP can be used for mild cases of Hemophilia A (stimulates release of Factor VIII / vWF).

31. All the following are true of antiphospholipid antibody syndrome (APAS) except:
    a. Classically has an elevated PTT (from lupus anticoagulant antibodies) that is not corrected with FFP (hypercoaguable with *elevated* PTT)
    b. Is associated with elevated anti-cardiolipin antibodies
    c. Patients are prone to spontaneous abortions
    d. Cardiolipin is a cell membrane phospholipid
    e. Is associated with elevated anti-lupus anticoagulant antibodies

    Answer d. Cardiolipin is a mitochondrial membrane phospholipid.

32. All of the following are true of hypercoaguable states except:
    a. Anti-thrombin III deficiency is associated with heparin resistance
    b. The mutation for Factor V Leiden is on protein C
    c. The MC acquired hypercoagulability disorder is smoking
    d. Hyperhomocysteinemia treatment is with folate and cyanocobalamin

    Answer b. Resistance to activated protein C (Factor V Leiden) is caused by a mutation on **Factor V**. *It is the MC congenital hypercoagulability disorder.*

33. The primary mechanism of uremia induced coagulopathy is:
    a. Preventing conversion of fibrinogen to fibrin
    b. Down regulation of the GpIb receptor
    c. Inhibition of von Willebrand factor (vWF) release
    d. Down regulation of the Gp IIb/IIIa receptor
    e. Inhibition of Anti-thrombin III

    Answer c. Uremia causes **inhibition of vWF release** and is the key dysfunctional element in **uremic coagulopathy**.

34. A 50 yo man on chronic hemodialysis is scheduled to undergo open inguinal hernia repair. Which of the following is the best therapy to help prevent intra-op bleeding:
    a. Hemodialysis
    b. Platelets
    c. DDAVP
    d. Factor VII concentrate

    Answer a. For non-acute situations, hemodialysis the day prior to surgery is the best preventative therapy for avoiding uremia and intra-op bleeding.

35. A 50 yo man on chronic hemodialysis presents with a clotted AV fistula graft and encephalopathy (BUN 125). You emergently place a temporary dialysis line which continues to bleed around the site. The best initial treatment for this patient is:
    a. Hemodialysis
    b. Platelets
    c. DDAVP
    d. Factor VII concentrate

    Answer c. The best acute treatment for bleeding associated with **uremia** is **DDAVP** (which causes release of vWF [and Factor VIII] from endothelium). If that fails, platelets should be given.

36. Prior to aortic valve replacement, you are unable to get the patient's activated clotting time (ACT) and PTT to an appropriate range that is safe for cardio-pulmonary bypass despite several rounds of heparin (ACT and PTT are normal). The patient was on heparin prior to surgery. The most appropriate next step is:
    a. Abandon surgery
    b. DDAVP
    c. Anti-thrombin III
    d. Factor VIII concentrate
    e. Cryoprecipitate

    Answer c. Pre-operative heparin therapy can decrease anti-thrombin III levels and cause relative **anti-thrombin III deficiency** resulting in **heparin resistance**. Tx is **recombinant anti-thrombin III**. If not available, **FFP** should be given (has highest concentration of AT-III).

    Anti-thrombin III deficiency can also present as **fresh red thrombus** following heparin administration for vascular procedures (eg fresh thrombus in an aortic graft after finishing the proximal anastomosis and moving the cross clamp)

37. After placing a left ventricular assist device (LVAD), diffuse bleeding occurs. Fibrinogen level is 20. The most appropriate next step is:
    a. FFP
    b. DDAVP
    c. Cryoprecipitate
    d. Factor VII concentrate
    e. Recombinant vWF:VIII

    Answer c. Cryoprecipitate has the highest concentration of **fibrinogen**. Normal fibrinogen levels should be > 100.

    Cryoprecipitate contains high concentrations of **Factor VIII, vWF,** and **fibrinogen**

38. The best treatment for thrombolytic overdose (eg urokinase, tissue plasminogen activator [tPA]) is:
    a. Aminocaproic acid (Amicar)
    b. FFP
    c. Packed red blood cells
    d. Cryoprecipitate

    Answer a. Thrombolytics work by converting plasminogen into plasmin. Plasmin then degrades fibrin. **Aminocaproic acid** (Amicar) works by binding plasminogen and preventing the conversion of plasminogen to plasmin.

    Fibrinogen levels < 100 are associated with increased risk and severity of bleeding. Tx with aminocaproic acid is indicated.

Prostatectomy or **TURP** can release **urokinase**, causing fibrinolysis and bleeding issues (eg persistent hematuria); Tx – aminocaproic acid (Amicar)

39. Which of the following would indicate disseminated intravascular coagulation (DIC), as opposed to simple fibrinolysis:
    a. Elevated D-dimer
    b. Elevated fibrin split products
    c. Decreased fibrinogen
    d. Decreased platelet count

    Answer d. Fibrinolysis is <u>not</u> associated with a decreased platelet count. DIC results in an elevated PT and PTT, decreased platelets, and decreased fibrinogen.

40. A 50 yo man is admitted for sigmoid diverticulitis (on CT scan). Despite fluid resuscitation and antibiotics he has the following lab values: BP 90/60, HR 105, WBC 20, PTT 100, platelets 35, INR 2.3, fibrinogen 40, elevated D-dimer, and elevated fibrinogen split products. The most essential step to improve this patient condition is:
    a. Rule out pulmonary embolism
    b. Colonoscopy
    c. FFP, cryoprecipitate, and platelets
    d. Sigmoidectomy

    Answer d. This patient has DIC based on lab values. Although blood products should be given pre-op, they will likely be soon consumed by the DIC process. The most important issue here is to remove the DIC source (ie sigmoidectomy for diverticulitis)

41. All of the following are true of deep venous thrombosis (DVT) except:
    a. The MC source of pulmonary embolism (PE) is ilio-femoral DVT
    b. The left leg develops DVT 2x more commonly than the right
    c. IVC filters should be placed above the renal veins
    d. An infected indwelling catheter with tip thrombosis requires removal
    e. An upper extremity DVT (eg arm swelling) related to an indwelling catheter is treated with catheter removal and heparin

    Answer c. **IVC filters** should be placed <u>below</u> the **renal veins**. If placed above renal veins, an embolus that clogs the filter can result in renal failure. HD catheters with infected thrombosis can't be salvaged (require removal).

42. All of the following are true of DVT risk except:
    a. The risk is elevated in pregnant patients compared to non-pregnant patients
    b. The risk is elevated in patients undergoing surgery for malignancy compared to those without malignancy
    c. The risk is elevated in patients undergoing open gastric bypass compared to those undergoing laparoscopic gastric bypass
    d. The risk is elevated in patients with Leiden Factor
    e. The best therapy for prevention of post-thrombotic syndrome is early thrombolytics

    Answer c. DVT risk is the same for patients undergoing open gastric bypass compared to laparoscopic gastric bypass. The pneumoperitoneum created intra-op (increasing risk of DVT) for patient undergoing laparoscopy is equally weighted by decreased ambulation post-op (increasing risk of DVT) in patients undergoing open surgery.

    Most adult surgery in-patients should receive DVT prophylaxis.

43. A 25 yo woman develops severe left leg pain and swelling to the level of her buttock. Her leg is massively swollen on exam with a blue appearance. Duplex U/S shows an

iliofemoral DVT. She still has motor and sensation in the extremity. The most appropriate next step is:

    a.   Open thrombectomy
    b.   Heparin only
    c.   Catheter directed thrombolytics
    d.   IVC filter

Answer c. This patient has **phlegmasia cerulea dolens**. This can result in leg gangrene so therapy is indicated. **Catheter directed thrombolytics** are superior to just heparin therapy alone for this condition.

44. Your patient has a recurrent pulmonary embolism despite appropriate anticoagulation and you decide to place an IVC filter. Pre-procedure U/S shows a ilio-caval DVT, the majority of which goes down the left common iliac vein. The most appropriate next step is:

    a.   Access the left femoral vein
    b.   Access the right femoral vein
    c.   Access the right internal jugular vein
    d.   Access the left internal jugular vein

Answer c. Patients with **iliocaval DVT** who require IVC filters should have them placed using the internal jugular vein as access (the right internal jugular vein is easier than the left for IVC filter placement).

45. You start Coumadin on a patient with a pulmonary embolus. Three days later, he starts sloughing off skin across his arms and legs. All of the following are true of this patients most likely condition except:

    a.   This is prevented by starting heparin before Coumadin
    b.   Patients with protein C deficiency are more susceptible
    c.   The skin sloughing is caused by skin necrosis
    d.   This patient most likely has hemophilia A

Answer d. Warfarin induced skin necrosis occurs when Coumadin is started without being on heparin 1st. It results from a relative hypercoaguable state because of the shorter half-life of protein C and S compared to factors II, VII, IX and X (Vit K dependent factors). Protein C and S decrease after Coumadin before the other factors decrease, resulting in a hypercoaguable state.

Patients with **protein C deficiency** are at increased risk for warfarin induced skin necrosis. It is prevented by starting heparin before giving Coumadin.

46. All of the following are true except:

    a.   Low molecular weight heparin (LMWH) binds Anti-thrombin III (AT-III) and neutralizes Factors IIa and X
    b.   LMWH is not reversed with protamine
    c.   Fondaparinux is a direct thrombin inhibitor
    d.   Argatroban works independently of AT-III
    e.   Dabigatran (Pradaxa, a direct thrombin inhibitor) requires dose adjustment for renal insufficiency

Answer a. LMWH (eg Lovenox) binds AT-III and inhibits **Factor Xa _only_**. **Unfractionated heparin** binds AT-III and inhibits Factors **IIa** and **Xa**.

47. A 50 yo woman receiving heparin suffers a small stroke. Her platelet count is 88 (baseline platelet count at admission was 225). Her PTT is 85. Which of the following is most accurate for diagnosing HIT in this patient:

    a.   IgG to heparin
    b.   Current platelet count of 88
    c.   PTT 85
    d.   Admission platelet count of 225

Answer a. **Antibodies to heparin** (most commonly IgG to heparin-PF4 complex) is the most accurate way of diagnosing HITT.

48. Which of the following is the best choice for continued anticoagulation in the above patient:
    a. Continued IV heparin with steroids
    b. Subcutaneous heparin
    c. Low molecular weight heparin (Lovenox)
    d. Argatroban

    Answer d. Direct thrombin inhibitors (eg Argatroban, Bivalirudin [Angiomax]) are the treatment of choice for suspected HITT.

    Argatroban is preferred for patients with renal insufficiency (has hepatic metabolism) and bivalirudin is preferred for patients with liver problems (has renal metabolism)

49. A 50 yo man is diagnosed with stage II colon CA. He had a drug-eluting coronary artery stent placed 1 month ago and is on clopidogrel (Plavix). The most appropriate next step is
    a. Surgery while on Plavix
    b. Hold the Plavix only and operate after 5-7 days
    c. Hold the Plavix, start a short-acting IIb/IIIa inhibitor, and operate in 5-7 days
    d. Hold the Plavix and only start the IIb/IIIa inhibitor if stent thrombosis occurs

    Answer c. Holding Plavix, starting a short-acting IIb/IIIa inhibitor, and operating in 5-7 days is appropriate. Abruptly stopping Plavix within the first year of drug-eluting stent placement is associated with stent thrombosis and acute myocardial infarction.

BLEEDING RISK
- ***History*** *and **Physical Exam** - best way to predict bleeding risk*
- **Normal circumcision** - does not rule out bleeding disorders; can still have clotting factors from mother (eg hemophilia A - factor VIII crosses placenta)
- Abnormal bleeding with **tooth extraction** or **tonsillectomy** - picks up 99% of patients with a bleeding disorder
- MCC of surgical bleeding - **incomplete hemostasis**
- **Warfarin, Plavix,** and **ASA** - hold for 5-7 days prior to major surgery

NORMAL COAGULATION / ANTI-COAGULATION
- Initial response to **vascular injury** (in order) – vasoconstriction, platelet adhesion, and thrombin generation
- **Coagulation Factors**
  - All are synthesized in the liver except **Factor VIII** (synthesized in endothelium)
  - **vWF** (cofactor for VIII) - also synthesized in endothelium
  - Exposed **collagen, prekallikrein, kininogen** and **Factor XII** initiate the intrinsic pathway
  - **Tissue factor** and **Factor VII** initiate in the extrinsic pathway
  - **Vit K dependent cofactors** - **II, VII, IX** and **X**; also **protein C** and **protein S**
    - Warfarin inhibits these factors
  - **Factor VII** - has shortest half-life
- **Prothrombin complex** (Xase complex)
  - Includes **Factor X, Factor V, calcium, platelet factor 3,** and **prothrombin**
  - Prothrombin complex forms on platelets; catalyzes formation of **thrombin**
- **Thrombin** *(Key to **coagulation cascade**)*
  - Converts **fibrinogen** to **fibrin** (and fibrinogen degradation products)
  - Activates **factors V** and **VIII**
  - Activates **platelets**
  - Generated on platelet surface (prothrombin complex above)
  - **Fibrin + platelets = platelet plug** (hemostasis)
- **vWF** - links **GpIb** on platelets to collagen

- **Fibrin** - cross-links platelets by binding **GpIIb/IIIa**
- **Anti-thrombin III** (AT-III, *Key to anticoagulation*)
  - Binds and inhibits **Factors IIa** (thrombin), **IX, X,** and **XI**
  - **Heparin** binds **AT-III** and increases activity (1000 x)
- **Protein C** - degrades **Factors V** and **VIII**, also degrades **fibrinogen**
- **Protein S** - protein C cofactor

- MC *congenital* hypercoaguable disorder - resistance to activated protein C (Leiden Factor V)
- MC *acquired* hypercoaguable disorder - smoking
- Key RFs for **venous thrombosis** (Virchow's triad) - stasis. endothelial injury, and hypercoagulability
- Key RF for **arterial thrombosis** - endothelial injury

COAGULATION FACTORS
- **Fresh frozen plasma** (FFP) - contains all coagulation factors
  - Corrects coagulopathy from <u>liver disease</u> or <u>warfarin</u> (high PT or INR)
  - Is frozen so it takes time to thaw; effects are <u>immediate</u> after infusion
- **Cryoprecipitate**
  - Has highest levels of **Factor VIII, vWF,** and **fibrinogen**
  - Good for patients with **low fibrinogen** (< 100)
  - Can be used for **vWD** and **Hemophilia A**
- **Vitamin K** (IV, IM, or oral) - IV requires <u>12 hours</u> for effect; used for <u>warfarin</u> reversal; may be hard to re-anticoagulate with warfarin after receiving Vit K
- **Prothrombin complex concentrate** (factors II, VII, IX and X) - prepared from human FFP; given as an injection (is <u>not</u> frozen)
  - Preferred Tx to **acutely reverse warfarin** for **bleeding** (eg intra-cranial hemorrhage, major GI bleeding)
    - Do <u>not</u> have to wait for thawing and has highest concentration of Vit K dependent co-factors (warfarin inhibits these)
    - If prothrombin complex <u>not</u> available, give **FFP** *and* IV **Vit K**
  - Also for patients on warfarin undergoing **emergency surgery**
- **DDAVP** - causes release of **VIII** and **vWF** from endothelium
  - Used for acute reversal of **uremic coagulopathy**
  - Can be used for von Willebrand disease *(Types I and II, <u>not</u> Type III)*

COAGULATION MEASUREMENTS
- **PT** (pro-thrombin time; INR) - used to follow **warfarin** Tx
  - *Best test for liver synthetic function*
  - Picks up **Factors I** (fibrinogen), **II** (prothrombin), **V, VII,** and **X**
- **PTT** (partial thromboplastin time) - used to follow **heparin** Tx (want PTT 60-90 sec)
  - Picks up **all factors** *except* **Factor VII** and **Factor XIII**
  - Can be used to follow argatroban and bivalirudin
- ACT (activated clotting time) - want ACT 150-200 for routine anticoagulation
  - Want act > 480 for cardiopulmonary bypass
- INR >1.5 - relative contraindication to performing surgical procedures
- INR >1.3 - relative contraindication to central line placement, percutaneous needle biopsies, and eye surgery

CONGENITAL BLEEDING DISORDERS
- **von Willebrand disease** (von Willebrand factor [vWF] problems)
  - *MC congenital bleeding disorder (AD)*
  - MC Sx: **epistaxis**: others - gum bleeding, heavy menstrual flow, ecchymosis
  - vWF production occurs in **endothelium**
  - vWF links **GpIb receptor** on **platelets** to **collagen**
  - Dx: PT normal, PTT normal or slightly prolonged
    - Positive ristocetin test; measurement of vWF protein levels, platelet function analyzer (PFA-100), prolonged bleeding time *(rarely used)*
  - Tx: **recombinant factor VIII:vWF** *(best Tx)*; **DDAVP** *(except* Type III); **cryoprecipitate** (highest vWF concentration of all blood products)

- **Type I** (MC type, 70%) - reduced quantity of vWF (mild Sx's)
- **Type II** - have enough vWF but doesn't work well
- **Type III** - almost no vWF, get **severe bleeding** (**DDAVP does _not_ work*)

- **Hemophilia A** (factor VIII deficiency, sex linked recessive)
  - MC Sx: **hemarthrosis**; others - muscle, GI tract, or brain hemorrhage
  - Factor VIII **crosses placenta** → newborns may not bleed at circumcision
  - **Spontaneous bleed** - occurs at levels < 1%
  - Dx: **prolonged PTT** and a normal PT
  - Tx: **recombinant Factor VIII** *(best Tx)* or **cryoprecipitate** (highest Factor VIII concentration of all blood products)
  - **Elective surgery** - need Factor VIII levels 100% pre-op
    - Need to keep levels at 80-100% for **14 days** after surgery
    - Monitor PTT every 8-12 hours
  - **Hemarthrosis** (bleeding in joint spaces) → **do _not_ aspirate*
    - Tx: **recombinant Factor VIII**, ice, and late range of motion exercises (well after the bleeding is controlled)
  - **Epistaxis, intracerebral hemorrhage**, contained **GI hemorrhage** (subcapsular liver/splenic hematoma; duodenal hematoma), **retroperitoneal hematoma,** or **hematuria** - Tx: **recombinant Factor VIII**
  - Development of **alloantibodies** can occur with _both_ recombinant and plasma derived factor VIII or factor IX (Tx for severe, life-threatening bleeding in patients with high Factor VIII or IX antibody titers - **recombinant factor VII** [7])
- **Hemophilia B** (factor IX deficiency, sex linked recessive) - Sx's _same as above_
  - Dx: **prolonged PTT** and normal PT
  - Tx: **recombinant factor IX** *(best Tx)* or **FFP**
  - Want peri-op levels similar Hemophilia A
  - Tx for severe, life-threatening bleeding in patients with high Factor IX antibody titers - **recombinant factor VII**
- **Platelet defect bleeding disorders**
  - **Bernard-Soulier syndrome** (GpIb receptor defect)
  - **Glanzmann thromboasthenia** (GpIIb/IIIa receptor defect)
  - Dx: platelet function analyzer (PFA-100), platelets aggregation studies, prolonged bleeding time
  - Tx: **platelets**

UREMIC COAGULOPATHY
- Occurs in patients on **dialysis** (BUN > 60-80); have bleeding problems
- *Uremia inhibits release of vWF (key problem)*
- Tx: **hemodialysis** _(best Tx: reverses uremia and coagulopathy)_
  - Hemodialysis the day before a procedure is usual
- *Acute reversal Tx* (eg bleeding patient) → give **DDAVP** (stimulates endothelial release of factor VIII and **vWF**; 30 minute time of onset, lasts 4 hours); give platelets if refractory

DIC (Disseminated Intravascular Coagulopathy)
- Consumption of blood products that results in bleeding
- MCC - **sepsis** (eg pneumonia, cholecystitis, diverticulitis)
- Dx: low platelets, low fibrinogen, high fibrin split products, high D-dimer
  - Prolonged PT and prolonged PTT
- Tx: need to correct the underlying cause (eg antibiotics for sepsis or removal of septic source)

CONGENITAL HYPERCOAGULABILITY DISORDERS
- Present as arterial or venous thrombosis / emboli (eg cold leg, PE, stroke)
- **Factor V Leiden Mutation** (resistance to activated protein C)
  - *MC congenital hypercoagulability disorder (5% of population)*
  - Mutation is on **Factor V**
- **Hyperhomocysteinemia** (MTHFR mutation _or_ folate, B6 or B12 deficiency)
  - **Hyperhomocysteinemia** → Tx: folate, pyridoxine, cyanocobalamin
- **Prothrombin gene mutation** (G20210A)
- **Protein C deficiency**

- Protein S deficiency
- Anti-thrombin III deficiency
  - *Causes **heparin resistance** (heparin will not increase PTT)*
  - Have to give recombinant **AT-III** 1st (or FFP), then heparin
  - **FFP** has highest concentration of AT-III of all blood products
  - Can develop after previous heparin exposure
- **Tx for all above** _except_ AT III deficiency and hyperhomocysteinemia → post-op **heparin**, then warfarin

WARFARIN-INDUCED SKIN NECROSIS
- Occurs when placed on Coumadin without being heparinized first
- Skin sloughs off extremities
- Due to **short half-life of proteins C and S** which are decreased before pro-coagulation factors; get hypercoaguable state → **thrombosis**)
- Patients with **protein C deficiency** are especially susceptible
- Tx: **heparin** if it occurs; prevent by starting heparin _before_ warfarin

HITT (Heparin-induced thrombocytopenia and thrombosis)
- **Anti-heparin antibodies** cause **platelet destruction** and at times activation with **thrombosis**
- **IgG** binds to **heparin** after formation of the heparin-platelet factor 4 complex
- Forms a **white clot**; can occur with just one low dose of heparin
- Clinical suspicion:
  1) **platelet drop** to < 100 or < 50% baseline _or;_
  2) arterial or venous **thrombosis / embolism** (cold leg, DVT, PE)
- Dx: **antibodies** to **heparin**
  - ELISA *(quickest to get)*
  - Serotonin Release Assay *(SRA; most specific but have to send out)*
- Tx: **stop** heparin and start **direct thrombin inhibitor** if the patient requires anticoagulation (eg **Argatroban, Bivalirudin**), then warfarin
- **Platelet transfusion** is _contraindicated_ with HITT - causes **thrombosis**
- **Argatroban** is a **direct thrombin inhibitor** and not dependent on AT-III

APAS (Anti-Phospholipid Antibody Syndrome)
- Sx's: **thrombosis** (venous or arterial) *and/or* **loss of pregnancy**
- Dx: high **anti-cardiolipin** *or* **lupus anticoagulant antibodies**
- **Cardiolipin** is a _mitochondrial_ **phospholipid**
- **Lupus anticoagulant antibodies** - prolong coagulation reactions
  - Patients have **hypercoagulability with elevated PTT** (that does not correct with FFP)
- Causes - primary or from autoimmune disease (eg SLE)
- Tx: **heparin,** then warfarin after surgery (lifelong)

DEEP VENOUS THROMBOSIS (DVT)
- Post-op **DVT prevention** - majority of adult surgery inpatients should receive **LMWH prophylaxis** unless contraindicated (in addition to early ambulation + sequential compression devices [SCD's])
  - SCDs - improve venous return but also induce **fibrinolysis** with compression (**release of tPA**)
  - Trauma patients with highest risk of DVT - **spinal cord injury**
- Post-op **DVT Tx** - **LMWH** *(preferred over unfractionated heparin* - therapeutic levels achieved quicker; stabilizes clot, prevents extension), then **direct thrombin inhibitor** *(preferred* eg Pradaxa, Xarelto) or warfarin
- Sx's: 50% are _asymptomatic_; pain, swelling, warmth, unexplained fever
  - MC DVT location – **calf**
  - MC location to result in PE – **Ilio-femoral**
  - **Left leg 2x** MC than right (left iliac vein compressed by right iliac artery)
- **Virchow's triad** - venous stasis, hypercoagulability, endothelial wall injury
- Dx: U/S

- **Phlegmasia alba dolens** (painful, swollen **white** leg) - less severe than below
- **Phlegmasia cerulea dolens** (painful, swollen **blue** leg) - more severe; can lead to **gangrene**; usually occurs with **iliofemoral** DVT
  - Tx: **catheter-directed thrombolytics**
  - Emergent **open balloon** or **percutaneous mechanical** (eg AngioJet) **thrombectomy** if extremity **threatened** (ie loss of sensation or motor function)
  - 50% of these patients have a **malignancy** somewhere
- **Post-thrombotic syndrome** - pain, heaviness, edema, ulcers
  - Long term Cx in patients with DVT
  - Prevented with use of **catheter-directed thrombolytics** for early DVT
- DVT and **pregnancy** - warfarin _contraindicated_ in pregnancy (teratogenic; Tx: **LMWH**)
  - Increased risk related to pressure on veins in pelvis / lower extremities and circulating hormones
- DVT and **gastric bypass surgery**
  - The higher the BMI, the greater the risk of DVT
  - No difference between laparoscopic and open procedures
  - Prevention - **LMWH** prophylaxis and **early ambulation**
  - PE is the MCC of death after gastric bypass (50% of post-op deaths)
- **Temporary IVC filters** (inferior vena cava; can be removed):
  - Indications:
    - PE with contraindications to anticoagulation
    - Documented PE while on anticoagulation
    - Recent pulmonary embolectomy
    - Free-floating IVC, ilio-femoral, or deep femoral DVT (_controversial indication_)
  - _Want to place IVC filter below **renal veins**_
  - **PE with IVC filter in place** - embolus comes from ovarian (gonadal) veins, IVC superior to filter, or SVC (superior vena cava; upper extremities)
  - **Free floating ilio-femoral DVT and need to place IVC filter** - enter the internal jugular vein, pass through the SVC and right atrium down to the IVC; place filter below renal veins
- **Hemodialysis catheter** (or an indwelling catheter)
  - **Tip thrombosis** - Tx: systemic **heparin** or **tPA down catheter**
  - If **infected** with thrombosis - Tx: **remove catheter**
  - **Upper extremity DVT** (ie arm swelling, Dx: duplex U/S) related to catheter - Tx: **remove catheter**, start heparin (then Coumadin)

CLOPIDOGREL (Plavix)
- Is a platelet **ADP receptor inhibitor** (prevents platelet cross-linking)
- Have a **prolonged bleeding time**
- Issues with **coronary stents** - _high risk of **stent thrombosis** (and myocardial infarction) if Plavix is stopped early after stent placement_
- **Elective surgery** recommendations:
  - **Bare metal** stents - Plavix for **6 weeks** before elective surgery
  - **Drug eluting** stents - Plavix for **1 year** before elective surgery
- **Emergency surgery** - operate on Plavix, have platelets available
- **Semi-urgent surgery** - stop Plavix **5-7 days** pre-op (takes this long to clear); bridge with short-acting IIb/IIIa inhibitors [eg eptifibatide (Integrilin)]
- Tx for bleeding associated with Plavix: **platelets**

HEPARIN
- **Unfractionated Heparin** (UFH)
  - Binds **AT-III** and inhibits **Factors IIa _and_ Xa**
  - Want PTT 60-90; 1/2 life is 60–90 minutes
  - Cleared by **reticuloendothelial system** (macrophages, spleen)
  - Indications - massive PE; bridge to oral therapy for various conditions
  - Can use in pregnancy (does not cross placental barrier; warfarin does)
  - **Pre-op** - hold heparin for 6 hours prior to surgery
    - Re-start heparin after 48 hours if not bleeding
  - Side effects: early - HITT, long term use - osteoporosis, alopecia

- Acute reversal Tx: **protamine** (binds and reverses heparin)
  - MC S/E – protamine reaction (1%); an anaphylactic reaction with hypotension and bradycardia (Tx: fluid resuscitation, epinephrine)
- **Low molecular weight heparin** (LMWH) and **Fondaparinux**
  - Indications - DVT and sub-massive PE (initial Tx); DVT prophylaxis
  - Do not need to monitor PTT
  - **LMWH** is a selective AT-III - **Xa inhibitor**
  - **Fondaparinux** is a **direct thrombin inhibitor**
  - LMWH has much smaller HITT risk compared to UFH
  - Fondaparinux has no HITT risk
  - *These are not reversed with protamine (non-reversible agents)*
  - DVT prophylaxis dose is higher in post-op **gastric bypass** patients compared to other post-op patients
  - Need dose adjustment for **renal insufficiency**

DIRECT THROMBIN INHIBITORS (Vit K antagonists)
- **Intravenous** - Argatroban, Bivalirudin (AngioMax)
  - Indications - HITT requiring continued anticoagulation, percutaneous coronary interventions
  - *Not reversible*
  - **Argatroban** has hepatic metabolism
  - **Bivalirudin** has renal metabolism
  - *Follow **PTT** for both (want PTT 60-90)*
- **Oral** - dabigatran (Pradaxa), rivaroxaban (Xarelto), apixaban (Eliquis)
  - Indications - DVT, PE, atrial fibrillation (not from heart valve problem)
  - *Not reversible*; hold Xarelto/Eliquis 24-48 hours before surgery; Pradaxa 3-5 days
  - Need dose adjustment for **renal insufficiency**
  - Do not need to follow INR
  - Oral direct thrombin inhibitors compared to Coumadin have the same efficacy with **less bleeding cx's**

WARFARIN (Coumadin; Vit K antagonist)
- Indications - mechanical valves, atrial fibrillation due to heart valve problem
- Acute reversal Tx (eg head or moderate to severe GI bleed): **prothrombin complex**
  - If not available, give FFP *and* IV Vit K
- Side-effects - bleeding cx's

THROMBOLYTICS (eg tissue Plasminogen Activator [tPA], streptokinase)
- Indications - usually for vessel **thrombosis** and **ischemia**
  - Given with heparin, usually for **8 - 24 hours** (*avoid* giving > 48 hours – significant bleeding risk)
  - **Thrombolytics** work by converting plasminogen into plasmin
  - Plasmin then degrades **Factors V and VIII, fibrinogen** and **fibrin**
- Follow **fibrinogen** levels → fibrinogen < **100** has a high bleeding risk and Tx with **aminocaproic acid** is indicated
- **Thrombolytic overdose** (fibrinogen < 100) - Tx: **aminocaproic acid** (Amicar; is an anti-fibrinolytic)
- **Prostate surgery** - can release **urokinase**, activates plasminogen → thrombolysis; Tx: **aminocaproic acid**
- *Absolute contraindications to thrombolytics:*
  - Active or recent **internal bleeding** or **known bleeding disorder**
  - **Intracranial pathology** (stroke, significant brain trauma, or neurosurgery within last 3 months; brain tumor)
  - **Aortic dissection**
- *Major contraindications to thrombolytics:*
  - Recent (< 10 days) surgery, organ biopsy, eye surgery, obstetric delivery, or major trauma
  - Left heart thrombus, active peptic ulcer, or uncontrolled severe HTN
  - Pregnancy

tPA (tissue Plasminogen Activator)
- Released from **endothelium**
- Induces **fibrinolysis** by converting **plasminogen** to **plasmin**
- **Plasmin** - degrades **Factors V** and **VIII** along with **fibrinogen** and **fibrin**
  - Lose platelet plug, get elevated fibrin degradation (split) products (FDPs or FSPs, eg **D-dimer**)
- **Alpha-2 antiplasmin** - natural inhibitor of plasmin, released from endothelium
- **Prostate surgery** (eg TURP, prostatectomy) can release **urokinase**; induces **fibrinolysis** (converts plasminogen to plasmin)
  - Sx's: **bleeding**
  - Tx: **aminocaproic acid** (inhibits plasmin)

PROSTACYCLIN (PGI$_2$)
- Released from **endothelium**
- **Inhibits platelet aggregation** and causes **vasodilation**
- *Increases **cAMP** in platelets*
- **ASA** irreversibly binds **cyclooxygenase**, but cyclooxygenase is **re-synthesized** in endothelium (has nuclear material unlike platelets) - result is <u>normal</u> PGI$_2$ production and **platelet inhibition**

THROMBOXANE (TXA$_2$)
- Released from **platelets**
- Causes **platelet aggregation** and **vasoconstriction**
- *Increases **calcium** in platelets* → exposes **GpIIb/IIIa** and **GpIb receptors** (induces **platelet binding**)
- **ASA** irreversibly binds **cyclooxygenase**, decreasing TXA production for the life of the platelet (7 days, platelets do not have nuclear material – can't re-synthesize cyclooxygenase) - result is <u>decreased</u> TXA$_2$ production and **decreased platelet aggregation**
- **ASA** - prolongs bleeding time
- **WBCs** - contain nuclear material; **RBCs** - <u>no</u> nuclear material; **platelets** - <u>no</u> nuclear material

Blood Products

50. A 21 yo female patient with blood type B requires pRBCs. Which of the following is the safest blood type to give her:
    a. Type A, Rh negative
    b. Type AB blood, Rh negative
    c. Type O blood, Rh negative
    d. Type A, Rh negative
    e. Type B, Rh positive

    Answer c. Type O blood (universal donor) contains no A or B antigens. Rh negative blood is indicated for females of pre-pubescent or of child-bearing age.

51. All of the following are true of acute hemolytic transfusion reactions except:
    a. Bilirubin is likely low
    b. Haptoglobin is likely low
    c. Free hemoglobin is likely high
    d. Volume resuscitation is the 1st step in management
    e. It is antibody mediated

    Answer a. Bilirubin would be elevated due to RBC hemolysis.

52. All the following are true of transfusion related acute lung injury (TRALI) except:
    a. Is caused by donor antibodies which bind recipient WBCs which then lodge in lung
    b. Tx is similar to ARDS
    c. Result in decreased capillary permeability
    d. Results in pulmonary edema

    Answer c. TRALI results in increased capillary permeability (and fluid leakage) and is caused by donor antibodies to recipient WBCs.

53. Prevention of febrile non-hemolytic transfusion reaction involves:
    a. Heating blood to destroy the white blood cells
    b. Prophylactic antibiotics
    c. NSAID's
    d. Leukocyte filter

    Answer d. Febrile non-hemolytic transfusion reaction is caused by **white blood cells** in donor blood and can be prevented by using a leukocyte filter during transfusion (the filter size is large enough to allow red blood cells through but small enough to trap white blood cells).

54. One week after RBC transfusion, your patient develops diffuse purpura and epistaxis. Her platelet count is 12 (starting platelet count 250). Which of the following is correct:
    a. Emergent platelet transfusion is indicated
    b. This is likely due to bacterial contamination
    c. This is likely a bone marrow problem
    d. Platelet alloimmunization likely occurred with a previous transfusion

    Answer d. Platelet alloimmunization likely occurred with a previous transfusion. This patient has **post-transfusion purpura**, in which the patient developed antibodies to platelets (from previous **transfusion** [platelets, or RBC / FFP contaminated with a few platelets] _or_ **pregnancies**). Subsequent transfusion (platelets or RBCs / FFP with platelet contamination) activates the reaction. Important to note that the reaction is against _all_ platelets, _including the patient's own platelets_.

    Tx: **immunoglobulin** _(primary Tx)_, plasmapheresis, _no further platelet transfusions_

55. All of the following are true of blood products except:
   a. The MCC of infectious related mortality following blood transfusion is hepatitis B
   b. The MC blood product containing bacterial contamination is platelets
   c. The MC bacterial contaminant is skin flora (eg staph epidermidis)
   d. Blood transfusion increases the risk of infection
   e. The MCC of transfusion related death is TRALI

   Answer a. The MCC of infectious related mortality following blood transfusion is bacterial contamination. The MC blood product to contain a **bacterial contaminant** is **platelets** because they are stored at room temperature (good medium for bacterial growth). TRALI recently replaced ABO incompatibility as the leading cause to transfusion related death.

BLOOD TRANSFUSION
- **Type O blood** (universal <u>donor</u>) - contains no A or B antigens
  - **Males** can receive Rh positive blood
  - **Females** who are pre-pubescent or of child-bearing age should receive Rh negative blood
- **Type AB blood** (universal <u>recipient</u>) - contains both A and B antigens; can only be used in an AB blood type patient
- **Type specific blood request** - assesses ABO compatibility; *but <u>not</u> minor antigens*
- **Type and screen** - looks for **preformed antibodies** to **minor HLA antigens**
- **Type and crossmatch** - same as type and screen and the blood bank will crossmatch the number of units requested
- MCC mortality from transfusion - **TRALI** (previously **clerical error** leading to **ABO incompatibility**)
- **Packed red blood cells** (pRBCs)
  - **1 unit of pRBCs** - should increase Hgb by 1 gm/dl (Hct by 3-4)
  - pRBCs are stored in **citrate** (CDPA) for preservation - citrate **binds Ca^{++}**
    Citrate causes **hypocalcemia** with **massive blood transfusion** ($\geq$ 10 units/24 hours or $\geq$ 5 units within 3 hours)
  - Stored pRBCs last **3 weeks**
  - **Storage effects** on pRBCs - $\downarrow$ 2,3 DPG, $\downarrow$ pH, $\uparrow$ K$^+$, and $\uparrow$ lactic acid
  - Trying to **raise Hgb without giving blood** (eg Jehovah's Witness with low Hct before surgery) $\rightarrow$ Tx: **Epoetin** and **Fe supplementation**
    Should raise hemoglobin 1-2 gm/dl after a week (Hct 3-5 after a week)
  - **Iron deficient anemia** (microcytic anemia) in **male** or **post-menopausal female** – need to screen for colon CA or another GI source of bleeding
  - **CMV negative pRBCs** (from CMV negative donors) - used for CMV sero-negative pregnancy, organ and bone marrow TXP candidates/recipients, HIV patients, and low birth weight infants
- **Platelets**
  - Platelet transfusion indications:
    1) **< 10,000** (very high risk of **spontaneous bleeding**)
    2) **< 20,000** with **infection** or **bleeding risk** (eg post-op patients)
    3) **< 50,000** with **active bleeding** or **pre-procedure**
  - *Contraindications* – TTP, HUS, HELLP, HITT (may need to give platelets to control severe bleeding with these syndromes)
  - **1 six pack of platelets** (1 unit) - should increase platelet count by 50,000
- **Fresh frozen plasma** (FFP)
  - Contains **all coagulation factors** (includes protein C, protein S, and AT-III)
  - Good for patients with deficiency of coagulation factors (eg dilutional coagulopathy with massive transfusion, DIC [controversial], liver disease, patients on warfarin, PT > 17 pre-procedure)
  - Can be used for **Hemophilia B**
- **Cryoprecipitate**
  - Has highest levels of **Factor VIII, vWF,** and **fibrinogen**
  - Good for patients with **low fibrinogen** (< 100; consider aminocaproic acid 1st)
  - Can be used for **vWD** and **Hemophilia A**

INFECTIOUS COMPLICATIONS FROM TRANSFUSION

- **Hep B** - 1: 200,000, **Hep C** - 1: 2,000,000, **HIV** - 1: 2,000,000
- Blood is also tested for syphilis, HTLV, and West Nile virus
- MC <u>contaminant</u> (of all viruses and bacteria) - **skin flora** (eg **staph epidermidis**); others - yersinia, pseudomonas, E. coli
- MCC of infectious-related <u>death</u> - **bacterial contamination** *(not viral)*
- MC <u>blood product</u> with bacterial contaminant - <u>platelets</u> (1:50,000)
  - Platelets are stored at **room temp** - good medium for bacteria growth
  - Platelets last for **5 days** at room temp
  - Not refrigerated because **half-life** would be decreased
  - Sx's of transfusion associated bacteremia (**within 90 minutes** of transfusion) – fever (> 39 C), shivering, tachycardia (> 120); Tx: broad spectrum antibiotics
- All blood products carry risk of **HIV** and **hepatitis** *except* **albumin** and **immunoglobulins** (these are heat treated)
- **Immune system** - blood product **transfusion** *alters* the immune system, placing patients at increased risk of **infection**

MASSIVE BLOOD TRANSFUSION EFFECTS

- **Dilution** of coagulation factors and platelets - causes **coagulopathy**
- **Hypocalcemia** - manifested as **hypotension** and **coagulopathy**
  - Calcium is required for clotting cascade
  - **Citrate** - used in stored blood; binds calcium; causes hypocalcemia
- **Hypothermia** (cold body temp) - causes **coagulopathy** (slows enzyme reactions)
  - Use **blood warmer** to help prevent
  - Best Tx for patient hypothermia - **warm air conduction** (Bair Hugger)

BLOOD TRANSFUSION REACTIONS - HEMOLYSIS

- **Acute hemolytic transfusion reaction** - caused by **ABO incompatibility**
  - Sx's: chills, rigors, fever, back pain, hematuria, tachycardia, shock
  - In anesthetized patients, can present as **diffuse bleeding** and **hypotension**
  - Can lead to renal failure, DIC, and shock
  - Caused by preformed **recipient antibodies** against donor RBC **ABO antigens**
  - Is a Type II Hypersensitivity Reaction
  - Dx:
    > <u>Low</u> haptoglobin (< 50 mg/dL; binds Hgb, then gets degraded)
    > High free hemoglobin (> 5 g/dL)
    > High unconjugated bilirubin
    > High lactate dehydrogenase (LDH)
  - Tx: stop transfusion; **fluids** and **pressors** (maintain urine output); HCO$_3^-$
- **Delayed hemolytic transfusion reaction** - from minor antigens
  - Sx's: mild jaundice; may go unnoticed (5-10 days after transfusion)
  - Caused by preformed **recipient antibodies** against donor RBC **minor HLA antigens**
  - Tx: observe if stable; type + screen (checks for HLA antigens) with future transfusions
- **Alloimmunity**
  - Body gains immunity against antigens of foreign blood products
  - 1% risk of developing alloimmunity with **RBC transfusion**
  - 25% risk of developing alloimmunity with **platelet transfusion**
  - Alloimmunity can develop against **RBCs** <u>or</u> **platelets**
  - Alloimmunization against **RBCs** - can cause **delayed hemolytic transfusion reaction** (see above); generally well tolerated
  - Alloimmunization against **platelets** can result in:
    1) **Refractoriness** to platelet transfusion (ie platelet count didn't rise as much as it should have after platelet transfusion)
    2) **Post-transfusion purpura** *(rare)* - antibodies to platelets develops (from previous **transfusions** [platelet, or RBC / FFP contaminated with a few platelets] <u>or</u> **pregnancies**). Subsequent transfusion (platelets or RBCs / FFP with platelet contamination) activates the reaction. *Is a life-threatening problem as the patient's antibodies turn against the patient's own* **platelets** *(not just the transfused ones)*. Severe thrombocytopenia

can occur (platelet count < 15), usually about a **week** after transfusion. This is more common in **women** (RF - multiple previous pregnancies) Tx: **immunoglobulin** *(primary Tx)*, plasmapheresis, *no further platelet transfusions*

■ Non-immune hemolysis - **from squeezing the blood bag**

BLOOD TRANSFUSION REACTIONS - OTHER
■ **Febrile non-hemolytic transfusion reaction**
  ● Sx's: **fevers** and **rigors** 0-6 hours after transfusion
  ● Caused by preformed **recipient antibodies** against **donor WBCs**
  ● Causes **cytokine release**
  ● Tx: stop transfusion; acetaminophen
  ● Use **WBC** (leukocyte) **filters** for subsequent transfusions (WBC filters are generally used for all transfusions)
■ **Urticaria** (rash)
  ● Reaction of **recipient antibodies** to **plasma proteins** in the blood product
  ● MCC - **IgA deficient patient** (with preformed **IgE antibodies** to IgA) receiving **IgA blood**; other allergens (consumed by the donor) - nuts, penicillin
  ● Tx: **histamine blockers** (diphenhydramine [Benadryl]), supportive
■ **Anaphylaxis** (rare) - urticaria, bronchospasm, hypotension, angioedema
  ● Same mechanism as urticaria above
  ● Can be an **airway emergency**
  ● Tx: **epinephrine** (Epi pen), fluids, steroids, histamine blockers
■ **Transfusion-related acute lung injury** (TRALI)
  ● Sx's: hypoxia, diffuse alveolar infiltrates, fever
  ● Non-cardiogenic pulmonary edema **< 6 hours** after transfusion
  ● <u>**Donor**</u> **antibodies** bind <u>**recipient**</u> **WBCs** which then lodge in the lung
  ● WBCs release mediators causing ↑ **capillary permeability**
  ● Results in non-cardiogenic **pulmonary edema** < 6 hours after transfusion
  ● Tx: similar to ARDS (may require intubation)

Immune System and Wound Healing

56. The key growth factor in wound healing is:
    a. PDGF
    b. PAF
    c. EGF
    d. FGF

    Answer a. PDGF is the key growth factor in wound healing.

57. All of the following participate in angiogenesis except:
    a. PDGF
    b. PAF
    c. Hypoxia
    d. FGF

    Answer b. PAF does not have angiogenesis properties. **Hypoxia** is the most potent stimulus for angiogenesis.

58. All of the following are chemotactic for inflammatory cells except
    a. IL-8
    b. LTB-4
    c. C5a and C3a
    d. TGF-beta

    Answer d. TGF-beta is not chemotactic for inflammatory cells. It is generally considered immunosuppressive.

59. All of the following are functions of the listed cytokine except:
    a. IL-6 increases hepatic acute phase proteins
    b. IL-8 induces PMN chemotaxis and angiogenesis
    c. IL-10 upregulates the inflammatory response
    d. IL-I induces fever

    Answer c. IL-10 down-regulates the inflammatory response.

60. All of the following hepatic proteins are increased during the acute phase response except:
    a. Albumin
    b. C reactive protein
    c. C3
    d. Fibrinogen

    Answer a. There is decreased synthesis of albumin, pre-albumin, and transferrin during the acute phase response.

61. Which of the following Infections is associated with defects in cell mediated immunity:
    a. Staph
    b. E. Coli
    c. Tuberculosis
    d. Proteus

    Answer c. Infections associated with **defects in cell mediated immunity** include **intra-cellular pathogens** (eg TB, other mycobacterium, viruses).

62. All of the following are true of cell adhesion molecules except
    a. Selectins are involved in rolling adhesion
    b. L-selectin binds E-selectin and P-selectin
    c. ICAM binds beta-2 integrin (CD 11/18) molecules
    d. P-selectin is located on leukocytes

Answer d. P-selectin is located on platelets.

63. All of the following are true of complement except:
    a. C5b, C6b, C7b, C8b and C9b form the membrane attack complex
    b. C1, C2, and C4 are found _only_ in the classic pathway
    c. C1 and C2 are anaphylatoxins
    d. Factors B, D, and P (properdin) are found _only_ in alternate pathway

    Answer c. C3a, C4a and C5a are **anaphylatoxins**.

64. All of the following are true of oxygen radicals except:
    a. The primary injuring mechanism of oxygen radicals is DNA damage
    b. Cellular defense against superoxide anion primarily involves superoxide dismutase
    c. Cellular defense against hydrogen peroxide primarily involves taurine
    d. Chronic granulomatous disease is caused by decreased superoxide radical (O_2^-) formation due to a defect in the NADPH-oxidase enzyme system

    Answer c. Cellular defense against hydrogen peroxide primarily involves peroxidase and catalase.

65. All of the following are true except:
    a. LTC_4, LTD_4 and LTE_4 (slow-reacting substances of anaphylaxis) cause bronchoconstriction and vasoconstriction, followed by increased permeability (wheal and flare)
    b. Thyroid hormone has a major role in inflammation and injury
    c. Dense granules have adenosine (as ATP, ADP), serotonin, calcium
    d. LTB_4 is chemotactic for PMNs and eosinophils

    Answer b. Thyroid hormone does _not_ have a major role in inflammation.

66. All of the following are true except:
    a. The most predominate cell in the 1st 24 hrs of a wound is PMNs
    b. The most predominant cell at days 3-4 after a wound is macrophages
    c. The order of cell arrival in wound is macrophages, platelets, PMNs, lymphocytes, and fibroblasts
    d. The most predominate cell type in a 7 day old wound is fibroblasts

    Answer c. The order of cell arrival in wound is platelets, PMNs, macrophages, lymphocytes, and fibroblasts.

67. All of the following are true except:
    a. The most predominant type of collagen in the body is Type I
    b. The most predominant type of collagen being synthesized in a healing wound in the 1st 24 hours is Type III
    c. The maximum collagen amount in a wound occurs at 3 weeks
    d. Maximum tensile strength of a wound occurs at 3 weeks

    Answer d. Maximum tensile strength occurs at 8 weeks. Although the maximum collagen amount occurs at 3 weeks, remodeling and cross-linking occur to increase tensile strength, which is maximum at 8 weeks.

68. All of the following are true except:
    a. The most important cell involved in wound healing is macrophages
    b. The most predominant collagen type in cartilage is Type II
    c. Vit A prevents the negative effects of steroids on wound healing
    d. Keloids are confined to the original scar area
    e. The best method for inhibiting keloid formation is steroid injection following keloid excision

    Answer d. Keloids are _not_ confined to original scar (hypertrophic scar tissue is).

69. Peripheral nerves regenerate at:
     a. 0.01 mm/day
     b. 0.1 mm/day
     c. 1 mm/day
     d. 5 mm/day

     Answer c. Nerves regenerate at **1 mm/day**.

70. The most important factor in the healing of wounds by secondary intention is:
     a. Tensile strength of the wound
     b. Epithelial integrity
     c. Platelet activating factor
     d. Prostacyclin

     Answer b. The most important factor in wound healing by **secondary intention** is **epithelial integrity**.

71. The most important factor in the healing of wounds by primary intention is:
     a. Tensile strength of the wound
     b. Epithelial integrity
     c. Platelet activating factor
     d. Prostacyclin

     Answer a. Wound healing by **primary intention** is dependent on the **tensile strength** of the wound. This is created by collagen cross-linking. Sutures hold the wound together until appropriate collagen deposition and cross-linking occurs.

72. A 21 yo man presents to the ED twelve hours after sustaining a large gluteal laceration. Other than dirt, you do not see any pus or signs of infection. Which of the following is most appropriate:
     a. Primary closure with suture
     b. No closure and let the wound granulate in on its own
     c. Delayed closure
     d. Primary closure with staples
     e. Wound vac only

     Answer c. Do not close wounds that are > 6 hours old (perform wound debridement, leave open, then close 48 hours later [delayed primary closure]).

73. Which of the following best prevents wound infection following an open wound injury:
     a. Prophylactic IV antibiotics
     b. Topical antibiotics
     c. Chlorhexidine skin preparation
     d. Wound vac
     e. Wound debridement

     Answer e. Wound debridement

74. A patient with a large open gluteal laceration wound injury returns to clinic and the wound is much smaller. This is primarily a result of:
     a. Lymphocytes
     b. Macrophages
     c. PMNs
     d. Myofibroblasts

     Answer d. Myofibroblasts participate in wound contraction.

75. All of the following are true except:

a. Natural killer are involved in T cell receptor and antigen-MHC class recognition
b. Newborn's innate immunity has poor phagocyte chemotaxis (eg PMNs, macrophages), making them susceptible to cutaneous infections
c. IL-2 is released from helper T cells and activates cytotoxic T and natural killer cells
d. Cytotoxic T cells (CD8) attack non-self antigens attached to MHC class I receptors

Answer a. Natural killer cells are not involved in antigen-MHC class recognition. They attack cells with low expression of MHC (missing self) and cells with bound antibody.

A newborn's innate immunity has **poor phagocyte chemotaxis** (PMNs and macrophages), making them susceptible to **cutaneous infections** (make sure you wash your hands).

76. Cachexia in patients with cancer is primarily the result of:
  a. IL-2
  b. IL-6
  c. IL-10
  d. TNF-alpha

Answer d. TNF-alpha promotes **cachexia** in patients with cancer.

77. Which is the primary antibody found in secretions from the gut:
  a. IgA
  b. IgG
  c. IgM
  d. IgD
  e. IgE

Answer a. IgA is the primary antibody found in gut secretions.

78. Which of the following is most effective in helping prevent osteoporosis:
  a. Vit C
  b. Vit K
  c. Vit A
  d. Vit D

Answer D. Vit D

INFLAMMATION
- **Injury** - leads to exposed <u>collagen</u> as well as <u>platelet-activating factor</u> (PAF) and <u>tissue factor</u> release from endothelium
- **Platelets bind collagen** - release growth factors (eg platelet-derived growth factor [PDGF]); leads to PMN and macrophage recruitment
- **Macrophages** - have the **dominant role** in **inflammation** and **wound healing**
  - Main producer of **growth factors** (PDGF) and **cytokines** (TNF-alpha and IL-1) which attract other inflammatory cells and fibroblasts
  - Involved in phagocytosis and remove debris (monocytes become macrophages)
  - Involved in both **cell-mediated** and **antibody-mediated immunity** (have Fc receptor for antibodies)
- **Order of cell arrival** in wound - Platelets, PMNs, Macrophages, Lymphocytes, Fibroblasts
- **Predominant cell type** by day:
  - **Days 0–2**   PMNs
  - **Days 3–4**   Macrophages
  - **Days 5 and on**   Fibroblasts
- **Wound healing stages**
  - **Inflammation** (PDGF, PAF) - *1ˢᵗ step in normal wound healing*

- **Proliferation** (PDGF, FGF, EGF)
- **Remodeling**
- **Cell mediated immunity**
  - Involves macrophages, cytotoxic T cells, and natural killer cells
  - Does not involve antibodies
  - **Intradermal skin test** (eg PPD for tuberculosis) - tests cell-mediated immunity
  - *Infections associated with defects in cell mediated immunity* - intra-cellular pathogens (eg TB, other mycobacterium, viruses)
- **Other cell types**
  - **Mast cells** - main cell type involved in Type I hypersensitivity reactions
  - **Basophils** - Type I Hypersensitivity reactions
  - **Eosinophils** - parasitic infections, Type I hypersensitivity reactions
- **Innate immune system** includes inflammation and complement

CYTOKINES
- Main cytokines released with **inflammation** - TNF-alpha (#1) and IL-1
  - Vast majority of cytokines are produced by **macrophages**
- **TNF-alpha** (tumor necrosis factor-alpha)
  - **Main source** - macrophages
  - ↑'s **cell adhesion molecules** (eg ICAM, selectins); is procoagulant
  - Activates **PMNs** and other **macrophages** → leads to **growth factor** production → **cell recruitment**
  - ↑ HR, ↑ cardiac output, ↓ SVRI → high concentration can cause myocardial depression, **circulatory collapse**, and **MSOF**
  - Causes **cachexia** in patients with CA
- **IL-1**
  - **Main source** - macrophages
  - Effects similar to TNF and synergizes TNF
  - Induces **fever** (is PGE_2 mediated in hypothalamus)
    - Raises thermal set point, causing fever
      - **NSAIDs** - ↓ fever by reducing PGE_2 synthesis.
  - **Alveolar macrophages** - cause fever with atelectasis by releasing **IL-1**
- **IL-6** - ↑ **hepatic acute phase proteins** (see below)
- **IL-8** - **PMN chemotaxis** (+ other inflammatory cells) and **angiogenesis**
- **IL-10** - down regulation inflammatory response (↓ TNF-alpha, IL-2, IL3, and interferons; down-regulates antigen presenting cells [APCs])
- **Interferons** - released by **lymphocytes** in response to **viral infection**; activate inflammatory cells, inhibit viral replication, upregulate MHC

GROWTH FACTORS
- **PDGF** (platelet-derived growth factor) - *key factor* in wound healing
  - **Chemotactic** for and activates **inflammatory cells**
  - **Chemotactic** for and activates **fibroblasts**
  - **Angiogenesis** and **epithelialization**
  - Chemotactic for **smooth muscle cells**
  - Accelerates **wound healing**
- **PAF** (platelet-activating factor)
  - Activates **platelets**; PAF is a **phospholipid**
  - Chemotactic and activates **inflammatory cells**
  - ↑s **adhesion molecule** expression
  - *Not stored,* generated by **phospholipase** in endothelium, other cells
- **FGF** (fibroblast growth factor) - chemotactic and activates **fibroblasts, angiogenesis, epithelialization**
- **EGF** (epidermal growth factor) - chemotactic and activates **fibroblasts, angiogenesis, epithelialization**
- **TGF-beta** (transforming growth factor-beta) - primarily **immunosuppressive** (inhibits lymphocytes and leukocytes)
- **Chemotactic** factors
  - For inflammatory cells - PDGF, PAF, IL-8, LTB-4, C5a and C3a
  - For fibroblasts - PDGF, FGF, EGF

- **Angiogenesis** factors - hypoxia (#1), PDGF, FGF, EGF, IL-8
  - Produced by **macrophages** and **platelets** in response to **hypoxia**
  - *Hypoxia is the most potent stimulus for angiogenesis*
  - PAF does <u>not</u> have angiogenesis properties
- **Epithelialization** factors - PDGF, FGF, EGF
- **PMNs** - last 2 days in tissue (last 7 days in blood)
- **Platelets** - last 7 days

HEPATIC ACUTE PHASE PROTEINS
- Proteins that are increased or decreased in response to **inflammation**
- **IL-6** - most potent stimulus
- **Increased synthesis** - <u>C-reactive protein</u> (an opsonin, activates complement), amyloid A and P, fibrinogen, haptoglobin, ceruloplasmin, alpha-1 antitrypsin, and C3 (complement)
- **Decreased synthesis** - albumin, prealbumin, and transferrin

CELL ADHESION MOLECULES
- **Selectins** - involved in **rolling adhesion** (1st step in transmigration process); **L-selectin** (on leukocytes) binds to **E-selectin** (endothelial) and **P- selectin** (platelets)
- **Beta-2 integrins** (CD 11/18 molecules)
  - Found on **leukocytes** and **platelets**
  - Involved in **anchoring adhesion** and transendothelial **migration**
  - Bind ICAM, VCAM, etc
- **ICAM, VCAM, PECAM,** and **ELAM**
  - Found on **endothelial cells**
  - Involved in **anchoring adhesion** and transendothelial **migration**
  - Bind **beta-2 integrin molecules** (above)

COMPLEMENT
- **Classic** pathway
  - Activation mechanisms:
    - 1) **Antigen-antibody complex** (IgG or IgM *only*) *or;*
    - 2) Direct binding of **pathogen** to C1
  - *Initial step* is formation of **C1 complex** (2 C1 molecules)
  - Factors **C1, C2,** and **C4** - found <u>only</u> in the classic pathway
- **Alternative** pathway
  - Activation mechanisms - **endotoxin, bacteria**, other stimuli
  - *Initial step* is **C3 activation**
  - *Factors B, D, and P (properdin)* - found <u>only</u> in alternative pathway
- **C3 activation** - common to and convergence point for both pathways
- **Mg**$^{++}$ required for both pathways
- **Products**:
  - **Anaphylatoxins** - C3a, C4a, and C5a; ↑ vascular permeability; bronchoconstriction; activate mast cells and basophils
  - **Cell membrane attack complex**: C5b-C9b (C5bC6bC7bC8bC9b)
    - Inserted into **pathogen cell membrane**, makes hole → cell lysis
    - Can also **attack normal cells infected with bacteria**
  - **Opsonization** - C3b and C4b; enhances **phagocytosis of antigen**
  - **Chemotaxis** of inflammatory cells (PMNs, macrophage) - C3a and C5a

OXYGEN RADICALS
- **Oxidants generated** in inflammation (oxidants and producers)
  - **Superoxide anion radical** (O_2^-)   NADPH oxidase
  - **Hydrogen peroxide** (H_2O_2)   Xanthine oxidase, NADPH oxidase
- **Cellular defenses** against oxidative species (oxidants and defense)
  - **Superoxide anion radical**   **Superoxide dismutase** (need Cu + Zn)
                                           Converts to hydrogen peroxide
  - **Hydrogen peroxide**   **Glutathione peroxidase, catalase**
- **Primary injuring mechanism of oxygen radicals** - DNA damage
- **Respiratory burst** (macrophages, PMNs) - releases <u>superoxide anion</u> and <u>hydrogen peroxide</u>; used to attack bacteria directly and cells infected with bacteria

- **Chronic granulomatous disease**
  - Defect in **NADPH-oxidase enzyme system** in PMNs and macrophages
  - Results in **decreased superoxide radical** (O_2^-) formation

PLATELET GRANULES
- **Alpha granules**
  - Aggregation Factors - platelet factor 4, vWF, fibrinogen, fibronectin
  - Beta-thromboglobulin - binds thrombin
  - PDGF and TGF-beta
  - Factors V and XIII
- **Dense granules** (ASC) - <u>A</u>denosine (as ATP or ADP), <u>S</u>erotonin, <u>C</u>alcium

LIPID MEDIATORS
- Mainly involved in **inflammation regulation**
- Initial substrate is **phospholipid essential fatty acids** (in cell membrane)
  - **Phospholipids** → (*phospholipase*) → **Arachadonic acid**
  - **Glucocorticoids** inhibit *phospholipase* and production of everything below
- Cyclooxygenase (COX) pathway (produces <u>prostaglandins</u>)
  - *PGI₂ (prostacyclin)* and **PGE₂**
    Systemic and pulmonary **vasodilation** (↓ SVR, ↓ PVR)
    ↓ platelet aggregation
    Bronchodilation
  - *TXA₂ (thromboxane), PGG₂, PGH₂,*
    Systemic and pulmonary **vasoconstriction** (↑ SVR, ↑ PVR)
    ↑ platelet aggregation
  - ASA inhibits cyclooxygenase
- Lipoxygenase pathway (produces <u>leukotrienes</u> and <u>lipoxins</u>)
  - Are **leukocyte derived** molecules
  - **Leukotrienes**
    LTC₄, LTD₄, LTE₄ - slow-reacting substances of anaphylaxis
    Bronchoconstriction
    Vasoconstriction followed by ↑ permeability (***wheal and flare***)
    LTB₄ - chemotaxis of PMNs and eosinophils
  - **Lipoxins** - anti-inflammatory (↓ chemotaxis, ↓ transmigration)

OTHER
- **Catecholamines** (neural response to injury) - peak 24-48 hrs after injury
- **Neuroendocrine response to injury**
  - **Afferent nerves** from site of injury stimulate ACTH, ADH, growth hormone, epinephrine, and norepinephrine release
- **Thyroid hormone** – does <u>not</u> play a major role in injury

WOUND HEALING
- **Wound healing phases**: 1) Inflammation, 2) Proliferation, and 3) Maturation and Remodeling
- **Inflammation** (1-10 d, see previous section)
- **Proliferation** (5 days to 3 weeks)
  - **Granulation tissue** [= vascularized **extracellular matrix (ECM)**]
    Provisional ECM - *hyaluronic acid* (primary component, is a <u>glycosaminoglycan</u>); produced by *fibroblasts*; undergoes neovascularization (**endothelial cells**)
  - **Epithelialization** (1-2 mm/day, requires **granulation tissue**)
    Keratinocytes (epithelial cells) from **hair follicles** *(#1 source)*, wound edges, and sweat glands **migrate** across granulation tissue
  - **Wound contraction** by myofibroblasts (peaks at **10-15 days**)
  - **Collagen deposition** by fibroblasts; provides **wound strength**
    Type I collagen predominant collagen <u>in wound</u> *(although **Type III** is predominant type synthesized in 1ˢᵗ 48 hours)*
- **Maturation and Remodeling** (3 weeks to 1 year)
  - **Maximum collagen synthesis** occurs at **3 weeks** → net amount then does not change although production and degradation occurs

- **Type III** collagen replaced with **Type I**
- **Cross-linking** occurs along **tension lines** which increases **tensile strength**
- Peak tensile strength occurs at **8 weeks** (80% normal, most it ever gets)

- **Macrophages** - the essential cell in wound healing (growth factors, cytokines)
- **Myofibroblasts**
  - Fibroblast with smooth muscle cell components (actin / myosin)
  - Communicate by **gap junctions**
  - Involved in **wound contraction** and healing by **secondary intention**
  - **Perineum** (more redundant tissue) - better wound contraction than leg
- **Peripheral nerves** - regeneration at **1 mm/day**
- **Zinc** - important in many enzyme systems of wound healing
- **Phosphate** - important for leukocyte **chemotaxis** and **phagocytosis** (low phosphate results in low ATP levels)
- **Vit C** is important for collagen synthesis and **wound healing**; Vit C deficiency can result in **scar dissolution**
- **Epithelial integrity** - most important factor in healing of **open wounds** (<u>secondary intention</u>); depends on **granulation tissue**
  - **Epithelial cell** (keratinocyte) **migration** occurs from **hair follicles** (#1 source), wound edges, and sweat glands - migration is dependent on **granulation tissue**
  - Unepithelialized wounds leak serum and protein → promotes **bacteria growth**
  - **Wound contraction** occurs with healing by secondary intention
- **Tensile strength** - most important factor in healing of **closed incisions** (<u>primary intention</u>)
  - Depends on **collagen deposition** and **cross-linking**
  - At 6 weeks - wound 60% original strength
  - At 8-12 weeks - wound **max tensile strength** (80% original strength)
  - **Submucosa** - strength layer of bowel
    - Weakest time point for small bowel anastomosis is **3-5 days**
- **Delayed primary closure** - leaving a wound open for **48 hours** (wet-to-dry dressing changes), making sure it is not infected, and then closing it
  - Good for **contaminated wounds** (eg open incision for ruptured appendicitis) and is thought to help prevent wound infection
  - There is a risk of **abscess** formation with this technique
- **Accelerated wound healing** - re-opening a wound results in quicker healing the 2nd time (healing cells are already present)
- **Open wound injury**
  - Do <u>not</u> close **infected** wounds (ie if pus is present)
  - Do <u>not</u> close wounds that are **> 6 hours** old (perform wound debridement, leave open, then close 48 hours later [delayed primary closure])
  - Perform **wound debridement** as soon as possible (*best* method for preventing wound infection - irrigation, removal of necrotic tissue)
  - Give **prophylactic antibiotics** (important to note these do <u>not</u> reach the source of wound infection, only the surrounding area)
  - *Topical antibiotics are <u>not</u> recommended*
  - **Tetanus** immunization status
- **Essentials** for open wound healing:
  - **Moist** environment (promotes cell migration; *avoid* wound desiccation)
  - **Oxygen delivery** - optimize fluids (no edema, no dehydration), no smoking, pain control, arterial revascularization if needed, supplemental oxygen
    - Want transcutaneous oxygen measurement (TCOM) **> 25 mm Hg**
  - **Avoid edema** (leg elevation if needed)
  - **Remove necrotic tissue**
  - Place **wound vac** or **wet to dry dressings**
- **Impediments** to wound healing:
  - **Bacteria > 10^5/cm^2** - bacteria prolong inflammation
  - **Devitalized tissue** and **foreign bodies** - inhibit granulation tissue
  - **Cytotoxic** and **chemotherapy** agents (eg 5-FU, methotrexate, cyclosporine) impair wound healing in the **1st 14 days** after injury
    - No effect on wound healing after 2 weeks
  - **Diabetes** - impedes inflammation (poor leukocyte chemotaxis)

- **Albumin < 3.0** - risk factor for poor wound healing (poor nutrition = poor wound healing)
- **Corticosteroids** - inhibit inflammatory cells and fibroblasts
  - Steroids decrease wound tensile strength due to poor collagen synthesis
    - **Vitamin A** (25,000 IU qd) - counteracts effects of steroids
- **Wound ischemia** (hypoxia) - can be due to fibrosis, pressure (sacral decubitus ulcer, pressure sores), poor arterial inflow (atherosclerosis), poor venous outflow (venous stasis), smoking, XRT, edema

- Wound vac _contraindications_ - malignant wounds; fistulas; osteomyelitis; anastomotic sites; wounds with necrotic eschar; placement on large blood vessels; placement over organs (eg liver, spleen, lung, heart) or nerves
- Diabetic foot ulcers - usually at 2nd **MTP joint** or **heel**; secondary to **neuropathy** (can't feel feet, pressure from walking leads to ischemia); can also occur on **toes**
- Leg ulcers - 90% from **venous insufficiency**; Tx: Unna boot (compressive dressing)
- Scars
  - Composed of proteoglycans, **hyaluronic acid**, and water
  - Scar revision - wait for 1 year to allow maturation; may improve with age
  - **Infants heal with little or no scarring**
- Denervation - has _no_ effect on wound healing
- Keloids - autosomal dominant; dark skinned patients
  - Collagen _goes beyond_ original scar
  - From **failure of collagen breakdown**
  - Tx: **intra-lesion steroid injection** after keloid excision _(best Tx)_; silicone infections, pressure garments, XRT
- Hypertrophic scar tissue - dark skinned patients; flexor surfaces of upper torso
  - Collagen _stays within confines_ of original scar
  - Often occurs in burns or wounds that take a long time to heal
  - From **hypervascularization**
  - Tx: **intra-lesion steroid injection**, silicone, pressure garments
- Vit C, Vit A, and Zinc - all important for wound healing
- Wound dehiscence RFs: **deep wound infection** (#1), poor nutrition, COPD (coughing), DM; these patients are at risk for **fascial dehiscence**
  - Tx: inspect fascia and make sure it's intact; antibiotics and wound vac usual
- Fascial dehiscence (Sx's - sudden leak of a large amount of **salmon colored fluid**; bulge under the skin incision [due to intestines])
  - Tx: _immediate_ operative re-exploration, place **retention sutures**
  - Small fascial dehiscence, late after surgery ($\geq$ 7 days) - consider conservative management (eg wet to dry dressing changes)
- Suture removal timing: **Face** - 1 week; **other areas** - 2 weeks
  - **Sutures** hold wound together until appropriate collagen deposition and cross-linking can occur

Collagen Types

I	**MC type in body**
	Skin, bone, tendons, **cornea** (not lens)
	Primary collagen in **healing wound**
II	MC collagen in **cartilage**
III	**Granulation tissue**; blood vessels, fetal skin
IV	**Basement membrane, eye lens**, glomeruli

Many other types

Collagen has **proline** every 3rd amino acid

Proline residues undergo hydroxylation _(prolyl hydroxylase)_ and **cross-linking** (requires _alpha_-ketoglutarate, Vit C, oxygen, and iron)

d-Penicillamine - inhibits collagen cross-linking

Vit C deficiency can result in **poor wound healing** and **scar dissolution** from lack of collagen synthesis

Cartilage - has _no_ blood vessels (get nutrients and oxygen by **diffusion**)

ADAPTIVE IMMUNE SYSTEM

- **Newborns** - innate immunity has **poor phagocyte chemotaxis** (PMNs and macrophages); susceptible to **cutaneous infections** → wash hands
- **Newborns** - have **IgG** (from mother through the placenta; is the <u>only</u> immunoglobulin [Ig] that crosses the placenta) and **IgA** (from breast milk); provide humeral immunity while newborn immune system develops
- **T cells** [produced in bone, maturation in Thymus, <u>all</u> have **T cell receptors** (CD3]
  - **Helper T cells (CD4)** - interact with **MHC class II** receptors (APC cells with attached antigen); functions include →
    - a) **IL-2** release - activates **cytotoxic T** and **natural killer cells** (cellular immune system)
    - b) **Interferon-gamma** release - activates **macrophages**
    - c) **IL-4** release - increases **B cell** antibody production (humoral immune system)

    Activated helper T cells differentiate into **Effector** and **Memory T cells**
  - **Suppressor T cells (CD4**; regulatory T cells) - **suppress immune response** and helps prevent autoimmunity; regulate CD4, CD8 cells
  - **Cytotoxic T cells (CD8)**; activated by **IL-2** (involved in cell-mediated immunity)

    Attacks antigens attached to **MHC class I** receptors (eg viral gene protein); release <u>perforin</u> and <u>granulysin</u> (creates pores)

    Cytotoxic T cells cause <u>nearly all</u> of liver injury from **HepB infection**
- **Natural killer cells** (activated by **IL-2**; involved in both cell-mediated and antibody-mediated immunity)
  - Attack **host cells** that have been infected by microbes

    Do not use MHC-antigen complexes

    Do not directly attack microbe
  - Attack cells with **low expression of MHC** (missing self)

    Occurs with cell infection (especially viral infection)
  - Can also attack cells with **bound antibody** (have Fc receptor)
- **B cells** (maturation in Bone)
  - Involved in **antibody-mediated immunity** (humoral immunity)
  - B cell encounters antigen (which binds IgD receptor on B cell), is activated by T helper cell (**IL-4**), and divides into many **plasma cells** (live 2-3 d), which secrete **antibodies** to the antigen
  - 10% of plasma cells become **memory B cells**

    Can be re-activated if the pathogen re-infects host

    IgG secreted (as opposed to IgM) with **re-infection** (class switching)
- **MHC classes** (major histocompatibility complex or HLA classes)
  - **MHC class I** (A, B, and C) - single chain with 5 domains

    Interacts with **CD8 cells** (mostly cytotoxic T cells)

    Class I MHC found on all nucleated cells (not RBCs)

    Cells present *endogenous antigen* (from cytosolic protein breakdown or endogenous antigen pathway [ie viral proteins produced in cell]) attached to MHC class I receptor

    Cytotoxic T cells → recognize and attack non-self antigens attached to **MHC class I** receptors
  - **MHC class II** (DR, DP, and DQ) - 2 chains with 4 domains each

    Interacts with **CD4 cells** (helper T cells and suppressor T cells)

    Class II MHC found on antigen presenting cells (APCs)

    APCs include dendritic cells, macrophages, and B cells

    ***Dendritic cells** are the most important **APC** (present antigen to T cells)*

    APCs present **exogenous antigen** (exogenous antigen pathway, eg phagocytosis of extra-cellular bacterial proteins) attached to MHC class II receptor when passing through lymph nodes

    Helper T cells are **activated** by MHC class II-antigen complex; then activate **macrophages** and **B cells**
- **Viral infection**
  - Endogenous viral proteins produced inside cell
  - Are bound to **MHC class I**

- **MHC class I - antigen complex** goes to cell surface, is recognized by CD8 cytotoxic T cells
- **Cytotoxic T cell** then **attacks the cell expressing the complex**
- Bacterial infection (extracellular pathogens)
    - **Dendritic cells** (APCs) engulf exogenous pathogens (eg bacteria, toxins) and migrate to T cell enriched lymph nodes
        APCs display non-self antigen coupled to **MHC class II** molecule
        This is recognized by **T Helper cells**
    - **T helper cells** then activate **macrophages** and **B cells**
- Adaptive immunity for cancer therapy *(→ IL-2 mediated)*
    - Convert harvested **lymphocytes** into **lymphokine-activated killer (LAK)** cells after exposure *in vitro* to tumor antigens and IL-2
    - Converts harvested **lymphocytes** into **tumor-infiltrating lymphocytes (TILs)** after exposure *in vitro* to tumor antigens and IL-2
    - IL-2 enhances endogenous T cell immune response to tumor
    - **Tumor vaccines** (ie CA antigens) are injected into the patient in an effort to stimulate **adaptive immunity against the tumor** (antigen engulfed by APCs, presented, etc)
    - Some success with melanoma for above

ANTIBODIES (immunoglobulins)
- **IgM**
    - *MC antibody in **spleen***
    - Responsible for the **primary immune response** (initial exposure to antigen)
    - **Largest antibody** - 5 domains and 10 binding sites (pentamer)
    - Activates **complement**
    - **Opsonization** for phagocytosis
    - *Does not cross the placenta*
    - **Primary antibody** against **A** and **B antigens on RBCs** (ABO blood type)
        Causes **clumping** of RBCs and **thrombosis**
    - *Lack of IgM after splenectomy results in **overwhelming post-splenectomy infection** (OPSI)*
- **IgG**
    - *MC antibody **overall** (75% of all immunoglobulins)*
    - Responsible for **secondary immune response**
    - Activates **complement** (takes 2 IgG's)
    - **Opsonization** for phagocytosis
    - **Crosses placenta** and provides protection in newborn period *(the only immunoglobulin able to do this)*
- **IgA**
    - *MC immunoglobulin in **mucosal linings*** (important in mucosal immunity)
    - Found in **secretions**, Peyer's patches in gut, lung, saliva, breast milk
    - IgA **binds pathogens** to prevent adherence and invasion (coats bacteria so that it cannot bind to mucosal epithelium)
- IgD - membrane-bound receptor found on B cells
- IgE - Type I Immediate Hypersensitivity Reactions, also **parasite** infections

- **IgM** and **IgG** are **opsonins**
- **IgM** and **IgG** activate (fix) **complement** (requires 2 IgG's or 1 IgM)
- **Variable region** - antigen recognition
- **Constant region** (Fc portion) - recognized by macrophages, PMNs, NK cells, eosinophils; Fc fragment does not have variable region
- All immunoglobulins have **2 binding sites** except IgM (has 10 binding sites)
- **Polyclonal antibodies** - have multiple binding sites to the antigen at multiple epitopes
- **Monoclonal antibodies** - have only one binding site to the antigen at only one epitope

OTHER
- **Primary lymphoid organs** - liver, bone, thymus
- **Secondary lymphoid organs** - spleen and lymph nodes
- **Immunologic chimera** - 2 different cell lines in one individual (eg allogenic bone marrow TXP recipient)

- **Mast cells** - main source of <u>histamine</u> in **tissues** other than stomach
- **Basophils** - main source of <u>histamine</u> in **blood**
    - Basophils are generally <u>not</u> found in tissue
- **Angiotensin-converting enzyme** (ACE; located in the **lung**) - inactivates bradykinin

HYPERSENSITIVITY REACTIONS

- **Type I** - **immediate hypersensitivity reaction** (bound **IgE**)
    - Ex: **allergic reactions** (eg bee stings, peanuts, lymphazurin blue dye for sentinel lymph node biopsy [SLNB]), **anaphylaxis,** and **asthma**
    - Provoked by **re-exposure**
    - **Mediator** - antigen interacts with **IgE** attached to **mast cells** (main cell involved) and **basophils**
    - **Response** - degranulation of mast cells and basophils
        - Main response factor: **histamine** (vasodilation, broncho-constriction)
    - **Effects**: bronchoconstriction, rhinorrhea, flushing, hypotension, dyspnea, angioedema (swelling of face, neck, and throat – can close off airway)
    - Tx: **Acute airway Tx** if necessary (angioedema)
        - *Epinephrine (primary Tx if severe)*, **anti-histamines** (diphenhydramine), **steroids**
- **Type II** - **antibody dependent cytotoxicity** (**IgG** or **IgM**)
    - Ex: **acute hemolytic transfusion reaction** and **hyperacute rejection after organ transplant**
    - **Mediator** - IgG or IgM; bind to **cell bound antigen** (or foreign cells with TXP hyperacute rejection or ABO-mismatched transfusion reaction)
    - **Response:**
        - 1) **Cell mediated immune response** to bound **IgG or IgM** via Fc receptor on macrophage, PMNs, NK cells, and eosinophils
        - 2) Bound IgM or IgG also activates **complement**
- **Type III** - **immune complex deposition**
    - Ex: **serum sickness** (eg anti-venom), **SLE**
    - **Antigen-antibody complexes** (IgG) are deposited in vessel walls and induces inflammation (rash, arthralgias, fever, adenopathy)
    - Tx: **corticosteroids, antihistamines**, possible **plasmapheresis**
- **Type IV** - **delayed type hypersensitivity reaction**
    - Ex: **PPD** (TB skin test), **contact dermatitis** (eg poison ivy), **chronic rejection**
    - Mediator - **T cell** mediated immune response *(antibody-independent response)*
    - Represents cell-mediated immunity *(is the only hypersensitivity reaction <u>not</u> involving antibodies)*
    - Takes **2-3 days** to develop (or years after TXP)
    - **Response** - APCs present MHC class II-antigen complex to **T helper cells** → create effector T helper cells → activate **macrophages** which destroy antigen

Transplantation

79. The MCC of nephropathy leading to kidney graft loss is:
    a. CMV
    b. HSV
    c. EBV
    d. BK polyomavirus

    Answer d. BK polyomavirus. 5% of renal grafts get BK virus associated nephropathy (BKVAN) and 80% of those patients lose their grafts.

80. Two hours after kidney TXP your patient is anuric. She was seronegative for CMV, positive for HepB surface antibody, and had a PRA of 70% prior to TXP. Organ ischmia time was 24 hours. The most appropriate next move is:
    a. Ganciclovir
    b. Lamivudine
    c. Re-exploration
    d. Duplex U/S

    Answer d. Anuria in the early post-op period is MC due to ATN (usually from graft ischemia), however, **vascular** and **anastomotic problems** should always be ruled out with duplex U/S (even though these Cx's are rare).

81. Monoclonal antibodies:
    a. Bind one epitope at one site
    b. Bind one epitope at multiple sites
    c. Bind multiple epitopes on a single antigen
    d. Bind multiple epitopes on multiple antigens

    Answer a. Monoclonal antibodies are all identical, so they bind **one epitope** at the exact same binding site. **Polyclonal antibodies** have multiple binding sites to the antigen at multiple epitopes.

82. Four days after orthotopic liver TXP, your patient is noted to have a steep rise in AST and ALT (400's) along with a rise in serum bilirubin (5.2). The next appropriate step is:
    a. Liver MRI
    b. CT scan
    c. Ultrasound (U/S) and biopsy (Bx)
    d. Re-transplant

    Answer c. The acute rise in LFTs could be due to acute rejection, hepatic artery thrombosis (or other vascular compromise), or infection (eg CMV, sepsis). To start, an **ultrasound** to look at the vascular connections and a **liver biopsy** to assess for rejection and CMV infection are needed. Blood cultures for infection are also indicated.

83. All the following are generally contraindications for donation in living donor kidney transplantation except:
    a. Duplicated urinary collecting system
    b. DM
    c. HIV
    d. Hep B

    Answer a. Duplicated urinary systems or collecting systems are not a contraindication to living related donor kidney TXP.

84. All of the following mechanisms are correct except:
    a. Cyclosporin binds cyclophilin protein, which inhibits calcineurin, and inhibits genes for cytokine synthesis (primarily **IL-2**)
    b. Azathioprine inhibits purine synthesis by way of 6-mercaptopurine which in effect inhibits T cells.

c. Sirolimus binds the FK binding protein and inhibits calcineurin protein
d. Tacrolimus binds the FK binding protein and inhibits calcineurin protein

Answer c. Sirolimus binds the **FK-binding protein** and that complex binds the **mammalian target of rapamycin** (mTOR). That complex inhibits the response to IL-2 and blocks activation of T-cells and B-cells.

85. Three weeks after kidney TXP, your patient presents with poor urine output and a creatinine of 2.0. You give a fluid challenge without an increase in urine output. U/S which shows a 4 x 4 x 4 cm hypoechoic mass and moderate hydronephrosis. The graft appears to have good perfusion. All of the following apply to the management of this patient's most likely condition except:
    a. Percutaneous drainage is the 1st option in management
    b. Peritoneal window should be performed if it recurs
    c. This complication usually occurs 3-4 weeks after transplant
    d. This complication is related to bleeding
    e. This is most likely a urine leak

Answer d. This patient has a lymphocoele that is obstructing his ureter. This complication usually occurs 3-4 weeks after TXP. Initial Tx is percutaneous drainage. If the lymphocele recurs, a **peritoneal window** should be performed to allow drainage into the peritoneum. A urine leak usually occurs early post-op (hours to days, not at 3 weeks).

86. Two months after kidney TXP, your patient develops respiratory symptoms requiring admission to the ICU. CXR shows diffuse infiltrates and bronchial washings show cells with inclusion bodies. Creatinine has risen from 1.4 to 2.0 The most appropriate Tx is:
    a. Gangciclovir
    b. Acyclovir
    c. Bactrim
    d. Penicillin

Answer a. CMV infection is the *MC infection among transplant patients* and forms characteristic **inclusion bodies** in cells. **Ganciclovir** is used to treat CMV infection.

87. All of the following are true of hyperacute rejection except:
    a. It is MC due to ABO incompatibility
    b. It is a Type II hypersensitivity reaction
    c. Successful Tx usually requires organ removal and re-transplantation
    d. Steroids are usually sufficient Tx

Answer d. Hyperacute rejection is most often due to ABO incompatibility and involves pre-formed recipient antibodies to donor antigens. Hyperacute rejection signs intra-op include the organ turning blue and mottled with interstitial hemorrhage, cyanosis, gross edema, and graft rupture. Tx is immediate removal of the organ and re-transplantation (or just removal if kidney)

88. The MC malignancy following transplantation is:
    a. Lung cancer
    b. Prostate cancer
    c. Breast cancer
    d. Skin cancer

Answer d. The MC malignancy following transplantation is **squamous cell skin cancer**.

89. A crossmatch is performed by:
    a. Mixing donor lymphocytes with recipient serum
    b. Mixing recipient lymphocytes with donor serum
    c. Mixing donor plasma with recipient serum

d.   Mixing recipient plasma with donor serum

Answer a. A **crossmatch** is performed by mixing donor lymphocytes (which contains the antigen) with recipient serum (which contains the antibody). A **positive cross-match** means that the recipient has preformed antibodies to donor antigens. **Hyperacute rejection** would likely occur if the transplant were to ensue.

90.   The principal cells involved in acute rejection is:
    a.   B cells
    b.   T cells
    c.   Macrophages
    d.   Platelets

Answer b. The principle cells involved in **acute rejection** is **T cells**.

91.   Post-transplant lymphoproliferative disorder has been most commonly linked to:
    a.   HSV
    b.   RSV
    c.   EBV
    d.   Influenza viruses

Answer c. Epstein Barr virus is implicated in development of post-transplant lymphoproliferative disorder.

92.   A 35 yo man POD #10 from a cadaveric renal transplantation develops a rise in creatnine. A fluid and lasix challenge has no effect The appropriate next step is:
    a.   Emergent re-operation
    b.   Angiography
    c.   OKT3
    d.   Ultrasound

Answer d. Elevated creatinine or decreased urine output (or any other signs of rejection) is an indication for **U/S** following kidney TXP. The U/S assesses vascular supply to the graft, looks for ureter compression, and can identify fluid collections consistent with either urine leaks, lymphocoeles, hematomas, or seromas. Kidney Bx can be performed at the same time.

93.   In the previous patient, U/S shows flow acceleration and narrowing at the level of the arterial anastomosis. The next appropriate step is:
    a.   Emergent re-operation
    b.   Angiography
    c.   OKT3
    d.   Biopsy

Answer b. Angiogram with angioplasty and stent placement is the Tx of choice for a tight arterial anastomosis following kidney TXP.

94.   Instead of the above, the U/S is normal. The most appropriate next step is:
    a.   Emergent re-operation
    b.   Angiography
    c.   OKT3
    d.   Biopsy

Answer d. If there is no mechanical problem with the graft, Bx should be performed.

95.   Biopsy in the above patient shows tubulitis. This is consistent with:
    a.   Acute rejection
    b.   Urinary tract infection
    c.   Chronic rejection

d. Renal vein thrombosis

Answer a. Lymphocytic **tubulitis** is consistent with **acute rejection**. A more severe acute rejection would involve vasculitis. Pulse steroids are indicated. You should follow creatnine and likely re-biopsy after 5-7 days.

96. Five days after kidney TXP, your patient has poor urine output despite fluid challenge and lasix. U/S shows a large fluid collection anterior to kidney. You aspirate the fluid and the creatinine is 20 (serum creatnine 0.8). The next step in management is:
    a. Explant the kidney
    b. Try to repair the cysto-ureteral anastomosis
    c. Place a stent and percutaneous drainage
    d. Nothing

    Answer c. The most appropriate Tx for a **urine leak** (in most instances) is percutaneous drainage and placement of a **ureteral stent** across the anastomosis (ie across the leak). Trying to redo the anastomosis is usually unsuccessful.

97. New proteinuria in a patient following kidney transplant is most consistent with:
    a. Acute rejection
    b. Urinary tract infection
    c. Chronic rejection
    d. Renal vein thrombosis

    Answer d. New proteinuria is consistent with **renal vein thrombosis**.

98. All of the following are true except:
    a. Cystic fibrosis requires <u>double</u> lung transplant
    b. Chronic allograft vasculopathy is the MCC of death after heart TXP
    c. Diabetic ESRD is the MC indication for combined kidney-pancreas TXP
    d. Bronchiolitis obliterans is the MCC of acute death after lung TXP
    e. Retinopathy stabilizes after kidney-pancreas TXP

    Answer d. Reperfusion injury is the MCC early death after lung TXP. Bronchiolitis obliterans is the MCC of late death after lung TXP.

99. The MCC of acute death in a living kidney donor is:
    a. Pulmonary embolism (PE)
    b. Hemorrhage
    c. Myocardial infarction
    d. Infection

    Answer a. The MCC of acute death in a living related kidney <u>donor</u> is **PE**. The MCC of death in a kidney TXP <u>recipient</u> is **myocardial infarction**.

100. All of the following are true of liver TXP except:
    a. Acute hepatic artery thrombosis after liver TXP usually resolves without Tx.
    b. Post-op lamivudine and adefovir reduce HepB re-infection to < 5%
    c. HepC is the MC indication for liver TXP and is the disease most likely to recur (re-infects almost all liver allografts)
    d. Primary sclerosing cholangitis recurrence is 20% after liver TXP

    Answer a. Acute hepatic artery thrombosis usually requires re-TXP.

101. A 50 yo man on cyclosporine and for a kidney TXP 3 months ago undergoes a difficult cholecystectomy requiring a biliary T-tube. Five days post-op he has an acute rise in creatnine and poor UOP. Given the most likely Dx, the most appropriate next step is
    a. Removal of T-tube
    b. Antibiotics
    c. Steroids

d. Ganciclovir

Answer c. Cyclosporine undergoes significant **entero-hepatic recirculation**. A biliary T-Tube would remove 90% of the cyclosporine and the patient would be subject to acute rejection, which would be treated with steroids.

102. All the following are true of renal TXP donor and recipient compatibility except:
  a. HLA-DR is the most important antigen in donor/recipient matching
  b. A blood type O recipient is compatible with a blood type AB donor
  c. Time on list, HLA matching, and PRA are used to decide kidney allocation in the US
  d. Better matching results in better long term function

Answer b. A blood type AB recipient is compatible with a blood type O donor.

TRANSPLANT IMMUNOLOGY
■ **Major transplant antigens** - <u>ABO</u> blood type and <u>MHC</u>
■ **MHC** (Major Histocompatibility Complex)
  ● Major factor leading to **acute** and **chronic rejection**
  ● HLA (Human Leukocyte Antigen) is the MHC form in humans
      HLA class I antigens: HLA -A, -B, and -C
      HLA class II antigens: HLA -DP, -DQ, and -DR
  ● HLA -A, -B, and -DR used for kidney allocation
      HLA-DR - *most important antigen* in donor / recipient matching
      Better HLA match = better long term function, less rejection
      Identical twin (paternal) organ TXPs do not undergo rejection
  ● **Time on list**, **HLA matching**, and **panel reactive antibody** (PRA) **results** - *criteria used for cadaveric kidney allocation in US;* special preference for <u>previous living kidney donor</u> status
■ **ABO blood compatibility**
  ● Generally need **ABO compatibility** for TXP
      ABO incompatibility would cause **hyperacute rejection** (Type II Hypersensitivity reaction)
  ● Recipient **AB blood type** (has <u>no</u> A or B antibodies) - can receive Type A, Type B, Type AB, or Type O organs
  ● Recipient **O blood type** (has antibodies to A + B antigens) - need Type O organ
■ **Crossmatch** (lymphocyte crossmatch)
  ● Detects **preformed recipient antibodies** by mixing recipient serum with donor lymphocytes → termed **positive crossmatch** *(would result in hyperacute rejection)*

REJECTION
■ **Hyperacute rejection** (minutes to hours after TXP)
  ● *Caused by **preformed recipient antibodies** to donor antigens*
  ● This should have been identified with the **crossmatch**
  ● MC problem - **ABO blood type incompatibility**
  ● Results in:
      1) **Type II Hypersensitivity Reaction**
      2) **Complement** activation (antibody binding) and **vessel thrombosis**
  ● Sx's: organ turns **blue and mottled**, hemorrhage, edema, rupture
  ● Tx: *remove organ* and *emergency re-transplantation* (if kidney, just remove organ)
■ **Acute rejection** (1 week to 6 months)
  ● ***Recipient T cells*** (cytotoxic and T helper) against donor HLA antigens; can occur with living related donors
  ● T cells need **1 week** for APC recognition, to differentiate, and to mount a response (reason for 1 week delay after TXP)
  ● Tx: **increase immunosuppression** (eg *pulse steroids [best initial Tx]*, thymoglobulin, organ preserved in 95%)
■ **Chronic rejection** (months to years)
  ● Chronic immune response to transplanted tissue

- *Acute rejection is a RF for chronic rejection*
- Major etiology - **MHC (HLA) incompatibility**
- Effectors: **T cells** (Type IV hypersensitivity), **B cells** (antibody production)
- *Is different from chronic allograft vasculopathy (see below)*
- Tx: ↑ **immunosuppression** (eg pulse steroids, thymoglobulin, maintenance drugs) → not effective long term
- **Re-transplantation** is the only definitive Tx
- ■ **Chronic Allograft Vasculopathy** (months to years)
  - **Fibrosis** or **accelerated atherosclerosis** of **internal blood vessels** of the transplanted tissue
  - Is a chronic rejection of **blood vessels**
  - *Main mechanism of chronic rejection after Heart TXP*
  - Tx: ↑ **immunosuppression** (eg pulse steroids, thymoglobulin, maintenance drugs) → not effective long term
  - **Re-transplantation** is the only definitive Tx

IMMUNOSUPPRESSIVE DRUGS
- ■ **Calcineurin Inhibitors**
  - **Cyclosporine** (Neoral, CSA)
    - Binds **cyclophilin protein**; cyclosporine-cyclophilin protein complex then inhibits **calcineurin protein**
    - Effect: **inhibits genes** for **cytokine synthesis** (eg **IL-2**, IL-4, interferon); blocks activation of **T-cells** and **B-cells**
    - S/Es: *nephrotoxicity*, hepatotoxicity, hemolytic-uremic syndrome (HUS), tremors, seizures, hirsutism, gingival hyperplasia
    - Undergoes **hepatic metabolism** and **biliary excretion**
    - *Undergoes significant enterohepatic re-circulation (reabsorbed in gut); a biliary drain (eg T-tube) decreases levels and can cause acute rejection*
    - Want trough level 200 - 300
  - **Tacrolimus** (Prograf, FK-506)
    - *MC primary maintenance immunosuppressive agent*
    - Binds **FK binding protein**; tacrolimus-FK binding protein complex then inhibits **calcineurin protein**
    - Effect: similar action as CSA (ie **inhibits genes** for **IL-2**, IL-4, INF-gamma), 50 x more potent
    - S/Es: nephrotoxic and others similar to CSA; *less* lipid, HTN, cosmetic problems; *more* diabetes
    - **Hepatic metabolism** (highly metabolized) – enterohepatic re-circulation much less of an issue
    - Want trough level 10 -15
    - *Fewer acute rejection episodes compared to cyclosporine*
- ■ **mTOR inhibitors**
  - **Sirolimus** (Rapamycin)
    - Binds **FK-binding protein** similar to tacrolimus, however the sirolimus-FK binding protein complex **inhibits mammalian target of rapamycin** (mTOR)
    - Effect: **inhibits response to IL-2** (blocks activation of T- and B-cells)
    - *Is not nephrotoxic (chief advantage over CSA and tacrolimus)*
    - S/Es: **interstitial lung disease**, thrombocytopenia
- ■ **Anti-proliferative agents**
  - **Mycophenolate** (MMF, Cellcept)
    - Inhibits de novo **purine synthesis**, which **inhibits T cells**
    - S/Es: **#1 GI intolerance** (N/V/D), #2 myelosuppression
    - Need to keep **WBCs > 3** while on this drug
- ■ **Steroids**
  - Inhibit **macrophages** and genes for **cytokine synthesis** (IL-1, IL-6)
  - S/Es: **Cushing's syndrome**
- ■ **Antibodies**
  - **Anti-thymocyte globulin** (ATG)
    - *Thymoglobulin* - rabbit antibodies; *Atgam* - equine antibodies

Polyclonal antibodies directed against antigens on T cells
Causes **complement dependent** opsonization of T cells
Is **cytolytic**
Used for **induction** or refractory **acute rejection**
Keep **WBCs > 3**
S/Es: **PTLD, myelosuppression, cytokine release syndrome** (SIRS reaction; need to pre-treat patient with steroids and antihistamines to prevent this)

- **Basiliximab** (Simulect) - IL-2 receptor inhibitor
  S/Es: **hypersensitivity reactions**
- **Monoclonal antibodies** are all identical, so they bind **one epitope** at the exact same binding site.
- **Polyclonal antibodies** have multiple binding sites to the antigen at multiple epitopes

■ **Induction agents** - steroids, thymoglobulin, atgam, and basiliximab
■ **Risks of long-term immunosuppression** - CA, cardiovascular disease, infection, osteopenia

TRANSPLANTATION RELATED MALIGNANCY
■ **MC malignancy following TXP -** skin cancer (MC squamous cell CA)
■ **Post-transplant lymphoproliferative disease** (PTLD)
  - Sx's - fever, adenopathy, mass lesions, SBO; usually in 1st year of TXP
  - 2nd MC malignancy following TXP; more common in **children** than adults
  - Highest risk - **small bowel TXP** (15% get this; lots of lymphoid tissue in small bowel)
  - *Caused by **Epstein-Barr virus** (EBV) mediated **B cell proliferation***
  - RFs - **cytolytic antibodies** (eg anti-thymocyte globulin [thymoglobulin, atgam]), patients with pre-TXP **seronegative EBV titers** who convert to **seropositive**
  - Mechanism - **immunosuppression** decreases **suppressor T cell population** so **B cell proliferation** after **EBV** infection goes unchecked → can progress to Non-Hodgkin's Lymphoma (**B cell**)
  - Dx: FNA or tissue Bx
  - Tx: significant lowering or **withdrawal of immunosuppression**
    Ganciclovir or **acyclovir**
    Rituximab (anti-CD 20, depresses B cells)
    CHOP-R (± XRT) for NHL

CMV INFECTION (Cytomegalovirus infection)
■ Found in and can be transmitted by **leukocytes** (use leukoreduced or CMV negative blood to prevent transmission)
■ *CMV is the MC infection in TXP recipients*
■ Can cause pneumonia, gastritis, colitis, ophthalmitis, and mononucleosis
■ MC manifestation - **febrile mononucleosis** (sore throat, adenopathy, malaise, myalgias, N/V)
■ Most deadly form - **CMV pneumonitis**
■ Dx: Bx - shows characteristic **cellular inclusion bodies**; CMV **serology**
■ Tx: **Ganciclovir** (inhibits DNA polymerase; S/Es - CNS toxicity, bone marrow suppression)
  - Reduce immunosuppression if possible
  - **CMV immunoglobulin** - given for severe infections and after TXP (along with ganciclovir) for CMV negative recipient with CMV positive donor; S/Es - N/V, flushing
■ **Varicella** (Zoster) - dissemination can be *life-threatening* (usually occurs in 1st year)
  - Tx: acyclovir, varicella immunoglobulin, ↓ immunosuppression, bronchoscopy to look for superinfection, respiratory isolation
■ **HSV** - Tx: acyclovir (inhibits DNA polymerase)
■ **EBV** - Sx's can range from mononucleosis, to B cell proliferation, to PTLD (see above)
■ **BK polyomavirus** - 5% of renal grafts get BK virus associated nephropathy (BKVAN) and 80% of those lose their grafts (MCC of graft loss due to nephropathy; Tx: **reduce immunosuppression** (many switch MMF out for Leflunomide)

KIDNEY TRANSPLANTATION

- **MC indication** - ESRD from diabetes
- *Not a contraindication* - HIV infection in recipient (many HIV to HIV, HepB to HepB, HepC to HepC transplants now performed)
- **Donor kidney** (cadaveric or living donor)
  - Can cold store for **48 hours**
  - **UTI in donor** - can still use kidney
  - **Acute ↑ in creatinine** (Cr; 1.0 - 3.0) - can still use kidney
- Attach to **iliac vessels** with **ureteral-bladder anastomosis**
- Cx's:
  - MCC post-op **Oliguria**   ATN (path - dilation + loss of tubules)
  - MCC post-op **Diuresis**   High urea and glucose before TXP
  - MCC new **Proteinuria**   Renal vein thrombosis (Dx – U/S)
  - MCC new onset **Diabetes**   S/E of steroids

  - **Urine leaks** *(MC complication)*
    - Sx's: ↓ed UOP <u>early</u> (**1st week**), ↑ed Cr
    - Dx: **Duplex U/S** - hypoechoic mass early; aspirate (fluid has high **Cr**)
    - Tx **percutaneous drainage** and **stent across anastomosis** *(best)*
  - **Renal artery stenosis** (or thrombosis) - *MC vascular Cx*
    - Sx's: ↓ed UOP, ↑ed Cr
    - Dx: **Duplex U/S** - shows flow acceleration, narrowing at anastomosis
    - Tx: **PTA** and **stent** (also the Tx for **renal vein stenosis**)
  - **Lymphocele** - MCC of **external compression** (MC **3 weeks** after TXP)
    - Sx's: ↓ed UOP <u>late</u> (from **compression of ureters**); ± pain
    - Dx: **Duplex U/S** - hypoechoic mass, hydronephrosis from ureter
      compression, good graft perfusion, fluid has normal Cr
    - Tx:
      - **1st** - percutaneous drainage (if that fails, some try leaving in
        externalized drain)
      - **2nd** - If above fails need **intra-peritoneal marsupialization**
        (<u>peritoneal window</u> - 95% successful) → drains through window
        into peritoneum and is re-absorbed
  - *Acute rejection*
    - Most commonly occurs between 1 week to 6 months
    - Dx: **Duplex U/S** and **renal Bx**
    - Path - **tubulitis** (**vasculitis** more severe form)
    - Tx: pulse steroids, other drugs
    - **Repeat Bx** after Tx to make sure rejection is cleared
  - **Chronic rejection** - usually occurs after 1 year; no good Tx
- MCC mortality after kidney TXP - **myocardial infarction**
- **5-year graft survival** – 75% (<u>cadaveric</u> 70%, <u>living donors</u> 80%)
  - Most fail from chronic rejection
- **Median patient survival** - 15-20 years (kidney TXP for ESRD extends patient survival **15 years**)
- **Recent kidney TXP,** now with **↑Cr** or poor UOP post-op →
  - DDx - acute rejection, vascular problem, urine leak with compression, lymphocele (late)
  - Initial Tx - **fluid** challenge and/or **Lasix** trial, check bladder catheter
  - Dx: **Duplex U/S** with **biopsy** *(best test)* - checks for vascular problem, urine leak, acute rejection, etc.
  - Tx: empiric ↓ in **CSA or FK** (these can be nephrotoxic), **pulse steroids** (often empiric); further Tx based on cause
- **Living kidney donors**
  - MC Cx - **wound infection** (1%)
  - MCC of death - **fatal PE** (0.05%)
  - The remaining kidney hypertrophies
  - Donor with **dual collecting systems** is <u>not</u> a contraindication to TXP

LIVER TRANSPLANTATION

- MC indication for <u>liver TXP</u> - **chronic hepatitis** from **Hep C**
  - MC indication in <u>children</u> - **biliary atresia**
- Some **hepatocellular CA** can undergo liver TXP
  - *Cannot* have metastases or vascular invasion; *No* cholangiocarcinoma
- *Not contraindications to liver TXP* - HIV, portal vein thrombosis, recipient age, prior ETOH abuse, hepatopulmonary syndrome, hepatorenal syndrome
- **Donor liver** (cadaveric or living related)
  - Can cold store for **24 hours**
  - **Macrosteatosis** (cadaveric)
    - Extracellular fat globules in liver allograft
    - Best overall predictor of **primary non-function**
    - If 60% of cross section is macrosteatotic in a potential donor, there is a 60% chance of primary non-function (60% is generally the cut-off when deciding whether or not to use the liver)
  - **Living related**
    - MC for **adult** donation - **right liver lobe** (segments 5, 6, 7 and 8)
    - MC for **pediatric** donation - **left lateral** (segments 2 and 3), sometimes left liver lobe (segments 2, 3 and 4)
    - Donor liver regenerates to 100% in **6-8 weeks**
- Cx's:
  - **Liver failure or problems post-op**
    - Dx: **Duplex U/S with Bx** (finds vascular problems, fluid collections, acute rejection, CMV infection, cholangitis, ect)
  - **Biliary leak** *(MC complication)* - Tx: **percutaneous drainage** and ERCP with sphincterotomy and **stent** (across leak if possible; usually temporary)
  - **Biliary stenosis** (dilated ducts on U/S) - Tx **ERCP dilatation** and stent (usually temporary)
  - **Primary non-function**
    - <u>*First 24 hours*</u>: bilirubin > 10, PT / PTT 1.5 x normal, bile output < 40 cc, metabolic acidosis
    - <u>*After 96 hours:*</u> lethargy, ↑ LFTs, renal failure (↑ K), respiratory failure
    - Tx: **emergent re-transplantation**
  - **Vascular Cx's**
    - **Early hepatic artery thrombosis**
      - **MC early vascular Cx**
      - Sx's: ↑ed LFTs, ↓ed bile output, **fulminant hepatic failure**
      - Dx: **duplex U/S**
      - Tx: Can try angio with PTA and stent or reoperate to repair anastomosis; *most often will need **emergent re-transplantation** for ensuing fulminant hepatic failure*
    - <u>**Late**</u> hepatic artery thrombosis results in biliary strictures and abscesses (<u>not</u> fulminant hepatic failure)
    - **MCC hepatic abscess** after liver TXP - late **hepatic artery thrombosis**
  - **Cholangitis** - see **PMNs** around portal triad, *not* mixed infiltrate (DDx vs. acute rejection, see below)
  - **Acute rejection**
    - T cell mediated against **blood vessels**, MC in 1st 2 months
    - Sx's: fever, jaundice, ↓ bile output
    - Dx: ↑ed WBCs, ↑ed LFTs; ↑ed PT; get duplex U/S and Liver Bx
    - Path (**portal triad** shows):
      - **Portal venous lymphocytosis**
      - **Endotheliitis** (<u>*mixed*</u> infiltrate, <u>not</u> just PMNs)
      - **Bile duct injury**
    - Tx: **pulse steroids**; other immunosuppressive agents
  - **Chronic rejection**
    - <u>***Very low** chronic rejection* with liver TXP – only 5% lifetime</u>
    - Path - disappearing bile ducts
    - RFs - high number of acute rejection episodes (biggest RF)

- **Recent liver TXP**, now with ↑ed LFTs or ↓ed bile output early post-op → Dx: **duplex U/S with liver Bx** (*best test*; will Dx vascular problem, acute rejection, primary non-function, bile leak)
- **5-year survival** - 70%
  - **Median Survival** - 15-20 years
  - **ETOH** - 20% will start drinking again (recidivism)
- **Living liver donor** – 10% complication rate (MC - bile leak)
  - Mortality < 1%
- **Hepatitis B recipient** - Tx: **Adefovir** and **lamivudine** (reverse transcriptase inhibitors) post-op to prevent re-infection → reduces re-infection rate to **< 5%**
- **Hepatitis C recipient**
  - *Disease most likely to recur in the new liver allograft*
  - Re-infects essentially all grafts; re-infection course is usually indolent (ie patients do not get acute hepatitis) although cirrhosis recurs in 15% after 5 years
  - Recurrence of HepC is the MCC of death and re-transplantation in these patients
  - Recent 90% Hepatitis C cure rates with **sofosbuvir** (Solvaldi) may change re-infection rate

HEART TRANSPLANTATION
- **Indications** - life expectancy < 1 year; can cold store heart for **6 hours**
- **Persistent pulmonary hypertension** after heart TXP (↑s mortality)
  - Tx: inhaled nitric oxide, ECMO if severe
- MCC **early mortality** (< 1 year) - infection
- MCC **late mortality** (> 5 years) - chronic allograft vasculopathy (accelerated atherosclerosis of small coronaries - can't use CABG)
- MCC **mortality overall** - chronic allograft vasculopathy
- **Acute rejection** - **peri-vascular infiltrate** with increasing grades of **myocyte inflammation** and **necrosis**
- High risk of **silent MI** due to **vagal denervation** after heart TXP
- **Median survival** - 10 years

LUNG TRANSPLANTATION
- **Indications** - life expectancy < 1 year; can cold store lung for **6 hours**
- Absolute indication for double-lung TXP (as opposed to single lung) - **cystic fibrosis**
  - MC lung infection with cystic fibrosis (often chronic)- **Pseudomonas aeruginosa**
- *Exclusion* criteria for using donor lungs - aspiration, moderate to large contusion, infiltrate, purulent sputum, $PO_2 < 350$ on 100% FiO_2
- MCC **early mortality** (< 1 year) - reperfusion injury (primary graft failure)
- MCC **late mortality** (> 1 year) - bronchiolitis obliterans
- MCC **mortality overall** - bronchiolitis obliterans
- **Acute rejection** - peri-vascular lymphocytosis
- **Chronic rejection** - bronchiolitis obliterans
- **Median survival** - 5 years

PANCREAS TRANSPLANTATION
- **MC indication** - type I diabetes and ESRD (usually combined with kidney)
- Need **donor celiac artery, SMA** (arterial supply to pancreas) and **portal vein** (for venous drainage); is attached to recipient **iliac vessels**
- Most use **enteric drainage** for the pancreatic duct (the donor pancreas and attached 2nd portion of duodenum is anastomosed to recipient small intestine)
- **Successful pancreas/kidney TXP** results in:
  - **Stabilization of retinopathy**
  - ↓ed **neuropathy** with ↑ed nerve conduction velocity
  - ↓ed **autonomic dysfunction** (↓ed gastroparesis)
  - ↓ed **orthostatic hypotension**
  - *No reversal of vascular disease*

Infection

103. All of the following are true of post-op fever except:
    a. Fever within 48 hours is MC due to atelectasis
    b. Fever after 48 hours is MC due to urinary tract infection
    c. Fever after day 5 is MC due to wound infection
    d. Abscess is MC within 3 days

    Answer d. Abscess is MC between days 7-10.

104. All of the following are true in prevention of surgical site infection (SSI) except:
    a. Antibiotics given within 1 hour prior to incision are used to prevent wound infection
    b. Blood glucose should be maintained between 80-120
    c. PaO_2 should remain high during the operation (use of 100% FiO_2)
    d. Warm IV fluids are the best method for preventing hypothermia
    e. Staph aureus is the MC organism in surgical site infections

    Answer d. Warm air conduction (eg Bair Hugger) is the best method for preventing hypothermia.

105. A 65 yo recent immigrant from Ukraine who is a poor historian of his multiple previous surgeries (some of which have been recent) presents with a sinus tract and drainage from the RLQ. CT scan shows a mass near the cecum. What is the most appropriate next step:
    a. Wound biopsy
    b. Antibiotics and drainage
    c. Chemo only
    d. Chemo-XRT
    e. Right hemicolectomy

    Answer a. A CA diagnosis has not been made at this point. A wound Bx of the obvious sinus tract is appropriate. This may represent infection or malignancy.

106. Wound biopsy in the above patient shows yellow-sulfur granules. The most appropriate next step is:
    a. Antibiotics (PCN) and drainage
    b. Chemo only
    c. Chemo-XRT
    d. Right hemicolectomy

    Answer a. Given the **yellow-sulfur granules**, this most likely represents **actinomyces** infection and antibiotics (**high dose PCN**) are appropriate. There is often an associated abscess which should be drained. Surgical resection of the associated mass is <u>not</u> indicated. Actinomyces infections can also present in **peri-oral** areas after trauma, tooth extraction, or in patients with poor dentition. They can also present in the **lung** as an abscess with sinus drainage.

107. All of the following are true of ventilator associated pneumonia (VAP) except:
    a. Initial Tx should include vancomycin for empiric Tx of MRSA
    b. Broncho-alveolar lavage cultures > 100,000 CFU/mL suggests VAP
    c. Routine ventilator circuit changes are indicated
    d. VAP is the MCC of infectious death in surgical patients
    e. It is related to duration of intubation

    Answer c. Routine circuit changes are <u>not</u> indicated (only with contamination).

108. All of the following are true of infections except:
    a. The internal jugular vein line site has the lowest infection rate for central lines
    b. Central lines are the MCC of blood stream infections

    c.   UTI is the MC acquired hospital infection
    d.   Bacteremia generally occurs 1 hour before fever

Answer a. Subclavian lines have the lowest infection rates.

109. A 65 yo man with severe type II DM presents with a chronic ulcer at his right 2nd MTP joint. There is mixed skin breakdown with mild purulence at the wound base in addition to mild surrounding erythema. All of the following are appropriate for this patient except:
    a.   Antibiotics
    b.   Debridement
    c.   Keeping the wound moist
    d.   Amputation

    Answer d. This patient is not presenting with a severe infection so an amputation is not indicated.

110. For the above patient, the best diagnostic test for organisms is:
    a.   Blood culture
    b.   Wound swab
    c.   Bone biopsy
    d.   Wound biopsy
    e.   Sputum culture

    Answer d. Wound Bx at the base of the wound is the best test for organisms.

111. For the above patient, the best diagnostic test for osteomyelitis is:
    a.   MRI
    b.   CT scan
    c.   Tagged WBC scan
    d.   Bone biopsy
    e.   Bone scan

    Answer a. MRI is the best diagnostic study for **osteomyelitis**. Bone scan is the best choice if the patient has hardware. Bone biopsy should be _avoided_ as this can lead to seeding of the bone marrow and osteomyelitis.

112. A 65 yo man with severe Type II diabetes presents to the ED with a mottled, cold right lower extremity with pus pouring out of an associated heel ulcer. He is extremely lethargic. His HR is 120 with a BP of 80/40. You start antibiotics and fluid resuscitation. The most appropriate next step is:
    a.   Amputation
    b.   Hyperbaric oxygen
    c.   Debridement
    d.   Insulin only
    e.   MRI

    Answer a. Amputation. This patient is in **septic shock** with an obvious source. The description of the **gangrenous extremity** indicates it is beyond salvage. Amputation is appropriate

113. A 65 yo man with severe Type II diabetes has severe edema, crepitus, and erythema in his lower extremity after stepping on a piece of glass. His vital signs are: BP 120/70, HR 90. The most appropriate next step is:
    a.   Amputation
    b.   Hyperbaric oxygen
    c.   Debridement
    d.   Insulin only
    e.   MRI

Answer c. Debridement. This presentation suggests **necrotizing fasciitis** and debridement with antibiotics is warranted (would not want to do an amputation here). The inoculation site can be small (eg stepping on a nail, glass, or piece of coral; a small foot ulcer). The infection can be caused by **strep pyogenes** (Group A beta-hemolytic strep), **MRSA**, or **mixed organisms**. Necrotizing fasciitis can also present as an **early post-op wound infection** (within 6 hours) following laparotomy (Sx's - erythema; crepitus; thin, grey, foul-smelling drainage).

114. A 50 yo diabetic patient presents with a severely swollen and inflamed left 2nd toe. There is frank pus coming out the end of the toe and red streaks going up his leg. The most appropriate next step in this patient is:
    a. Antibiotics only
    b. Debridement only
    c. Ray amputation and antibiotics
    d. Antibiotics and debridement
    e. Hyperbaric oxygen therapy

    Answer c. Ray amputation and antibiotics

115. Six hours after a penetrating farming accident to the lower extremity, your patient is confused, has a fever of 41 C, and develops gray, foul smelling, 'dishwater' drainage from his wound. You feel crepitus.. All of the following are true except:
    a. GPRs on gram stain would be consistent with the most likely diagnosis
    b. Alpha toxin is the greatest source of morbidity and mortality
    c. This patient requires emergent debridement
    d. The patient requires broad-spectrum antibiotics *only*

    Answer d. This presentation is classic for **clostridium perfringens myonecrosis** infection. The patient needs emergent **wound debridement** and **antibiotics**.

116. A 50 yo diabetic man has significant tenderness and drainage of pus from the scrotum and perineal area. The most important next step is:
    a. Antibiotics
    b. Emergent debridement
    c. Wound vac
    d. Percutaneous drain
    e. Blood sugar control

    Answer b. Fournier's Gangrene refers to a **perineal** necrotizing fasciitis that is **polymicrobial**. Emergency **wound debridement** is the most important step in treatment. **Antibiotics** are also indicated. Fournier's can occur in diabetic patients, after urologic / perineal procedures, after trauma, or in patient's with a peri-rectal abscess. One should try and preserve the testicles if possible during debridement.

117. A 50 yo man develops abdominal pain, fever, and profuse foul diarrhea after being hospitalized for pneumonia (BP 80/30, HR 120). He is diffusely tender but does not have peritoneal signs. His WBCs are 52. You start aggressive fluid resuscitation. All of the following are true of this patient's likely condition except:
    a. IV vancomycin is the treatment of choice
    b. ELISA for toxin A + B is the most rapid test for the condition
    c. A high WBC is consistent with the condition
    d. Vancomycin PO is treatment of choice in pregnant women

    Answer a. Given recent antibiotics for pneumonia, severe diarrhea, and extremely elevated WBCs, the most likely diagnosis in this patient is **pseudomembranous colitis**. **Flagyl** (IV or PO), **PO vancomycin,** or **Fidaxomicin** (Dificid) can be used for treatment. *IV vancomycin is not effective for Clostridium difficile colitis.*

118. In the above patient, antibiotics for pneumonia are discontinued and IV Flagyl is started. Three days later, however, his diarrhea is the same. He is less tender. His colon is normal caliber on X-ray. What is the most appropriate next step:
    a. Colectomy
    b. Neostigmine
    c. Soap suds enema
    d. Endoscopic decompression
    e. Change antibiotics

    Answer e. Change antibiotics (switch to PO vancomycin or Dificid). If one antibiotic fails to control the infection it should be switched out to another one.

119. Instead of the above, antibiotics for pneumonia are discontinued and IV Flagyl is started. Three days later, however, his pain and tenderness increase and his colon is significantly dilated. What is the most appropriate next step:
    a. Colectomy
    b. Neostigmine
    c. Soap suds enema
    d. Endoscopic decompression
    e. Change antibiotics

    Answer a. Colectomy (with ileostomy). Toxic megacolon can occur with C. difficile colitis and total abdominal colectomy is indicated. C. difficile toxic megacolon carries a significantly high mortality rate (25% in some series).

120. All of the following are true except:
    a. Spontaneous bacterial peritonitis (SBP) is MC poly-organismal
    b. IV albumin increases survival in patients with SBP
    c. Fungal infection of peritoneal dialysis catheters requires removal
    d. Peritoneal fluid with WBCs > 500 or PMNs > 250 suggest SBP
    e. SBP in children MC occurs in the setting of nephrotic syndrome

    Answer a. SBP is MC <u>mono-organismal</u> (MC - E. coli; children - strep pyogenes). <u>Poly-organismal</u> infection suggests secondary bacterial peritonitis (eg perforated viscous).

121. A 55 yo man with ESRD undergoing peritoneal dialysis (PD) develops severe, diffuse abdominal tenderness and fever. The effluent is murky and almost opaque. Which of the following organisms are most likely involved:
    a. E. coli and Klebsiella
    b. Klebsiella and Serratia
    c. Staph aureus and pseudomonas
    d. Enterococcus and yeast
    e. Bacteroides fragilis and E. coli

    Answer c. *Staph aureus* and **pseudomonas** are most likely to cause <u>severe</u> pain with PD catheter-related **peritonitis**. *Staph epidermidis* is the MC organism involved in infected peritoneal fluid associated with PD catheters, however, it is more likely to cause <u>mild</u> pain.

122. For the above patient, all of the following are appropriate steps at this time except:
    a. Send the fluid for gram stain and culture
    b. Start IV vancomycin and gentamicin
    c. Administer intra-peritoneal vancomycin and gentamicin
    d. Stop peritoneal dialysis and start hemodialysis
    e. Administer intra-peritoneal heparin

    Answer d. You should continue peritoneal dialysis at this point with antibiotics given in the dialysate as well as systemically. ESRD patients have limited venous access sites so starting hemodialysis at this point is not indicated. **Exit**

site (> 95% salvage rate) and **tunnel infections** (70% salvage rate) are also initially treated conservatively (ie without PD catheter removal) with antibiotics and local wound care.

123. A 55 yo man with ESRD and a right sided permacath (tunneled central venous access catheter) develops erythema (0.5 cm rim) and purulence localized to the exit site. The most appropriate next step is:
    a.   Topical antibiotics with systemic antibiotics if infection worsens or is refractory
    b.   Change line over a wire and antibiotics
    c.   Remove the catheter, place a new catheter at a new site, and antibiotics
    d.   Observation only

    Answer a. This is most likely an **exit site infection** so topical antibiotics only are indicated at this stage. Avoidance of mechanical trauma is necessary in these patients (stabilize the catheter). If the infection worsens or is refractory, systemic antibiotics are indicated.

124. Instead of the above, U/S shows the catheter floating in fluid with purulent drainage out of the exit site. The most appropriate next step is:
    a.   Antibiotics only
    b.   Change line over a wire and antibiotics
    c.   Remove the catheter, place a new catheter at a new site, and antibiotics
    d.   Observation only

    Answer c. This is a **tunnel infection** so removing the catheter is appropriate here (note this is different from a PD catheter tunnel infection above).

125. Instead of the above, the exit site and U/S look normal however the patient has had recurrent fevers. Blood cultures are positive for staph epidermidis. The most appropriate next step is:
    a.   Antibiotics only
    b.   Change line over a wire and antibiotics
    c.   Remove the catheter, place a new catheter at a new site, and antibiotics
    d.   Observation only

    Answer b. This patient most likely has a **catheter-related blood stream infection**. In patients _without_ ESRD simply removing the catheter all together or removing the catheter with placement in a new site is appropriate. Because the patient has **ESRD**, _conservation of access sites is appropriate_. Changing the line over a wire at the same site and antibiotics are appropriate (80% salvage rate).

126. A 55 yo man with ESRD has a left arm AV fistula graft. He presents with erythema and localized purulence over a previous puncture site. The most appropriate next step is:
    a.   Antibiotics only
    b.   Close the wound and antibiotics
    c.   Local debridement and antibiotics
    d.   Partial graft resection, bypass through non-infected area, and antibiotics
    e.   Whole graft resection and antibiotics

    Answer c. Local debridement (drainage, wet to dry dressings) and systemic antibiotics are appropriate for an AV fistula graft **access site infection**.

127. Despite appropriate therapy, the patient above develops increased pus drainage from the site. At exploration, you find a deep infection involving a graft segment, however, the areas proximal and distal to the site are scarred in and attached to the surrounding soft tissue. The most appropriate next step is:
    a.   Antibiotics only
    b.   Close the wound and antibiotics
    c.   Local debridement and antibiotics
    d.   Partial graft resection, bypass through non-infected area, and antibiotics

e.   Whole graft resection and antibiotics

Answer d. Partial graft resection, bypass through non-infected area, and antibiotics are appropriate for a **localized graft infection**.

128. Despite appropriate therapy, the above patient's condition worsens. An U/S shows the majority of the graft floating in fluid. The most appropriate next step is:
    a.   Antibiotics only
    b.   Close the wound and antibiotics
    c.   Local debridement and antibiotics
    d.   Partial graft resection, bypass through non-infected area, and antibiotics
    e.   Whole graft resection and antibiotics

Answer e. Whole graft resection and antibiotics are indicated for **tunnel infections** or infection at an **anastomosis** (risk of severe hemorrhage).

129. A 22 yo with acute myelogenous leukemia (AML) is undergoing chemotherapy and is at his nadir (WBC 2) when he develops significant RLQ pain and tenderness with a fever to 103 F. CT scan shows pneumatosis intestinalis throughout his cecum. The most appropriate next step is:
    a.   Cecostomy
    b.   Cecal resection and ileostomy
    c.   Right hemicolectomy
    d.   Antibiotics only
    e.   Cecal stent

Answer d. Antibiotics only. **Neutropenic typhlitis** (enterocolitis) is inflammation that occurs when WBCs are low. It is often associated with chemotherapy at its nadir. Patients may have pneumatosis intestinalis, although it is not in itself a surgical indication. Tx - **broad spectrum antibiotics**; surgery reserved for cases of free perforation (Tx: cecal or colonic resection)

130. All of the following are true except:
    a.   Enterococcus is sensitive to most cephalosporins
    b.   Proteus produces urease
    c.   Staph Aureus in the MC organism in VAP
    d.   The MC fecal bacteria is bacteriodies fragilis

Answer a. Enterococcus is resistant to _all_ cephalosporins.

131. Which of the following is true:
    a.   Hepatitis A can cause hepatoma
    b.   Hepatitis E can cause hepatoma
    c.   Acute fulminant liver failure is common for hepatitis C
    d.   Hepatitis E causes acute hepatitis in pregnancy

Answer e. Hepatitis E causes acute hepatitis in pregnancy. Hepatitis A and hepatitis E do not cause chronic hepatitis or hepatoma. Hepatitis C rarely causes acute fulminant hepatic failure.

132. All of the following are true except:
    a.   Elevated anti-HBs antibodies only suggests previous HepB infection
    b.   High anti-HBc, anti-HBe, and anti-HBs antibodies and <u>no</u> HBs antigens suggests patient had infection, recovery, and subsequent immunity
    c.   HepC is the most common viral infection leading to liver TXP
    d.   Combined HepB + HepD infection has the highest mortality for viral hepatitis

Answer a. Elevated **anti-HBs antibodies** only suggests HepB immunization.

133. All of the following are true of HIV except:

a. CMV colitis complications (bleeding, perforated ulcer) are the MC indication for laparotomy in HIV patients
b. The MC CA in HIV patients requiring surgery is lymphoma (for bleeding or perforation)
c. Kaposi's sarcoma is most commonly treated non-operatively
d. The MC solid organ lymphoma in HIV patients is colon

Answer d. The MC **solid organ lymphoma** in HIV patients is **stomach** (usually NHL, presents as bleeding, perforation, or pain).

GUT FLORA
- **Stomach** - almost sterile, few GPCs, some yeast
- **Proximal small bowel** - 10^5 bacteria, mostly GPCs
- **Distal small bowel** - 10^7 bacteria; GPCs, GPRs, GNRs
- **Colon** - 10^{11} bacteria; 99% **anaerobes**; a few GNRs and GPCs
- MC organism overall in gut (also MC fecal bacteria) - **Bacteroides fragilis**
- MC GNR in gut and MC aerobic organism in gut - **E coli**
- MC GPC in gut - **enterococcus**
- GPCs - **exotoxins**
- GNRs - **endotoxins**

IMPORTANT ORGANISMS
- **Staph aureus** (coagulase positive)
  - Has **exoslime biofilm** - adhere to prosthetic material
  - **Resistant to PCN** due to **beta-lactamase**
  - **MRSA** (methicillin resistant staph aureus) - resistance due to **altered penicillin binding protein** (Tx: vancomycin first line)
- **Staph epidermidis** (coagulase negative)
  - Have **exoslime biofilm** - adhere to prosthetic material (eg PD catheter)
- **Enterococcus faecalis** - common in gut (95% of population)
  - *Resistant to all cephalosporins*
  - **Vancomycin resistant enterococcus** (VRE)
    Resistance from **mutation in cell wall binding protein**
    Tx: Synercid or Linezolid
- **Pseudomonas aeruginosa** - have alginate mucoid layer (biofilm), colonize tubes
- **Anaerobes** outnumber aerobic bacteria in colon (1000:1); anaerobes need **low oxygen content** (lack superoxide dismutase and catalase, making them vulnerable to oxygen radicals)

NOSOCOMIAL INFECTIONS
- Infections acquired in hospital (> 48 hours after admission or within 30 days of discharge)
- 35% of all nosocomial infections can be prevented
- **Hand-washing** before patient contact is the most effective way of preventing nosocomial infections
- **Contact precautions** - gown / gloves are removed inside out and left in patient's room
- **Highest risk** for hospital acquired infection - patients with **burn wounds**
- **Nosocomial Infections:** SSI, VAP, CRBSI, UTI (MC)
- **Malnutrition** - MC immune deficiency; leads to infection

FEVER (after surgery)
- MC fever source within **48 hours** — **Atelectasis**
- MC fever source **48 hours - 5 days** — **Urinary tract infection**
- MC fever source after **5 days** — **Wound infection**

Fever Source	MC Time Frame (post-op day)
Atelectasis	1-2
UTI	3-5
Wound infection, medications, DVT	5-7
Abscess	7-10

SCIP AND PROPHYLACTIC MEASURES (surgical care improvement project)
- **Pre-op**
  - *Avoid* elective operations if patient has an **active infection**
  - **Stop tobacco** (causes poor healing although has <u>not</u> been shown to reduce pulmonary Cx's)
  - **Clippers** to remove hair (<u>not</u> shaving)
  - **Shower** night before with antibiotic soap
- **Chlorhexidine gluconate** skin prep *(better coverage and fewer wound infections compared to betadine)* and **ioban skin drape** (iodophor)
- **Prophylactic antibiotics** (are used to **prevent surgical site infection**)
  - Should be given **within 1 hour** prior to incision (ensures appropriate blood levels)
  - Should be stopped **within 24 hours** of end operation time (prevents the development of antibiotic resistance)
- **FiO₂ 100%** while in OR (want pO_2 high, inhibits bacteria)
- **OR temperature** - should be kept warm at **70 F**
- Keep **patient warm** - warm air conduction *(best method, eg Bair Hugger)*; *avoid* hypothermia which promotes infection
- **Glucose management** - should be maintained between **80-120** (prevents hyperglycemia which promotes infection)
- **Beta-blocker** and **DVT prophylaxis**
- **Sterile dressing** for 24-48 hours
- **Remove urinary catheter** on POD 1 or 2

SURGICAL SITE INFECTION (SSI)
- ***Staph aureus*** - MC organism overall in SSI
- ***E. coli*** - MC **GNR** in SSI
- ***B. fragilis*** - MC **anaerobe** in SSI
  - Anaerobe growth indicates necrosis or abscess (only grows in low redox state)
- **Dx of SSI** - need **≥ 10⁵ bacteria** (less if foreign body present)
- **RFs**: long operations, advanced age, chronic disease (eg COPD, renal failure, liver failure, diabetes), malnutrition, immunosuppression, obesity, ASA class, hypothermia

SSI Incidence
Clean (eg inguinal hernia):	1-2%
Clean contaminated (prepped elective bowel resection)	4%
Contaminated (stab wound to colon with repair)	8%
Gross contamination (perforated appendix)	30%

- **Surgical infections** within **48 hours** of procedure:
  - **Injury to bowel** with leak
  - **Invasive soft tissue infection** - *S. aureus* and beta-hemolytic strep; can present within hours post-op (produce exotoxins)

URINARY TRACT INFECTION
- *MC **infection** in surgery patients*
- **#1 RF** - **urinary catheters** (MC infection - **E. coli**)
- Early removal (POD 1 or 2) of urinary catheters decreases UTI

VENTILATOR ASSOCIATED PNEUMONIA (VAP)
- *MCC of **infectious death** in surgical patients*
- RFs: *prolonged intubation* (#1), advanced age, pre-existing lung disease, immunosuppression, malnutrition, burns, ARDS
- From **aspiration** of exogenous or endogenous microbes in **oropharynx**
- Sx's: **fever**, purulent sputum, hypoxia
- Dx: Labs - ↑ed WBCs, CXR - **new unilateral infiltrate**
- **Measures to reduce VAP**:
  - Minimize duration of intubation (risk increases 1% / day)
  - Barrier techniques by staff; wash hands
  - Elevate head of bed 30 degrees
  - Ventilator circuit change <u>only</u> if contaminated

- Adequate drainage of oral and sub-glottic secretions
- Oral hygiene (chlorhexidine rinse) and nasal mupirocin (Bactroban)
- Daily sedation withdrawal - wake patient up
- Tracheostomy when ventilation is needed for > 7 days
- *Avoid* nasal intubation (sinusitis → pneumonia)
- *Avoid* unnecessary antibiotics and transfusions
- Stress ulcer prophylaxis with PPI
- Blood sugar control (80-120)
- Measures that do not reduce VAP:
  - Gut decontamination
  - Routine ventilator circuit changes (only change if contaminated)
- **VAP pathogens**
  - #1 ***Staph aureus***, #2 *Pseudomonas aeruginosa*, #3 *E. coli*
  - **GNRs** - MC class of organism in VAP
- Sx's of VAP: fever, purulent sputum, new infiltrate on CXR, high WBCs
- Tx: **Vancomycin** (cover MRSA) + (**fluoroquinolone**, 3rd generation cephalosporin, or anti-pseudomonal PCN - all cover pseudomonas) until sensitivities back; need **2 weeks** of antibiotics
- **Hospital acquired pneumonia** (**nosocomial** or **aspiration** while in hospital)
  - Pathogens - same as VAP pathogens
  - Tx: same as VAP
- **Community aspiration pneumonia**
  - MC site - **superior segment of RLL** (right lower lobe)
  - MC organism - **strep pneumonia**; others - staph aureus, **anaerobes**
  - Tx: (3rd gen cephalosporin or fluoroquinolone) ± (clindamycin or Flagyl)
  - **Lung abscess** can form (MC location - **superior segment of RLL**); Tx - *antibiotics only (not percutaneous drainage)*

CENTRAL LINE INFECTIONS
- Sx's: fever, site erythema, ↑ed WBCs; can lead to blood stream infection (see below)
- #1 ***Staph epidermidis***, #2 Staph aureus, #3 yeast (*Candida albicans*)
- **Femoral lines** at *highest risk* for central line infection
- **Subclavian lines** have the *lowest risk* of central line infection (preferred route of central venous access)
  - *Contraindications* to subclavian line - coagulopathy or low platelets (incompressible area); patients in whom a pneumothorax would be life-threatening
- The **longer** a central line is in → the greater the **infection risk**
- Prevention of central line infections: wash hands, **chlorhexidine** for skin prep, barrier precautions when inserting (ie mask, shield, and gown), remove line when unnecessary
- If worried about **central line infection**, best to pull out the central line and place peripheral IVs if the central line is not needed
  - If central line is still needed temporarily, best to place it at a **new site**

BLOOD STREAM INFECTION (bacteremia)
- MCC of blood steam infection - **central line infection**
- MC organism - ***Staph epidermidis*** *(coagulase negative staph)*
- Tx: **remove central line** unless used for dialysis (see below)
  - Antibiotics for **2 weeks** (include vancomycin for MRSA until cultures and sensitivities back)
- **Optimal glucose levels** in a septic patient: 80 - 120 mg/dL

HEMODIALYSIS CATHETER / SUBCUTANEOUS PORT INFECTIONS
- **Higher infection rate** compared to AV fistulas and grafts
- **Exit site infection** (erythema and purulence at exit site) - Tx: topical **antibiotics** and avoidance of mechanical trauma if mild; if severe start systemic **antibiotics**
- **Tunnel infection** (above *plus* fluid collection deep to cuff site or pus drainage through the exit site) - Tx: **catheter removal** and IV antibiotics
- Catheter-related **blood stream infection** - Tx: **catheter exchange** over a wire and IV antibiotics (80% salvage rate; important for dialysis patients)

ABSCESSES

- Intra-abdominal abscesses usually contain anaerobic and aerobic bacteria
    - MC bacteria: <u>GPC</u> - Enterococcus faecalis, <u>GNR</u> - E. coli, <u>anaerobic</u> - B. fragilis
- A surgical-associated abscess usually occurs **7-10 days** after operation
- Tx: **drainage** for majority (usually the most important Tx; usually percutaneous for intra-abdominal abscess)
- **Broad spectrum antibiotics** indicated for: diabetes, cellulitis, sepsis (eg fever, elevated WBC), or bioprosthetic hardware (eg mechanical valves, hip replacements)
    - Include **Flagyl** for anaerobes
- Special cases:
    - **Lung** abscess - Tx: **antibiotics _only_** *(treats 95%)*; rarely need drainage
        - MCC of lung abscess - **aspiration**
    - **Splenic** abscess - Tx: **percutaneous drain** if <u>uniloculated</u>, **splenectomy** if <u>multiloculated</u>
        - MC source - **endocarditis** or **IVDA** (mortality rate 30%)
    - **Pancreatic** abscess - Tx: **open debridement** (*classic answer* as drains generally do <u>not</u> work)
    - **Peri-rectal or peri-anal** abscess - open drainage
    - **Epidural** abscess - open drainage
    - **Retropharyngeal** abscess - *airway emergency*, open drainage
        - Can lead to **mediastinitis**
    - **Parapharyngeal** abscess - watch airway, open drainage
        - Can lead to **mediastinitis**
    - **Liver** abscess - variety of causes and Tx (see Liver chapter)
    - **Suppurative flexor tenosynovitis** (flexor tendon sheath in finger) - Tx: need axial longitudinal drainage (see Orthopaedics chapter)

GRAM NEGATIVE SEPSIS

- **MC organism** - E. coli
- **Endotoxin** (lipopolysaccharide [LPS], **lipid A** portion) is released
    - **Lipid A** is the most potent trigger of **TNF-alpha** release
    - **TNF-alpha** (from macrophages) → activates inflammatory, complement, and coagulation cascades (microthrombi); high TNF-alpha levels leads to **SIRS**
- **Hyperglycemia** occurs with sepsis
    - **Early**: ↓ insulin, ↑ glucose (impaired utilization)
    - **Late**: ↑ insulin, ↑ glucose (due to insulin resistance)

NECROTIZING SOFT TISSUE INFECTIONS

- Can be caused by beta-hemolytic **_Strep pyogenes_** (group A), **_Staph aureus_**, **_Clostridium perfringens_**, or mixed organisms
- RFs: diabetes, peripheral arterial disease, poor hygiene, ETOH abuse
- Can present **quickly** after surgical procedures or injury (within **6 hours**)
- Earliest Sx: **pain out of proportion to skin findings**
- Later Sx's: skin erythema, blistering, edema, and crepitus; sepsis with lethargy and N/V; WBCs > 20-30
- **Necrotizing fasciitis**
    - **Inoculation site** can be small (eg stepping on a nail, glass, or coral; a small foot ulcer); spreads along fascial plane
    - Can present within **6-8 hours** of **trauma or surgery** (*rapid* wound infection)
    - Sx's: N/V, fever, mental status changes (lethargy)
    - Skin can look **normal** in the early stages (infection starts and spreads along **fascia**, then moves to soft tissue, often <u>spares</u> muscle)
        - *Initially may have pain out of proportion to apparent cellulitis (is initially a deep infection)*
    - Skin progresses to **pale red** with **blisters** as infection spreads
    - Can have '**dish-water**' colored fluid drainage, foul smelling
    - Organisms
        - **Type I** - <u>poly-microbial</u> (GPCs GNRs, anaerobes); surgery related
        - **Type II** - <u>mono-microbial</u> (2 types)
            - 1) **Strep pyogenes** (Group A beta hemolytic strep)

'Flesh eating strep'; MC mono-microbial cause

Release **exotoxins** (**A** + **C** → SIRS syndrome) - these are the major of source of **morbidity** and **mortality**

Infection → Fever → SIRS → MSOF → death

2) **Staph aureus** (especially **MRSA**) - also has **exotoxins**

Wound Bx for Type II shows GPCs with paucity of PMNs

- Tx: **emergency debridement** (clinical Dx enough for surgical exploration; debride fascia and soft tissue)

  Broad spectrum **antibiotics** until organism(s) identified

  Strep pyogenes - high dose PCN G + clindamycin

  MRSA - vancomycin

- **Clostridial myonecrosis** (gas gangrene; *C. perfringens*)
  - Occurs in **necrotic muscle** (anaerobe; needs low O_2 environment)
  - Can occur with **farming injuries**
  - Infection can spread **early** and **rapidly**
  - Sx's: acute onset of pain; may <u>not</u> show skin changes initially

    Lethargy and mental status changes

    Progressive crepitus, edema, erythema, and bullae

    Thin, gray, foul-smelling drainage; 'dishwater' fluid
  - X-ray: **gas dissecting into muscle**
  - **Alpha toxin** inserts in cell membrane, creates gap, then cell lysis

    Is the major of source of **morbidity** and **mortality**
  - Gram stain shows GPRs *without* WBCs
  - Tx: **emergency debridement** (clinical Dx enough for surgical exploration; debride muscle and fascia); high-dose penicillin and clindamycin
- **Fournier's gangrene**
  - Severe **necrotizing fasciitis** in perineal and scrotal region
  - Sx's: pain and redness in scrotum, penis, labia, and/or perineum; crepitus
  - Foul smelling grey discharge
  - RFs: diabetes, ETOH abuse, poor hygiene
  - Common etiologies - perianal abscess, perineal trauma / surgery, episiotomy following vaginal delivery, urogenital surgery or injury
  - **Polymicrobial** (GPCs, GNRs, and anaerobes)
  - Mortality rate - 25%
  - Tx: **emergency debridement** (clinical Dx enough for surgical exploration; debride fascia and soft tissue; try to preserve <u>testicles</u> if possible); broad spectrum antibiotics (cover aerobes and anaerobes)

OSTEOMYELITIS
- MC in **diabetic foot infections** (eg malperforans ulcer at 2nd MTP joint, heel ulcer)
- MC organism - *Staph aureus*
- Dx: **MRI** *(most sensitive test)*; if hardware is present (eg pacemaker, metal hip replacement, mechanical valve) get 3-phase bone scan (Technetium-99)
- Bone Bx itself may *increase* the risk of osteomyelitis in patients with diabetic foot infections and ulcers *(<u>avoid</u> bone Bx in these situations - can seed the bone)*
- Tx: antibiotics (6 weeks); possible bone / cartilage debridement (eg 2nd MTP cartilage)

SPONTANEOUS BACTERIAL PERITONITIS (SBP, primary bacterial peritonitis)
- Sx's: **fever** and **abdominal pain** in a patient with **cirrhosis** and **ascites**
  - Mental status changes (eg lethargy) can occur if septic (may be the only Sx)
  - In children, most often occurs in the setting of **nephrotic syndrome**
- Mortality rate - up to 25%
- RFs: low protein ascites (< 1 g/dL), previous SBP, current variceal GI bleeding
- Secondary to decreased host defenses (intra-hepatic shunting, impaired bactericidal activity in ascites); <u>not</u> due to transmucosal migration
- Fluid cultures are negative in many cases
- Dx: **paracentesis** *(best test)* and examine peritoneal fluid (*<u>any</u> are diagnostic* → **WBCs** > 500, **PMNs** > 250, or **positive cultures**)
  - MC organism - *E. coli* (50%); others - Strep pneumoniae, Klebsiella pneumoniae
  - MC organism in <u>children</u> - *strep pyogenes* (Group A strep)

- Should be **mono-microbial** → if not, worry about secondary bacterial peritonitis and intra-abdominal source (eg viscous perforation → would need exploratory laparotomy)
  - Tx: **ceftriaxone** or other 3rd generation cephalosporin; patients usually respond in **48 hours**; if not getting better → confirm Dx by repeating paracentesis or exploratory laparotomy if suspected intra-abdominal source (eg perforated diverticulitis)
    - **Albumin** infusion _decreases_ mortality in high risk patients (eg those with elevated BUN or Cr)
  - **Weekly prophylactic antibiotics** (fluoroquinolones; eg **norfloxacin**) are indicated after an episode of **SBP**
  - Patients with **bleeding esophageal varices** should receive **prophylactic norfloxacin** (these patients are at high risk for SBP)
  - Liver transplant is <u>not</u> an option with active SBP

PERITONEAL DIALYSIS CATHETER - RELATED INFECTIONS
- Can have exit site infection, tunnel infection, or peritonitis
- MC organisms for all - *Staph aureus (MC for exit site and tunnel infection)* **pseudomonas**, and *Staph epidermidis (MC for peritonitis; usually from 'touch-contamination')*
- **Exit site infection** - erythema and <u>localized</u> purulence
  - Tx: <u>topical</u> **antibiotics** and local wound care if mild; avoid mechanical trauma; start <u>systemic</u> **antibiotics** if severe or refractory
- **Tunnel infection** - erythema and purulent <u>drainage</u> from exit site
  - U/S shows **fluid collection** around the catheter
  - Tx: **tunnel exploration** (drainage of abscess, wet to dry dressings) and systemic antibiotics (70% salvage rate); *note this Tx is different from a tunnel infection associated with an AV graft which requires graft removal (see below)*
- **Peritonitis** - cloudy dialysate fluid, abdominal pain, and fever
  - Tx: leave catheter in and start **intra-peritoneal vancomycin / gentamicin** _and_ **IV antibiotics**; increase <u>dwell time</u> and give intra-peritoneal <u>heparin</u> (decreases fibrin blockage of catheter)
  - The **intra-peritoneal** antibiotics are more effective than the IV antibiotics
  - Need **removal of catheter** for peritonitis that lasts **> 5 days**
  - *Staph aureus* and **pseudomonas** are more likely to cause <u>severe</u> **pain**
  - *Staph epidermidis* more likely to cause <u>mild</u> **pain** (*MC organism for PD catheter related peritonitis*; some can be treated as an outpatient)
  - **Fungal infections** are very hard to treat (usually require catheter removal)
  - **Fecal peritonitis** requires **laparotomy** to find perforation

AV GRAFT INFECTIONS (dialysis graft infections)
- **Access site abscess** (superficial infection) - patients have erythema and localized purulence over a previous puncture site
  - Tx: **local debridement** (drainage, wet to dry dressings) and systemic antibiotics
- **Localized graft infection** - is a deep infection that involves a portion of the AV graft, however, the areas proximal and distal to the infection site are well incorporated and not infected
  - Tx: resect involved **graft segment** (local wet to dry dressing changes) and **bypass** area using proximal and distal graft sites well away from infected area
- **Tunnel infection** (U/S shows graft floating in fluid)**, multiple abscesses** throughout the graft, or infection at an **anastomosis** → *are all indications for* **graft resection**

PSEUDOMEMBRANOUS COLITIS
- MCC - *Clostridium difficile*
- Sx's: foul, watery, green, mucoid diarrhea; abdominal pain and cramping; fever; can also occur in absence of diarrhea
  - Can occur up to 3 weeks after a single dose antibiotics
  - Normal colonic flora altered by **antibiotics**, allowing overgrowth of C. difficile
- RFs: elderly, ICU patients, nursing home residents
- Can have really **elevated WBCs** (30-40s)
- PMN inflammation of mucosa / submucosa (pseudomembranes, plaques)
- Dx: ELISA for **toxin A** or **B** *(most expeditious test; are C. difficile toxins)*

- May need to send sample multiple times (false negative rate 15%) → if clinical suspicion is high, treat the patient without relying on ELISA
- Cell culture cytotoxin assay is most accurate but takes too long (24-48 hours)
- Fecal leukocytes - not specific enough
- **Toxins A + B** kill mucosal cells, **toxin A** is more damaging
- Mucosal inflammation with **yellow pseudomembranes**
- Tx: **fluid resuscitation**; stop other antibiotics and avoid anti-motility drugs
    - Oral - **vancomycin**; IV - **Flagyl** (metronidazole; oral Flagyl for mild cases)
    - If a patient fails to respond to PO vancomycin, then IV Flagyl should be started and vice versa
    - **Fidaxomicin** (Dificid) - as effective as vancomycin; less recurrences
    - *IV vancomycin is not effective*
    - *Avoid colonoscopy if the colon is dilated (risk of perforation)*
- **Fulminant colitis** (in 1%; life-threatening; toxic megacolon / colitis) – includes *any* of the following:
    - 1) Uncontrolled sepsis *or:*
    - 2) Significant distension (> 10-12 cm) with worsening Sx's or localized peritonitis despite antibiotics *or:*
    - 3) Perforation *or:*
    - 4) Diffuse peritoneal signs (diffuse rebound or guarding)
    - Tx: **total abdominal colectomy** and **ileostomy** *(for any above – is life-saving)*
    - High mortality with C. difficile toxic megacolon (40%; **NAP1** strain very virulent)
- **Pregnancy** with pseudomembranous colitis - Tx: **oral vancomycin** (no systemic absorption; is very effective although expensive)

NEUTROPENIC TYPHLITIS (or enterocolitis)
- Follows chemotherapy when WBCs are low (nadir)
- Can mimic surgical disease
- May have pneumatosis intestinalis *(not a surgical indication)*, fat stranding, thickened cecum / colon
- Tx: **broad spectrum antibiotics**; patients will improve when WBCs increase; *surgery only for free perforation*
    - Granulocyte colony stimulating factor (**GCSF**) is used to increase WBCs

VIRAL HEPATITIS
- ***All hepatitis viruses*** *(A, B, C, D+B, and E)* can cause:
    - 1) ***Acute hepatitis*** and:
    - 2) ***Fulminant hepatic failure*** (although rare for HepC)
- **HepE** causes acute hepatitis in **pregnancy**
- **HepB, HepC** and **HepD** can also cause **chronic hepatitis** and **hepatoma**
- HepA and HepE do *not* cause chronic hepatitis or hepatoma

- **HepB** (DNA)
    - The only **DNA** hepatitis virus (proteins: **s** = surface, **e** = envelope, **c** = core)
    - Infection - Anti-HBc **IgM** highest in first 6 months, then **IgG** takes over
    - HepB Vaccination - have increased **anti-HBs** antibodies only
    - *Ex:* ↑ed *anti-HBc, anti-HBe* and *anti-HBs* antibodies and *no* HBs antigens→ *patient had infection, recovery, and subsequent immunity*
- **HepD** (RNA) - **cofactor** for HepB
    - **HepB + HepD** has the **highest overall mortality rate** for all hepatitis infections (20%; die from cirrhosis or hepatocellular CA)
- **HepC** is the most common viral infection leading to liver TXP
- *No surgery in setting of **acute hepatitis*** *(viral or ETOH; has a very high mortality)*

HIV (Human Immunodeficiency Virus)
- Loss of **cell mediated immunity** due to low **T helper cell** (CD4) counts; then susceptible to **opportunistic infections**
- Is an **RNA virus** that has a **reverse transcriptase** to make DNA that gets incorporated into host genome
- **Testing**: ELISA (looks for antibodies), then Western Blot (detects HIV protein)
- Tx: **HAART** (Highly Active Anti-Retroviral Tx) $\geq$ 3 drugs in $\geq$ 2 classes

- **Post-exposure prophylaxis** (eg needle stick from HIV patient)
  1) **Begin HAART Tx <u>immediately</u>** (within 1 hour)
  2) Usually **4 weeks** of Tx; ELISA at time of exposure and at 4 weeks
- **Bactrim** or **pentamidine** used for prophylaxis against PCP

HIV AND SURGERY
- **Infection** (opportunistic) - MC indication for laparotomy in HIV (MC - **CMV**)
- **Malignancy** - 2nd MC reason for laparotomy in HIV (MC - **lymphoma**)
- **CMV colitis** - MC intestinal manifestation of AIDS
  - MC infection in HIV requiring **laparotomy** (usually for bleeding or perforation)
  - Sx's: can present with pain, bleeding, or perforation from ulcer
  - Tx: **ganciclovir**; surgery for perforation or refractory bleeding
- **Kaposi's Sarcoma** - purple nodules with ulceration; highly **vascular lesion**
  - *MC malignancy in HIV patients*
  - <u>*All*</u> *are caused by* **human herpes virus 8** (HHV 8)
  - From **lymphatic endothelium** that forms vascular channels
  - <u>*Rarely*</u> *need surgery*
  - <u>*Rarely*</u> *a cause of death in AIDS (slow growing; goal here is* ***palliation****)*
  - MC sites - oral and pharyngeal mucosa; others skin, respiratory or GI
  - Sx's: bleeding, dysphagia
  - Tx: primary goal is **palliation** (<u>not</u> surgery); exception - severe intestinal hemorrhage (rare)
    - **HAART** (triple HIV Tx) shrinks AIDS-related Kaposi's (*Best Tx*)
    - Local Tx (for bleeding) - XRT, intra-lesional vinblastine, cryosurgery
- **Lymphoma**
  - MC malignancy in HIV requiring **laparotomy** (usually for bleeding or perforation)
  - MC location - **stomach**; followed by rectum
  - Mostly non-Hodgkin's (B cell)
  - Tx: chemotherapy (CHOP-R); surgery for refractory bleeding or perforation
- **Anal CA** (MC - squamous cell CA) - increased in HIV (due to **HPV**)
- **Condylomata acuminata** (anogenital warts) - can grow very rapidly with HIV (felt to be low grade **verrucous CA** due to HPV) - Tx: **laser fulguration**
- **GI bleeds**
  - **Lower GI bleeds** are more commob than upper GI bleeds in HIV patients
  - **Upper GI bleeds** - <u>Kaposi's sarcoma</u> (MC), lymphoma
  - **Lower GI bleeds** - <u>CMV</u> (MC), HSV

FUNGAL INFECTION
- MC organism in **fungemia** (fungal blood stream infection) - *Candida albicans*
  - RFs - prolonged antibiotics
  - Empiric Tx: **Anidulafungin** (Eraxis, *best Tx*) or liposomal amphotericin
- **Candiduria** - typically from colonization of catheter
  - Tx: **remove catheter**, do <u>not</u> need anti-fungals
- *Actinomyces* (anaerobe; <u>not</u> a true fungus) - often associated with poor dentition
  - Can cause **tortous abscesses** in head/neck (MC), chest, and abdomen
  - Often **confused with malignancy** (eg tortuous abscess in cecum)
  - Path - shows **yellow sulfur granules**
  - Tx: **drainage** and **PCN-G**
- *Nocardia* (anaerobe; <u>not</u> a true fungus) - pulmonary and CNS Sx's
  - Tx: **drainage** and **Bactrim** (sulfonamides)

OTHER INFECTIONS
- **Brown recluse spider bites** - Tx: oral **dapsone** initially and WTD dressings; <u>*avoid early surgery*</u>; possible resection and skin graft <u>*late*</u>
- **Acute septic arthritis** - *Gonococcus*, staph aureus
  - Tx: **open drainage**, vancomycin and 3rd generation cephalosporin until cultures show organism
- **Diabetic foot infections** (mixed) - staph, strep, GNRs, and anaerobes
  - Best test for organism in diabetic foot infection - **Bx of wound base**
  - Tx: broad-spectrum antibiotics (eg Unasyn, Zosyn)
  - Increased infection risk in **diabetics** due to →

1) **PMN dysfunction** (glycosylation ↓s chemotaxis)
2) **↓ed blood flow** - arteriopathy (narrowing of small blood vessels)
3) **Glycosylation** of **RBCs** impairs oxygen delivery
4) **Neuropathy** - patients don't realize the wound (delayed Dx)
- Consider **MRI** in these patients to rule-out osteomyelitis

■ **Human bites** - are poly-microbial
- MCC - **closed fist injury** (hitting someone in teeth)
- MC organism - ***Strep pyogenes*** *(other strep species)*
- ***Staph aureus*** - can cause serious bite wound infections
- **Eikenella** - *only found in human bites*; risk of permanent joint injury
- Tx: broad-spectrum antibiotics (eg Augmentin), tetanus

■ **Cat** and **dog bites** - are poly-microbial
- ***Pasteurella multocida*** - MC organism; *only found in cat / dog bites*
- Tx: broad-spectrum antibiotics (eg Augmentin), tetanus

■ **Impetigo, erysipelas, cellulitis, folliculitis, furuncle** and **carbuncle**
- **MC organism** - staph; others - strep
- **Folliculitis** - infection of hair follicle; Tx: antibiotics
- **Furuncle** - boil (abscess of hair follicle); Tx: drainage and antibiotics
- **Carbuncle** - a multi-loculated furuncle (often with sinuses); RFs: **DM**
  Tx: drainage and antibiotics

■ **Sinusitis**
- RFs: nasoenteric tubes, intubation, severe facial fractures
- Usually polymicrobial
- Dx: CT head shows air-fluid levels in the sinus
- Tx: broad-spectrum antibiotics; *rare to have to tap sinus*

■ **Proctitis** (inflammation of the rectum)
- **Infectious proctitis** - MCC STD's (#1 **gonorrhea**, #2 chlamydia)
- Proctitis can also occur in the setting of **inflammatory bowel disease** or **XRT**

INFECTIONS AND MOST COMMON BACTERIA

SSI	Staph aureus
SSI (GNR)	E. coli
SSI (anaerobe, ie abscess)	B. fragilis
VAP	Staph aureus
Nosocomial pneumonia	Staph aureus
Lung abscess	Staph aureus
Central line	Staph epidermidis
Catheter related blood stream	Staph epidermidis
AV graft	Staph epidermidis
SBP	E. coli
UTI	E. coli
Liver abscess (pyogenic)	E. coli
Biliary infections (eg cholangitis)	E. coli

TETANUS PROPHYLAXIS

Previous Vaccines	Clean, minor wounds	Contaminated wounds*
Unknown or < 3	Td only, <u>No</u> TIG	Td and TIG
3 or more^	<u>No</u> Td**, <u>No</u> TIG	<u>No</u> Td^^, <u>No</u> TIG

* Contamination with dirt, feces, soil, or saliva; also puncture wounds, avulsions, GSW, crush, burns, frostbite, or > 6 hours old
^ Give fourth dose if only 3 give so far
** Yes if > 10 years since last dose
^^ Yes if > 5 years since last dose
Td (tetanus toxoid)
TIG (tetanus immune globulin) - give only to patients with contaminated wounds who lack appropriate immunizations *(given **IM**, inject **near the wound**)*

Antibiotics

134. The best initial therapy for candidemia is:
    a. Amphotericin
    b. Voriconazole
    c. Fluconazole
    d. Caspofungin

    Answer d. Caspofungin

135. The best initial therapy for an *Acinetobacter* infection is:
    a. Ampicillin / Sulbactam
    b. Cefazolin
    c. Cefoxitin
    d. Ticarcillin
    e. Vancomycin

    Answer d. Ticarcillin

136. The best initial therapy for ESBL (extended spectrum beta-lactamase) E. Coli is:
    a. Ceftriaxone
    b. Meropenem
    c. Linezolid
    d. Ampicillin
    e. Gentamicin

    Answer b. Meropenem

137. The best initial therapy for an *Enterococcus* infection is:
    a. Ceftriaxone
    b. Meropenem
    c. Linezolid
    d. Ampicillin
    e. Vancomycin

    Answer d. Ampicillin

138. The best initial therapy for vancomycin-resistant enterococcus (VRE) is:
    a. Ceftriaxone
    b. Meropenem
    c. Linezolid
    d. Ampicillin
    e. Gentamicin

    Answer c. Linezolid

139. The best therapy for MRSA infection is:
    a. Vancomycin
    b. Meropenem
    c. Linezolid
    d. Ampicillin
    e. Gentamicin

    Answer a. Vancomycin

140. The best therapy for a vancomycin-resistant MRSA infection is:
    a. Ceftriaxone
    b. Meropenem
    c. Linezolid
    d. Ampicillin
    e. Gentamicin

Answer c. Linezolid.

141. All of the following are true except:
    a. Erythromycin is considered bacteriostatic
    b. Mechanism of action for fluoroquinolones is inhibition of DNA gyrase
    c. Mechanism of action for rifampin is inhibition of the 50s ribosome
    d. Mechanism of action for metronidazole is oxygen radical production

Answer c. Rifampin inhibits RNA polymerase.

142. All of the following are true except:
    a. MRSA MC develops from plasmids to beta-lactamase
    b. Aminoglycoside resistance is from decreased active transport due to modifying enzymes
    c. PCN resistance is from plasmids for beta-lactamase
    d. Ceftriaxone can cause gallbladder sludging and cholestatic jaundice

Answer a. MRSA develops from **mutation in cell wall binding proteins**.

143. All of the following are true except:
    a. The most likely antibiotic to cause erythema multiforme is bactrim
    b. Carbapenems can induce seizures
    c. Cilastatin increases the half-life of carbapenems
    d. Extended spectrum PCNs are implicated in tendon ruptures
    e. Vancomycin can cause red-man syndrome due to histamine release

Answer d. Fluoroquinolones are implicated in **tendon ruptures**.

144. Appropriate vancomycin peak and trough values are:
    a. Peak 20-40, trough 5-10
    b. Peak 5-10, trough < 1
    c. Peak 40-80, trough 20-40
    d. Peak < 1, trough 5-10

Answer a. The appropriate peak (20-40) and trough (5-10) values for **vancomycin** are important in patients with renal failure.

The appropriate peak (5-10) and trough (< 1) values for **gentamicin** are also important in patients with renal failure.

145. All of the following are true except:
    a. Prophylactic antibiotics are given within 1 hour of incision are primarily used to prevent surgical site infections
    b. Prophylactic antibiotics are discontinued within 24 hours primarily to decrease the spread of resistant organisms
    c. The most effective non-invasive mechanism of warming a patient in the OR is warm air conduction
    d. A blood glucose of 150-250 is optimal for preventing surgical site infections

Answer d. A blood glucose of 80-120 is optimal for preventing surgical site infections.

146. A patient on gentamicin has a peak level of 80 and a trough of < 1. The most appropriate management is:
    a. Continue current dosing
    b. Decrease dose but maintain frequency
    c. Decrease dose and decrease frequency
    d. Maintain dose and decrease frequency

Answer b. To decrease the **peak** level of a drug, one needs to decrease the dose of the drug (the peak level is taken 1 hour after dosing). To decrease the **trough** of a drug, you need to increase the interval at which the drug is given (decrease frequency or longer time between doses).

MECHANISM OF ACTION
- **Inhibitor of DNA gyrase** (topoisomerase) - Quinolones
- **Inhibitor of RNA polymerase** - Rifampin
- Produces **oxygen radicals** that breakup DNA - Metronidazole (Flagyl)
- **Sulfonamides** - has a PABA analogue which inhibits purine synthesis
- **Trimethoprim** - inhibits dihydrofolate reductase (inhibits <u>purine</u> synthesis)
- *Bacteriostatic* antibiotics:
  - Chloramphenicol, tetracycline, clindamycin, macrolides (eg erythromycin) - *all have <u>reversible</u> ribosomal binding*
  - Bactrim (trimethoprim-sulfa)
  - Other antibiotics are considered *bactericidal*
- **Aminoglycosides** - have irreversible binding to ribosome and are considered **bactericidal**

MECHANISMS OF ANTIBIOTIC RESISTANCE
- MC method of antibiotic resistance - **transfer of plasmids** between organisms
  - MC type - Beta lactamase plasmids
- **PCN, cephalosporin, monobactam,** and **carbapenem resistance** - all due to **beta lactamase** type plasmids
  - <u>Exception</u> - MRSA (see below)
- **Gentamicin** resistance - due to **modifying enzymes** leading to **decreased active transport** into cell
- **MRSA** (methicillin-resistant staph aureus) - due to mutation in **cell wall binding proteins**
- **VRE** (vancomycin-resistant enterococcus) - due to mutation in **cell wall binding proteins**
- **Penicillin (PCN)**
  - GPCs - *Clostridium perfringens*, beta-hemolytic strep
  - <u>Not</u> effective against Staph or Enterococcus
- **Oxacillin, nafcillin,** and **methicillin**
  - **Anti-staph** penicillins *(Staph <u>only</u>)*
- **Ampicillin** and **amoxicillin**
  - Same as penicillin but also picks up *Enterococcus*
- **Unasyn** (ampicillin/sulbactam) and **Augmentin** (amoxicillin/clavulanic acid)
  - Broad spectrum - pick up **GPCs** (staph and strep), **GNRs,** ± anaerobic
  - Effective for *Enterococcus*
  - <u>Not</u> effective for *Pseudomonas*, *Acinetobacter*, or *Serratia*
  - Sulbactam and clavulanic acid are beta-lactamase inhibitors
- **Ticarcillin** and **piperacillin** (anti-pseudomonal PCN)
  - GNRs - enterics; gets *Pseudomonas*, *Acinetobacter*, and *Serratia*
  - Side effects: **inhibit platelets**; high salt load
- **Timentin** (ticarcillin/clavulanic acid) and **Zosyn** (piperacillin/tazobactam)
  - Broad spectrum - pick up **GPCs** (staph / strep), **GNRs,** and **anaerobes**
  - Effective for *Enterococcus*
  - Effective for *Pseudomonas*, *Acinetobacter*, and *Serratia*
  - Side effects: **inhibit platelets**, high salt load
- **First-generation cephalosporins** (cefazolin, cephalexin)
  - GPCs - staph and strep
  - <u>Not</u> effective for *Enterococcus*
  - Ancef (cefazolin) has longest half-life → best for prophylaxis
  - 1% of patients with a PCN allergy have cephalosporin allergy
- **Second-generation cephalosporins** (cefoxitin, cefotetan)
  - GPCs, GNRs, ± anaerobic coverage; lose some staph activity
  - <u>Not</u> effective for *Enterococcus*
  - <u>Not</u> effective for *Pseudomonas*, *Acinetobacter*, or *Serratia*
  - Effective only for community-acquired GNRs

- Cefotetan has longest half-life → best for prophylaxis
- **Third-generation cephalosporins** (ceftriaxone, ceftazidime)
  - GNRs mostly, ± anaerobic coverage
  - <u>Not</u> effective for *Enterococcus*
  - Some effective for *Pseudomonas*, *Acinetobacter*, and *Serratia* (ceftazidime)
  - Side effects: **cholestatic jaundice**, gallbladder sludging (ceftriaxone)
- **Monobactams** (aztreonam)
  - GNRs; picks up *Pseudomonas*, *Acinetobacter*, and *Serratia*
- **Carbapenems** (meropenem, imipenem) - given with cilastatin
  - Broad spectrum - **GPCs, GNRs**, and **anaerobes**
  - <u>Not</u> effective for **MEP**: MRSA, *Enterococcus, and Proteus*
  - Cilastatin - prevents renal hydrolysis of drug and increases half-life
  - Side effects: **seizures**
- **Bactrim** (Trimethoprim / sulfamethoxazole)
  - GNRs, ± GPCs
  - <u>Not</u> effective for *Enterococcus*
  - <u>Not</u> effective for *Pseudomonas*, *Acinetobacter*, or *Serratia*
  - Side effects (numerous): teratogenic, allergic reactions, renal damage, erythema multiforme, hemolysis in G6PD-deficient patients
- **Quinolones** (ciprofloxacin, levofloxacin, norfloxacin)
  - Some **GPCs,** mostly **GNRs**
  - <u>Not</u> effective for *Enterococcus*
  - Effective for *Pseudomonas*, *Acinetobacter*, and *Serratia*
  - Same efficacy PO and IV
  - Side effects - **tendon ruptures** (tendonitis; especially with steroid use)
- **Aminoglycosides** (gentamicin, tobramycin)
  - GNRs
  - Good for *Pseudomonas*, *Acinetobacter*, and *Serratia*
  - <u>Not</u> effective for anaerobes (needs O_2 to work)
  - Side effects: reversible **nephrotoxicity**, irreversible **ototoxicity**
  - Resistance due to modifying enzymes leading to **decreased active transport**
- **Vancomycin** (glycopeptides)
  - GPCs (including *Enterococcus*), **MRSA**, *Clostridium difficile* (with PO intake)
  - Side effects: HTN, **Redman syndrome** (histamine release), nephrotoxicity, ototoxicity
  - Resistance develops from change in **cell wall binding sites**
- **Linezolid** (oxazolidinone; can be given **IV** or **oral**)
  - GPCs; includes **MRSA** and **VRE**
- **Synercid** (a streptogramin; quinupristin-dalfopristin; **IV** <u>only</u>)
  - GPCs; includes **MRSA** and **VRE**
- **Clindamycin** (macrolide)
  - **Anaerobes**, some GPCs
  - Good for aspiration pneumonia
  - Can be used to treat *C. perfringens*
  - Side effects: pseudomembranous colitis
- **Metronidazole** (Flagyl)
  - **Anaerobes**
  - Active agent - **ferredoxin** (creates oxygen radicals that disrupt DNA)
  - Side effects: disulfiram-like reaction (N/V with ETOH), **peripheral neuropathy** (long term use)
- **Anti-fungal drugs**
  - Need fungal coverage for: positive blood cultures, 2 sites other than blood, endophthalmitis, or prolonged antibiotics and failure to improve
  - **Candiduria Tx-** *remove urinary catheter only (no anti-fungals needed)*
  - **Prolonged broad-spectrum antibiotics** or **candidemia** → Tx: anidulafungin (Eraxis; less toxicity than liposomal amphotericin)
  - **Candida endophthalmitis** → Tx: liposomal amphotericin
  - Invasive **Aspergillosis** → Tx: voriconazole
  - **Fungal sepsis** other than Candida / Aspergillus → Tx: liposomal amphotericin
  - Anidulafungin (Eraxis), micofungin, or caspofungin
    - *1st line therapy* for suspected **candidemia**

Inhibits **cell wall synthesis** (inhibits **glucan synthase**)
S/Es → **very few S/Es** and equally effective as amphotericin
Spontaneous degradation - safe with renal or hepatic disease

- **Amphotericin** (polyene)
    - *Creates channels by binding **ergosterol** in cell wall (increases cell membrane permeability, causes cell lysis)*
    - S/Es: renal toxicity, hypotension, fever, ↑ed LFTs, anemia, ↓s K
        - S/Es less with **liposomal variant** (liposomal amphotericin B)
        - Used less since introduction of less toxic drugs with equal efficacy

■ Broad-spectrum antibiotics can lead to **superinfection**
■ Effective for ***Enterococcus*** - ampicillin or amoxicillin
- For severe infections - vancomycin, Timentin / Zosyn
- *Enterococcus is resistant to <u>all</u> cephalosporins*

■ Effective for **VRE** (vancomycin-resistant enterococcus) - Linezolid, Synercid
■ Effective for ***Pseudomonas, Acinetobacter,*** and ***Serratia*** - ticarcillin/piperacillin, Timentin/Zosyn, 3rd generation cephalosporins, aminoglycosides (gentamicin/tobramycin), meropenem/imipenem, or fluoroquinolones
■ Effective for **MRSA** (methicillin-resistant staph aureus) - vancomycin, Linezolid, Synercid, topical mupirocin (Bactroban; apply to nares, burn wound infections)
■ Effective for **ESBL** (extended spectrum beta-lactamase) - **carbapenems** *(1st line Tx)*
■ Appropriate **drug levels**:
- **Vancomycin**: peak 20 - 40 ug/ml; trough 5 - 10 ug/ml
- **Gentamicin**: peak 6 - 10 ug/ml; trough < 1 ug/ml
- **Peak too high** → decrease amount of each dose
- **Trough too high** → decrease frequency of doses (increase time interval between doses)

■ **Anti-septic** - antimicrobial that kills and inhibits organisms on body (skin)
- **Iodophors** (eg Betadine) - GPCs, GNRs, <u>poor</u> fungi
- **Chlorhexidine gluconate** (eg Hibiclens) - GPCs, GNRs, and fungi
    - *<u>Better coverage</u>* overall compared to betadine type drugs

■ **Disinfectant** - antimicrobial that kills and inhibits organisms on inanimate objects
■ **Sterilization** - all organisms killed (eg autoclave)

Pharmacology

147. A patient with a Type B aortic dissection being transitioned to oral medications has decreased response to hydralazine despite being effective with the first 3 doses. This is an example of:
    a. Hyperactivity
    b. Tachyphylaxis
    c. Addiction
    d. High potency
    e. High efficacy

    Answer b. Tachyphylaxis (tolerance after only a few doses)

148. Prevention of post-op ileus is best accomplished with which of the following:
    a. Lomotil
    b. Loperamide
    c. Famotidine
    d. Alvimopan

    Answer d. Alvimopan, a mu-opioid receptor antagonists, is used for treatment and prevention of post-op ileus.

149. All of the following are true of gadolinium except:
    a. It is used in MRI
    b. The MC side effect is nausea
    c. It is safe in patients with renal insufficiency
    d. Systemic fibrosis can occur

    Answer c. Gadolinium should not be used in patients with **renal insufficiency** (GFR < 60) as **acute renal dysfunction** and/or **nephrogenic systemic fibrosis** can occur from gadolinium deposition.

150. A drug that is given demonstrates first order elimination kinetics. All of the following are true except:
    a. A fixed ratio of the drug is eliminated over time
    b. Increasing the dose will increase the amount eliminated
    c. The enzyme and elimination systems involved in removing the drug are likely <u>not</u> saturated
    d. Zero order elimination kinetics is exponential.

    Answer d. In **first order elimination kinetics** a <u>fixed ratio</u> of the drug is eliminated over time. Increasing the amount of the drug in the body will increase the amount eliminated.

    In **zero order elimination kinetics** a <u>fixed amount</u> of the drug is eliminated regardless of the dose. This is considered linear and the elimination systems involved in removal of the drug are likely **saturated**.

151. All of the following are complications of ketorolac (Toradol) except:
    a. Bleeding
    b. Renal insufficiency
    c. Ulcers
    d. Peripheral neuropathy

    Answer d. Side effects of **ketorolac** (and other NSAIDS) include **bleeding**, **renal insufficiency** (caution in patients aged > 65 or with elevated creatinine), and **ulcers**.

    Peripheral neuropathy is a side effect of **metronidazole**

152. All of the following are true except:

a. Drugs that readily distribute into fat have a high volume of distribution
b. Hoffman elimination relies on kidney metabolism
c. Tachyphylaxis is tolerance to a drug after only a few doses
d. Hydrophilic drugs are more likely to be excreted in unaltered form

Answer b. Hoffman elimination does not rely on organ metabolism. These drugs can be used in patients with liver or kidney failure without toxic buildup of metabolites (eg **cisatracurium** undergoes Hoffman elimination).

153. All of the following are true except:
    a. Over-diuresis with Lasix can result in metabolic alkalosis
    b. The cytochrome p-450 system is the primary mechanism for most drug metabolism
    c. Over-diuresis with acetazolamide can result in metabolic acidosis
    d. Furosemide doses > 100 mg can result in ototoxicity
    e. Over-diuresis with spironolactone can result in hypokalemia.

Answer e. Over-diuresis with spironolactone Tx results in hyperkalemia.

154. The most common reaction to iodine is:
    a. Nausea
    b. Hypotension
    c. Loss of consciousness
    d. Cardiac arrest

Answer a. The MC reaction to iodine is **nausea**. The MC life-threatening reaction is **dyspnea**.

PHARMACOKINETICS
- **Absorption**
  - **Sublingual** and **rectal medications** - do not pass through the liver first so do not undergo first pass metabolism (these drugs have **higher bioavailability**)
  - **Skin** - drugs with **high lipid solubility** have better absorption through epidermis
  - **CSF** - absorption usually restricted to non-ionized, **lipid soluble** drugs
- **Kinetics**
  - *Zero order kinetics* - **constant amount** of drug eliminated regardless of dose (increasing dose will not increase amount eliminated)
    Enzyme and elimination systems are saturated
  - *1st order kinetics* – amount of drug eliminated is proportional to dose (increasing dose will **increase** amount eliminated); fixed ratio of drug is eliminated
    Enzyme and elimination systems are likely <u>not</u> saturated
  - Need **5 half-lives** for a drug to reach steady-state
  - **Volume of distribution** = amount of drug in body divided by amount of drug in plasma (blood)
    Drugs with a high volume of distribution have higher concentrations in the **extra-vascular compartment** (eg fat) compared to the intra-vascular compartment
  - **Bioavailability =** fraction of unchanged drug reaching systemic circulation (considered to be 100% for IV drugs, less for PO)
- **Drug Effects**
  - **Hyperactive** - effect at an unusually low dose
  - **Tachyphylaxis** - tolerance after only a few doses
  - **Potency** - dose required for effect (smaller dose for effect = higher potency)
  - **Efficacy** - ability to achieve result without untoward effect
  - **Tolerance** - progressive decline in potency with continued usage
  - **Addiction** - psychological compulsion to take drug
  - **Physical dependence** - physiological effects occur when drug is stopped
- **Drug metabolism**
  - Converts **lipophilic** (more lipid soluble) compounds into more readily excreted **hydrophilic** polar products (more water soluble)
  - 99% of the time this is associated with **detoxification** of drug

- **Primary system** - hepatocyte **smooth endoplasmic reticulum** _and_ **cytochrome P-450** mono-oxygenase system
  - **Phase I** - demethylation, oxidation, reduction, hydrolysis
  - **Phase II** - conjugation reactions
    - **Glucuronic acid** (MC) and **sulfates** are attached to the drug
    - Forms **water-soluble metabolite** (usually inactive) → then undergoes excretion
  - Drugs excreted in bile may become **deconjugated** in intestines with **re-absorption**, some in active form (eg cyclosporine) → process is termed **entero-hepatic recirculation**
  - Patient with a **biliary drainage tube** that bypasses the intestines will not have this reabsorption [eg kidney TXP patient requiring bile duct T-tube has acute rejection episode (↑ Cr, ↓ UOP) due to low cyclosporine levels] Tx: **pulse steroids**
- **Hoffman degradation** _(does not rely on organ metabolism)_ - these drugs can be used in patients with liver or kidney failure without worry about toxic buildup of metabolites; drug is metabolized in the blood (eg **cisatracurium**)

- **Drug Elimination**
  - **Kidney** - most important organ for eliminating most drugs (glomerular filtration and tubular secretion)
  - **Biliary system** - may have entero-hepatic recirculation (see above)
  - **Polar drugs** (ionized) - more **water soluble** and more likely to be eliminated in unaltered form
  - **Non-polar drugs** (non-ionized) - more **lipid soluble** and more likely to be metabolized before excretion

- **Important drug interactions**
  - **Albumin** - largely responsible for binding drugs (PCNs and Warfarin are 90% bound)
  - **Sulfonamides** (eg Bactrim) - displace unconjugated bilirubin off albumin in newborns; causes **kernicterus** (brain damage)

GI DRUGS
- **Promethazine** (Phenergan, anti-emetic) - dopamine receptor blocker
  - S/Es: **tardive dyskinesia**, Tx: diphenhydramine (Benadryl)
- **Metoclopramide** (Reglan, prokinetic) - dopamine receptor blocker; increases gastric and gut motility
- **Erythromycin** - acts on **motilin receptor** (pro-kinetic)
- **Loperamide** - slows gut motility by binding **mu opioid receptors**
- **Lomotil** (diphenoxylate and atropine) - slows gut motility
- **Famotidine** - histamine H_2 receptor blockers; ↓s stomach acid
- **Proton pump inhibitors** (eg Omeprazole) block H^+/K^+ ATPase of parietal cell (final pathway for H^+ release); ↓ stomach acid
- **Megestrol** (Megace) - increases appetite in patients with advanced CA
- **Octreotide** - long-acting **somatostatin analogue**; decreases gut secretions and decreases GI blood flow
- **Alvimopan** and **methylnaltrexone** - mu-opioid receptor antagonists; used for treatment and prevention of **post-op ileus**; for short-term use only; S/E - risk of **myocardial infarction** with long-term use

DIURETICS
- **Loop diuretics** [eg **furosemide** (Lasix), bumetanide (Bumex)]
  - Over-diuresis causes **metabolic <u>alkalosis</u>** and <u>**hypokalemia**</u>
  - Lasix S/Es – **ototoxicity** (keep dose ≤ 100 mg)
- **Thiazide** [eg hydrochlorothiazide (HCTZ)]
  - Over-diuresis results in **metabolic <u>alkalosis</u>**
- **Carbonic anhydrase inhibitor** [eg acetazolamide (Diamox)]
  - Over-diuresis results in **metabolic <u>acidosis</u>** and <u>**hypokalemia**</u>
- **Potassium sparing diuretics** (eg spironolactone)
  - Over-diuresis results in **metabolic <u>acidosis</u>** and <u>**hyperkalemia**</u>

INFLIXIMAB (Remicade)
- **Antibodies** to **TNF-alpha** (given IV or IM)
- Used for **inflammatory bowel disease** (Crohn's Disease, Ulcerative Colitis)
- _Contraindications_ - allergy to rodents, active infection, CHF
- S/Es: **infection risk** (MC serious complication)
  - _MC serious infection_ → _tuberculosis_ (↑ed re-activation and ↑ed **incidence** of acquiring TB)
  - PPD placed before starting drug
  - When treating patients with Infliximab who have a positive PPD, **isoniazid** should be started as well

GADOLINIUM (Gd)
- Used in MRI as a contrast agent
- MC side effect: **nausea**
- _Do not use with **renal insufficiency** (GFR < 60) → can get buildup of **Gd** resulting in acute renal dysfunction or nephrogenic systemic fibrosis_
- S/Es: 1) **Acute renal dysfunction**
       2) **Nephrogenic systemic fibrosis** (fibrosis of skin, joints, eyes, organs); from **Gd deposition**

IODINE CONTRAST
- MC side effect - **nausea**; (others - urticaria, itching, heat)
- MC side effect requiring medical Tx (MC life-threatening S/E) - **dyspnea**

NSAIDs (non-steroidal anti-inflammatory drugs)
- **Non-selective COX inhibitors** (cyclooxygenase inhibitors)
  - Types: naproxen, ketorolac (Toradol), ibuprofen, indomethacin, ASA
  - Inhibit both **constitutive** (COX-1) and **inducible** (COX-2) **cyclooxygenase**; results in inhibition of **prostaglandin** synthesis (all are reversible _except_ ASA)
  - S/Es (dose dependent):
    1) **GI bleeding** (gastric ulcers and gastritis)
       Inhibition of prostaglandin synthesis leads to **decreased mucus production** (↓ed protection)
       PPIs can be given for protection
    2) **Renal insufficiency**
       Inhibition of prostaglandin synthesis leads to **vasoconstriction of renal afferent arterioles**
       Prostaglandins usually keep the arterioles vasodilated
       Refrain from use in patients with an **elevated creatinine**
  - **ASA** (_irreversible_ non-selective COX inhibitor)
       S/Es (ie poisoning) - headaches, N/V
       1st - respiratory alkalosis, **2nd** - metabolic acidosis
- **Selective COX-2 inhibitors** (celecoxib)
  - **Inhibit inducible form of cyclooxygenase** (COX-2)
  - Expressed at sites of inflamed tissue
  - **Fewer ulcers** and **less renal failure** than non-selective COX inhibitors
  - S/Es: **increased risk of cardiovascular events** (2-3 x, eg MI, stroke)

Anesthesia

155. All of the following are true except:
    a.   The MCC of post-op hypoxia is atelectasis (alveolar hypoventilation)
    b.   The MCC of post-op hypercarbia is poor minute ventilation
    c.   The most effective way to prevent peri-operative hypothermia is warm IV fluids
    d.   Bipolar cautery is the safest method of electrical surgical dissection

Answer c. The most effective way to prevent peri-operative **hypothermia** is warm air conduction (eg Bair Hugger).

156. Severe hallucinations are a common side effect of:
    a.   Ketamine
    b.   Etomidate
    c.   Propofol
    d.   Sodium thiopental

Answer a. Severe hallucinations are a side effect of **ketamine**.

157. All of the following are true of rapid sequence intubation in a patient with congestive heart failure (CHF) and small bowel obstruction except:
    a.   Pre-oxygenation is the first step
    b.   Paralytic is given before induction
    c.   Cricoid pressure can help reduce risk of aspiration in patients with small bowel obstruction
    d.   Etomidate is fast acting, has the least amount of cardiovascular side effects, and works well as an induction agent for RSI.
    e.   Nitrous oxide should be avoided in patients with bowel obstruction as it diffuses into closed spaces and increases risk of perforation.

Answer b. The induction agent is given before the paralytic.

158. Prior to performing a lung resection, the anesthesiologist attempts to intubate the patient but he is not sure if the tube is in the trachea. The best determinant of esophageal versus tracheal intubation is:
    a.   Breath sounds
    b.   Gastric sounds
    c.   Opinion of the anesthesiologist
    d.   End tidal CO_2

Answer d. The most sensitive test as to whether or not the endotracheal is placed correctly is **end tidal CO_2**.

159. Histamine release is characteristic of:
    a.   Meperidine
    b.   Fentanyl
    c.   Sufentanil
    d.   Morphine

Answer d. Morphine has a characteristic histamine release which can cause **hypotension**.

160. Seizures in patients with acute renal failure is characteristic of which drug:
    a.   Meperidine
    b.   Fentanyl
    c.   Sufentanil
    d.   Morphine

Answer a Meperidine in acute renal failure can result in buildup of normeperidine analogues which can cause **seizures**.

161. An overdose of fentanyl is treated with:
    a. Flumazenil
    b. Narcan
    c. Neostigmine
    d. Edrophonium

    Answer b. All narcotic agent overdoses (eg morphine, fentanyl, Demerol, sufentanil, Percocet, etc.) can be treated with **Narcan** (naloxone).

162. All of the following are contraindications to succinylcholine except:
    a. Renal failure
    b. Burn patients
    c. Spinal cord injury
    d. Elderly

    Answer d. Succinylcholine in not contraindicated in the elderly.

163. Metabolic acidosis is a specific risk for which of the following agents:
    a. Etomidate
    b. Sevoflurane
    c. Ketamine
    d. Propofol
    e. Precedex

    Answer d. Propofol

164. Malignant hyperthermia is MC is related to a defective receptor (ryanodine receptor) on the sarcoplasmic reticulum that controls calcium release. The 1st sign of malignant hyperthermia after succinylcholine in an intubated patient is:
    a. Fever
    b. Rigors
    c. Increase in end-tidal CO_2
    d. Tachycardia

    Answer c. Increase in **end-tidal CO_2**

165. The most appropriate first step in the treatment of malignant hyperthermia is:
    a. Dantrolene
    b. Dopamine
    c. Dobutamine
    d. Lasix and potassium

    Answer a. Malignant hyperthermia can be triggered by either succinylcholine or inhalation anesthetics (sevoflurane, isoflurane, etc.). **Dantrolene** is the most effective Tx.

166. Cisatracurium is metabolized by:
    a. Liver
    b. Kidney
    c. Plasma cholinesterase
    d. Hoffman degradation

    Answer d. Cisatracurium undergoes **Hoffman degradation** (degraded in blood) which makes it ideal for patients with either renal failure or liver failure.

167. Two days after a severe inhalational injury, you have trouble oxygenating your patient so you decide to paralyze her with pancuronium. The MC side effect of this drug is:
    a. Fever
    b. Hypotension
    c. Increased intracranial pressure

d.   Tachycardia

Answer d. The MC S/E of pancuronium is **tachycardia**.

168. All of the following are true except:
    a.   Neck muscles and face are the 1st to relax with paralytics
    b.   Diaphragm muscles are last to relax with paralytics and 1st to recover with paralytics
    c.   Non-depolarizing paralytics can be reversed with neostigmine
    d.   Depolarizing paralytics can be reversed with atropine

Answer d. Depolarizing paralytics cannot be reversed (are metabolized by pseudocholinesterases). Patients with **atypical pseudocholinesterases** have prolonged paralysis.

169. A severe overdose of Ativan (lorazepam) is treated with:
    a.   Flumazenil
    b.   Narcan
    c.   Neostigmine
    d.   Edrophonium

Answer a. Severe overdoses of benzodiazepines (Ativan, Valium, Versed) are treated with **flumazenil**.

170. Which is the appropriate maximal dose of lidocaine for a 70 kg male:
    a.   70 cc of 1% lidocaine
    b.   49 cc of 1% lidocaine with epinephrine
    c.   7 cc of 1% lidocaine
    d.   49 cc of 1% lidocaine
    e.   17 cc of 1% lidocaine with epinephrine

Answer b. 0.5 cc/kg for 1% lidocaine or **0.7 cc/kg** for 1% lidocaine with epinephrine is indicated. Half these amounts are appropriate if 2% lidocaine is used.

171. Of the anesthetics listed below, the one most likely to cause an allergic reaction is:
    a.   Lidocaine
    b.   Bupivicaine
    c.   Mepivicaine
    d.   Procaine

Answer d. Ester type local anesthetics, such as procaine, cocaine, and tetracaine are more likely to cause allergic reactions because of their PABA analogue.

Amide type local anesthetics (all have "i" in 1st part of their name) such as lidocaine, bupivacaine, and mepivacaine rarely cause allergic reactions.

172. All of the following are true of local anesthetics except:
    a.   These agents work by increasing the action potential threshold in peripheral nerves
    b.   They work better in acidic environments
    c.   They can cause seizures
    d.   The first symptom of lidocaine toxicity is peri-oral paresthesias (numbness and tingling)

Answer b. Local anesthetics work <u>poorly</u> in **acidic environments** (which makes it hard to anesthetize infected wounds).

173. When starting a CABG procedure, the monitor shows ventricular fibrillation and you confirm there is no pulse. The most appropriate next step is:

    a. Epinephrine
    b. Atropine
    c. Defibrillation
    d. Lidocaine

Answer c. Emergent electrical defibrillation (360 joules) is indicated for ventricular fibrillation (always confirm there is no pulse - avoids shocking someone due to EKG artifact).

174. The above patient now has pulseless electrical activity (PEA) for which you start CPR. In addition to epinephrine, which of the following can be used as a bolus:
    a. Levophed
    b. Vasopressin
    c. Dobutamine
    d. Milrinone

Answer b. ACLS guidelines approves vasopressin (single dose) for PEA codes.

175. The above patient now has: SBP 65 and HR of 35. The most appropriate next step is:
    a. Levophed
    b. Atropine
    c. Defibrillation
    d. Lidocaine

Answer b. Atropine is used for bradycardia and hypotension.

176. The MCC of intra-op bradycardia is:
    a. Undiagnosed heart block
    b. Inhalational anesthesia
    c. Myocardial infarction
    d. Urinary retention
    e. Gastric distension

Answer b. Inhalational anesthesia

177. A 25 yo man is having a laceration closed using local anesthesia. During the case, he becomes asystolic and you start CPR. The most appropriate next step is:
    a. Epinephrine
    b. Atropine
    c. Defibrillation
    d. Lidocaine

Answer a. Epinephrine. Inadvertent intravenous injection of local anesthetic can result in bradycardia (Tx: atropine) or even asystole (Tx: epinephrine).

178. POD #7 following aortic valve replacement your patient has 3rd degree heart block. The most appropriate next step is:
    a. Pacemaker
    b. Beta-blocker
    c. Amiodarone
    d. Calcium channel blocker

Answer a. Pacemaker is indicated for patients with persistent 3rd degree heart block. They are also indicated for Type II 2nd degree heart block.

179. On POD #3 following a 3 vessel CABG, your patient goes into atrial fibrillation. The best initial drug to give is:
    a. Lidocaine
    b. Amiodarone
    c. Beta-blocker
    d. Calcium channel blocker

Answer b. Amiodarone is the best initial agent for atrial fibrillation.

Amiodarone is also the best drug for stable patients with ventricular tachycardia (so you don't have to shock the patient).

180. All of the following are contraindications to spinal anesthesia except:
    a. Cirrhosis
    b. Hypertrophic cardiomyopathy
    c. Elevated ICP
    d. INR 1.3

    Answer d. INR of 1.3 is not a contraindication to spinal anesthesia.

181. A patient undergoing lung resection has an epidural placed containing morphine and bupivicaine. All of the following are true concerning the epidural except:
    a. Respiratory depression is most likely due to the morphine
    b. Hypotension and bradycardia are most like due to the bupivicaine
    c. Epidurals are well tolerated in patients with hypertrophic cardiomyopathy
    d. Spinal headaches can often be treated with a blood patch

    Answer c. Hypertrophic cardiomyopathy is a contraindication to epidurals because they cause a decrease in afterload, which can be catastrophic in patients with dilated cardiomyopathy (the ventricle will collapse on itself usually at the level of the septum).

    Hypotension and bradycardia which occur with epidurals are almost always related to the local anesthetic (bupivicaine) placed in the epidural.

    Interestingly, although morphine can cause hypotension when given systemically, it does not occur with epidural infusion (likely because the CSF does not contain histamine releasing mast cells). Respiratory depression is related to morphine in epidurals. Many centers place Dilaudid (hydromorphone) in epidurals to avoid this side-effect.

182. A 65 yo man on dialysis for renal failure undergoes an elective abdominal aortic aneurysm repair. This patients ASA class is:
    a. II
    b. III
    c. IV
    d. V

    Answer c. Class IV

183. Which of the following represents the highest cardiac risk for patients undergoing non-cardiac surgery:
    a. Recent MI
    b. Previous stroke (no residual deficits)
    c. S3 gallop
    d. Peripheral arterial disease

    Answer c. S3 gallop represents **uncompensated CHF**, which is the highest risk factor on the Goldman criteria (11 points). **Creatinine > 2** is also a cardiac RF for patients undergoing non-cardiac surgery.

184. A 45 yo woman is undergoing colectomy for ulcerative colitis. She has not taken prednisone for 4 months (she was taking 20 mg/day). What is most appropriate for her peri-op steroid management:
    a. No steroids
    b. 50 mg hydrocortisone intra-op, then 20 mg prednisone daily with taper
    c. 320 mg hydrocortisone intra-op, then 20 mg prednisone daily with taper

     d.   500 mg hydrocortisone intra-op, then 20 mg prednisone daily with taper
     e.   No intra-op steroids, 20 mg prednisone daily with taper

Answer a. No steroids. Patients who have been off steroids for > 3 months do not need peri-op steroid prophylaxis.

185. Instead of the above, she has been on 40 mg of prednisone a day. What is most appropriate for her peri-op steroid management:
     a.   No steroids
     b.   50 mg hydrocortisone intra-op, then 25 mg q8 x 1 day, then 40 mg prednisone daily with taper
     c.   500 mg hydrocortisone intra-op, then 125 mg q8 x 1 day then 40 mg prednisone daily with taper
     d.   No intra-op steroids, 40 mg prednisone daily with taper

Answer b. 50 mg hydrocortisone intra-op, then 25 mg q8 x 1 day, then 40 mg prednisone daily with taper.

186. Instead of the above, she has been on 80 mg of prednisone a day. What is most appropriate for her peri-op steroid management:
     a.   No steroids
     b.   320 mg hydrocortisone intra-op, then 80 mg prednisone equivalent daily with taper
     c.   500 mg hydrocortisone intra-op, then 80 mg prednisone equivalent daily with taper
     d.   No intra-op steroids, 80 mg prednisone daily with taper

Answer b. 320 mg hydrocortisone intra-op, then 80 mg prednisone daily with taper. *High dose steroids intra-op (ie 500 mg hydrocortisone) are <u>not</u> recommended for peri-op prophylaxis.*

187. An 75 yo woman has rest pain in her left lower leg despite maximal medical therapy. Angiogram shows a good distal target with anterior tibial runoff below the ankle to the dorsalis pedis artery. She has an elevated Cr (2.0), COPD, diabetes, and previous stroke (no residual deficits). Which of the following is most appropriate concerning her risk of major adverse cardiovascular events (MACE) prior to lower extremity bypass:
     a.   A METs score of 7 should prompt cardiac catheterization
     b.   A METs score of 7 should prompt dobutamine thallium scan
     c.   A METs score of 3 requires no further testing
     d.   A METs score of 3 should prompt dobutamine thallium scan

Answer d. A METs score < 4 should prompt dobutamine thallium scan. METs (**metabolic equivalent of task**) is a measure of energy costs of physical activity. Patients with a high combined peri-op MACE risk (co-morbidities + high risk surgery) should have METs calculated. METs < 4 should have pharmacologic testing (eg dobutamine-thallium scan). METs $\geq$ 4 should proceed with surgery without further testing.

It has been difficult to show benefit from pre-op cardiac revascularization prior to non-cardiac surgery in terms of preventing MACE.

188. All of the following are true of myasthenia gravis except:
     a.   The ocular muscles are the most commonly involved muscles
     b.   Myasthenia crisis can be precipitated by stress and is usually treated with steroids, Mestinon, plasmapheresis, and possible intubation
     c.   The most accurate and sensitive test for myasthenia gravis is the EMG "jitter" test
     d.   Emegency surgery is often indicated for myasthenia crisis

Answer d. Surgery is not indicated for myasthenia crisis (should be treated medically).

INHALATIONAL INDUCTION AGENTS (volatile anesthetics)
- Cause unconsciousness (anesthesia), amnesia, and some analgesia (pain relief)
- Blunt hypoxic drive (respiratory depression)
- Are short-acting (5-10 minutes)
- Most have myocardial depression, ↑ cerebral blood flow, and ↓ renal blood flow
- **Sevoflurane** (MC inhalational induction agent) - fast, minimal laryngospasm; good for **mask induction**
- **Desflurane** - most rapid onset / offset of all volatile anesthetics; has a **pungent odor** so is not used for induction; usually reserved for **maintenance anesthesia**
- **Nitrous Oxide** (NO_2) - fast, **minimal myocardial depression**; tremors at induction
  - Diffuses into closed spaces (do not use with small bowel obstruction or pneumothorax)
  - Is generally used in combination (carrier) with sevoflurane or desflurane
- MCC of intra-op **bradycardia** - **inhalational anesthesia** (Tx: **Atropine**)
- Volatile anesthetic **hepatitis** - fever, eosinophilia, jaundice, ↑ed LFTs
  - Repeated exposure to volatile anesthetics may increase risk

INTRAVENOUS INDUCTION AGENTS
- **Propofol** *(MC IV induction agent)* - unconsciousness, anesthesia, and amnesia, *not analgesic*; rapid on/off
  - Side effects: **hypotension** (MC), respiratory depression, irritation with infusion
  - **Propofol infusion syndrome** *(rare);* occurs with long term use → causes **metabolic acidosis** (and subsequent renal failure, cardiac failure, death); increased risk in **children**
  - *Contraindications* - egg allergy, pregnancy, Parkinson's
  - *Avoid* prolonged use in children
- **Etomidate** - unconsciousness, anesthesia, and amnesia, *not analgesic*
  - Has **fewest cardiac effects** - good for patients with cardiac disease (eg CHF, angina); fast acting
  - Often used for **rapid sequence intubation**
  - Side effects - **adrenocortical suppression** with continuous infusions
- **Dexmedetomidine** (Precedex)
  - Provides anesthesia and analgesia *without* blunting hypoxic drive (no respiratory depression); good for **early extubation protocols** (eg cardiac surgery)
  - Mechanism - CNS alpha-2 receptor agonist
  - Side effects - BP lability (usually hypotension)
- **Ketamine** - places patient in a cataleptic state (amnesia, analgesia)
  - No respiratory depression
  - Good for **children**
  - Mechanism - causes dissociation of thalamic and limbic systems
  - Side effects: **hallucinations**, catecholamine release (↑ end-tidal CO_2, tachycardia), ↑ airway secretions, and ↑ cerebral blood flow
  - *Contraindications* - **head injury**
- **Rapid sequence intubation** - used in patients at risk for **aspiration**
  - RFs for aspiration - recent oral intake, GERD, delayed gastric emptying (gastroparesis), pregnancy, bowel obstruction
  - Sequence:
    1) **Pre-oxygenation** (tight fitting mask)
    2) **IV induction agent** (eg Etomidate - fast acting)
    3) **IV paralytic** (eg succinylcholine - fast acting)
    4) **Cricoid pressure** to reduce risk of aspiration with intubation

MUSCLE RELAXANTS (paralytics)
- **Diaphragm** - last muscle to go down and 1st muscle to recover from paralytics
- **Neck muscles and face** - 1st to go down and last to recover from paralytics
- **Succinylcholine** - the only depolarizing agent; fast, short acting; get fasciculations
  - Depolarizes the neuromuscular junction
  - Metabolism - degradation by **plasma pseudocholinesterases**
  - Depolarizing paralytics **cannot be reversed**
  - S/E's:
    Malignant hyperthermia (MH; autosomal dominant)

From defect in **calcium metabolism** (MC - ryanodine receptor in sarcoplasmic reticulum); Ca is released and causes **muscle excitation-contraction syndrome**

*1st sign is <u>increased</u> **end-tidal CO_2**;* then fever, tachycardia, rigidity, acidosis, hyperkalemia, creatinine kinase elevation, and myoglobinemia

Rhabdomyolysis can lead to **myoglobin release**

Tx: **dantrolene** (*best Tx*; 10 mg/kg) inhibits Ca release; cooling blankets, HCO_3^-, supportive care (follow glucose, K), oxygen, stop all anesthetics

MH can be caused by **succinylcholine** or **inhaled anesthetics** (volatile anesthetics); Sx's can occur as late as 24 hours

Intravenous anesthetics do <u>not</u> trigger the reaction (consider for future surgeries, eg propofol)

Hyperkalemia - depolarization **releases K^+** (can cause hyperkalemia)

Do <u>not</u> use in patients with **neurologic issues** (eg neuromuscular disorders, spinal cord injury) - all have up-regulation of **acetylcholine** (Ach) **receptors** in muscle which dramatically increases potassium release; can lead to cardiac arrest

Do <u>not</u> use in patients with **massive trauma** or **large burns** (increased potassium release from tissue injury)

Do <u>not</u> use in patients with **acute renal failure**

Open-angle glaucoma can become closed-angle glaucoma

Increased intra-cranial pressure - <u>avoid</u> in patients with head injury

Atypical pseudocholinesterase - causes prolonged paralysis (Asians)

<u>Not</u> reversible (have to wait until metabolized)

- ■ **Non-depolarizing agents**
  - ● Inhibit neuromuscular junction by competing with acetylcholine (ACh) at the ACh receptor (competitive antagonists)
  - ● **Cisatracurium** - undergoes **Hoffman elimination** (breaks down on its own in <u>blood</u> - not metabolized by kidney or liver)

    Good for patients with **liver failure** or **renal failure**
  - ● **Pancuronium** - slow acting, long-lasting; metabolism - <u>renal</u>

    MC side effect - **tachycardia** (<u>no</u> hypotension)
  - ● **Rocuronium** - the **fastest acting** non-depolarizing agent, metabolism - <u>hepatic</u>
  - ● **Reversing drugs** for non-depolarizing agents:

    Neostigmine or **edrophonium** - block **acetylcholinesterase,** increasing acetylcholine

    Atropine or <u>glycopyrrolate</u> should be given with reversal agents to counteract the effects of generalized acetylcholine overdose (eg salivation, diarrhea)

LOCAL ANESTHETICS

- ■ **Mechanism** - increase **action potential threshold**, preventing Na influx (makes it harder to have an action potential occur so the pain sensation is not transmitted)
- ■ **Neuro blockade**: sensory > motor
- ■ **Infected tissues** - hard to anesthetize secondary to **acidosis**
- ■ **Length of action** - bupivacaine > lidocaine > procaine
- ■ Side effects (or accidental intra-venous administration): **CNS** (tremors, tinnitus seizures) and **cardiac** (bradycardia, hypotension, asystole, cardiac arrest)
- ■ **Bupivacaine** (maximum dose 2 mg/kg; 3 mg/kg with epinephrine)
- ■ **Lidocaine** (maximum dose 5 mg/kg; 7 mg/kg with epinephrine)
  - ● Easier - 0.5 cc/kg of 1% lidocaine, 0.7 cc/kg of 1% with epinephrine
- ■ Can re-administer local anesthetic after **2 hours**
- ■ **Epinephrine** allows higher doses to be used; anesthetic stays local
  - ● No epinephrine with arrhythmias, unstable angina, uncontrolled hypertension, poor collaterals (penis / ear), placental insufficiency
- ■ **1st sign of toxicity** - peri-oral paresthesias (tingling, numbness)
- ■ *<u>Overdose</u>* of local anesthetic (cardiac Sx's) - Tx: **atropine** *(best for bradycardia)* or **epinephrine** *(best for asystole)*

- **Allergic reactions**
  - **Amides** (all have an "i" in first part of name) - lidocaine, bupivacaine, mepivacaine; *rare* allergic reactions
  - **Esters** - tetracaine, procaine, cocaine; increased **allergic reactions** (bronchospasm, pruritus); secondary to **PABA analogue**

NARCOTICS (OPIOIDS)
- **Types** - morphine, fentanyl, meperidine (Demerol), codeine, hydromorphone (Dilaudid), oxycodone (Percocet), hydrocodone (Vicodin), dextropropoxyphene (Darvocet)
- Effects - **analgesia** (blunt sympathetic response; euphoria), respiratory depression (decreased CO_2 drive), no cardiac effects (although morphine causes hypotension due to histamine release), miosis
- All act on **μ-opioid receptor** in CNS
- **Liver metabolism** and **kidney excretion**
- *Overdose* of narcotics - Tx: **naloxone** (Narcan, works for all)
  - Place patient on drip for oral overdose
- **Morphine** S/E's - constipation, histamine release (causes **hypotension**), decreases coughing
- **Demerol** S/E's - tremors, fasciculations, convulsions (**seizures**)
  - No histamine release (no hypotension)
  - **Seizures** (normeperidine analogues) - *avoid* in patients with **renal failure**; careful with total amount given for other patients
  - *Avoid* in patients on **MAOI** (mono-amine oxidase inhibitors) → can cause **hyperpyrexic coma** (high fever; Serotonin Release Syndrome in CNS → severe fever, tachycardia, seizures, coma)
- **Fentanyl** - fast acting; 80× strength of **morphine** (does not cross-react in patients with morphine allergy); no histamine release
- **Sufentanil** and **remifentanil** - very fast-acting with short half-lives
- *Most potent narcotic – **sufentanil** (10x potency of fentanyl)*
- Careful with opioid and benzodiazepine combinations (**synergistic effect**)
- **Methadone** - simulates morphine, less euphoria

BENZODIAZEPINES
- Effects - anxiolytic, anticonvulsant, amnesic; not analgesic; respiratory depression
- Mechanism - bind **GABA receptor** (most prevalent inhibitory brain receptor)
- Metabolism - **hepatic**
- **Versed** (midazolam) - short acting; contraindicated in pregnancy
- **Valium** (diazepam) - intermediate acting; lot of metabolites, not used as drip
- **Ativan** (lorazepam) - long acting
- *Overdose* of benzodiazepines - Tx: **flumazenil** (competitive inhibitor; may cause seizures; contraindicated if elevated ICP or status epilepticus)

EPIDURAL AND SPINAL ANESTHESIA
- **Epidural anesthesia**
  - Allows **analgesia** by sympathetic denervation (sensory blockade) with motor function still intact; also causes vasodilation
    - Pain receptors affected much more than motor receptors
    - Does not provide good paralysis
    - Good for **post-op pain control**
    - Lowers respiratory and cardiac complications in post-op patients
    - Does not influence mortality
  - Anesthetic is placed outside dura, in the epidural space
    - **Finding epidural space** - loss of resistance with injection
    - **Bloody tap** - insert at new level
  - *Avoid* insertion at **T-5** or higher - affects cardiac nerves (**bradycardia**)
  - Location of epidural for **thoracotomy**: T6 - T9
  - Location of epidural for **colectomy**: T8 - T10
  - **Morphine** component Cx's - **respiratory depression**
    - Tx for **respiratory depression** - turn epidural off, possible intubation
    - Use **hydromorphone** (Dilaudid) instead of morphine to avoid this

Although morphine can cause hypotension when given systemically, it does not occur with epidurals because the CSF does not contain histamine releasing mast cells

- **Lidocaine** component Cx's - ↓ed **heart rate** and **blood pressure**
  - Tx for **acute hypotension** and **bradycardia** - turn epidural down and give fluids; phenylephrine and atropine if severe
  - Make sure hypotension not due to another source (eg post-op bleeding)
- **Decreased leg motor function** (usually unilateral and due to a malpositioned catheter off to one side; foot should feel **warm**) - Tx: turn epidural down and monitor
- **Epidural hematoma** - sudden **localized back pain** at epidural site followed 1-2 hours later by **loss of sensation** and **motor in extremities**; may also have loss of bowel and bladder function; Dx - MRI, Tx - emergent decompressive laminectomy
- **Spinal headaches** - caused by CSF leak after spinal or epidural
  - Headache gets **worse** sitting up
  - Tx: rest, fluids, caffeine, analgesics; **blood patch** to site if it persists > 24 hours
- **Urinary retention** - all patients need a bladder catheter
- **Epidural abscess** - requires open drainage
- *Contraindications* to epidural anesthesia:
  - **Hypertrophic cardiomyopathy** (sympathetic denervation decreases afterload and causes LV outflow tract collapse)
  - **Cyanotic heart disease** (decreased afterload shunts blood away from lungs and causes hypoxia)
  - **Aortic stenosis** (decreased afterload impairs coronary blood supply and causes hypotension)
  - **Cirrhosis** (bleeding risk → risk of epidural hematoma)
  - **Systemic infection** or at site (worry about epidural abscess)
  - **Coagulopathy** (INR > 1.5, low platelets, uremia, heparin; all have increased bleeding and epidural hematoma risk)
  - **Anatomic abnormalities** (eg spina bifida, meningomyelocele)
  - **Elevated ICP**
  - Severe **hypovolemia** (can worsen hypotension)

- **Spinal anesthesia** - injection into subarachnoid space
- **Sensory** *and* motor blockade (sensory blockade is above motor)
- Lasts up to **2 hours**
- Must be injected **below L2** to avoid hitting **spinal cord**
- Given as **one-shot only** (not infused like epidural)
- *Can perform any surgery below the umbilicus* with spinal anesthesia *alone* (eg C-sections, hernia, ortho, appendectomy, hysterectomy)
- **Caudal block** - through sacrum; good for pediatric hernias, perineal surgery
- Contraindications same as epidural anesthesia

Surgical Procedure and
Risk of Major Adverse Cardiovascular Event (MACE)

High risk (> 5%)
  Emergent operations (especially in elderly)
  Aortic, peripheral, and other major vascular surgery *(except CEA)*
  Long procedure with large fluid shifts
Intermediate risk (1-5%)
  CEA
  Head and neck surgery
  Intra-peritoneal and intra-thoracic surgery
  Orthopedic surgery
  Prostate surgery
Low risk (< 1%)
  Endoscopic procedures
  Superficial procedures
  Cataract surgery
  Breast surgery

PERI-OP CARDIOVASCULAR EVENTS (MI, stroke, CHF, and sudden death)
- **Co-morbidities** with a **high risk** of cardiovascular event:
  - **CHF** (pulmonary edema, S3 gallop, jugular venous distension [JVD])
  - **Ischemic heart disease** (previous MI, angina, Q waves on EKG)
  - **Cerebrovascular disease** (previous TIA or stroke)
  - **Diabetes** (or insulin resistance)
  - **Renal insufficiency** or **failure** (pre-op **creatinine > 2.0**)
- Highest RFs for **cardiovascular events**:
  #1 **uncompensated CHF** (or cardiogenic shock; Sx's - JVD, high CVP, or S3 gallop)
  #2 **recent MI**
- Patients with **elevated risk** (combined co-morbidity and procedure risk) - figure out **metabolic equivalent of task** (METs) →
  - If **< 4 METs** (only slow walking, light calisthenics, light effort on stationary bike) → obtain **pharmacologic testing** (eg dobutamine-thallium scan)
  - If ≥ **4 METs** → no further testing and proceed with surgery
  - Has been hard to show benefit from pre-op revascularization in patients undergoing non-cardiac surgery
- **Beta-blocker** - best single agent to prevent peri-op cardiovascular events
- Wait **6-8 weeks after MI** before elective surgery (eg cholecystectomy)
  - 10% mortality for elective surgery if < 6-8 weeks after MI
- **Peri-op myocardial infarction** (MI)
  - Sx's: chest pain, hypotension, tachycardia, change in EKG
  - Dx: EKG, cardiac enzymes
  - Tx (BMOAN): **beta-blocker, morphine, oxygen, ASA, NTG** (sublingual)
  - **ST elevation MI** (STEMI) or patient **unstable** → go to cardiac cath lab for coronary angiogram and possible intervention

PAIN MANAGEMENT
- **Pain scale** of 1-10; should be kept in the **1-3 range** (PCA effective)
- Sx's of **inadequate pain control** - tachycardia, HTN, diaphoresis, tachypnea, splinting (poor inspirations on incentive spirometer)
- **Visceral pain** - internal organs; Tx: opioids
- **Somatic pain** - skin and musculoskeletal; well localized; Tx: NSAIDs, opioids
- Appendicitis starts out as **visceral pain** (peri-umbilical) with obstruction of the appendix lumen; as inflammation occurs in the RLQ and involves the abdominal musculoskeletal wall, **somatic pain** occurs
- _Contraindications_ to PCA (patient controlled analgesia)
  - Age < 5
  - Those who are confused or have learning difficulties
  - Poor manual dexterity
  - Critically ill

END TIDAL CO_2
- Best determinant of esophageal vs tracheal intubation - **end-tidal CO_2** ($ETCO_2$)
  - Reflects exchange of CO_2 from blood to alveolus
- Intubated patient undergoing surgery with sudden transient **rise in $ETCO_2$**
  - Dx: most likely **hypoventilation** (poor minute ventilation)
  - Tx: ↑ tidal volume or ↑ respiratory rate
  - If laparoscopic procedure and patient has _hypotension_ - CO_2 embolus will cause a _transient_ rise followed quickly by a _precipitous drop_ in $ETCO_2$ (CO_2 embolus is MC associated with a **drop in $ET-CO_2$**)
  - Rise in $ETCO_2$ can also be caused by **malignant hyperthermia**
- Intubated patient with sudden **drop in $ETCO_2$**
  - Dx: likely became **disconnected from the vent**
  - Could also be due to **PE**, an **air embolism** through a central line, or a CO_2 **embolism** during a laparoscopic procedure (all would also have **hypotension**)
- **Endotracheal tube** - should be placed 2 cm above the carina

ASA CLASS (American Society of Anesthesiologists)
- **Class I** - healthy patient
- **Class II** - mild disease without limitation (eg HTN, DM, obesity, smokers)
- **Class III** - severe disease (eg stable angina, previous MI, moderate COPD)
- **Class IV** - disease is a severe constant threat to life (eg unstable angina, renal or liver failure, severe COPD)
- **Class V** - moribund patient (eg ruptured AAA, saddle pulmonary embolus)
- **Class VI** - organ donor

NON-INVASIVE CARDIAC TESTING
- Looking for areas of **ischemia** (ie decreased thallium uptake) with either:
  - 1) the heart under **stress** (eg Dobutamine or walking) *or*
  - 2) **coronary vasodilatation** (eg adenosine or dipyridamole)
  - Above is termed **reversible ischemia**
- **Positive stress test** = chest pain, ST changes, hypotension, or areas of reversible ischemia → all indications for **coronary angiogram** (cardiac catheterization)

CORONARY ANGIOGRAM INDICATIONS (invasive testing; cardiac catheterization)
- 1) **Positive non-invasive cardiac testing**
- 2) **Acute ST elevation MI** (STEMI) – standard is 90 minutes from ED arrival to PTCA time (termed door to balloon time); **STEMI's** should undergo **stenting** if technically feasible
- 3) **Non-ST elevation MI** - usually get cardiac cath before discharge

ACLS DRUGS
- **Epinephrine** - best drug for PEA or asystole code; best drug after failed defibrillation for ventricular tachycardia or ventricular fibrillation code
- **Atropine** - best drug for symptomatic bradycardia (increases heart rate)
- **Amiodarone** - best drug for converting acute atrial fibrillation to normal sinus rhythm; also used for ventricular arrhythmias (ventricular tachycardia, ventricular fibrillation after cardioversion)
- **Magnesium** - can be used to Tx torsades de pointes (ventricular tachycardia)
- **Ventricular fibrillation Tx**: *immediate electrical cardioversion*

PERI-OP STEROID MANAGEMENT

Pre-op dose (prednisone)	Stress (surgery)	Treatment
< 10 mg/day	Assume normal physiologic response to surgery	Usual morning dose No additional steroids
10-59 mg/d	<u>Minor</u> (eg lap choly)	Usual morning dose **25** mg hydrocortisone at induction
	<u>Moderate</u> (eg colon surgery)	Usual morning dose **50** mg hydrocortisone at induction, then 25 mg q8 x 1 day, then usual home dose
	<u>Major</u> (eg esophagectomy)	Usual morning dose **100** mg hydrocortisone at induction, 50 mg q8 x 1 day, then taper dose by ½ daily until maintenance equivalent dose is achieved
≥ 60 mg/day	Assume adrenal suppression	Give usual prednisone dose in IV form until PO intake (if taking 60 mg prednisone / day will need 240 mg hydrocortisone / day [or 80 mg q8])

- **< 3 months** since stopping steroids - treat as if on steroids
- **> 3 months** since stopping steroids - <u>no</u> peri-op steroids necessary
- After surgery, patients on steroids can often undergo a prednisone taper and come off steroids (eg resection for ulcerative colitis, thymectomy for myasthenia gravis)

- *High dose steroids (eg 500 mg hydrocortisone) are <u>not</u> recommended for prophylactic management; **low dose steroids** are recommended for prophylaxis under certain circumstances (as described above)*
- **Steroid potency**
  - 1× - hydrocortisone
  - 4× - prednisone, prednisolone
  - 5× - methylprednisolone
  - 30× - dexamethasone

OTHER
- MCC **post-op hypoxemia** - <u>alveolar hypoventilation</u> (causes **atelectasis**), results in V/Q shunt
- MCC **post-op hypercarbia** - <u>poor minute ventilation</u>
- MC PACU Cx - **nausea** and vomiting
- Safest electrosurgical setting - **bipolar cautery**, use to avoid lateral thermal injury and arcing (short circuit created between tips of instrument)

MYASTHENIA GRAVIS
- Sx's: **ocular muscles** MC involved; general skeletal weakness in 90%
- Dx: **EMG** *(best test,* Jolly test) - shows **jitter** (non-uniform NMJ destruction)
- Path: **antibodies to ACh receptors at NMJ** → ACh receptors get destroyed
  - Myeloid cells in thymus my serve as Ag source
- Tx:
  - **Cholinesterase inhibitors** (<u>*best Tx*</u>; pyridostigmine [Mestinon])
    S/Es - salivation, diarrhea, bradycardia
    Cholinergic crisis - too much ACh (see below)
  - Steroids, plasmapheresis (removes antibodies), immunoglobulin
- **Thymectomy** for myasthenia gravis:
  - **Indications** - <u>thymomas</u> or <u>severe</u> disease (80% get improvement)
  - Thymus receives branches from **inferior thyroid artery** and **internal mammary artery**
  - *Need to give **post-op steroids** following thymectomy - avoids **Addisonian crisis** (acute adrenal insufficiency)*
- **Myasthenia Crisis** (too <u>little</u> ACh)
  - **Respiratory failure** - caused by infection, stress, sepsis
  - *<u>NO surgery</u> - no role for emergency thymectomy*
  - Tx: **pyridostigmine** (Mestinon), plasmapheresis, steroids; poss. intubate
- **Cholinergic Crisis** (too <u>much</u> ACh)
  - Overdose of cholinesterase inhibitor
  - Causes too much ACh at NMJ - results in **depolarization blockade**
  - **Effects** - paralysis, respiratory failure, salivation, sweating
  - May need intubation to allow it to wear off

Patient Safety, Outcomes, Ethical-Legal

189. All of the following are true except:
    a.   The ACS NSQIP collects outcome data to measure and improve surgical quality in U.S
    b.   GAP protection seeks structured handoffs and checklists for patient transfers and transfer of patient care between caregivers
    c.   A sentinel event is an unexpected occurrence involving death or serious injury, or the risk thereof; hospital undergoes root cause analysis to prevent
    d.   A time-out should just verify the patient and procedure

    Answer d. The **time out** before the incision is made should include the following: verifying <u>patient</u>, <u>procedure</u>, <u>position</u> <u>site + side</u>, and availability of <u>implants</u> or <u>special requirements.</u>

190. The leading cause of adverse events is:
    a.   Inadequate communication between health care providers
    b.   Depression
    c.   Emergency surgery
    d.   Diverse patients
    e.   Unfamiliar setting

    Answer a. Inadequate communication between health care providers

191. An 85 yo trauma patient has fixed pupils at 6 mm, has negative corneal reflexes, a weak gag reflex at intubation with decerebrate posturing, Kussmaul breathing, and a large intra-cerebral hemorrhage (5 cm midline shift) on head CT after a fall at a nursing home. The most appropriate next step is:
    a.   Emergent craniotomy
    b.   Morphine and Ativan
    c.   Contact next of kin with recommendation for withdrawal of support
    d.   Contact next of kin with recommendation for craniotomy
    e.   Place PEG tube and tracheostomy only

    Answer c. The prognosis is very grim for the above patient. This prognosis, and a recommendation, should be provided by the physician.

192. A 65 yo woman is brought in for a fall and is found to have breast CA with diffuse metastases to her lung, liver, and head. The family and patient demand surgery to remove all tumor sites and "want everything done". The most appropriate next step is:
    a.   Metastatectomies for all tumor sites
    b.   Refuse and sign off on the consult
    c.   Consult palliative care and hold a family meeting to discuss palliative options
    d.   Call risk management

    Answer c. Consult palliative care and hold a family meeting to discuss palliative options

193. You operate on a 55 yo man for a ruptured AAA who fails to wake up after surgery. Head CT shows massive bilateral infarcts. The patient's wife expired some time ago. Which party should be informed of the prognosis and decide on next steps:
    a.   The patient's father
    b.   The patient's sister
    c.   The patient's daughter
    d.   The patient's brother
    e.   The case should be taken to court

    Answer c. The patient's daughter as she is next of kin

194. You finish your off-pump coronary artery bypass procedure in an elderly, widowed man from a nursing home and notice a mass in his left lower lobe with another small mass attached to his right atrium. Both come back as lung adenocarcinoma. His eldest son doesn't want you to tell him because of his age and he should make decisions for him as he knows the patient's wishes. His brother does want you to tell him because he knows him best and would know what he wants. The most appropriate next step is:
   a. Don't tell him and let his eldest son make decisions on his care because he is next of kin
   b. Bring in the ethics committee
   c. Talk to the patient and see if he wants to know your findings
   d. Bring in palliative care
   e. Tell him based on his brothers decision because he is next of kin

   Answer c. Talk to the patient and see if he wants to know you findings. Unlike the previous question, there is no indication the patient is unable to make decisions for himself

195. You explain the diagnosis and the implications of chemo-XRT to the above patient. Chemo-XRT in this patient is an example of:
   a. Autonomy
   b. Beneficence
   c. Justice
   d. Equal rights
   e. Double effect

   Answer e. Double effect

196. The above patient refuses further treatment. Abiding to his decision represents:
   a. Autonomy
   b. Beneficence
   c. Justice
   d. Equal rights
   e. Double effect

   Answer a. Autonomy (self-determination)

197. A 25 yo suicidal patient who lacks insurance stabs himself in the thigh. Treating his wound regardless of his insurance status is an example of:
   a. Autonomy
   b. Paternal effect
   c. Justice
   d. Double effect

   Answer c. Justice (fairness) – treating like cases alike.

198. The above patient wakes up and tries to stab himself with a large bore needle. You order restraints despite the patient's wishes. This is an example of
   a. Autonomy
   b. Paternal effect
   c. Justice
   d. Double effect

   Answer b. Paternal Effect

199. A 80 coherent man from a nursing home has multiple sclerosis and persistent chest pain from a 99% left main coronary artery stenosis that is not amenable to stenting. The pain occurs everyday, is incapacitating, and he would like something done if possible. You feel you can get him through coronary artery bypass grafting (CABG) with acceptable risks however you find a DNR order in his EMR. The most appropriate next step is:
   a. Bring in the ethics committee

b. Form a peri-op agreement that is acceptable for both the patient and cardiac team
c. Bring in palliative care
d. Bring in risk management

Answer b. Form a peri-operative plan that is acceptable for both the patient and cardiac team.

200. Which of the following is the most appropriate:
a. Phenergan 25 mg PO QID PRN
b. Phenergan 25 mg PO q.i.d. PRN
c. Phenergan 25 mg po qid PRN
d. Phenergan 25 mg PO qid PRN
e. Phenergan 25 mg p.o. QID PRN

Answer d. Phenergan 25 mg PO qid PRN

201. A patient is undergoing left lower lobectomy for lung CA. Which of the following is appropriate?
a. An X on the right chest by the nurse
b. An X on the right chest by the surgeon
c. An X on the left chest by the patient
d. Initials on the left chest by the nurse
e. Initials on the left chest by the surgeon

Answer e. Initials on the left chest by the surgeon

202. A 15 yo Jehovah's witnesss boy has hypotension and a hemoglobin of 5.5 following traumatic splenectomy. His parents refuse pRBC transfusion. You should
a. Transfuse anyway
b. Not transfuse
c. Give lacatated ringers
d. Give iron and epogen
e. Obtain a court order and transfuse

Answer e. Obtain a court order and transfuse. Althought the parents have the right to express relgious freedom for themselves they are required to act in the child's best interest (not exposing the child to risk of illness or death).

203. Having a retained towel after assisting with laparotomy closure is a example of:
a. Latent error
b. Failure of gap protection
c. Something that could be prevented with the time-out
d. Ethical issues in surgery

Answer a. Latent error is an error due to **systems** or **routines** that are formed in such a way that humans are pre-disposed to making these errors (eg using a towel, which is not counted at the end of the case, to pack bowel during a laparotomy pre-disposes it to being left in the patient)

PATIENT SAFETY
- **JCAHO prevention of wrong site / procedure / patient**:
  - Pre-op verification of **patient** and **procedure**
  - Operative **site** and **side** (**surgeon's initials** and marking if left or right or multiple levels; must be visible after the patient is prepped)
  - **Time out** before incision made (verifying patient, procedure, position site + side, and availability of implants or special requirements)
- **Promoting Culture of Safety**
  - Confidential system of reporting errors
  - Emphasis on learning over accountability
  - Flexibility in adapting to new situations or problems

- RFs for **retained object** after surgery (MC sponge) - emergency procedure, unplanned change in procedure, obesity, towel used for closure
- **Sentinel Event** (JCAHO) - unexpected occurrence involving death or serious injury, or the risk thereof; hospital undergoes **root cause analysis** to prevent and minimize future occurrences (eg **wrong site surgery**)
- **GAP protection technique** - gaps in care (eg change in care-giver, divisions of labor, shift changes, transfers) can lead to loss of information and error
  - Prevention - **structured handoffs** and **checklists** (face to face if possible); standardizing orders; reading back orders if verbal
- **Latent Error** - error due to **systems** or **routines** that are formed in such a way that humans are pre-disposed to making these errors (eg using a towel, which is not counted at the end of the case, to pack bowel during a laparotomy pre-disposes it to being left in the patient)
- **Human Factors** associated with **injury**:
  - Insufficient training and experience; fatigue, depression, burnout
  - Diverse patients, unfamiliar setting, time pressure
  - Failure to acknowledge medical errors
- **Human Factors** associated with **injury prevention:**
  - People are supportive of one another
  - People trust one another
  - People have friendly, open relationships emphasizing credibility and attentiveness
  - Work environment is resilient and emphasizes creativity and goal achievement, providing strong feelings of credibility and trust
- Ineffective injury prevention strategies
  - Assigning blame to "incompetent" health care providers after an event
  - Assigning blame to patient's co-morbidities (eg obesity, COPD) after adverse outcome
  - Not reporting adverse outcomes
  - Hierarchical structure in O.R. instead of team approach
- **Ethical Issues** in injury prevention - failure to report an **adverse event to family** due to concerns over malpractice litigation
- **Inadequate communication** between healthcare providers is the leading cause of adverse events
- **Most important measure of injury outcome**:
  - Individual - ability to return to work and/or activities of daily living:
  - System - prevention of similar adverse events in the future

CORE ETHICAL PRINCIPALS

- **Autonomy** - self-rule or self determination; entails the ability of a person to make a choice free from external constraints (eg family pressure)
- **Beneficence** - the duty to do good
- **Double effect** - when both good and harmful effects accompany an action (eg chemotherapy); the balance should favor the good effects
- **Justice** - like cases should be treated alike; no special preference
- **Non-maleficence** - duty to not inflict harm
- **Paternal effect** - weighs beneficence/non-maleficence over autonomy (eg preventing a patient from committing suicide)
- **Respect for Human Rights**

SURGICAL OUTCOMES

- **National Surgical Quality Improvement Program** (NSQIP) - seeks to collect outcome data to measure and improve surgical quality in the U.S.; outcomes are reported as observed vs expected ratios (O:E ratios)
- **Higher volume hospitals** are associated with lower mortality for abdominal aortic aneurysm repair and for pancreatic resection
- **Process Measures** - eg hand washing %, extubation times, pre-op beta-blocker use, antibiotics before incision; process measures should be linked to a desired outcome measure (eg hand-washing and nosocomial infection)
- **Outcome Measures** - eg mortality; stroke, infection, and pneumonia rates

DNR STATUS
- Patients with terminal illness may at times benefit from surgery although the procedure may not affect the natural history of the underlying disease (eg bowel obstruction in patients with advanced malignancy)
- Policies that either completely suspend or completely enforce DNR orders may not appropriately address the patient's right to self-determination
- Best approach is to discuss with the patient the peri-operative risks and approach to potentially life-threatening problems; the results of these discussions are passed on to the anesthesiologist and operative team

ADVANCED ORAL DIRECTIVES
- **Advanced oral directives** take precedence in cases where the patient is otherwise not able to make informed decisions about their care
- The next order of precedence is a **living will**
- Next is durable **power of attorney** (eg wife or husband; can also be designated by the patient)
- **Hierarchy** for **power of attorney**
    1) Spouse
    2) Adult son or daughter
    3) Either parent
    4) Adult brother or sister
    5) Guardian

MEDICAL ABBREVIATIONS
- Times: three times a day - tid; twice a day - bid (all lower case, no periods)
- Amounts: milligrams - mg; micrograms - mcg; grams - g (all lower case)
- Morphine - MSO4
- As needed - PRN
- Nausea and vomiting - N/V
- By mouth - PO

Fluids and Electrolytes

204. All of the following would contribute to high serum osmolarity except:
    - a. Hyperglycemia
    - b. Hypernatremia
    - c. Hyperkalemia
    - d. Azotemia

    Answer c. Potassium does not contribute to serum osmolarity.

    Serum osmolarity = $(2 \times Na^+) + (glucose/18) + (BUN/2.8)$

205. Aggressive fluid resuscitation with dextran (hetastarch) can result in:
    - a. Bleeding
    - b. Metabolic acidosis
    - c. Renal failure
    - d. Seizures

    Answer a. Bleeding (coagulopathy)

206. A ventilated patient has the following arterial blood gas values: pH 7.50, CO_2 55, HCO_3^- 35. This condition is most likely caused by:
    - a. Poor minute ventilation
    - b. Aggressive NG tube suctioning
    - c. Renal failure
    - d. Severe sepsis

    Answer b. The ABG presented suggests a **metabolic alkalosis**. Of the items listed, NGT suctioning is most likely to cause a metabolic alkalosis.

207. A ventilated patient has the following arterial blood gas values: pH 7.50, CO_2 24, HCO_3^- 18. This condition is most likely caused by:
    - a. Low minute ventilation
    - b. NGT suctioning
    - c. Renal failure
    - d. High minute ventilation

    Answer d. The ABG presented suggests a **respiratory alkalosis**. Of the items presented, high minute ventilation is the most likely cause. You correct this by either decreasing respiratory rate or decreasing tidal volume.

208. A ventilated patient has the following arterial blood gas values: pH 7.25, CO_2 70, HCO_3^- 35. This condition is most likely caused by:
    - a. Poor minute ventilation
    - b. NGT suctioning
    - c. Renal failure
    - d. Severe sepsis

    Answer a. The ABG presented is most consistent with a **respiratory acidosis**. Of the items listed, poor minute ventilation is most likely to give you a respiratory acidosis. You correct this by either increasing respiratory rate or tidal volumes.

209. A ventilated patient has the following arterial blood gas values: pH 7.26, CO_2 28, HCO_3^- 18. This condition is most likely caused by:
    - a. Poor minute ventilation
    - b. NGT suctioning
    - c. Renal failure
    - d. High minute ventilation

    Answer c. This is most consistent with **metabolic acidosis**. Of the items listed, **renal failure** is most likely to give you a metabolic acidosis (with high anion gap).

210. A 70 kg man with an isolated closed head injury is intubated and paralyzed. His vent settings are tidal volume 200, RR 10, FiO_2 100%, PEEP 5, and pressure support 10. This is most likely to result in:
- a.　pH 7.4, CO_2 40, HCO_3^- 24
- b.　pH 7.5, CO_2 30, HCO_3^- 16
- c.　pH 7.25, CO_2 60, HCO_3^- 32
- d.　normal blood gas values

Answer c. pH 7.25, PCO_2 60, HCO_3^- 32. Minute ventilation (RR x tidal volume) should be between 5-10 L/minute. The above minute ventilation is only 2 L/minute. This would result in **respiratory acidosis**.

211. A 70 kg man with an isolated closed head injury is intubated and paralyzed. His vent settings are tidal volume 700, RR 30, FiO2 100%, PEEP 5, and pressure support 10. This is most likely to result in:
- a.　pH 7.4, CO_2 40, HCO_3^- 24
- b.　pH 7.5, CO_2 30, HCO_3^- 16
- c.　pH 7.25, CO_2 60, HCO_3^- 32
- d.　normal blood gas values

Answer b. pH 7.5, PCO_2 30, HCO_3^- 16. Minute ventilation is 21 L/minute and would result in **respiratory alkalosis**.

212. All of the following are consistent with chronic renal failure except:
- a.　Hypophosphatemia
- b.　Metabolic acidosis
- c.　Hyperkalemia
- d.　Hypermagnesemia
- e.　Chronic dialysis generally results in hypocalcemia

Answer a. Chronic renal failure results in **hyperphosphatemia**.

213. The composition of lactated ringers is:
- a.　Na 154, Cl 109, K 4, Ca 2.7, HCO_3 28
- b.　Na 130, Cl 103, K 4, Ca 2.7, HCO_3 28
- c.　Na 154, Cl 109, K 4, Ca 4, HCO_3 28
- d.　Na 130, Cl 109, K 4, Ca 2.7, HCO_3 28

Answer d. Lactated ringers has Na 130, Cl 109, K 4, Ca 2.7, HCO_3 28

214. The composition of 3% saline is:
- a.　Na 154, Cl 154
- b.　Na 308, Cl 308
- c.　Na 513, Cl 513
- d.　Na 130, Cl 109, K 4, Ca 2.7, HCO_3 28

Answer c. Na 513, Cl 513

215. Following esophageal resection and placement of a spit fistula in the neck, your patient loses about 1 liter of saliva per day. This is most likely to result in:
- a.　Hypocalcemia
- b.　Hypomagnesemia
- c.　Hyponatremia
- d.　Hypokalemia
- e.　Hypophosphatemia

Answer d. Saliva has the highest K concentration in the body.

216. A 50 yo man develops massive vomiting for 3 days related to a large obstructive gastric CA. Which of the following is the most appropriate fluid resuscitation:

    a. Normal saline
    b. Lactated ringers
    c. 0.45% normal saline
    d. 0.2% normal saline
    e. D51/2 NS with 20 mEq K

Answer a. Normal saline. Correcting the chloride level is the most important part of fluid resuscitation in patients with gastric outlet obstruction.

217. *Before resuscitation*, the above patient most likely had a:
    a. Metabolic Alkalosis
    b. Metabolic Acidosis
    c. Respiratory Alkalosis
    d. Respiratory Acidosis

Answer a. Metabolic alkalosis

218. *Before resuscitation*, the above patient most likely had which of the following lab values
    a. Hyperchloremia, hyperkalemia
    b. Hypochloremia, hyperkalemia
    c. Hyperchloremia, hypokalemia
    d. Hypochloremia, hypokalemia

Answer d. Hypochloremia, hypokalemia, metabolic alkalosis

219. Fluid resuscitation with lactated ringers in the above patient would most likely cause:
    a. Continued metabolic alkalosis
    b. Metabolic acidosis
    c. Respiratory alkalosis
    d. Respiratory acidosis

Answer a. Continued metabolic alkalosis. Lactated ringer's carries a significant amount of HCO_3^- which will further worsen the metabolic alkalosis.

220. Pyloric stenosis is most likely to result in:
    a. Metabolic alkalosis
    b. Metabolic acidosis
    c. Respiratory alkalosis
    d. Respiratory acidosis

Answer a. Pyloric stenosis results in hypokalemic, hypochloremic, metabolic alkalosis (similar to gastric outlet obstruction). Appropriate fluid resuscitation in children with pyloric stenosis is with normal saline.

221. A 50 yo woman with Crohn's disease develops a very high output small bowel fistula. Which of the following is the most appropriate fluid resuscitation:
    a. Normal saline
    b. Lactated ringers
    c. 0.45% normal saline
    d. 0.2% normal saline
    e. D51/2 NS with 20 mEq K

Answer b. Lactated ringers. A significant amount of HCO_3^- is lost with high output small bowel fistulas.

222. *Before resuscitation*, the above patient most like had a:
    a. Metabolic acidosis
    b. Metabolic alkalosis
    c. Respiratory acidosis
    d. Respiratory alkalosis

Answer a. Metabolic acidosis (with a normal anion gap)

223. Fluid resuscitation with normal saline in the above patient would most likely cause:
   a. Hyperchloremic metabolic acidosis
   b. Hyperchloremic metabolic alkalosis
   c. Hypochloremic metabolic acidosis
   d. Hypochloremic metabolic alkalosis
   e. Normal electrolyte balance

   Answer a. Fluid resuscitation with non-bicarbonate solutions in this scenario will result in hyperchloremic metabolic acidosis. Although not given, her chloride level is also likely very high making normal saline a poor choice.

224. Eight hours *after* normal saline fluids, the above patient is most likely to have which of the following ABG values:
   a. pH 7.35, CO_2 32, HCO_3 16
   b. pH 7.45, CO_2 42, HCO_3 26
   c. pH 7.55, CO_2 32, HCO_3 16
   d. pH 7.35, CO_2 52, HCO_3 32
   e. pH 7.35, CO_2 52, HCO_3 32

   Answer a. pH 7.35, CO_2 32, HCO_3 16. In an effort to correct the pH, the patient will blow off CO_2 with a subsequent drop in HCO_3^-.

225. A 22 yo woman in the ICU for 3 weeks following a MVA develops significant diarrhea as a result of C. difficile colitis. The most appropriate fluid resuscitation is:
   a. Lactated Ringers
   b. Normal saline
   c. 3% normal saline
   d. Packed red blood cells
   e. Albumin

   Answer a. Lactated Ringers. Normal saline resuscitation or any non-bicarbonate solution for massive diarrhea would result in hyperchloremic metabolic acidosis (with a normal anion gap) so it is <u>not</u> indicated.

226. Which of the following lab values would be most likely in the above patient *before* resuscitation:
   a. Na 130, K 2.5, pH 7.30, HCO_3 18
   b. Na 150, K 2.5, pH 7.30, HCO_3 30
   c. Na 150, K 4.5, pH 7.30, HCO_3 18
   d. Na 150, K 2.5, pH 7.50, HCO_3 30

   Answer b. Na 150, K 2.5, pH 7.30, HCO_3 30. The potassium level would be very low in this patient (you lose a lot of potassium with diarrhea). Na would likely be high due to dehydration and pH would likely by low due to loss of HCO_3^- (this patient would have hyperchloremic metabolic acidosis before resuscitation).

227. The following are the initial fluids used to Tx each dehydration category except:
   a. Sweat loss (eg runner that collapses on hot day) - normal saline bolus
   b. Gastric loss from pyloric stenosis - normal saline bolus
   c. Bile duct fistula - normal saline bolus
   d. Pancreatic fistula - lactated ringers bolus

   Answer c. Initial fluid for dehydration due to a bile duct fistula is lactated ringers.

228. A 30 yo man suffers an isolated closed head injury (CHI). In the ED, he has low urine output and a sodium of 120. His CVP is 15. The most appropriate next step is:
   a. Dialysis
   b. D5-water
   c. Desmopressin

d. Tolvaptan
e. Water restriction and Lasix

Answer d. This patient has **SIADH** related to a CHI. The urine in this patient would be very concentrated (ie high urine specific gravity, high urine osmolality). Chronic Tx for SIADH includes fluid restriction (1st) and then diuresis, however, for _acute_ SIADH **Tolvaptan** is recommended.

Caution should be used when correcting this patient's sodium as **central pontine myelinolysis** can occur if it is corrected too fast.

229. A 30 yo man suffers an isolated closed head injury (CHI). After arriving at the ED, the patient starts making a very significant amount of urine. His Na is 155. The most appropriate next step is:
     a. Dialysis
     b. D5-water
     c. Desmopressin
     d. Tolvaptan
     e. Water restriction and Lasix

     Answer c. This patient has diabetes insipidus related to a CHI. The urine in this patient would be very dilute. Chronic Tx includes free water, however, for _acute_ diabetes insipidus **Desmopressin** (anti-diuretic hormone) is indicated.

     Caution should be used when correcting this patient's sodium as brain swelling can occur if it is corrected too fast.

230. All of the following are true of hyponatremia in chronic liver failure except:
     a. The hyponatremia is related to fluid overload
     b. ADH is usually high in these patients
     c. Aldosterone is usually low in these patients
     d. Severe hyponatremia should be corrected slowly to avoid central pontine myelinolysis

     Answer c. Aldosterone tends to be high in patients with liver failure and hyponatremia.

231. All of the following are indicated to tumor lysis syndrome except:
     a. Pre-chemo hydration prevention
     b. Rasburicase
     c. Loop diuretic
     d. Aggressive calcium replacement
     e. Pre-chemo sevelamer chloride

     Answer d. Ca replacement should be _avoided_ to prevent Ca-PO$_4$ precipitation and associated **renal failure**.

232. A 55 yo woman with breast CA develops confusion, somnolence, and a shortened QT on EKG. Her serum calcium is 15 The next appropriate step is:
     a. Mithramycin
     b. Beta-blockade
     c. Calcium
     d. IV fluids and Lasix
     e. Alendronate

     Answer d. Intravenous fluids (1st) and **Lasix** (2nd) - _this is the first-line therapy for severe hypercalcemia_

233. For the above patient, the best drug to give next is:
     a. Alendronic acid
     b. Cinacalcet

c.   Calcitonin
d.   Calcium channel blocker
e.   Beta-blocker

Answer c. Calcitonin. Calcitonin is faster acting than alendronic acid. Calcium channel blockers and beta-blockers are not effective.

234. A 60 yo woman undergoes parathyroidectomy for a parathyroid adenoma. Seven days post-op she develops peri-oral tingling and numbness and has noticed a twitching in her face. All of the following are true except:
    a.   Bone hunger likely accounts for her problem
    b.   The treatment is calcium
    c.   A magnesium level is important in this patient
    d.   This is caused by hypercalcemia

Answer d. This patient has **hypocalcemia** likely from **bone hunger**.

235. All of the following are true except
    a.   The MCC of significant hypophosphatemia is renal failure
    b.   The MCC of significant hypocalcemia is previous thyroid surgery
    c.   The MCC of significant hypomagnesemia is massive diuresis
    d.   The MCC of significant hypokalemia is over-diuresis

Answer a. The MCC of significant **hypo-phosphatemia** is **re-feeding syndrome**.

236. A 35 yo woman suffering from Crohn's disease is admitted to the hospital for control of a high output fistula. She was started on TPN some time ago. She now has tremors, confusion, hyperreflexes, tetany, and a prolonged Q-T interval This is associated with which of the following metabolic disorders?
    a.   Hyperkalemia
    b.   Hypomagnesemia
    c.   Hypermagnesemia
    d.   Hypercalcemia

Answer b. Hypomagnesemia. The Sx's are similar to hypocalcemia. 50% of patients with hypomagnesemia also have hypokalemia or hypocalcemia.

237. The best Tx for symptomatic hypermagnesemia is:
    a.   Potassium chloride
    b.   Calcium gluconate
    c.   Potassium phosphate
    d.   Sodium Chloride

Answer b. Calcium gluconate

238. A 55 yo patient with severe pancreatitis has the following lab values: Amylase 850, Lipase 900, LDH 600, AST 400, triglycerides 2200, glucose 140, WBC count 22, Na 125. All of following are true except:
    a.   This patient's hyponatremia is from over-resuscitation
    b.   This patient's hyponatremia is from hyperlipidemia
    c.   There is no specific treatment for this patient's for hyponatremia
    d.   Tx of the underlying pancreatitis corrects the problem

Answer a. This patient has **pseudo-hyponatremia** as a result of **hyperlipidemia** associated with pancreatitis. The elevated lipids draw fluid into the intravascular compartment creating pseudohyponatremia. No specific Tx (other than treating the underlying disorder) is necessary.

239. The initial Tx of choice for hyperkalemia with peaked T waves is:
    a.   Insulin and glucose

b. Calcium gluconate
c. Kayexalate
d. Dialysis

Answer b. Although all of these agents are used for **hyperkalemia**, a patient that is having arrhythmias as a result of the hyperkalemia should receive **calcium gluconate** 1st to stabilize cardiac muscle cell membranes.

240. A 55 yo severely malnourished patient starts tube feeding. Re-feeding syndrome results in all of the following except:
    a. Hypokalemia
    b. Hypomagnesemia
    c. Hyponatremia
    d. Hypophosphatemia

Answer c. Re-feeding syndrome can result in **low K, Mg** and **PO4.** It occurs in the severely malnourished when they start receiving nutrition. Re-feeding syndrome is prevented by starting nutrition at a low rate initially (10-15 kcal/kg/day). Phosphate is replaced with **potassium phosphate.**

241. The most important electrolyte to monitor in the above patient is:
    a. Potassium
    b. Calcium
    c. Magnesium
    d. Phosphate

Answer d. Phosphate is responsible for the majority of deleterious effects associated with re-feeding syndrome.

242. Which of the following abnormalities can cause prolonged ventilation:
    a. Hypokalemia
    b. Hypomagnesemia
    c. Hyponatremia
    d. Hypophosphatemia

Answer d. Hypophosphatemia can result in prolonged ventilation due to relative **ATP insufficiency** (need PO4 to convert ADP to ATP).

243. Severe hypophosphatemia can result in all of the following except:
    a. Respiratory failure
    b. Encephalopathy
    c. Muscle weakness
    d. Hypercortisolism

Answer d. Severe hypophosphatemia is not associated with hypercortisolism

244. All of the following are true except:
    a. Hyperosmolar, hyperglycemic, non-ketotic syndrome can result in cerebral edema, seizures, coma and respiratory arrest
    b. DKA results in hypokalemia
    c. DKA occurs almost exclusively in Type I DM
    d. Initial Tx for DKA is fluid hydration and insulin

Answer b. DKA results in hyperkalemia.

GENERAL
- **Protein** - main determinant of intravascular and interstitial compartment *oncotic* **pressure**
- **Na+** - main determinant of intracellular and extracellular *osmotic* **pressure**
- **Volume overload** - MCC is iatrogenic; 1st sign is **weight gain**
  - 3rd **space fluid** (edema) is in the **interstitial space**

- **0.9% normal saline**: Na 154 and Cl 154
- **3% saline**: Na 513 and Cl 513
- **0.45% saline**: Na 77 and Cl 77
- **Lactated Ringer's** (LR; ionic composition of plasma): Na 130, K 4, Ca 2.7, Cl 109, bicarbonate (HCO_3; as lactate) 28
- Normal **serum osmolality**: 280 - 295
  - $= (2 \times Na) + (glucose/18) + (BUN/2.8)$
  - _High_ serum osmolality suggests dehydration or diabetes insipidus
  - _Low_ serum osmolality suggests fluid overload or SIADH
- **Water** shifts from areas of low solute concentration (low osmolarity) to areas of high solute concentration (high osmolarity) to achieve **osmotic equilibrium**
- Normal **urine specific gravity**: 1.002 - 1.028
  - _High_ urine specific gravity (high urine osmolality) suggests dehydration or SIADH
  - _Low_ urine osmolality suggests fluid overload or diabetes insipidus
- **ADH** (anti-diuretic hormone; vasopressin) reabsorbs water; collecting ducts
- **SIADH** - syndrome of inappropriate anti-diuretic hormone (too much ADH; see below)
- Normal K^+ **requirement**: 0.5 - 1.0 mEq/kg/day
- Normal Na^+ **requirement**: 1 - 2 mEq/kg/day
- **Hemodialysis** (HD) can remove **K, Ca, Mg** and PO_4; also **urea** and **Cr**

ESTIMATES OF VOLUME REPLACEMENT
- 4 cc/kg/h for 1st 10 kg
- 2 cc/kg/h for 2nd 10 kg
- 1 cc/kg/h for each kg after that
- Best indicator of adequate volume replacement (non-trauma patients) - **urine output** (0.5 cc/kg/hr; _for trauma patients use serum lactate < 2.5_)
- **Replacement fluids** after **major adult gastrointestinal surgery**
  - During operation and 1st 24 hours - use **LR**
  - After 24 hours - switch to **D5 ½ NS with 20 mEq K**
  - D5 ½ NS @ 125/h provides 150 g glucose per day (525 kcal/day)
  - 5% dextrose stimulates **insulin release** (↑s glucose and amino acid uptake, ↑s protein synthesis, and prevents protein catabolism)
- **Open abdominal operations** - fluid loss is **0.5 - 1.0 L/hr** unless there is a measurable blood loss
- Usually do <u>not</u> replace blood loss unless it's **> 500 cc**
- **Insensible fluid losses** - 10 cc/kg/day (75% sweat and 25% respiratory; fluid loss is hypotonic)
- Significant 3rd **spacing of fluid** (interstitial space) occurs after major surgery

GI FLUID / ELECTROLYTE LOSSES AND REPLACEMENT
- **Stomach** (eg NG tube, gastric outlet obstruction, pyloric stenosis) - lose H and Cl
  - Results in _metabolic alkalosis_
  - Replacement with **normal saline** until patient is resuscitated, then switch to D5 ½ NS with 20 mg K
- **Pancreas** (eg high output pancreatic fistula) - lose HCO_3
  - Results in _metabolic acidosis_
  - Replacement with **lactated ringers**
- **Bile** (eg PTC tube with high output) - lose HCO_3
  - Results in _metabolic acidosis_
  - Replacement with **lactated ringers**
- **Small intestine** (eg high output ileostomy or fistula) - lose HCO_3
  - Results in _metabolic acidosis_
  - Replacement with **lactated ringers**
- **Large intestine** (eg massive diarrhea) - lose K and HCO_3
  - Results in _metabolic acidosis_
  - Replacement with **lactated ringers**
- **GI fluid losses** - should generally be replaced **cc/cc**
- **Dehydration** (eg marathon runner) - Tx: replacement with **normal saline**
- **Urine output** - should be kept at least 0.5 cc/kg/h; should <u>not</u> be replaced, usually a sign of normal post-op recovery
- _Never bolus normal saline with K added (risk of cardiac arrest)_

	Normal Fluid Secretion (cc/d)	Electrolyte Loss	Maintenance IVFs*
Sweat	300-500	**Water**, some NaCl	**Normal Saline**
Saliva	Normally negligible	K^+ (highest K concentration in body)	**1/2 NS with 20 mEq K^+**
Stomach	1000-2000	H^+ and Cl^-	**D5 1/2 NS with 20 mEq K^+** (eg gastric outlet obstruction)
Pancreas	500-1000	HCO_3^-	**LR** (eg fistula)
Biliary System	500-1000	HCO_3^-	**LR** (eg fistula)
Small Intestine	*Fluid absorption unless fistula*	HCO_3^-, ± K^+	**LR**** (eg fistula)
Large Intestine	*Fluid absorption unless diarrhea*	HCO_3^- and K^+	**LR***** (eg diarrhea)

*Above are **maintenance fluids,** not resuscitation IVFs for dehydration (see above)
**May need additional HCO_3^- replacement
***May need additional K^+ replacement

SODIUM (normal 135-145)
- **Hypernatremia** - usually from **dehydration** related to poor PO intake; others - over-diuresis, diabetes insipidus
  - Sx's: restlessness, irritability, weakness, ataxia, seizures
  - Tx: correct with **D5 water**
  - Correct Na slowly to avoid **brain swelling** (< 0.7 meg/L/hr)
- **Hyponatremia** - usually from **fluid overload** (iatrogenic); others - SIADH, following TURP when using water irrigation instead of normal saline
  - Sx's: headaches, lethargy, N/V, seizures, coma
  - Tx: **water restriction** (1st), then **diuresis**
  - Correct Na slowly to avoid **central pontine myelinolysis** (≤ 0.5 mEq/L/hr)
  - **Hyperglycemia** (eg glucose > 400 with DKA) and **hyperlipidemia** (eg triglycerides > 1000 with acute pancreatitis) cause **pseudo-hyponatremia** → no specific Tx is needed, just Tx the underlying disease
- **Diabetes insipidus** (patients have low ADH) - patients lose water
  - Sx's: **copious urine output**
  - Have **hypernatremia**, high serum osmolarity, and low urine osmolality (dilute urine)
  - Can occur with head injury, ETOH
  - **Chronic Tx**: replace free water with D5-water
  - **Acute Tx** (eg head trauma) - **desmopressin** (closely monitor Na levels and do not correct Na too quickly to prevent brain swelling)
- **SIADH** (syndrome of inappropriate ADH) - patients have high ADH and retain water
  - Sx's: **poor urine output** and fluid overload (*without* edema)
  - Have **hyponatremia**, low serum osmolarity, and high urine specific gravity (concentrated urine); also have ↑ed **urine cAMP** (ADH acts on distal tubules to reabsorb water - **cAMP** mediated)
  - Can occur with **head injury**,
  - **Chronic Tx**: fluid restriction (1st), then diuresis
  - **Acute Tx** (eg head trauma) - **conivaptan** or **tolvaptan** (ADH receptor antagonists; closely monitor Na levels and do not correct too quickly to prevent central pontine myelinolysis)

POTASSIUM (normal 3.5-5.0)
- **Kidneys** regulate serum K^+
- **Hyperkalemia** - EKG has peaked T waves; usually have **renal failure**; Tx →
  - ½ amp **calcium gluconate** *(1st drug to give; membrane stabilizer that helps prevent arrhythmias)*
  - 1 amp **sodium bicarbonate** (alkalosis causes K to enter cell in exchange for H)
  - 1 amp **50% dextrose** and 10 U **insulin** (K driven into cells with glucose)
  - **Kayexalate**
  - Other - Lasix, albuterol
  - **Dialysis** if refractory
  - **EKG** - initial peaked T waves deteriorates to **ventricular fibrillation** (shock at 360 joules)
  - **Pseudo-hyperkalemia** - hemolysis of blood sample
- **Hypokalemia** - T waves disappear on EKG; usually occurs with **excessive diuresis**
  - Other causes - poor intake (eg TPN), GI loss (gastric outlet obstruction, diarrhea)
  - Tx: **potassium chloride** (10 mEq ↑s serum K by 0.1 mEq/L)
  - May need to replace **Mg** before you can correct K
  - **Diabetic ketoacidosis** (DKA) can cause severe hypokalemia (lose K in urine)
    - Tx: **fluid resuscitation** and **insulin**; potassium replacement

CALCIUM (normal 8.5-10.0; normal ionized 1.0-1.5)
- Ca is absorbed in GI tract (**calcium binding protein**) and reabsorbed in kidney (regulated primarily by **PTH**)
- **Hypercalcemia** - ulcers, kidney stones, pancreatitis, depression, bone loss
  - **Primary hyperparathyroidism** - MC benign cause and MCC overall
  - **Breast CA** - MC malignant cause of hypercalcemia
  - MCC of **hypercalcemic crisis** - undiagnosed **hyperparathyroidism** with stressor (eg surgery, trauma)
    - As a group, **hypercalcemia of malignancy** is #1
  - Hyperparathyroidism and malignancy account for 90% of all cases of hypercalcemia (see Parathyroid chapter)
  - Tx for **hypercalcemic crisis** (Ca > 13; lethargy, N/V, hypotension, arrhythmias):
    - *Normal saline* at 200-300 cc/h *(1st)* and *Lasix (2nd)* - best initial Tx
    - For **malignant disease** → calcitonin (*best early drug*, quick onset), alendronic acid (*good long term drug*, very effective but *slow* onset); these drugs primarily inhibit osteoclast bone resorption
    - **Dialysis** if refractory to above
    - No lactated Ringer's (contains Ca)
    - No thiazide diuretics (these retain Ca)
    - If due to hyperparathyroidism → parathyroidectomy *after* recovery
    - CA causing malignant hypercalcemia is usually unresectable
  - MC CA causing hypercalcemic crisis - **breast CA** (PTH-rp [related peptide])
  - CA with the **highest risk** of hypercalcemic crisis - #1 **parathyroid CA**, #2 squamous cell CA of the lung
- **Hypocalcemia** (Ca usually < 8 for Sx's) - **perioral tingling / numbness** *(1st symptom, ie paresthesias)*, hyperreflexia, facial twitching, carpopedal spasm, tetany, irritability, confusion, prolonged Q-T interval; can occur after parathyroidectomy
  - **MCC hypocalcemia** - previous thyroid surgery (ie parathyroids were devascularized, resulting in hypoparathyroidism)
  - Other causes - massive blood transfusion, pancreatitis
  - Tx:
    - Mild Sx's - PO **calcium carbonate**
    - Severe Sx's - IV **calcium gluconate**
    - Vit D long term (calcitriol)
  - May need to correct **Mg** before being able to correct calcium
  - **Hypoproteinemia** (decreased albumin) causes *artificially* **low Ca;** for every 1 g decrease in protein, add 0.8 to Ca level
  - Hypocalcemia can occur after surgery for **hyperparathyroidism**
    - Caused by *bone hunger* (*early*, bone repleting lost supply) or *failure of parathyroid remnant or graft* (*late*)
    - Remember to give Ca after parathyroid surgery

MAGNESIUM (normal 2.0-2.5)

- **Hypermagnesemia** - causes lethargic state and Sx's similar to hypercalcemia; usually occurs in **renal failure** patients taking magnesium antacids or laxatives
  - > 10 → complete heart block; > 13 → risk for cardiac arrest
  - Tx: **calcium gluconate** *(best Tx, competitive Mg antagonist)*, diuretics, dialysis
- **Hypomagnesemia** - Sx's similar to hypocalcemia (eg paresthesias, tetany); can occur with **chronic TPN** without mineral replacement (eg short gut, Crohn's) or **excessive diuretics** *(massive diuresis)*
  - Sx's start when Mg < 1
  - Tx: **magnesium sulfate**

PHOSPHATE (normal 2.5-4.5 mg/dl)

- **Hyperphosphatemia**
  - MCC - **renal failure**
  - Sx's: majority asymptomatic; may have Sx's associated with hypocalcemia (see above)
  - Tx: **sevelamer chloride** (Renagel; phosphate binder in gut), low phosphate diet (eg avoid dairy), dialysis (removes PO_4^-)
- **Hypophosphatemia**
  - Usually due to PO_4^- shift from extra-cellular to intra-cellular
  - MCC - **re-feeding syndrome** *(often have ETOH abuse)*
  - Many ICU patients have hypophosphatemia but re-feeding syndrome is the MCC of significant hypophosphatemia
  - Sx's: **muscle weakness** (lack of PO_4^- for ATP production), **failure to wean from the ventilator** (decreased ATP production), **infection risk** (poor leukocyte chemotaxis from low ATP), **encephalopathy**
  - Tx: **potassium phosphate**

METABOLIC ACIDOSIS

- **Anion gap = Na - (HCO_3^- + Cl); normal is < 10-15**
  - The gap is caused by unmeasured acid anions
- **High anion gap** metabolic acidosis etiologies (all are **gaining acid**) - "MUDPILES" = methanol, uremia, diabetic ketoacidosis, paraldehydes, isoniazid, lactic acidosis, ethylene glycol, salicylates; other – hyperparathyroidism
- **Normal anion gap** metabolic acidosis etiologies:
  1) **Loss of HCO_3^-** (eg PTC tube, ileostomies, pancreatic fistulas, diarrhea) *or*;
  2) Rapid **IV fluid replacement** with **non-bicarbonate containing solutions** (eg normal saline, ½ normal saline) → causes a **dilutional acidosis**
- Tx: fix the underlying cause; keep pH > 7.20 with bicarbonate (severely decreased pH can cause cardiovascular instability)

METABOLIC ALKALOSIS

- Usually a **contraction metabolic alkalosis** (eg NG tube suction, gastric outlet obstruction, pyloric stenosis)
  - Results in **hypochloremic, hypokalemic, metabolic alkalosis**
  - Tx: **normal saline** (need to correct the Cl deficit)
- Mechanism of **hypochloremic, hypokalemic, metabolic alkalosis** with paradoxical aciduria
  - Causes - gastric fluid loss with NG tube, **gastric outlet obstruction**
  - Loss of Cl^- and H ion from stomach (**hypochloremic alkalosis**)
  - Water loss causes kidney to reabsorb Na (+ water) in exchange for K^+ (Na/K ATPase) resulting in **hypokalemia**
  - K^+/H^- exchanger in kidney activated (reabsorbs K, excretes H)→ **paradoxical aciduria**
  - Tx: fluid resuscitation with **normal saline** (key is to replace the Cl- deficit)

RESPIRATORY ACIDOSIS / ALKALOSIS

- **Respiratory Alkalosis** - from hyper-ventilation (eg anxiety attack)
- **Respiratory Acidosis** - from poor minute ventilation (eg COPD exacerbation)

Acid-Base Balance

Condition	pH (7.4)	CO_2 (40)	HCO_3^- (24)
Respiratory acidosis	↓	↑*	↑=
Respiratory alkalosis	↑	↓*	↓=
Metabolic acidosis	↓	↓=	↓*
Metabolic alkalosis	↑	↑=	↑*

( ) - normal mean value (all have a 4)
* Indicates primary problem
= Indicates the compensation to get pH back to normal

- **Normal Values:**
  - **pH**: 7.35-7.45 (7.4)
  - CO_2: 35-45 (40)
  - HCO_3^-: 22-26 (24)
- **Lung** (respiratory compensation) controls pH through CO_2 **regulation** (*rapid process, takes minutes*)
- **Kidney** (renal compensation) controls pH primarily through HCO_3^- **regulation** (carbonic anhydrase mediated, *slow → takes hours to days*)
- Unusual causes of **metabolic acidosis** - primary hyperparathyroidism, spironolactone, lactulose, sulfamylon (mafenide acetate)
- Unusual causes of **metabolic alkalosis** - hyperaldosteronism, furosemide (Lasix)

TUMOR LYSIS SYNDROME
- Rapid **tumor lysis** following **chemotherapy** leads to **acute metabolic disarray**
- Destroyed cells release **purines** and **pyrimidines** (→ *metabolized to uric acid*)
  - **K** and PO_4 are also leaked from cells
- Leads to acute **renal failure** from calcium-phosphate crystal deposition, (uric acid less of a problem since Rasburicase) and **arrhythmias** (primarily due to K)
- RFs: **lymphomas** and **leukemias**; chemotherapy (can also occur following XRT)
- Path: ↑ **uric acid**, ↑ **K**, and ↑ PO_4; can also have ↓ **Ca**
- Tx: *pre-hydration (best Tx) prior to chemo (give volume if it occurs - normal saline)*
  - **Allopurinol** (decreases uric acid production)
  - **Rasburicase** (converts uric acid to inert metabolite allantoin)
  - Give **phosphate binding antacids** before chemo (eg sevelamer chloride)
  - **Loop diuretic** (eg furosemide)
  - **Sodium bicarbonate** (HCO_3; alkalinizes urine, prevents uric acid precipitation)
  - **Dextrose 50%** and **insulin** for severe hyperkalemia
  - **Hemodialysis** if previous fail
  - *Avoid giving Ca (can cause Ca-PO_4 precipitation)*

OTHER
- **Contrast dyes** - Tx: **pre-hydration** *(best prevents renal damage)*
  - HCO_3 and *N*-acetylcysteine other options
- **Myoglobinemia** (eg severe trauma, rhabdomyolysis) - converted to ferrihemate in acidic environment, which is toxic to renal cells
  - Tx: **hydration** *(best)*, alkalinize urine with HCO_3

Nutrition

245. Over-feeding patients in the intensive care unit is most likely to result in:
     a. Prolonged intubation
     b. Hypoglycemia
     c. Renal failure
     d. Hypokalemia

Answer a. Overfeeding can lead to high carbohydrate build-up and increased CO_2 production. This makes the lungs work harder to get rid of CO_2, which can tire patients out, and result in **prolonged ventilation**.

246. All of the following are true except:
     a. Respiratory quotient is CO_2 production over O_2 consumption
     b. A respiratory quotient < 0.7 indicates starvation
     c. The respiratory quotient of fat = 0.7
     d. Excess carbohydrates are converted to amino acids

Answer d. Over-feeding with carbohydrates results in conversion of carbohydrates to fat. This conversion causes an increase in CO_2 production compared to O_2 consumed, thus RQ will increase.

Conversely, **under-feeding** results in breakdown of fat and glycogen stores which does not increase CO_2. Oxygen consumption increases during starvation. In this situation, the RQ will decrease.

247. A patient with a severe emphysema requires TPN. The solution should contain:
     a. High fat
     b. Low fat
     c. Low carbohydrates
     d. High carbohydrates
     e. Low protein

Answer c. Low carbohydrates are beneficial as it avoids CO_2 build-up in patients with severe emphysema.

248. A 55 yo man with a recent 20% weight loss has a gastric CA you feel is resectable. What is the most effective way of avoiding electrolyte imbalances in this patient:
     a. Starting TPN at a low rate
     b. Starting TPN at a high rate
     c. Removing calcium from the TPN
     d. Removing potassium from the TPN
     e. Removing magnesium from the TPN

Answer a. Starting TPN at a low rate avoids re-feeding syndrome.

249. Pre-op TPN for the above patient is associated with:
     a. Increased ICU time
     b. Decreased survival
     c. Increased incidence of infectious complications
     d. Decreased incidence of non-infectious complications

Answer d. Patients with *severe* **malnutrition** (> 15% weight loss over the last 6 months) have *decreased* post-op non-infectious complications (eg prolonged ventilation, renal failure, anastomotic leaks) when given pre-op TPN.

Patients with *severe* malnutrition pre-op should preferentially be given enteral feeds over TPN if possible (enteral feeding decreases *overall* complication rate, including non-infectious *and* infectious complications).

250. For the above patient, instead of a 20% weight loss, his weight loss is 10% in the last 6 months. Pre-op TPN is now associated with:
   - a. Increased ICU time
   - b. Increased survival
   - c. Increased incidence of infectious complications
   - d. Decreased incidence of non-infectious complications

Answer c. Patients with _simple_ malnutrition (< 15% weight loss over the last 6 months) have increased peri-op infections when given pre-op TPN _(should be avoided)_. Patients with _simple_ malnutrition do _not_ benefit from pre-op nutrition.

251. The above patient undergoes resection, the most appropriate time to start nutrition is:
   - a. Day of surgery
   - b. POD #1
   - c. POD #2
   - d. With flatus
   - e. With bowel movement

Answer a. Day of surgery

252. The best method for nutrition in the above patient is:
   - a. Oral intake
   - b. TPN
   - c. J-tube feeding
   - d. G-tube feeding

Answer c. J-Tube feeding (start at a low rate 20-25 cc/hour). G-tube would not be appropriate given the recent gastric resection. TPN should be avoided if possible. Oral intake should be avoided this soon after upper GI surgery (start with clear liquids on POD 2 or 3). Feeding the gut avoids bacterial translocation (caused by mucosal atrophy) and avoids Cx's associated with TPN (eg electrolyte problems, infection risk).

253. A patient receives a 1000 cc bag of TPN which contains 10% dextrose and 7% protein. In addition, this patient receives 250 cc of a 20% fat emulsion solution. How many calories does this approximately represent?
   - a. 1070 calories
   - b. 1420 calories
   - c. 1820 calories
   - d. 2220 calories

Answer a.
A 1000 cc bag of 10% dextrose is equal to 100 gm of dextrose (0.10 x 1000 = 100 gm), which is 340 calories (100 gm x 3.4 calories/gm).

A 1000 cc bag of 7% protein is equal to 70 gm of protein (0.07 x 1000 = 70 gm), which is 280 calories (70 gm x 4 calories/gm).

A 250 cc bag of 20% fat emulsion is equivalent to 50 gm of fat (0.20 x 250 = 50), and 50 gm of fat is equivalent to 450 calories (50 gm x 9 calories/gm).

Then just add them up 340 + 280 + 450 = 1070 calories.

254. All of the following are true except:
   - a. Intestinal medium and short chain fatty acids enter the circulation through lymphatics
   - b. Chylomicrons contain primarily triacylglycerides (TAGs)
   - c. Linoleic acid is an essential fatty acid
   - d. Lipoprotein lipase is located on endothelium and clears chylomicrons from blood

Answer a. Intestinal **medium** and **short chain fatty acids** enter the circulation through the **portal vein.** Conversely, **chylomicrons** and **long chain fatty acids** enter the circulation through **lymphatics** (terminal lacteals; these feed into the the thoracic duct).

255. All of the following are true of carbohydrate metabolism except:
  a. The first enzyme in carbohydrate digestion is amylase
  b. Skeletal muscle contains the majority of the body's glycogen stores
  c. Skeletal muscle is abundant in glucose-6 phosphatase
  d. The body's glycogen stores are depleted 18-24 hours after fasting

Answer c. Skeletal muscle lacks **glucose-6 phosphatase**, thus glucose from glycogen breakdown **stays in muscle** (glucose-6 can't be released). **Fat** is the main energy source after 24 hours of starvation or major stress. The first enzyme in carbohydrate digestion is **salivary amylase**.

256. All of the following are true of protein metabolism except:
  a. The first enzyme in protein digestion is pepsin
  b. Leucine is both a branched chain and essential amino acid (AA)
  c. Glutamine is the MC AA in the blood stream and tissues
  d. Pancreatic proteases are not required for protein absorption

Answer d. Pancreatic proteases are required for protein absorption. Stomach pepsin is the 1st enzyme in protein digestion (not essential for protein absorption).

257. All of the following are true of nutrition sources except:
  a. The primary source for colonocytes is short chain fatty acids (butyrate)
  b. The primary source for small bowel is glutamine
  c. The primary source for most cancer cells is glutamine
  d. During prolonged starvation, the brain switches from glucose to glutamine

Answer d. Brain switches from glucose to ketones with prolonged starvation.

258. Which of the following lab values is most predictive of post-op mortality?
  a. Low sodium
  b. Low potassium
  c. Low transferrin
  d. Low albumin

Answer d. Low albumin (< 3.5) has been directly correlated with increased morbidity and mortality following operative procedures.

259. Ileal resection can result in all of the following except:
  a. Decreased B_{12} and folate uptake, resulting in megaloblastic anemia
  b. Decreased bile salt uptake which can cause osmotic diarrhea (bile salts) and steatorrhea (decreased fat uptake)
  c. Increased bile salt uptake which can result in the formation of gallstones
  d. Ca oxalate kidney stones (hyperoxaluria)

Answer c. Ileal resection does not result in increased bile salt resorption. It does result in decreased bile salt uptake and the formation of **gallstones**.

260. The strongest layer of the bowel wall is:
  a. Mucosa
  b. Submucosa
  c. Muscularis
  d. Serosa

Answer b. The strongest layer of the bowel wall is the **submucosa**. This is where you want your sutures when doing a hand sewn bowel anastomosis. The time point at which small bowel is weakest is **3-5 days**.

261. A 35 yo woman suffering from Crohn's disease on chronic TPN is admitted for hair loss, skin lesions on her extremities and peri-orificial areas, diarrhea, and wasting of body tissues. This is associated with which of the following?
   a. Copper deficiency
   b. Zinc deficiency
   c. Phosphate deficiency
   d. Chromium deficiency
   e. Vitamin K deficiency

   Answer b Zinc deficiency is associated with poor healing, hair loss, diarrhea, extremity and peri-oral skin lesions, and body wasting.

262. Instead of the above, the patient has easy bruising, epistaxis, and gum bleeding. This is associated with which of the following?
   a. Copper deficiency
   b. Zinc deficiency
   c. Phosphate deficiency
   d. Chromium deficiency
   e. Vitamin K deficiency

   Answer e. Vitamin K deficiency results in coagulopathy.

263. All of the following are true except:
   a. Glutamine is the MC substrate for gluconeogenesis
   b. Fatty acids cannot be used for gluconeogenesis
   c. Glutamine is to MC amino acid released from catabolism of skeletal muscle
   d. Steatorrhea from obstructive jaundice can result in deficiency of fat soluble vitamins (A, D, E, K) which can result in complications such as bleeding

   Answer a. Alanine is the MC (and important) substrate for **gluconeogenesis**.

264. A 22 yo man is HD #4 following a 30% BSA 2nd and 3rd degree burn. This patient most importantly needs:
   a. High glucose support
   b. High protein support
   c. High lipid support
   d. Growth hormone
   e. Glutamine

   Answer b. Patients with *extensive* **healing issues** (eg severe burns, necrotizing fasciitis) have **high protein requirements** required for healing.

265. A 55 yo man is undergoing elective colon CA resection that involves the sigmoid colon. Which of the following is true of this patient:
   a. This patient should have over-night fasting
   b. A post-op clear liquid diet (ad lib) should be started within 24 hours
   c. A bowel prep is recommended
   d. A nasogastric tube should be placed
   e. An epidural should be avoided

   Answer b. A post-op **clear liquid** diet (ad lib) should be started within **24 hours** after colon or rectal surgery (see Colon and Rectum chapter).

266. Instead of the above, the patient is undergoing low anterior resection and a temporary ileostomy is planned. Which of the following is true in this patient:
   a. This patient should have over-night fasting
   b. A bowel prep is recommended
   c. A nasogastric tube should be placed
   d. An epidural should be avoided

Answer b. A bowel prep is recommended if undergoing rectal surgery and an ileostomy is planned (see Colon and Rectum chapter).

267. All of the following are part of the metabolic syndrome except:
   a.   Obesity
   b.   Hypothyroidism
   c.   Insulin resistance
   d.   Elevated triglycerides

Answer b. Hypothyroidism is <u>not</u> part of the metabolic syndrome.

NUTRITION REQUIREMENT
- **Calories:**

Fat	9 calories/g
Protein	4 calories/g
Oral carbohydrates	4 calories/g
Dextrose	3.4 calories/g

- **Caloric need**: 25 calories/kg/day (70 kg male → 1500-1700 calories/d)
- **Nutritional requirements** for average healthy adult male (use for **TPN calculations**)
  - **50% carbohydrate** calories
  - **30% fat** calories - provides essential fatty acids
  - **20% protein** calories (1 g/kg/day) - provides essential amino acids (AAs)
- **Increased caloric requirements** - up to 30 calories/kg/day
  - Increase calories for **trauma, surgery**, and **sepsis** (stress factors)
  - <u>Protein</u> requirement also increases with above
- **Burns** - start nutrition early for severe burns (for $\geq 2^{nd}$ degree burns over $\geq$ 20% BSA)
  - <u>Calories</u>: 25 calories/kg/day + (30 calories/day × % burn)
  - <u>Protein</u>: 1 g/kg/day + (3 g × % burn)
  - **Protein** is very important in burn wound healing
- **Large wounds** require significant **protein** ($\geq$ 1.5 g/kg/day) for wound healing
- <u>Never</u> exceed 3000 calories/d (avoids over-feeding and increased CO_2 production)
- **Central line** total parenteral nutrition (TPN) - is <u>glucose</u> based
- **Peripheral line** parenteral nutrition (PPN) - is <u>fat</u> based (high glucose concentration can damage veins)
- **Energy expenditure**
  - Much of energy expenditure is used for **heat production**
  - **Harris-Benedict equation** calculates basal metabolic rate from **weight, height, age**, and **gender**

PRE-OPERATIVE NUTRITIONAL ASSESSMENT
- Normal **albumin** level: 3.5 - 5.5
- Pre-op signs of ***severe* malnutrition**:
  - Acute weight loss (**> 15% body weight** within 6 months)
  - **Albumin < 2.5**
- **Low albumin** (< 3.0) - very strong RF for post-op **morbidity / mortality**
- <u>Acute</u> indicators of nutritional status (eg post-op patients with questionable intake) - **pre-albumin** (#1), retinal binding protein, transferrin
- **Approximate half-lives**
  - Albumin   18 days
  - Transferrin   8 days
  - Prealbumin   2 days

PERI-OPERATIVE NUTRITION SUPPORT
- *Only **severely** **malnourished** patients* undergoing <u>major</u> non-cardiac thoracic or abdominal procedures benefit from **pre-op nutrition** (7-10 days best) →
  - Pre-op **enteral nutrition** *decreases* <u>overall complications</u> (non-infectious and infectious) and <u>length of stay</u> (LOS); is preferred over parenteral nutrition (avoids bacterial translocation in gut and TPN issues)
  - Pre-op **parenteral nutrition** *decreases* <u>non-infectious complications</u> (eg renal failure, anastomotic leak, prolonged ventilation); give if not able to feed the gut

- *Normal* and **simply malnourished** patient groups should <u>not</u> have surgery deferred for pre-op nutrition
  - Pre-op parenteral nutrition (TPN) in **normal** or **simply malnourished** groups (ie <u>not</u> severely malnourished) causes *higher* <u>infectious complications</u>
- **Post-op nutrition** - for *all surgical groups* (ie normal, malnourished, and severely malnourished) using **enteral nutrition** (eg J-tube feeding, PO intake) **within 24 hours** of major GI surgery *decreases* <u>overall complications</u> (infectious and non-infectious) and <u>length of stay</u>
- Mortality is <u>not</u> influenced by either pre-op or post-op nutrition

RESPIRATORY QUOTIENT (RQ)
- Ratio of CO_2 produced to O_2 consumed - is a measurement of energy expenditure (RQ = CO_2 / O_2)
- **RQ > 1** = lipogenesis (ie **over-feeding**)
  - Sx's - ↑ed RR, ↑ed CO_2; ↑ed metabolic rate
  - High carbohydrate intake leads to CO_2 **buildup** and **failure to wean from the ventilator** (lungs working hard to get rid of CO_2, RF - COPD)
  - High CO_2 is produced when excess carbohydrates are converted to fat
  - Tx: *decrease* carbohydrates and caloric intake
- **RQ < 0.7** = ketosis and fat oxidation (ie **starving**)
  - Results in a *reduced* metabolic rate
  - Fat utilization does <u>not</u> ↑ CO_2
  - O_2 consumption does ↑ with starvation
  - Tx: *increase* carbohydrates and caloric intake
- Pure **fat** utilization - RQ = 0.7
- Pure **protein** utilization - RQ = 0.8
- Pure **carbohydrate** utilization - RQ = 1.0
- Balanced feeding - RQ = 0.825

POSTOPERATIVE PHASES
- **Diuresis phase** - post-op days 2-5
- **Catabolic phase** - post-op days 0-3 (negative nitrogen balance)
- **Anabolic phase** - post-op days 3-6 (positive nitrogen balance)

RE-FEEDING SYNDROME
- Occurs when feeding after prolonged starvation or malnutrition (**ETOH abuse** often a contributing factor); MC occurs on **Day 4** of re-feeding
- Sudden shift from fat metabolism to carbohydrate metabolism
- Results in decreased **K, Mg,** and **PO_4** (all move intracellular along with glucose)
- Causes CHF, profound weakness, encephalopathy, cardiac arrhythmias, and failure to wean from the ventilator *(most of the effects are due to low PO_4 → lack of ATP)*
- Prevent this by starting to re-feed at a **low rate** (10-15 calories/kg/day) and monitoring electrolytes *(especially **phosphate**)* with replacement

NITROGEN BALANCE
- **6.25 g of protein** contains **1 g of nitrogen**
- **N balance** = (N in - N out) = ([protein/6.25] - [24-hour urine N + 4 g])
  - **Positive N balance** - more protein ingested than excreted (anabolism, protein synthesis)
  - **Negative N balance** - more protein excreted than taken in (catabolism, protein breakdown)

ENTERAL TUBE FEEDING
- **Standard tube feeds** (eg Jevity) have 1-1.5 calories/cc
  - **Diarrhea** - Tx: **slow rate,** add **fiber** (bulk) to slow transit time, use **less concentrated** feeds (prevents osmotic diarrhea)
  - **High gastric residuals** (stomach tube feeds; > 250 cc over 4 hours)
    Tx: **Reglan** (metoclopramide) or erythromycin
  - **Aspiration** of tube feeds can occur
  - **Renal formulation** (Nepro) - low in K and PO_4; also low in protein

- Try to feed **gut** (rather than use TPN) to avoid **bacterial translocation** (caused by bacterial overgrowth and increased permeability due to starved enterocytes and mucosal atrophy)
- Early **enteral feeding** (< 24-48 hours) <u>reduces ICU stay</u> and <u>improves survival</u> in **critically ill** non-surgical patients on mechanical ventilation or multiple pressors (eg pancreatitis, sepsis, ARDS, head injury, burns)
- **PEG tube** - consider when regular feeding not possible or predicted to not occur for > 4 weeks

CENTRAL VENOUS TPN (general composition)
- **50% calories** as **dextrose**
  - Consists of a 25% dextrose solution
- **30% calories** as **fat** (lipids; 500 cc of 10% lipid solution contains 550 calories)
  - **Lipids** are given <u>separately</u> from TPN
  - 10% lipid solution contains 1.1 calories/cc; 20% lipid solution has 2 calories/cc
- **20% calories** as **protein** (1 g protein/kg/day, 20% essential AAs)
  - Usually use a 10% amino acid solution
- **Electrolyte solution** (Na, Cl, K, Ca, Mg, PO_4, and acetate)
  - Na^+ - 2 mg/kg/day; K^+ - 1 mg/kg/day
  - **Acetate** - buffer to ↑ pH of solution (prevents metabolic acidosis)
- **Vitamins** and **minerals**
  - **Vit K** is added separately (can get **coagulopathy** if not added)
  - **Zinc deficiency** can occur if minerals are not added (Sx's - poor wound healing, hair loss, diarrhea, peri-oral skin lesions, weight loss from poor appetite)
- **ETOH abuse** - add thiamine and folate
- **Total volume** = 2-3 liters / day usual (apx. rate → 100-150 cc/hr)
- **Indications for TPN** - short gut, high output fistulas, when enteral feeding can't be used

- **Branched-chain AAs** - leucine, isoleucine, valine ("LIV")
  - Are essential AAs; metabolized in **muscle**; important fuel in patients with **liver failure**
- <u>Limit protein intake</u> in patients with **liver failure** and **renal failure** to avoid **ammonia** (encephalopathy) and **urea buildup**, respectively
- **Essential fatty acids** - linolenic, linoleic; important for immune system

- **Stopping TPN** - cut rate in ½ for 1-2 hours 1st (avoids hypoglycemia)
- **Short term TPN** - complicated by issues associated with **indwelling catheters** (eg line sepsis, pneumothorax)
- **Long term TPN** - can eventually lead to **cirrhosis**

Vitamin and Mineral Deficiencies

Deficiency	Effect
Zinc	Poor wound healing, hair loss, skin lesions, diarrhea, weight loss (loss of appetite)
Phosphate	Weakness (failure to wean off ventilator), encephalopathy, CHF
Cobalamin (B_{12})	Megaloblastic anemia, peripheral neuropathy, beefy tongue
Folate	Megaloblastic anemia, glossitis
Vitamin A	Night blindness
Vitamin K	Coagulopathy
Vitamin D	Rickets, osteomalacia, osteoporosis
Vitamin E	Neuropathy

- **Transferrin** – <u>transporter</u> of iron; **Ferritin** – <u>storage</u> form of iron

FAT AND CHOLESTEROL DIGESTION
- **Triacylglycerides** (TAGs), **cholesterol**, and **lipids** are digested
  - Broken down by pancreatic **lipase**, **cholesterol esterase**, **phospholipase** and **bile salts** → form **micelles** and **free fatty acids** (FFAs) in the intestinal lumen

- **Micelles**
  - Aggregates of bile salts, **long- chain FFAs**, **monoacylglycerides** and **cholesterol**; also contain **fat-soluble vitamins** (A, D, E, K)
  - Enter enterocyte by **fusing with membrane**
  - Bile salts - help form **micelles** (↑s absorption area for fats)
- **Medium-** and **short- chain FFAs** - enter enterocyte by **simple diffusion** (these are not found in micelles)
- Micelles and medium- / **short- chain FFAs** enter **enterocytes**
  - **TAGs are re-synthesized** in intestinal cells and placed in **chylomicrons**
  - **Chylomicrons** then enter <u>lymphatics</u> (terminal lacteals → thoracic duct); chylomicrons contain - **90% TAGs** + 10% phospholipids, proteins, cholesterol
  - **Long-chain FFAs** - enter <u>lymphatics</u> along with chylomicrons
  - **Medium-** and **short- chain FFAs** - enter **portal system** (same as AAs and carbohydrates)
- The majority of **body cholesterol** is **synthesized in liver**; 95% of the cholesterol released into bile is **reabsorbed** (termed entero-hepatic recirculation)
- **LDL receptors** are located on cells at **clathrin coated pits** - bind LDL, then endocytosis
- <u>Essential</u> fatty acids – linolenic (omega 3) and **linoleic** (omega 6)
  - Needed for **prostaglandin** synthesis (long-chain fatty acids)
  - Important for **immune cells**

CARBOHYDRATE DIGESTION
- **Carbohydrates** are the body's key source of **energy**
  - Glucose is the prime energy source for the **brain**
  - **Glucose** either: 1) enters **glycolysis pathway** to produce **energy** (ATP), 2) is stored as **glycogen** or; 3) is converted to **fat** in adipose tissue
- Digestion begins with **salivary amylase**, then pancreatic amylase and intestinal brush border <u>disaccharidases</u> (maltase, sucrase, lactase)
- **Disaccharides**
  - **Sucrose** = fructose + glucose
  - **Lactose** = galactose + glucose
  - **Maltose** = glucose + glucose
- **Transport**
  - **Glucose** and **galactose** - absorbed from gut by secondary active transport (Na⁺ gradient); released into **portal vein**
  - **Fructose** - absorbed by facilitated diffusion; released into **portal vein**
- **Glucose** ingestion causes **insulin release** from beta cells in **pancreas,** which results in cellular uptake of circulating glucose
- **Primary storage area for glucose** (as glycogen) - **skeletal muscle** (#1), liver
- **Glucagon** - has opposite effect of insulin, causes breakdown of glycogen to glucose
- **Cellulose** (fiber) - non-digestible carbohydrate chains

PROTEIN DIGESTION
- Digestion begins with **stomach pepsin**, then pancreatic proteases (eg trypsinogen, chymotrypsinogen, and pro-carboxypeptidase)
  - Pepsin is not required for digestion
  - **Pancreas proteinases** are required for digestion
- **Trypsinogen** is released from pancreas and activated by **enterokinase** (which is released from the duodenum)
  - Other pancreatic proteases are then activated by trypsin
  - Trypsin can also **auto-activate** other trypsinogen molecules
- **Protein** is broken down to AAs, di-peptides, and tri-peptides
  - These are absorbed by **secondary active transport** (Na⁺ gradient) into enterocytes (primarily **jejunum**) and released as free AAs into the **portal vein**
  - They are then taken up by various cells under the influence of **insulin**
  - During **stress**, protein is shunted to the **liver** for **gluconeogenesis**
- **Liver** is the prime regulator of **AA production** and **breakdown**
- *Nonessential* AAs - those that begin with **A, G,** or **C** plus **serine, proline, tyrosine,** and **histidine**

- *Essential* AAs – leucine, isoleucine, valine, lysine, methionine, phenylalanine, threonine, and tryptophan
- **Branched-chain AAs** (are essential AAs) - leucine, isoleucine, valine ("LIV")
  - Can be metabolized in **muscle** (only AAs metabolized outside liver)
  - Important source of **protein** with **chronic liver disease** (controversial; studies show improved albumin, less encephalopathy, and improved survival)
- Majority of protein breakdown from skeletal muscle during catabolism is in the form of **glutamine** (#1) and **alanine**
- **Glutamine**
  - MC AA in **bloodstream** and **tissue**
  - MC AA **released from muscle** during catabolism
  - Can be used as an **energy source** (TCA cycle, see below)
  - Can be used for **gluconeogenesis** (see below)
  - Primary AA used in the **urea cycle** (see below)
  - Enhances **immune function** by **inhibiting small bowel mucosal breakdown** (main fuel for small bowel enterocytes) and **preventing bacterial translocation**
- Need to limit protein intake with **liver failure** to avoid **ammonia buildup** and worsening **encephalopathy**
- Need to limit protein intake with **end stage kidney disease** (to limit **urea buildup**)

NORMAL MAJOR FUEL SOURCE (non-stress, non-starvation)
- **Stomach, small bowel** enterocytes, **pancreas, spleen** - glutamine
- **Liver** - amino acids
- **Large bowel colonocytes** - short chain fatty acids (eg butyrate, acetate)
- **Heart** - short chain fatty acids
- **Skeletal muscle, brain,** and **kidney** - glucose
- **Peripheral nerves, adrenal medulla, RBCs, PMNs** - obligate glucose use
- **MC primary fuel for neoplastic cells** - glutamine (glucose #2)
- **Glutamine, ketones** and **short chain FFAs** - can enter TCA cycle for NADP, NADPH, and FADH synthesis → eventual ATP production

CORI CYCLE
- Glucose is utilized and converted to **lactate** in muscle
- **Lactate** then goes to liver and is converted back to **pyruvate** and eventually **glucose** via gluconeogenesis
- **Glucose** is then transported back to muscle

UREA CYCLE
- Accounts for 90% of all nitrogen loss
- **Glutamine** is principal NH_3^+ donor to remove **excess ammonia** from the body in the form of **urea**; reactions occur and urea is formed in **liver**; urea is removed by **kidney**

RESPONSE TO STARVATION AND MAJOR STRESS
- **Major stresses** - major surgery, trauma, sepsis
- **Glycogen stores**
  - Depleted after **18-24 hours** of starvation or major stress
  - 2/3 stored in **skeletal muscle** (#1 glycogen storage site) and 1/3 in **liver**
    Liver is the source of systemic glucose in times of stress
    Skeletal muscle lacks **glucose-6-phosphatase** (found only in **liver**); glucose-6-phosphate stays in muscle after breakdown from glycogen and is utilized there (*cannot* be released into circulation)
  - Body **switches to fat** after glycogen stores run out (fat is the largest potential energy source in the body)
- **Adipose stores**
  - **Fat** is main energy source with **starvation** and **major stress**
  - Fat is broken down to acetyl-CoA or succinyl-CoA which enter the Krebs cycle
- **Krebs cycle** (citric acid cycle) produces NADPH, NADH and FADH from **FFAs, lactate** (pyruvate), and **AAs** (AAs and pyruvate are converted to acetyl-CoA 1st)
- **Electron transport chain** - NADPH, NADH, and FADH are used to produce **ATP**; occurs on inner mitochondrial membrane
- **Gluconeogenesis** (formation of glucose)

- **Precursors** - **#1 alanine** (primary substrate for gluconeogenesis, simplest precursor), lactate, pyruvate, glycerol, other AAs
- Gluconeogenesis primarily occurs in **liver**
- Occurs to a much greater degree with **major stress** than with starvation
- Fatty acids are <u>not</u> used in gluconeogenesis because Acetyl-CoA <u>cannot</u> be converted back to pyruvate

- **Simple Starvation**
  - Causes *decreased* **metabolic rate**
  - ↓ed insulin, ↑ed glucagon
  - **Fat** is major energy source with ↑↑ed **ketone production**
  - ***Protein is conserved*** - gluconeogenesis doesn't occur until late
- **Major stress**
  - *Increases* **catecholamines, cortisol, and cytokines** → all *increase* **metabolic rate**
  - ↓ed insulin and ↑ed glucagon
  - **Fat** is main energy source, however, significant ***protein breakdown*** and **gluconeogenesis** occur (*catecholamine + cortisol effect*)
  - Hepatic **urea** formation and **negative nitrogen balance** also occur with protein breakdown
- **Brain** - switches to <u>ketones</u> as energy source (from fatty acid breakdown)

METABOLIC SYNDROME (need 3) - all related to obesity
- **Obesity** (waist circumference > 40 inches men, > 35 inches women)
- **Insulin resistance** (fasting glucose > 100)
- **Elevated TAGs** (> 100)
- **Reduced HDL** (< 50)
- **HTN** (> 130/85)

SPECIFIC DEFICIENCIES
- **Cachexia** - anorexia, weight loss, wasting; *mediated by **TNF-alpha***
- **Kwashiorkor** - protein deficiency
- **Marasmus** - starvation

- Vitamin important for **wound healing** - **Vit C**
- **Vit K deficiency** - coagulopathy (bleeding); elevated INR (PT)
  - Most Vit K produced by **bacteria** in the intestines
- **Vit D deficiency** - increased risk of **osteoporosis** and **fractures**; osteomalacia, rickets
- **Trace element deficiencies** - often associated with long term TPN
  - **Zinc deficiency** - causes **poor healing**, hair loss, diarrhea, skin lesions on extremities and peri-oral areas, body wasting

STEATORRHEA
- Can occur with <u>obstructive jaundice</u> (lack of bile acids in bowel), <u>terminal ileum resection</u> (can't reabsorb bile acids), <u>short-gut syndrome</u> (bile acids not reabsorbed), and <u>chronic pancreatitis</u> (lack of pancreatic enzymes)
- Causes <u>deficiency</u> of **fat soluble vitamins** (A, D, E, K) and **essential fatty acids** (important in immune function and inflammation)

COMPLICATIONS AFTER TERMINAL ILEUM RESECTION
- Can also occur with severe **terminal ileum inflammatory bowel disease** (becomes non-functional for absorption)
- Complications include:
  1) ↓ed **B-12** and **folate uptake** can result in **megaloblastic anemia**
  2) ↓ed **bile salt uptake** causes osmotic **diarrhea** (bile salts) and **steatorrhea** (↓ed fat uptake) in colon
  3) ↓ed **bile salt uptake** can result in the formation of **gallstones**
  4) ↓ed **oxalate binding to Ca** secondary to increased intra-luminal fat → oxalate then gets absorbed in colon → released in urine → **Ca-oxalate kidney stones** (hyperoxaluria)

Oncology

268. All of the following are true except:
     a. Ebstein Barr Virus (EBV) is associated with nasopharyngeal CA
     b. The src family of proto-oncogenes code for tyrosine kinases
     c. The ras family of proto-oncogenes code for G proteins
     d. p53 is primarily involved in angiogenesis

     Answer d. p53 is primarily involved in cell cycle regulation and **apoptosis**.

269. All of the following are true except:
     a. The MC metastasis to the small bowel is lung CA
     b. The MC metastasis to an axillary node is lymphoma
     c. The most important prognostic factor for sarcomas devoid of metastases is tumor grade
     d. The most important prognostic factor for breast CA devoid of systemic metastases is nodal status

     Answer a. The MC metastasis to the **small bowel** is **melanoma**. Notably, these metastases are most likely to cause bowel obstruction from **intussusception** (not tumor filling the lumen).

270. All of the following mechanisms are true except:
     a. Taxol stabilizes microtubules
     b. 5-FU inhibits thymidylate synthetase
     c. Taxol can cause neuropathy
     d. Etoposide is an anti-metabolite

     Answer d. Etoposide blocks DNA unwinding and replication by inhibiting **topoisomerase**.

271. All of the following toxicities are true except:
     a. Cardiotoxicity at doses greater then 500 mg/m^2 is characteristic of Adriamycin (doxorubicin)
     b. Pulmonary fibrosis is characteristic of bleomycin
     c. Ototoxicity is characteristic of cisplatin
     d. Hemorrhagic cystitis is characteristic of etoposide

     Answer d. Hemorrhagic cystitis is a side effect of **cyclophosphamide**. This is prevented with the use of **mesna** during chemotherapy.

272. All of the following are true of directed immunotherapy for CA except:
     a. This takes advantage of body's adaptive immune system
     b. T Killer cells cannot be tumor specific
     c. It can involve harvesting T cells
     d. IL-2 is added to T cells to form T killer cells (LAK cells)

     Answer b. T killer cells can be made to be tumor specific by adding tumor antigen. T-cells are harvested, **IL-2** is added as well as the tumor antigen to form tumor specific T killer cells. These cells attack the tumor. Has been used for melanoma with some success

273. All of the following are true of XRT for tumor therapy except:
     a. Tumor cells are most sensitive to XRT during the M stage of the cell cycle
     b. The main target of XRT is DNA
     c. Damage is primarily due to formation of oxygen radicals
     d. Large sarcoma are generally considered extremely radiosensitive

     Answer d. Large sarcomas are considered radio-resistant (sarcomas are considered radio-resistant, large tumors are also radio-resistant due to *lack of oxygen* within the tumor).

274. All of the following are true of PET scan except:
     a.   18-fluoro deoxyglucose is injected IV
     b.   PET detects fluorodeoxyglucose molecules (FDG-6-phosphate)
     c.   PET is good in detecting brain metastases
     d.   The test may not work well in diabetics

    Answer c. Due to the high glucose metabolism in the brain, PET has not been accurate for the detection of metastases to the brain. MRI is generally indicated for the detection of brain metastases.

275. All of the following are true of sentinel lymph node biopsy except:
     a.   Lymph nodes staining blue after lymphazurin blue dye should be resected
     b.   The sentinel lymph node is the hypothetical first lymph node(s) reached by cancer cells from a tumor
     c.   The lymph node with the highest gamma count should be resected
     d.   Lymph nodes within 10% of the highest gamma count should be resected
     e.   Patients with clinically positive nodes should undergo SLNB

    Answer e. Patients with **clinically positive nodes** should undergo **formal lymph node dissection.**

276. The most sensitive test for detection of metastases to the liver is:
     a.   CT scan
     b.   MRI
     c.   PET scan
     d.   Intra-op U/S
     e.   Tagged RBC scan

    Answer d. Intra-op U/S

277. The genes involved in development of colon CA include the following except:
     a.   APC
     b.   p53
     c.   DCC
     d.   Ret
     e.   K-ras

    Answer d. Ret is not routinely involved in the development of colon CA.

278. A phase II clinical trial:
     a.   Evaluates whether or not a drug is safe and at what dose
     b.   Evaluates whether or not the drug is effective
     c.   Evaluates whether or not the drug is better than existing therapy
     d.   Involves implementation and marketing

    Answer b. Phase II trials evaluate whether or not the drug is effective.

MOST COMMONS
- **Cancer #2 cause of death in US** (#1 - heart disease)
- **MC CA in women** - breast CA
- **MCC of CA death in women** - lung CA
- **MC CA in men** - prostate CA
- **MCC of CA death in men** - lung CA

ONCOGENESIS (cancer transformation)
- **Retroviruses** can contain **oncogenes**
  - **Epstein-Barr** - Burkitt's lymphoma (8:14 translocation, B cell, mandible); nasopharyngeal CA; post-transplantation lymphoproliferative disease (PTLD)
  - **HPV** - cervical CA
  - **Hep-B, -C,** and **-D** - hepatocellular CA

- **Tumor Suppressors** - have 1 or both of the following functions
    - 1) **Inhibit cell cycle**
    - 2) **Induce apoptosis** (programmed cell death)
- Generally need multiple oncogenic gene transformations and mutations in tumor suppressors to get cancer

PROTO-ONCOGENES (human genes with malignant potential)
- Can be converted to oncogenes and promote CA
- **Growth factors** (eg **c-*sis*** - platelet derived growth factor)
- <u>**Cytoplasmic**</u> tyrosine kinases (eg ***src*** family)
- <u>**Receptor**</u> tyrosine kinases (PDGF receptor, EGF receptor, VEGF receptor)
- **GTPase proteins** (G proteins; eg ***ras*** family) - are usually transmembrane
    - **k-ras** oncogene - protein is a **GTPase** involved in signal transduction and cell cycle regulation; involved in colon CA
- **Transcription factors** (eg ***myc*** family)

TUMOR SUPPRESSOR GENES (normal protein function listed)
- **APC** (adenomatous polyposis coli) - involved in **cell cycle regulation** and **cell adhesion**
- **p53** - involved in **cell cycle regulation** and **apoptosis** (normal gene induces cell cycle arrest and programmed cell death; abnormal gene allows unrestrained cell growth)
- **DCC** (Deleted in Colorectal Cancer) - transmembrane receptor involved in **apoptosis**
- **BRCA 1 and 2** - involved in **DNA damage repair** and **apoptosis**
- **SWI/SNF** (SWItch/Sucrose Non-Fermentable) - involved in **DNA re-modeling**; mutation of this gene is found in *20% of all human malignancies*

CANCER IMMUNOLOGY
- **Natural killer cells** can independently attack tumor cells (can attack cells without MHC expression)
- **Cytotoxic T cells** need MHC complex to attack tumor; tumor antigens are random unless viral-induced tumor
- **Cytotoxic T cells** can be made to be tumor specific by adding tumor antigen
    - T-cells are harvested, **IL-2** is added as well as tumor antigen to form tumor specific cytotoxic T cells
    - These are then injected and attack the tumor; some success with melanoma

CANCER SPREAD
- **Resection of a normal organ to prevent cancer**
    - **Breast** - BRCA I or II with strong family history
    - **Thyroid** - RET proto-oncogene with family history of MEN or thyroid CA
    - **Other** (although organ not totally normal)
        Undescended testicle in adults (testicular CA)
        Porcelain gallbladder → gallbladder CA
- **MC CA in suspicious <u>axillary</u> lymph node** - lymphoma
- **Lymph nodes** have poor barrier function → better to view them as signs of **probable systemic metastasis**
- **Sentinel lymph node biopsy** - *no role for clinically palpable nodes* → you need formal lymphadenectomy
- **MC metastasis to small bowel** - <u>melanoma</u> (causes **intussusception**)
- **Krukenberg tumor** - gastric CA metastasis to the ovary (also colorectal CA)
- **Most successfully cured <u>isolated</u> metastases with surgery** (5-year survival)
    - **Germ cell** (eg testicular CA) to lung, **75% 5-YS** *(best)*

CHEMOTHERAPY AGENTS
- **Cell cycle-nonspecific agents** (all involved in DNA cross-linking and binding)
    - Act at *all phases* of the cell cycle
    - **Linear** response to cell killing (increase in dose increases killing)
    - Are all **alkylating agents** - add **alkyl groups** to DNA (forms a **covalent bond**)
        Cisplatin (platinum) - nephrotoxic, neuropathy, **ototoxic**
        Carb<u>o</u>platin (platinum) - **<u>bone</u>** (myelo-) suppression

Oxaliplatin (platinum) - nephrotoxic, neuropathy, ototoxic (all less than cisplatin); cold sensitivity; used in **colon CA**

Cyclophosphamide - **acrolein** is the active metabolite

S/Es: **hemorrhagic cystitis**

Mesna can help with hemorrhagic cystitis

Busulfan and **bleomycin**: S/Es - pulmonary fibrosis

Streptozocin (nitrosurea) - used for **pancreatic islet cell tumors**; is a 'Glucose mimic' to islet cells only → kills islet cells

- **Cell cycle–specific agents**
  - Act at **specific stages** of cell cycle (S or M); only cells <u>at that stage</u> affected; exhibit a **plateau** in cell-killing ability (at a certain point, increasing the dose doesn't change the killing rate)
  - **S Phase** (interfere with DNA replication and DNA <u>synthesis</u>)

    Methotrexate - inhibits <u>dihydrofolate reductase</u> (DHFR), which inhibits purine and DNA synthesis

    S/Es: renal toxicity, radiation recall

    Leucovorin rescue (tetrahydro-folic acid) - reverses effects of methotrexate

    5-Fluorouracil (5-FU) - inhibits <u>thymidylate synthase</u> (TS), which inhibits purine and DNA synthesis

    Leucovorin - increases toxicity of 5-FU

    Gemcitabine - inhibits <u>thymidylate synthase</u>

    Etoposide - interferes with DNA replication by <u>inhibiting topoisomerase</u>

    S/Es: bone marrow suppression

    Topoisomerase normally unwinds DNA for DNA duplication

    Doxorubicin (Adriamycin) - <u>DNA intercalator</u>

    S/Es: **cardiomyopathy** (CHF) secondary to O_2 **radicals** at doses > **500 mg/m^2**

  - <u>M</u> phase (<u>m</u>icrotubule <u>m</u>odulators - arrest <u>m</u>itosis)

    Alkaloids

    Vincristine (microtubule inhibitor) - **peripheral neuropathy**, neurotoxic

    Vinblastine (microtubule inhibitor) - **bone** (myelo) suppression

    Taxanes (docetaxel, paclitaxel [Taxol]) - promote **microtubule formation** and **stabilization** that cannot be broken down; S/E - **neuropathy**

HORMONAL THERAPY

- **Selective Estrogen Receptor Modulators** (SERMs)
  - **Tamoxifen** - treatment and prevention of <u>breast CA</u>

    Preferred for **pre-menopausal**: 1) **prevention** of breast CA for high risk patients <u>and</u>; 2) **treatment** of **receptor positive breast CA** (or unknown status)
  - **Raloxifene** - preferred for **prevention** of **post-menopausal breast CA** in high risk patients; also decreases fractures post-menopause
  - S/Es: **DVT** (1%), **endometrial CA** (0.1%) - *all less with Raloxifene*
- **Aromatase Inhibitors** (anastrozole, letrozole)
  - Block conversion of androgens to estrogen
  - Preferred <u>treatment</u> for **post-menopausal receptor positive breast CA** (or unknown receptor status)
  - S/Es: **fractures** (2x more common than SERMs)
- **GnRH analogues** (gonadotropin releasing hormone; eg leuprolide): ↓s FSH and LH → ↓s testosterone; used for hormone sensitive <u>prostate CA</u>
- **Anti-androgens** (eg flutamide, bicalutamide) - inhibit androgen receptors (testosterone and DHT receptors); used in <u>prostate CA</u>

MONOCLONAL ANTIBODY THERAPY

- **Trastuzumab** (Herceptin) - blocks **HER/neu receptor**, used for <u>breast CA</u>; **HER/neu** (Human Epidermal Growth Factor Receptor Tyrosine Kinase)
- **Bevacizumab** (Avastin) - binds **VEGF** protein and **inhibits angiogenesis**; used in <u>lung CA</u> and metastatic <u>colorectal CA</u>

RECEPTOR TYROSINE KINASE INHIBITORS (multi-RTKI)
- **Imatinib** (Gleevec)
  - Binds **c-kit** (stem cell growth factor receptor)
  - Used for malignant GIST tumors (very effective)
  - S/Es: CHF (uncommon)

IMMUNOTHERAPY
- **IL-2**: for metastatic melanoma or renal cell CA, can use as single Tx
- **Vaccines to prevent CA** - HepB vaccine, HPV vaccine (Gardasil)

OTHER AGENTS
- **Mitotane** (DDD) - cytolytic for adrenal cortex
  - **Use** - unresectable or metastatic adrenocortical CA
- **Octreotide** - used for pancreatic islet cell tumors (including gastrinoma) and carcinoid syndrome
- **Levamisole - anti-helminthic drug** that increases immunity against CA
- *Least* myelosuppression - bleomycin, vincristine, busulfan, cisplatin, hormonal Tx, monoclonal antibody Tx

RADIATION THERAPY (XRT, ionizing radiation)
- **M phase** - most vulnerable stage of cell cycle for XRT
- Most **damage** done by formation of **oxygen radicals** → maximal effect with **high oxygen levels**
- Main target is **DNA** - oxygen radicals **damage DNA**; with damaged DNA, the cell is **no longer able to divide** successfully
- **Higher energy** radiation has **skin-preserving effect** (maximal ionizing potential not reached until deeper structures)
- **Very radio-sensitive tumors** - seminomas, lymphomas
  - The more frequently the cells **divide**, the more **sensitive to XRT**
- **Very radio-resistant tumors** - epithelial, sarcomas
  - **Large tumors** - less responsive to XRT due to **lack of oxygen in the tumor**
- **Brachytherapy** - source of radiation in or next to tumor (Au-198, I-128); delivers high, concentrated doses of radiation
- **Gamma knife** - high intensity **cobalt XRT** directed at brain tumors
- **XRT sensitizers** (enhance effect) - oxygen, chemotherapy, hyperthermia
- *XRT can be used for **painful bony metastases***

TUMOR MARKER HALF-LIVES
- **PSA** should fall to zero after **6 - 8 weeks** following prostatectomy (short half life of 2-3 days but has to go to zero as even microscopic amounts can be detected)
- **CEA** should fall to normal level (< 2.5 ng/dl) after **4 weeks** following colon CA resection (half life of 5 days)
- **AFP** should fall to normal level (< 10 ng/dl) after **4 weeks** following orchiectomy for non-seminomatous testicular CA (half life of 5 days)

TUMOR LYSIS SYNDROME (see Fluids and Electrolytes chapter)

PET *(positron emission tomography)*
- **18-FDG** (fluorodeoxyglucose) metabolized to **FDG-6-phosphate** by **hexokinase**
- PET detects **FDG-6-phosphate** molecules
- 5-10% false positive rate (**inflammatory disease** - histoplasmosis, TB)
- 5-10% false negative rate (**slow metabolizing tumors** - carcinoid, bronchoalveolar lung CA)
- Accuracy for **brain** low because of **increased glucose uptake in brain**
- Test may not work in **diabetics** or with **hyper-insulinemia**
  - Hyperglycemia competes with 18-FDG uptake
  - Insulin promotes 18-FDG uptake into normal cells

SLNB (sentinel lymph node biopsy)

- **Sentinel lymph node** - hypothetical first lymph node(s) reached by cancer cells from a tumor
- **Lymphazurin blue dye** and **technetium labeled sulfur colloid radiotracer** used; are injected around primary tumor area; need 1-4 hours for uptake → dye and radiotracer travel to sentinel node(s)
- **Type I hypersensitivity reactions** (1%) can occur with lymphazurin blue dye
- Usually find 1-3 nodes; send for permanent
- **All blue nodes** and **nodes within 10%** of highest gamma count node should be taken
- *Can't find dye or gamma counts in OR→ need **formal lymph node dissection***
- *Tumor found in **lymphatics** along path to nodes → **formal lymph node dissection***
- *Tumor found in **lymph nodes** at pathology → all get **formal lymph node dissection***
- *Patients with **clinically positive nodes** should undergo **formal lymph node dissection***
- For a high gamma count outside area you were expecting (eg you are performing SLNB for breast CA and the supra-clavicular region lights up), you should take those lymph nodes if it is at least 10% of the highest count node
- **MC uses** - breast CA and melanoma

HEPATIC METASTASES

- **Intra-op U/S** - most sensitive for picking up intra-hepatic metastases: **3-5 mm** resolution
- **Conventional U/S**: 5-10 mm
- **CT scan**: 5-10 mm
- **MRI**: 5-10 mm

OTHER

- Most important prognostic factor of **breast CA** devoid of systemic metastasis - **nodal status**
- Most important prognostic factor of **sarcoma** devoid of systemic metastasis - **tumor grade**
- **Ovarian CA** - one of the few tumors for which **surgical debulking** improves chemotherapy (not seen in other tumors, see Gynecology chapter)
- **Colon CA** - genes involved in development include **APC, p53, DCC**, and **K-ras**
- **Colon CA** does not usually go to bone
- **Curable solid tumors with chemo only** - lymphoma
- **T-cell lymphomas** - HTLV-1; mycosis fungoides (skin lesions; Sezary cells)
- **Core needle biopsy** (CNBx) - gives architecture
- **Fine needle aspiration** (FNA) - gives cytology (just cells)

TYPES OF THERAPY

- **Induction** - initial Tx; often used for advanced disease (eg metastatic lung CA) or when no other better treatment exists (eg lymphoma)
- **Primary** (neo-adjuvant) - administration of an agent before another therapy
  - Chemo usually given 1st, followed by another (secondary) therapy (XRT, surgery, or both)
- **Adjuvant** (secondary) - administration of an agent after another therapy (eg chemo given after another Tx is used [XRT, surgery, or both])
- **Salvage** - for tumors that fail to respond to initial chemotherapy

DEFINITIONS

- **Hyperplasia** - increased number of cells
- **Metaplasia** - replacement of one tissue with another (with GERD squamous epithelium in esophagus can change to columnar epithelium → Barrett's esophagus)
- **Dysplasia** - altered size, shape, and organization (Barrett's Dysplasia)

CLINICAL TRIALS

- Phase I - is it safe and at what dose?
- Phase II - is it effective?
- Phase III - is it better than existing therapy?
- Phase IV - implementation and marketing

Trauma

279. A 26 yo woman is involved in a severe MVA. She is hypotensive (BP 70/40, HR 120), intubated, and has a mildly distended abdomen. She also has a pelvic fracture. She has had 2 liters of LR and you start transfusing 2 units of pRBCs. Her BP goes to 80/40. The most appropriate next step in management is:
   a. Abdomen and Pelvic CT
   b. Angiogram
   c. FAST scan
   d. Exploratory laparotomy

   Answer c. This is a very frequent occurrence in busy trauma centers. Put simply, in a hypotensive patient, you need to figure out if the bleeding is from the abdomen, pelvis, chest, or extremities. The first test should be a **FAST scan** - if **positive**, go to the OR for laparotomy.

   If FAST is **negative** (and you are reasonably sure the source of the bleed is not the chest - usually assessed by exam and CXR) place an external fixator in ED if ortho is standing there and waiting, but otherwise go to **angiography** ASAP for embolization of pelvic vessels. Wrapping a sheet tightly around the pelvis can be used to temporarily tamponade pelvic bleeding while waiting for angiography.

280. The above patient's BP falls again (65/40). Volume resuscitation should be:
   a. Lactated Ringers
   b. 5% albumin
   c. 3% normal saline
   d. Normal saline (0.9%)
   e. pRBCs

   Answer e. pRBCs (once you start giving pRBCs, don't go back to LR)

281. FAST scan is positive in the above patient and while in the OR, you give another 4 units of pRBCs. At this point, FFP and platelets should be given in this patient:
   a. For an elevated PT or PTT
   b. With a ratio of pRBCs, FFP, and platelets at 1:1:1
   c. For a platelet count < 100
   d. For a fibrinogen level < 100
   e. For diffuse bleeding sites

   Answer b. Hemostatic resuscitation is appropriate for massive transfusion (apx. defined as $\geq$ 4 units in first hour) with a ratio of pRBCs, FFP, and platelets at 1:1:1. This *prevents* **coagulopathy** and *improves* **oxygenation**.

282. You perform a splenectomy in the above patient for a Grade V hilar injury and bring the patient to the ICU. What is the best measure of adequate resuscitation in this patient?
   a. Lactate
   b. Respiratory rate
   c. Blood pressure
   d. Heart rate
   e. Urine output

   Answer a. Serum lactate (< 2.5) is the best measure of adequate resuscitation in trauma patients (*not urine output*).

283. A 21 yo woman with a GSW in the left flank presents with a BP of 75 despite 2 L of crystalloid. You start giving pRBCs. The most appropriate next step is:
   a. FAST scan
   b. Abdominal CT
   c. Laparotomy
   d. Laparoscopy

Answer c. Penetrating abdominal injury in an unstable patient requires emergent laparotomy (**flank** and **low back** injuries can damage **retroperitoneal structures** [eg aorta, IVC] as well as enter the **peritoneum**).

284. You perform a FAST scan on an unstable patient involved in a MVA which shows a large fluid collection in the peri-splenic space. The patient is hypotensive despite blood resuscitation. The patient has a blown pupil (6 mm) on the right along with head trauma. The most appropriate next step in management is:
    a. Head CT
    b. Abdominal CT
    c. Head and abdominal CT
    d. Go to OR

    Answer d. A positive FAST scan in a hypotensive patient means you go to the OR for laparotomy. In the ABC's scheme you need to take care of C (circulation) before assessing the head injury. While in the OR, a **Burr hole** should be placed to decompress the side of the head with the blown pupil. This is placed 5 cm anterior and 5 superior to the external auditory canal (frontal bone).

285. All of the following are true of maxillofacial trauma except:
    a. The MCC of traumatic facial nerve injury is temporal bone fracture
    b. A Le Fort III fracture is across the orbital walls
    c. Malocclusion is the best indicator of mandibular injury
    d. Nasoethmoid fractures with CSF leak should undergo immediate repair
    e. The MC injured major nerve with temporal bone fracture is cranial nerve VII

    Answer d. Nasoethmoid Fx with **CSF leak** is initially treated conservatively (consider a lumbar catheter to drain CSF - helps close leak).

286. All of the following are true of epistaxis except:
    a. Posterior bleeds are more life-threatening
    b. Pressure and packing usually controls anterior bleeds
    c. Angio-embolization of the superior thyroid artery may be necessary for posterior bleeds
    d. Anterior bleeding is usually from Kiesselbach's Plexus

    Answer c. Angio-embolization of the **internal maxillary** or **ethmoidal artery** may be necessary for posterior bleeds.

287. A patient with a CHI is having difficulty maintaining his airway so you intubate him. Head CT shows loss of sulci and compression of cisterns and ventricles so you place an intra-cerebral pressure (ICP) catheter. All of the following are true of cerebral perfusion pressure (CPP) except:
    a. In general, a cerebral perfusion pressure of 60 or better is sufficient
    b. CPP = mean arterial pressure – intracranial pressure
    c. Mannitol can help lower intra-cranial pressure
    d. Hypoventilation benefits these patients

    Answer d. Relative hyperventilation for modest cerebral vasoconstriction (pCO_2 30–35) limits brain edema and lowers ICP.

288. All of the following are true except:
    a. Subdural hematomas are MC from torn bridging veins
    b. Loss of consciousness, then lucid interval, followed by neurologic deterioration is classic for epidural hematoma
    c. A blown (dilated) pupil with head injury is from compression of CN II (2)
    d. Diffuse axonal injury indicates a poor prognosis
    e. Epidural hematomas are most commonly from injury to the middle meningeal artery

    Answer c. A **blown pupil** from head injury is due to compression of **CN III** (3).

289. A 50 yo woman on warfarin for a left ventricular assist device (LVAD) you implanted 1 year ago trips on a step. She is brought to the ED by family. She has a small area of ecchymosis on her right temple and has trouble remembering the event. She is neurologically intact now. Head CT is normal. The most appropriate next step is:

    a.   Discharge
    b.   Observe only
    c.   Observe and repeat head CT in 8 hours
    d.   FFP and Vit K
    e.   Craniotomy

Answer c. Observe and repeat head CT in 8 hours. Patients on warfarin (or other anticoagulation) are high risk for **intra-cranial bleeding** with head trauma.

290. After 8 hours, the repeat head CT in the above patient shows a right sided 8 mm intra-cerebral hematoma. The most appropriate next step is:

    a.   Discharge
    b.   Observe only
    c.   Observe and repeat head CT in 8 hours
    d.   FFP and Vit K
    e.   Craniotomy

Answer d. Reverse anticoagulation with **FFP** and **Vit K** is appropriate here. The bleeding site can *expand rapidly* if warfarin is not reversed *(is life-threatening)*.

291. Instead of the above, the patient becomes progressively lethargic during observation and you order a STAT head CT which shows a right sided 15 mm wide subdural hematoma. Along with reversing anticoagulation with FFP and Vit K, which of the following is most appropriate in this patient:

    a.   Observation
    b.   Repeat head CT in 8 hours
    c.   Craniotomy
    d.   Burr hole

Answer c. Craniotomy. In general a Burr hole is not as effective as craniotomy for drainage of a subdural hematoma and wouldn't control vessels that were still bleeding. Given the choice, craniotomy is preferred.

292. A 25 yo man involved in a MVA will open his eyes only to painful stimuli, does not form words but mumbles, and withdraws to pain. All of the following are true except:

    a.   Blunt injury carries a worse prognosis compared to penetrating injury give equal GCS scores
    b.   His GCS is 8
    c.   Motor score carries the most prognostic significance
    d.   Head CT is indicated

Answer a. Penetrating head injury carries a worse prognosis compared to blunt injury give equal GCS scores. Open eyes to painful stimuli is 2, incomprehensible sounds is 2, and withdrawals from pain is 4. 2 + 2 + 4 = 8

293. What is the most important next step in the above patient:

    a.   Head CT
    b.   FAST scan
    c.   DPL
    d.   Laparotomy
    e.   Intubation

Answer e. Intubation. GCS of **10 or lower** is an indication for intubation *(should be performed before going to CT scan)*

294. A 20 yo woman involved in a MVA is stable and complains of right anterior neck pain after hitting the steering wheel. Ecchymosis and a small hematoma are present in that area. The most appropriate next step is:
   a.   Plain films of the neck
   b.   Neck MRI
   c.   Neck CT angio
   d.   Observation
   e.   Formal cerebral angiogram

   Answer c. Neck CT angio is appropriate for asymptomatic blunt neck trauma.

295. Instead of the above, the patient has C-spine tenderness. The most appropriate next step is:
   a.   Plain films of the neck
   b.   Neck MRI
   c.   Neck CT
   d.   Observation
   e.   Formal cerebral angiogram

   Answer c. Neck CT is most appropriate for C-spine evaluation _(not plain films)_.

296. The above patient has pre-vertebral soft tissue swelling on neck CT scan. You do not see any fractures (Fx's) or dislocations. The most appropriate next step is:
   a.   MRI
   b.   PET scan
   c.   Cervical spine x-rays
   d.   Close observation

   Answer a. Patients with **pre-vertebral cervical soft tissue swelling** or with **neurologic deficits without bony injury** are at high risk for ligamentous injury or occult Fx. The best study to check for this is an **MRI.**

297. A 22 yo man is stabbed in the left mid-neck with an ice pick and has been coughing up blood tinged sputum. The most appropriate next step is:
   a.   Go the OR for neck exploration
   b.   Formal angiogram
   c.   Neck CT scan
   d.   Immediate intubation
   e.   Observation

   Answer a. Explore in the OR. This is worrisome for a **tracheal injury.** **Symptomatic penetrating neck injuries** should be explored. Also, any **Zone II penetrating neck injury** is also an indication for exploration.

   Endotracheal **intubation** of this patient is best achieved in the OR. There are no signs of losing or lost airway at this stage (eg no stridor or respiratory distress - so there is no need for ED cricothyroidotomy) but this can change _dramatically_ after rapid sequence intubation (RSI). The best move is to get these patients in the OR for intubation unless there is an airway issue in the ED. Be prepared in the OR for a change in airway status after RSI (ie need for cricothyroidotomy).

298. Instead of the above, the patient has _right_ sided arm and leg weakness. The most appropriate next step is:
   a.   Go the OR for neck exploration
   b.   Formal angiogram
   c.   CT scan
   d.   MRI
   e.   Observation

Answer a. This is worrisome for a <u>left</u> **carotid artery injury** and neuro deficit. Exploration is indicated. Either primary repair or an interposition graft can be used with open repair of carotid artery injuries.

299. A 21 yo man suffers a right sided GSW just above his right clavicle. The patient's initial SBP is 65, responds to 2 L lactated ringers, and now has a SBP of 90. The most appropriate next step is:
    a. Exploration through neck incision
    b. Median sternotomy
    c. Bronchoscopy, EGD, and arteriogram
    d. Observation only

    Answer b. This patient is obviously bleeding. Tx for **symptomatic Zone I neck** injuries is exploration. Zone I neck exploration with a vascular injury is achieved with a **median sternotomy** to get proximal control of the blood vessels.

    If the patient were <u>asymptomatic</u>, **bronchoscopy, EGD,** and **arteriogram** would be indicated.

300. All of the following are true except:
    a. Zone II penetrating neck injuries are usually explored
    b. Aortic transection at the ligamentum arteriosum is best approached with median sternotomy
    c. Zone I neck vascular injury is best approached with median sternotomy
    d. Zone III extends from the angle of the mandible to the base of the skull
    e. Proximal left subclavian artery injuries are best approached with median sternotomy and trap-door incision

    Answer b. Left thoracotomy is the open approach for **aortic transection** at the ligamentum arteriosum (MC area for aortic transection). The majority of aortic transections are now repaired with **endografts**.

    For access to the <u>proximal</u> left subclavian artery, **median sternotomy** with left **trap-door incision** (dividing the sternum at the 2nd intercostal space and raising the 1st and 2nd ribs) is indicated. The <u>distal</u> left subclavian artery is accessed best through a **left thoracotomy**.

301. A 25 yo woman involved in a MVA develops new left sided weakness on HD #2. Head CT was negative at the initial trauma work-up. Her other studies were negative as well. The most appropriate next step should be:
    a. Head MRI
    b. Repeat Head CT
    c. Head and neck CT angio
    d. EEG
    e. Neurology consult

    Answer c. This scenario is suspicious for **blunt neck vascular trauma**, which often occurs with **hyper-extension** (often with no physical signs of trauma on the neck itself) or with a **direct blow** to the neck. These injuries can involve the **carotid** or **vertebral arteries** and manifest themselves as **dissections** or **wall disruptions**.

302. Head and neck CT angio in the above patient shows an isolated right carotid artery dissection with patent antegrade flow. The most appropriate Tx for this injury is:
    a. Observation
    b. Open repair
    c. Endovascular stent placement
    d. Anticoagulation therapy

    Answer c. Because this patient is **symptomatic** (eg stroke symptoms) and there is **still residual flow**, endovascular placement of a **covered stent** across the dissection is appropriate (open repair if that fails). Similarly for **carotid thrombosis** (which can occur from dissection or wall disruption), if **symptomatic** and there is **still antegrade flow**, repair is indicated (either with an endovascular stent or open repair).

If the carotid artery were **completely occluded** (ie a completed stroke, no antegrade flow), *anti-coagulation only* (heparin or Plavix) would be indicated (to prevent distal propagation of thrombosis) for both carotid **dissection** and carotid **wall disruption**.

The initial Tx of <u>asymptomatic</u> carotid artery **dissections** is **anti-coagulation only**. This is done in an effort to prevent thrombotic and embolic events.

The initial Tx for <u>asymptomatic</u> carotid artery **wall disruption** (and not completely occluded) is **covered stent** or **open repair** (high risk of developing pseudoaneurysm or other Cx's late).

303. A 24 yo man is stabbed in the chest with an ice-pick just to the left of midline at the 5th intercostal space. The patient's airway is intact, he is breathing spontaneously, and his blood pressure is 120/80 with a heart rate of 90. He has 2 large bore IVs placed. CXR shows a left pneumothorax so you place a chest tube. Which of the following is the most appropriate next step in this patient's work-up:
    a. Careful observation only
    b. Pericardial window, esophagoscopy, and bronchoscopy
    c. Median sternotomy and exploration
    d. Chest CT

    Answer b. Pericardial window, esophagoscopy, and bronchoscopy are appropriate for penetrating "box" injuries. Some groups are using FAST scan as opposed to pericardial window when assessing for hemopericardium.

304. A 21 yo patient has a persistent pneumothorax following a MVA despite 2 good chest tubes. Which of the following is the most appropriate next step:
    a. CT scan of chest
    b. Increase suction from 20 to 40 cm H_2O
    c. Bronchoscopy
    d. Thoracotomy

    Answer c. Persistent pneumothorax despite 2 well placed chest tubes raises the suspicion of either a mucus plug (or foreign body) obstructing the airway or a tracheo-bronchial injury. **Bronchoscopy** is best for Dx.

305. A 23 yo involved in a MVA has a Grade V splenic laceration with active blush, an aortic transection, a pelvic Fx, and a severe pulmonary contusion. The patient is hypotensive (SBP 80) despite 4 units pRBCs. Which is most appropriate next step:
    a. Splenectomy
    b. Aortic transection repair
    c. ICU management
    d. Angio
    e. CT scan

    Answer a. You should address other life-threatening injuries (eg bleeding spleen above, a significant subdural hematoma, an unstable patient from a pelvic fracture) *before* an aortic transection. Once the patient is completely stable, the aortic transection is addressed *(this may take 24-48 hours)*.

    Patients with aortic transections who reach the hospital alive have **contained aortic transections** (the adventitia is intact, otherwise the patient would have exsanguinated). Although there is still a risk of rupture, it is low. Other life-threatening injuries should be addressed first.

The pelvic Fx above could be a significant source of bleeding, however, the bleeding splenic laceration takes precedence at this stage.

306. A 65 yo man has 4 left sided rib fractures at 2 sites along each rib with paradoxical chest wall motion and poor oxygenation All of the following are true except:
    a.   Mechanical impairment is the biggest factor for his poor oxygenation
    b.   This patient may require intubation
    c.   Paravertebral nerve block or epidural catheter reduces pain and improves oxygenation in these patients
    d.   A PA catheter can help manage fluid status

Answer a. The underlying **pulmonary contusion** is the biggest impairment to respiratory impairment, not the mechanics of the **flail chest** itself.

307. A 22 yo man is involved in a MVA and has a significant hemothorax for which you place a chest tube. All of the following are true of hemothorax except:
    a.   Lung inflation generally worsens bleeding
    b.   The most important RF for empyema after chest trauma is retained hemothorax
    c.   Drainage of > 1500 cc of blood after initial chest tube placement is an indication for OR thoracotomy
    d.   Unresolved hemothorax despite 2 well placed chest tubes requires VATS drainage when the patient is stable
    e.   Drainage of 250 cc/hr over 4 consecutive hours is an indication for OR thoracotomy

Answer a. Lung inflation decreases bleeding by compressing the bleeding area.

308. The above patient is stable after chest tube drainage of 500 cc. He also has a sternal fracture and an elevated troponin I. Which of the following is most appropriate:
    a.   Admit to cardiac monitoring unit for 24 hours
    b.   Cardiac left heart and coronary catheterization
    c.   Go to the OR for left thoracotomy
    d.   Dobutamine ECHO
    e.   Follow creatine kinase (CK) enzymes and troponins

Answer a. Cardiac telemetry for 24 hours is most appropriate for suspected **cardiac contusion** (RF - sternal fracture). Patients with both a **normal EKG** _and_ a **normal troponin I** are essentially ruled-out for a blunt cardiac injury. If either the **EKG** _or_ the **troponin I** is _abnormal_, telemonitoring for 24 hours is indicated. An EKG other than normal sinus rhythm (NSR) is considered _abnormal_.

309. You are in the OR performing a left thoracotomy in a patient (BP 70/40, HR 120) with a GSW to the chest. A massive amount of blood is coming from deep in the lung parenchyma. You try to suture ligate the area and attempt pulmonary tractotomy, however, blood keeps welling up to fast. The most appropriate next step is:
    a.   Pneumonectomy
    b.   Lobectomy
    c.   Angio-embolization
    d.   Clamp the pulmonary hilum

Answer d. Clamping the pulmonary hilum will control the bleeding and allow visualization for repair of the injury.

Pulmonary tractotomy basically consists of using a pulmonary stapler to staple through the lung to get to the **bleeding source** and also staple the bleeding area. This technique can also take care of **air-leaks** (best with bovine pericardium-lined staple rows).

310. You are in the OR performing a left thoracotomy in a patient (BP 70/40, HR 120) with a GSW to the chest. You open the pericardium and find a hole in the left ventricle with a large amount of blood exiting with systole. Your first move is:
    a. Dissect out the groin for cannulation
    b. Clamping the left ventricle
    c. Digital compression
    d. Place an endograft

    Answer c. Digital compression (put your finger in the hole). Then place an interrupted suture with pledgets to close the hole. Try to place the suture under major coronary arteries if they are in proximity of the hole.

311. A 21 yo man involved in a MVA is struggling for air, has tracheal deviation to the right, and left sided subcutaneous emphysema. He has the following vital signs: HR 130, BP 70/50, RR 40. You cannot hear any left sided breath sounds. Your next move is:
    a. Intubation
    b. Left tube thoracostomy
    c. Left thoracotomy
    d. Go to the OR

    Answer b. This patient has a **tension PTX**. A chest tube is indicated.

312. All of the following are true of tracheo-bronchial injuries except:
    a. They are more common on the right
    b. Breathing may be worsened after chest tube placement
    c. Is one of the very few conditions in which clamping the chest tube may be beneficial
    d. Approach to the proximal left mainstem (< 1 cm from the carina) is best carried out through a left thoracotomy

    Answer d. Approach to the proximal left mainstem bronchus (< 1 cm from carina) is right thoracotomy *(aorta is in the way on the left)*.

313. A 25 yo man comes to your office 3 months after a MVA with left chest pain. CXR shows air-fluid levels in the chest. The most appropriate next step is:
    a. Exploration through the abdomen
    b. Exploration through the chest
    c. Chest tube
    d. Percutaneous drain

    Answer b. The acute Tx of a **diaphragmatic injury** is to go through the **abdomen** for repair. With **delayed presentation** (> 1 week), go through the **chest** because adhesions to the lung will have developed which you must take down through a chest incision. Often, a sheet of **PTFE** (Gore-Tex) is used to repair the diaphragm.

314. A 25 yo man shot in the right chest above the nipple loses his pulse in the ED (BP 50/0). The most appropriate next step is:
    a. Left thoracotomy
    b. Right thoracotomy
    c. Median sternotomy
    d. Angio-embolization

    Answer a. Even though the patient was shot in the right chest, ED left thoracotomy is indicated. You should open the pericardium (anterior to the phrenic nerve) and clamp the descending thoracic aorta (watch out for the esophagus which is anterior to the descending thoracic aorta).

315. You open the pericardium and clamp the aorta in the above patient (BP now 80/40). The heart feels empty and you do not find any pericardial or left chest blood. The most appropriate next step is:

      a.   Chest CT
      b.   Median sternotomy in the OR
      c.   Clamshell
      d.   Trap-door
      e.   Endograft placement

Answer c. The **clamshell incision** basically involves bilateral thoracotomies that are taken across the sternum. The exposure with this incision is excellent (jack-knife the bed a little to open the space up). This will access the right chest which is the most likely location for the bleeding source.

316. A 25 yo man involved in an MVA. CT scan shows an isolated large splenic subcapsular hematoma (BP 90/70). The most appropriate next step is
      a.   Laparotomy
      b.   Embolization
      c.   ICU observation
      d.   Percutaneous drainage

Answer c. Observation

317. Instead of the above, CT scan shows a splenic subcapsular hematoma with an arterial pseudoaneurysm. The most appropriate next step is:
      a.   Laparotomy
      b.   Embolization
      c.   ICU observation
      d.   Percutaneous drainage

Answer b. Embolization. Arterial pseudoaneurysms can rupture.

318. Instead of the above, CT scan shows a grade II splenic injury with active contrast extravasation. The most appropriate next step is:
      a.   Laparotomy
      b.   Embolization
      c.   ICU observation
      d.   Percutaneous drainage

Answer b. Embolization. For this and the previous question, if the patient were unstable (SBP < 90 despite 2 L LR), splenectomy would be indicated.

319. Instead of the above, CT scan shows a grade IV splenic injury with a large perisplenic hematoma (first BP 70/40, now 90/60 after 2 L LR). The most appropriate next step is:
      a.   Laparotomy
      b.   Embolization
      c.   ICU observation
      d.   Percutaneous drainage

Answer c. Close ICU observation. The CT finding of a large hematoma is worrisome as there was likely a significant amount of bleeding at some point which could recur.

320. The above patient becomes persistently hypotensive in the ICU despite 4 units of pRBCs (BP now 70/40). What is the most appropriate next step:
      a.   Laparotomy
      b.   Embolization
      c.   Continued ICU observation
      d.   Percutaneous drainage

Answer a. This patient has failed conservative management. Because the patient is **unstable**, emergency exploration is warranted.

321. What is the most appropriate procedure for the above patient:

a. Revascularize the spleen
b. Partial splenectomy
c. Damage control packing
d. Splenectomy

Answer d. Splenectomy. Splenic salvage is not indicated in unstable patients.

322. Which of the following splenic injuries is most likely to undergo successful conservative management?
    a. Hilar transection
    b. Presence of a pseudoaneurysm
    c. 2 cm splenic fracture
    d. 4 cm intraparenchymal hematoma
    e. 5% surface area subcapsular hematoma

    Answer e. 5% surface area subcapsular hematoma. The lower the grade, the more likely conservative management will work.

323. Which of the following splenic injuries is least likely to undergo successful conservative management?
    a. Completely shattered spleen
    b. Presence of a pseudoaneurysm
    c. 2 cm splenic fracture
    d. 4 cm intraparenchymal hematoma
    e. 5% surface area subcapsular hematoma

    Answer a. Completely shattered spleen. The higher the grade, the less likely conservative management will work.

324. All of the following are true of splenic injuries except:
    a. Hemodynamic instability is a contraindication to splenic salvage
    b. A large fluid collection 5 days following splenectomy that is high in amylase requires re-operation
    c. Immunizations should be given 2 weeks after a traumatic splenectomy
    d. Stable subcapsular hematomas (ie no pseudoaneurysm or contrast extravasation) should be left alone

    Answer b. Pancreatic leak after splenectomy should be treated with percutaneous drainage _only_ (95% successful).

325. A 25 yo man is shot in the abdomen and you explore him. He has a severe anterior liver injury that you try to repair but blood keeps welling up out of the liver bed and you cannot control it. You perform a Pringle maneuver which is:
    a. Clamping of the portal triad
    b. Clamping the IVC
    c. Placing an atrio-caval shunt
    d. Packing off the area and heading to the ICU

    Answer a. The **Pringle maneuver** involves clamping the portal triad which is located in the hepato-duodenal ligament. The Pringle maneuver will <u>not</u> control bleeding from the hepatic veins or IVC (located posterior to liver).

    The portal triad structures include the **portal vein** (posterior), **common bile duct** (lateral), and the **proper hepatic artery** (medial). The portal triad enters the liver at **segments IVb** and **V.**

326. A 25 yo woman involved in a MVA is persistently hypotensive despite 2 L of LR and 2 units pRBCs (SBP 70). FAST scan is positive for intra-abdominal fluid. The most appropriate next step is:
    a. Laparotomy
    b. Embolization

    c.   ICU observation
    d.   Percutaneous drainage

Answer a. Emergency laparotomy

327. In the above patient, intra-op there is severe venous bleeding from the posterior liver. The Pringle maneuver fails to control the bleeding. You attempt repair for 1 hour, but, blood keeps welling up and you are not successful. The most appropriate next step is:
    a.   Liver resection
    b.   Damage control
    c.   Atrio-caval shunt
    d.   Argon beam

Answer b. This patient likely has injury to the hepatic vein(s) where they enter the IVC or the retrohepatic IVC itself. These are hard to fix and are associated with high mortality. In general for liver injuries, if bleeding is not controlled after reasonable effort, go with **damage control peri-hepatic packing** (lots of packs). Then consider angio-embolization if arterial bleeding is suspected, otherwise, go to the ICU for **hemostatic resuscitation**. If packing fails to control the bleeding (uncommon), place an **atrio-caval shunt** (eg 32 Fr chest tube) and repair injury. Supra-hepatic IVC control may require **median sternotomy** (open pericardium).

328. The above patient survives and the packs are removed the next day. You find some bleeding areas which you suture ligate. The patient has a prolonged recovery period. On POD #21 she is noted to have abdominal pain and severe hematemesis. She has 2 large bore IVs in place and you send a type and screen for 6 units of blood. Her hematocrit (Hct) is 21 so you transfuse 2 units of pRBCs. The most appropriate next step in this patient's management is:
    a.   Exploratory laparotomy
    b.   EGD
    c.   Angiography
    d.   TIPS procedure

Answer b. EGD is the best initial Dx test for patients with an upper GI bleed.

329. EGD in the above patient shows blood coming out of the Ampulla of Vater (hemobilia). The most appropriate next step in management is:
    a.   Exploratory laparotomy
    b.   ERCP with stent
    c.   Angiography
    d.   TIPS procedure

Answer c. This patient has **hemobilia** from a **vascular to bile duct fistula** (usually hepatic artery to bile duct). These usually arise from an hepatic artery pseudoaneurysm that erodes into the bile duct. Tx is **angio-embolization**.

330. A 25 yo woman is shot in the right flank. In the OR, she has significant blood in the peritoneum and a GSW wound to segment 6. You do not see any active bleeding. The most appropriate next step is:
    a.   Segment 6 segmentectomy
    b.   Explore segment 6
    c.   Pack the GSW with omentum
    d.   Place a drain in GSW
    e.   Observation

Answer e. Because the area has stopped bleeding, no further Tx is necessary. Try to avoid messing with the area, which could disrupt the clot that has formed and cause it to bleed again.

331. A 25 yo man involved in an MVA has a CT scan that shows a grade III liver injury with an arterial pseudoaneurysm (BP 90/60). The most appropriate next step is:

a. Laparotomy
b. Embolization
c. ICU observation
d. Percutaneous drainage

Answer b. Angio-embolization.

332. Instead of the above, CT scan shows a grade III liver injury with active contrast extravasation. The most appropriate next step is:
    a. Laparotomy
    b. Embolization
    c. ICU observation
    d. Percutaneous drainage

    Answer b. Angio-embolization. For this and the previous question, if the patient were unstable (SBP < 90 after 2 L LR), laparotomy would be indicated.

333. Instead of the above, CT scan shows a grade V liver injury with a large hematoma (initial BP 70/40, now BP 90/60 after 2 L LR). The most appropriate next step is:
    a. Laparotomy
    b. Embolization
    c. ICU observation
    d. Percutaneous drainage

    Answer c. ICU observation. The CT finding of a large hematoma is worrisome as there was likely significant bleeding at some point which could recur.

334. In the ICU, the above patient drops her BP, which improves with pRBCs, but then drops again after 1 hour. You have given her 6 units of pRBCs (BP 90/40) for these transient drops in BP. The most appropriate next step
    a. Laparotomy
    b. Angio-embolization
    c. Continued ICU observation
    d. Percutaneous drainage

    Answer b. This patient has failed conservative management. Because the patient is a **transient responder**, angio-embolization is warranted.

335. Concerning traumatic pancreatic injuries, all of the following are true except:
    a. The main concern is to figure out whether or not the duct is involved
    b. Edema, hematoma, fluid, and fat necrosis are worrisome for injury
    c. Trauma Whipples have an operative mortality similar to elective procedures
    d. For pancreatic duct injury, the cut-off between distal pancreatectomy and Whipple is duct injury in relation to the superior mesenteric vein

    Answer c. Mortality is 50% for a trauma Whipple *(trauma Whipples should be avoided - better to go with staged repair).*

336. A 25 yo man suffers a GSW through the pancreas neck. He now has severe venous bleeding posterior to the pancreas which you cannot control. The most appropriate next step in this patient's management is:
    a. Portal vein ligation
    b. Whipple
    c. Transect the pancreas
    d. Splenectomy

    Answer c. Access to this portion of the **portal vein** is obtained by transecting the **pancreas neck** (need distal pancreatectomy with that move).

337. A 25 yo man has a perpendicular pancreatic fracture on CT scan after a fall. The fracture is through the pancreas neck and the pancreas is completely divided. The most appropriate next step is:

    a. Whipple
    b. Percutaneous drainage
    c. ICU observation
    d. Pancreatic stent
    e. Distal pancreatectomy

Answer e. Distal pancreatectomy (the pancreatic duct was transected)

338. A 25 yo man suffers a GSW to the right flank. During laparotomy, you notice bile stained fluid in the right upper quadrant. The most appropriate next step is:

    a. Endoscopy
    b. Gastrostomy
    c. Whipple
    d. Kocher maneuver

Answer d. The most appropriate move is to perform a **Kocher maneuver** which entails mobilizing the duodenum (colon hepatic flexure must be taken down first) and examining the duodenum, the portal triad, and the pancreas head. Findings requiring Kocher maneuver include para-duodenal (1st or 2nd) hematomas, bile staining, sucus drainage, or fat necrosis.

339. A 25 yo man suffers an abdominal GSW. At laparotomy there is a large segment of wall missing from the 2nd portion of the duodenum immediately adjacent to the ampulla. You make an attempt at bringing the duodenum together for a primary transverse closure, however, there is significant tension. The most appropriate next step is:

    a. Resection and primary anastomosis
    b. Whipple
    c. Jejunal serosal patch
    d. Drainage only
    e. Longitudinal primary closure

Answer c. Repair with **jejunal serosal patch** (not mucosal). Resection and primary anastomosis is generally not possible in the 2nd portion of the duodenum due to the location of the Ampulla of Vater. Longitudinal closure would narrow the lumen too much.

340. Instead of the above, the medial 2nd portion of duodenum is completely disrupted and the Ampulla of Vater is beyond repair. The most appropriate next step at this time is:

    a. Resection of the injured duodenum and primary anastomosis
    b. Whipple
    c. Primary repair
    d. Drainage and damage control surgery

Answer d. Drainage and **damage control surgery**. Single stage trauma Whipple has an extremely high mortality and should be _avoided_. **Damage control surgery** initially with **staged Whipple** (24-48 hours later) has the lowest mortality. These patients almost always have severe associated injuries.

341. Instead of the above, there is a 1.9 cm diameter hole in the anterior wall of the 3rd portion of the duodenum. The most appropriate next step is:

    a. Resection and primary anastomosis
    b. Whipple
    c. Primary repair
    d. Drainage only

Answer c. Primary repair with transverse closure is appropriate for this small hole.

342. Instead of the above, there is a 85% circumferential lesion of the 1st portion of the duodenum. The most appropriate next step is:
   a. Resection and primary anastomosis
   b. Whipple
   c. Primary repair
   d. Drainage only

   Answer a. Resection and **primary anastomosis** (duodeno-duodenostomy) is necessary for a lesion involving **> 75%** the circumference of the duodenal wall.

343. Instead of the above, there is a 1.5 cm hole in the anterior wall and a corresponding 1.5 cm hole in the posterior wall of the distal 4th portion of the duodenum. The most appropriate next step is:
   a. Resection and primary anastomosis
   b. Whipple
   c. Primary repair
   d. Drainage only

   Answer a. Resection of injured duodenum and **primary anastomosis** (likely a duodeno-jejunostomy for this scenario) is indicated. Primary closure is contraindicated with that much damage as it would almost certainly result in significant luminal narrowing (*contraindications to primary repair - repair that would result in bowel with < 50% normal circumference or < 1/3 normal bowel luminal diameter*).

344. A 15 yo old boy is struck in the abdomen when he goes over the handle bars on his bike. You get an abdominal CT with IV and oral contrast and you cannot identify any abnormality. The next day, you try to feed the child clears but he vomits twice. His abdomen also feels somewhat more distended compared to yesterday. The most appropriate next step in management is:
   a. Repeat abdominal CT
   b. Zofran (ondansetron)
   c. Phenergan (promethazine)
   d. Exploratory laparotomy

   Answer a. (see below)

345. You repeat the child's CT scan with oral and IV contrast and identify a hematoma in the third portion of the duodenum. You do not see any extravasation of contrast at the site. The most appropriate next step is:
   a. Exploratory laparotomy, evacuate the clot, close the duodenum
   b. Percutaneous evacuation of the clot
   c. NG tube suction and TPN
   d. Whipple

   Answer c. The first issue is that if a trauma patient has a change in clinical status or is failing to progress normally (eg N/V with clears), you need to repeat appropriate studies. Pancreatic injuries, small bowel tears, duodenal injuries, and diaphragmatic injuries can present late.

   Duodenal hematomas can occur as a delayed presentation in trauma. The 1st step is to make the Dx. This is probably best done with an **UGI contrast study** (will show a "stacked coin" or a "coiled spring" appearance) although abdominal CT scan with oral and IV contrast can pick these injures up. Tx is **NPO and TPN** for up to **3 weeks.** The **vast majority** of para-duodenal hematomas resolve with **conservative Tx.**

   If there were a free contrast leak from the duodenal injury, open repair would be required.

346. A 25 yo man suffers a close range shotgun blast to the right flank. At exploration you find extensive damage and devascularization throughout the right colon with significant sucus spillage and peritonitis. The most appropriate next step is:
   a. Right hemicolectomy only
   b. Right hemicolectomy, long Hartman's pouch, cecostomy
   c. Packing only
   d. Primary repair and place drains
   e. Total abdominal colectomy

Answer a. Although in the past diversion was considered necessary for right colon injuries, either **primary repair** _or_ **resection and anastomosis** _without diversion_ are now considered adequate (essentially right colon and transverse colon injuries are treated like small bowel injuries). Given this patient sustained extensive right colon damage, Tx is right hemi-colectomy (not primary repair)

347. A 25 yo man suffers a close range shotgun blast to the left flank. At exploration you find left colon damage (40% circumference with gross contamination and peritonitis). The patient has required 8 units of pRBCs. The most appropriate next step is:
   a. Left hemicolectomy only (colo-colic anastomosis)
   b. Left hemicolectomy (colo-colic anastomosis) and diverting loop ileostomy
   c. Packing only
   d. Primary repair without diversion
   e. Total abdominal colectomy

Answer d. _Primary repair **without** diversion is the procedure of choice for all non-destructive left colon lesions (ie < 50% circumference and **not** associated with significant devascularization)._ This includes patients with associated issues such as hypotension, gross contamination, peritonitis, delay in surgery, other critical injuries, large transfusion requirement, etc.

348. A 25 yo man suffers a shotgun blast to the left flank. At exploration you find left colon damage (70% circumference) and _gross_ contamination. Considerable time has elapsed between injury and exploration (8 hours). The most appropriate next step is:
   a. Left hemi-colectomy only (colo-colic anastomosis)
   b. Left hemi-colectomy (colo-colic anastomosis) and diverting loop ileostomy
   c. Packing only
   d. Primary repair and place drains
   e. Total abdominal colectomy

Answer b. The indication for **resection** and **primary anastomosis** (as opposed to primary repair) for left colon injuries is a **destructive injury** (ie > 50% circumference lesions or those with significant colon devascularization).

Indications for diversion **loop ileostomy** following **left sided colon resection** for trauma include: **gross contamination** (eg peritonitis), > 6 hours has elapsed between injury and repair, significant comorbidities, or > 6 units pRBCs have been given.

If this patient was in **shock**, an **end colostomy** with **Hartman's pouch** would be indicated (avoids left colon anastomosis with shock which would be at risk of breaking down; also a leak in a patient already in shock would be devastating).

349. A 25 yo man suffers a GSW wound to his rectum. You inspect the area with proctoscopy and are unable to reach the low rectal, extra-peritoneal, 4 cm laceration. The most appropriate next step is:
   a. APR
   b. Observation and antibiotics only
   c. End colostomy near the lesion
   d. Cut through the low anterior rectum to get to the extraperitoneal injury for primary repair
   e. Pre-sacral drainage and antibiotics

Answer c. Rectal injuries that are <u>inaccessible</u> (too high for trans-anal repair and too low for easy repair via laparotomy) or have <u>extensive local damage</u> beyond primary repair should undergo ***proximal diverting end colostomy <u>only</u>***. In 6-8 weeks the area heals and definitive hook-up can be performed.

350. A 25 yo man suffers a GSW to the lower abdomen. On exploration, the left ureter above the pelvic brim is transected with a 1 cm segment missing. The most appropriate management of this injury is:
    a. Ureterocystostomy
    b. Trans uretero-ureterostomy
    c. Uretero-ureterostomy
    d. Externalized urinary diversion
    e. Nephrectomy

    Answer c. (see below)

351. A 25 yo man suffers a GSW to the lower abdomen. On exploration, the left ureter below the pelvic brim is transected with a 1 cm segment missing. The most appropriate management of this injury is:
    a. Ureterocystostomy
    b. Trans uretero-ureterostomy
    c. Uretero-ureterostomy
    d. Externalized urinary diversion
    e. Nephrectomy

    Answer a. (see below)

352. A 25 yo man suffers a GSW wound to the lower abdomen. On exploration, the left ureter above the pelvic brim is transected with a 2.5 cm segment missing. He also has a nearby left colon injury with stool spread throughout the abdomen and peritonitis. The most appropriate management of this injury is:
    a. Ureterocystostomy
    b. Trans uretero-ureterostomy
    c. Re-anastomosis
    d. Externalized urinary diversion
    e. Nephrectomy

    Answer d. Full transection ureteral injuries can be divided into **high/middle** (*above* pelvic brim) and **lower** injuries (*below* pelvic brim).

    Complete transections *below* the **pelvic brim** (lower injuries) are always treated with **re-implantation into bladder** because a ureterocystostomy anastomosis has much higher success rate than a ureteroureterostomy anastomosis (especially after trauma).

    Injuries *above* the **pelvic brim** are handled in one of 2 ways:
    1) If there is just a short segment missing (≤ **2 cm**), go ahead and mobilize as much ureter as you can without devascularizing it and perform re-anastomosis; place a ureteral stent and leave drains

    2) If > **2 cm** is missing, externalized urinary diversion is indicated (either with a percutaneous nephrostomy tube and tie off both ends of the ureter or with an externalized catheter tied to the proximal ureteral segment). At a later date, a urologist can perform a trans ureteroureterostomy or place an ileal conduit. One could argue performing the anastomosis at this time but with the area covered in stool it would be inappropriate. An unstable patient would be another reason to delay repair.

    Partial transection ureteral injuries can be repaired over a stent.

Ureter injuries can occur with **pelvic tumor resections, LAR's,** and **APR's**. Some place pre-op ureteral stents to help avoid injury for difficult dissections (eg retroperitoneal fibrosis, inflammatory aneurysms, perforated diverticulitis), *although this does not always help avoid injury.*

353. A 25 yo man suffers a significant pelvic fracture and has hematuria. You get a retrograde cystourethrogram and the bladder has extra-peritoneal contrast extravasation. The most appropriate therapy for this patient is:
    a. Foley drainage for 7 days
    b. Open repair
    c. Nothing
    d. Partial cystectomy
    e. Supra-pubic cystostomy

    Answer a. The most appropriate Tx for an ***extra*-peritoneal bladder rupture** is urinary catheter drainage for 7 days.

354. Instead of the above, the bladder has intra-peritoneal contrast extravasation. The most appropriate therapy for this patient is:
    a. Foley drainage for 7 days
    b. Open repair
    c. Nothing
    d. Partial cystectomy
    e. Supra-pubic cystostomy

    Answer b. The most appropriate Tx for an ***intra*-peritoneal bladder rupture** is laparotomy with primary surgical repair.

355. Instead of the above, the patient has significant extravasation of contrast in the perineum. The most appropriate therapy for this patient is:
    a. Foley drainage for 7 days
    b. Open repair
    c. Nothing
    d. Partial cystectomy
    e. Supra-pubic cystostomy

    Answer e. **Urethral injuries** require percutaneous drainage (supra-pubic cystostomy) and **late repair** (wait 2-3 months). *Early repair of injuries to the urethra result in a high stricture rate.*

356. You clamp the infra-diaphragmatic aorta in a persistently hypotensive patient with a penetrating Zone I supramesocolic hematoma, perform a Mattox maneuver, and find the left renal vein is completely avulsed from its connection with the IVC. The most appropriate step is:
    a. Oversew the renal vein and ligate IVC connection
    b. Perform primary repair
    c. Left nephrectomy
    d. Pack and go to the ICU

    Answer a. The **left renal vein** has adrenal and gonadal vein collaterals making ligation at the IVC connection relatively safe (indicated for this persistently hypotensive patient). The **right renal vein** has no collaterals and requires repair.

357. You explore a trauma patient following an MVA and find a severe hepatic fracture with ongoing bleeding and a large left zone II expanding hematoma with a completely avulsed left renal artery on inspection. The patient also has a blown left pupil and head trauma. With hemostatic resuscitation the patient's pressure is 70/40 (2 L LR, 6 units pRBCs, 2 units FFP, and 2 units platelets). The most appropriate next step is:
    a. Pack everything and go to the ICU for resuscitation
    b. Left nephrectomy
    c. Angio-embolization

d.   Head CT

Answer b. In this severe scenario, **left nephrectomy** will likely be life-saving so it is warranted and is the most appropriate next step. A Burr hole in the OR should also be considered (left blown pupil). If the liver bleeding cannot be controlled intra-op, damage control packing (with possible angio-embolization) followed by resuscitation in the ICU is indicated.

358. A stable 25 yo man involved in an MVA has fractured left posterior ribs and no left renal uptake of contrast on CT scan. The most appropriate next step is:
     a.   Chest tube
     b.   Open repair
     c.   Angiography
     d.   Nephrectomy

Answer c. This patient has obstructed flow to the left kidney which may be caused by an **intimal flap** or other correctable lesion. **Immediate angiogram** should be performed with possible **stenting of the left renal artery.**

359. A stable 25 yo man involved in an MVA has fractured left posterior ribs and a full thickness cortical laceration that almost reaches the renal pelvis on CT scan. The next appropriate step is:
     a.   Ureteroscopy and stent
     b.   Nephrectomy
     c.   Open exploration and primary repair
     d.   Observation
     e.   Partial nephrectomy

Answer d. Observation. The vast majority of kidney injuries can be observed. The only indication for _acute_ surgery is ongoing hemorrhage in an unstable patient.   •

360. A 25 yo man suffers a GSW to the medial thigh. Exam demonstrates no pulse or doppler signal in the extremity. The most appropriate next step is:
     a.   Observation
     b.   Heparin
     c.   Open exploration
     d.   Formal angiogram
     e.   CT angiogram

Answer c. Open exploration in the OR

361. Instead of the above, exam demonstrates a weak pulse and an ABI of 0.6. The most appropriate next step is:
     a.   Observation
     b.   Heparin
     c.   Open exploration
     d.   Formal angiogram
     e.   CT angiogram

Answer e. CT angiogram

362. Instead of the above, exam demonstrates an ABI of 0.9. The most appropriate next step is:
     a.   Observation
     b.   Heparin
     c.   Open exploration
     d.   Angiogram
     e.   CT angiogram

Answer a. Observation and discharge from the ED. Patients with an ABI ≥ 0.9, no major/minor signs of vascular trauma, and no fracture should undergo observation (no further work-up and discharge from the ED). The exception to this rule is patients with posterior knee dislocations (all need formal angiogram).

363. Instead of the above, the entrance wound is near the femoral triangle. Exam demonstrates leg weakness and an ABI of 1.0. The most appropriate next step is:
    a. Observation
    b. Heparin
    c. Open exploration
    d. Formal angiogram
    e. CT angiogram

    Answer a. Injury to an anatomically related nerve is <u>not</u> considered an indication for CT angiogram. Injury in close proximity to a vessel is likewise <u>not</u> an indication for CT angiogram. Observation and discharge from the ED is appropriate if this patient's clinical status remains the same.

364. All of the following are indications for CT angiogram of an extremity except:
    a. ABI < 0.9
    b. History of severe blood loss from the injury
    c. Large hematoma
    d. Obvious thrill and bruit

    Answer d. Bruit or thrill is an indication for OR exploration, not CT angio.

365. A 25 yo man suffers a posterior knee dislocation with loss of pulse. The most important next step is:
    a. Go to the OR for revascularization
    b. Reduction
    c. Heparin
    d. Formal angiogram
    e. CT angiogram

    Answer b. The most important step at this point is to reduce the dislocation.

366. You are able to get the knee back in place in the above patient and a pulse is now present. The most appropriate next step in this patient's management is:
    a. Nothing else
    b. Heparin
    c. Open exploration
    d. Formal angiogram
    e. CT angiogram

    Answer d. Posterior knee dislocations have a high incidence of popliteal artery injury. **Formal angiogram** is mandatory for <u>*all*</u> posterior knee dislocations.

367. Non-operative management is most appropriate for which of the following:
    a. Intimal flap in a popliteal artery that is not flow limiting
    b. Cold foot after external fixation of a femur fracture
    c. Large traumatic AV fistula
    d. Pulsatile bleeding from a thigh stab wound

    Answer a. An intimal flap in the popliteal artery that is not flow limiting can be treated conservatively (Tx: ASA or Plavix).

368. A 25 yo man suffers a close range shotgun blast to his thigh with 5 cm of superficial femoral artery missing. The most appropriate bypass conduit is:
    a. Saphenous vein from contralateral leg
    b. Saphenous vein from the same leg
    c. Radial artery

d.   Gore-Tex (PTFE)
e.   Dacron (woven polyester)

Answer a. Avoid further damage to the leg and take vein from the other side. Avoid artificial material here as well.

369. All of the following arteries can generally be ligated in the acute trauma setting except:
a.   The right subclavian artery
b.   The right internal carotid artery
c.   The anterior tibialis artery
d.   The radial artery

Answer b. The right internal carotid artery ligation would be at high risk for **stroke** (20%). This artery needs to be repaired.

The **subclavian arteries** can generally be ligated in the trauma setting although an attempt at repair should be made. Issues with **stroke** (1-2%) can come up as patients with an incomplete Circle of Willis may be dependent on a vertebral artery (which come off the subclavian arteries).

Either the **ulnar** or **radial artery** can be ligated as long as the other one has a pulse. An attempt at repair should be performed, however, as 1-2% of the population has an incomplete palmar arch and hand ischemia could occur.

Either the **anterior tibialis** or the **posterior tibialis** can be ligated as long as there is a pulse in the other vessel (ie dorsalis pedis or posterior tibialis). An attempt at repair should be performed as 1-2% of the population has an incomplete pedal arch and in rare circumstances foot ischemia can occur. The peroneal artery can almost always be ligated in trauma settings.

370. All of the following are true of hip dislocations except:
a.   Closed reduction with conscious sedation should be performed in the ED as soon as the patient is stable
b.   Anterior dislocations are associated with femoral artery injuries
c.   Posterior dislocations are associated with sciatic nerve injuries
d.   Bed rest and skeletal traction are the best Tx for hip dislocation

Answer d. Hip dislocations are especially susceptible to **avascular necrosis**. **Closed reduction** should be performed in the ED as soon as the patient is stable (< 24 hours).

371. A 35 yo man suffers a severe left leg soft tissue crush injury and tibial plateau fracture after being pinned underneath a car. The patient initially does not have a pulse in the foot but after placing a traction splint, a pulse is restored. All of the following are true of the above patient except:
a.   He is at increased risk for popliteal artery injury
b.   This patient is at risk for compartment syndrome
c.   This patient is at increased risk for rhabdomyolysis and acute renal failure
d.   Concomitant major arterial, venous, and nerve injury do not increase his risk of requiring amputation

Answer d. Combined major arterial, venous, and nerve injury increase the risk for requiring amputation.

372. At laparotomy following a GSW, you identify a zone I retroperitoneal hematoma. The hematoma is at the level of the diaphragm. The most important next step for proximal aortic control is:
a.   Through a left thoracotomy
b.   At the diaphragmatic hiatus
c.   Just below the left renal vein at transverse mesocolon base
d.   At the aortic bifurcation

Answer a. Aortic control through a **left thoracotomy**. *Always obtain **proximal vascular control** first.* For direct aortic injury or injury to the takeoffs of its major branches, clamping the aorta **proximal** *(first priority)* to the injured area is the best method to control bleeding and allow repair. Clamping the aorta distal to the injured area helps control back-bleeding.

373. Instead of the above, the zone I retroperitoneal hematoma is at the level of the transverse mesocolon. The most important next step for proximal aortic control is:
    a. Through a left thoracotomy
    b. At the diaphragmatic hiatus
    c. Just below the left renal vein at transverse mesocolon base
    d. At the aortic bifurcation

    Answer b. Aortic control at the diaphragmatic hiatus

374. Instead of the above, the zone I retroperitoneal hematoma is below the transverse mesocolon and extends to the left. The most important next step for aortic control is:
    a. Through a left thoracotomy
    b. At the diaphragmatic hiatus
    c. Just below the left renal vein at transverse mesocolon base
    d. At the aortic bifurcation

    Answer c. Aortic control just below left renal vein at transverse mesocolon base

375. Instead of the above, the zone I retroperitoneal hematoma is below the transverse mesocolon and extends to the right. Your perform a Cattell maneuver and find a through and through injury to the infra-renal IVC with a large amount of dark blood welling up. The most important next step is:
    a. Clamp the proximal and distal IVC
    b. Median sternotomy for atrio-caval shunt
    c. Sponge stick compression
    d. Ligate the IVC

    Answer c. The best method for controlling bleeding from the IVC is to take sponge-sticks and compress the IVC proximal and distal to the area. Clamps require more time for mobilization of the IVC and can be damaging to the IVC.

    Repair of the posterior IVC wall is performed through the opening in the anterior wall.

376. A patient undergoes splenectomy following a MVA. He is now stable. While in the OR, you find a left sided zone II retroperitoneal hematoma. Intra-op IVP demonstrates an intact kidney system. The left colon also looks intact. What is the most appropriate next step:
    a. Angio-embolization
    b. Place drain in hematoma
    c. Observation only
    d. Mattox maneuver and exploration of hematoma

    Answer c. Observation

377. All of the following are true of retroperitoneal hematomas except:
    a. All Zone I hematomas (both penetrating and blunt) should be explored
    b. Blunt zone III hematomas should be explored
    c. Penetrating zone II injuries should be explored
    d. Blunt zone II injuries are usually observed
    e. Penetrating zone II injuries should be explored

Answer b. Blunt **zone III** retroperitoneal hematomas should *not be explored*. If a blunt zone III hematoma is expanding due to pelvic fracture, pack the area, place external fixator, and go to angiography for embolization.

Penetrating **zone III** retroperitoneal hematomas should be **explored** (proximal vascular control at the aortic bifurcation or common iliac artery first). If having trouble with exploration, go with angio-embolization as a back-up.

Blunt **zone II** retroperitoneal hematomas are **observed** unless there is an expanding or pulsatile perirenal hematoma or a colon injury.

Penetrating **zone II** retroperitoneal hematomas are *generally* **explored.**

All **Zone I** retroperitoneal hematomas (both penetrating and blunt) are **explored.**

378. A 25 yo woman at 12 weeks pregnancy is involved in a high speed MVA with airbag deployment. She is alert, had no loss of consciousness, has a BP of 120/70, and has no signs of external trauma. Which of the following is most appropriate:
    a.   Abdominal and pelvic CT scan
    b.   Observation only
    c.   FAST scan
    d.   Laparotomy
    e.   DPL

    Answer c. FAST scan is an excellent method of screening **pregnant patients** with significant mechanism capable of severe injury but who show no external signs of trauma. This avoids any radiation risk.

379. A 25 yo pregnant woman at 34 weeks has a fracture of her 5th metacarpal after tripping over a step. She is hypotensive in the ED. The most appropriate next step is:
    a.   Roll her to the left
    b.   Roll her to the right
    c.   Place head down
    d.   Place feet down

    Answer a. Roll her to the **left** to relieve compression off the **IVC**.

380. A 25 yo woman at 27 weeks pregnancy suffers a GSW to the abdomen. Intra-op you discover a 3 cm long tangential uterine wall laceration. You do not see any amniotic fluid leakage. She is otherwise stable. What is the most appropriate next step:
    a.   C-section
    b.   Hysterectomy
    c.   Leave alone
    d.   Primary repair

    Answer d. Primary repair. This would be at significant risk for uterine rupture with contractions if it were left alone. Chromic sutures are often used.

381. A 25 yo pregnant woman at 30 weeks suffers a significant fall (BP 100/70 and HR 100 after 2 L LR). FAST scan shows a peri-hepatic fluid collection. What is the most appropriate next step:
    a.   Observation
    b.   Obtain a Kleihauer-Betke test
    c.   Place a drain
    d.   CT scan
    e.   Go to the OR

    Answer d. CT scan of the abdomen. Given the positive FAST scan, this patient is at increased risk for severe intra-abdominal injury and a CT scan is warranted.

Pregnancy should not lead to "underdiagnosis" or "undertreatment" due to unfounded fears of fetal effects (rads < 5-10 that occur with a CT scan have not been shown to have a negative impact on fetus, especially after the 1st trimester).

382. A 25 yo pregnant woman at 26 weeks has a pubic rami fracture following a high speed MVA (BP 110/70, HR 100). Which of the following is the best indication for continuous fetal monitoring (4-24 hours):
    a.   A displaced pubic rami fracture and pelvic hematoma
    b.   Hematocrit 27
    c.   A fetal heart rate of 160
    d.   3 contractions per hour
    e.   High amylase

    Answer e. High amylase. **Elevated trauma labs** are an indication for continuous fetal monitoring. **Vaginal bleeding** or **≥ 4 contractions per hour** are also indications for continuous fetal monitoring.

383. A 25 yo woman at 32 weeks pregnancy in being monitored in the ICU following an MVA that resulted in a severe CHI and multisystem trauma. She has a fetal monitor and uterine tocodynamometer in place. Lactate is 1.5 after resuscitation. Which of the following is the best indication to proceed with caesarean section (C-section):
    a.   Late decelerations
    b.   Fetal HR 120
    c.   3 contractions per hour
    d.   Pelvic hematoma
    e.   Elevated AST

    Answer a. Late decelerations is an indication of inadequate fetal oxygenation (perfusion) and **C-section** is warranted. This could be caused by inadequate resuscitation, however, the patient's lactate is 1.5.

384. The order of preference for fluid access in a child ≤ 5 years of age is:
    a.   Antecubital fossa, intraosseous of the proximal tibia, saphenous vein, intraosseous at the distal femur
    b.   Antecubital fossa, intraosseous of the proximal tibia, intraosseous at the distal femur, saphenous vein
    c.   Antecubital fossa, saphenous vein, intraosseous at the distal femur, intraosseous of the proximal tibia
    d.   Antecubital fossa, saphenous vein, intraosseous of the proximal tibia, intraosseous at the distal femur

    Answer d. Antecubital fossa, saphenous vein, intraosseous of the proximal tibia, intraosseous at the distal femur. At times in children, venous access cannot be achieved and the intraosseous route is needed.

385. All of the following are true of electrical injuries except:
    a.   Cataracts can occur
    b.   Bone has the highest electrical resistance
    c.   The MCC of early death is brain injury
    d.   Compartment syndrome can occur in these patients

    Answer c. MCC of early death is cardiac arrest from **ventricular fibrillation**.

386. All of the following are true except:
    a.   Tx for Brown Recluse spider bites is Dapsone
    b.   Thyroid hormone is released as part of the flight or fight response
    c.   The MCC of airway obstruction is the tongue
    d.   Head injury is the MCC of death after reaching the ED alive

    Answer b. Thyroid hormone is <u>not</u> involved in fight or flight response.

ACUTE TRAUMATIC COAGULOPATHY / HEMOSTATIC RESUSCITATION

- **Coagulopathy** occurs in **severely injured** trauma patients *prior* to resuscitation and arriving at the hospital
  - Can result in **massive transfusion**; increases morbidity and mortality
  - **Hemostatic resuscitation** is indicated for patients receiving $\geq$ **4 units** pRBCs in the *first hour or $\geq$* **10 units** pRBCs within 24 hours (approximate indications)
- **Damage control surgery** (for severely injured trauma patients):
  - Early control of **bleeding** (surgical and/or interventional) and **contamination** with *delay* in definitive surgery until patient is stabilized
  - Give **blood products** to ensure oxygenation and correct coagulopathy *(not give continued lactated ringers)*
  - **Hemostatic resuscitation** - give RBCs : FFP : platelets in a ratio of **1:1:1**
  - *Limit* crystalloid solutions to avoid hemodilution (initial 2 L LR *only*)
  - Allow **permissive hypotension** (SBP > 70) until hemorrhage controlled (after that want SBP > 90)
  - Early correction of **hypothermia / acidosis / hypocalcemia**
  - *Exceptions* - traumatic brain injury patients (want SBP > 90 initially)

INITIAL EVALUATION

- **Blunt trauma**
  - *Stable* patient $\rightarrow$ normal work-up
    - Stable with pelvic Fx - continue full workup before addressing pelvis
  - *Unstable* patient $\rightarrow$ (SBP < 90 despite 2 L of LR) $\rightarrow$ **FAST scan** (or DPL)
    - If **positive FAST** (bleeding from **abdomen**) $\rightarrow$ OR (for laparotomy)
    - If **negative FAST** $\rightarrow$ need to find the source of bleeding:
      - **Pelvic Fx** (exam, PXR)
      - **Chest** - hemorrhage, tension PTX, tamponade (exam, CXR)
      - **Extremity** bleeding - lacerations or femur fractures
      - **Neurogenic** shock (lateral c-spine in ED) - rule-out above 1st
    - If **pelvic Fx** and **negative FAST** (and not bleeding from chest or extremity)
      1) **Stabilize pelvis** (cross pelvis with sheet or place external fixator if ortho is there)
      2) **Go to angio** for **embolization** *(do not wait for ortho)* - they can meet you in angio

- **FAST scan** (focused abdominal sonography for trauma)
  - Used in hypotensive patients (SBP < 90) with blunt trauma
  - U/S looks for fluid in perihepatic fossa, perisplenic fossa, pelvis, and pericardium
  - Obesity can obstruct view
  - May not detect free fluid < 50-80 mL
  - Need **laparotomy** (or pericardial window) if FAST scan is **positive** and patient is **persistently hypotensive** (ie **unstable**; SBP < 90 after 2 L of LR)
  - **FAST scan misses** - *retroperitoneal bleeding, hollow viscous injury*

- **Diagnostic peritoneal lavage** (DPL)
  - Used in hypotensive patients (SBP < 90) with blunt trauma
  - Positive if >10 cc blood, >100,000 RBCs/cc, food particles, bile, bacteria, >500 WBC/cc
  - Need **laparotomy** if DPL is **positive** and patient is **unstable**
  - DPL needs to be supraumbilical if pelvic fracture is present
  - **DPL misses** - *retroperitoneal bleeds, contained hematomas*

- **CT scan** - indicated for **blunt trauma** with: abdominal pain / tenderness, need for general anesthesia, closed head injury, intoxication, significant mechanism (although not in pregnancy, use FAST scan), paraplegia, distracting injury, or hematuria
  - Patients with a negative DPL will need an abdominal CT scan
  - **CT scan misses** (false negatives) - *hollow viscous injury, diaphragm injury*

- **Penetrating abdominal** injury: if *unstable* or high velocity GSW → laparotomy
- **Possible penetrating abdominal** injury: knife or low-velocity GSW and patient *stable* → local exploration and observation if fascia not violated; if fascia was violated, can perform diagnostic laparoscopy to see if peritoneum was violated; need laparotomy if peritoneum was violated
- **Penetrating tangential flank** or **low back** (ie not sure if retroperitoneal structures were injured or peritoneum was entered): *unstable* → **laparotomy**; *stable* → **CT scan** to follow trajectory, possible laparotomy based on findings
- **Penetrating chest injury** and patient is ***stable*** (SBP ≥ 90) - start with a **CXR** (place chest tube if pneumothorax or hemothorax)
  - Penetrating **"box" injuries** - borders are clavicles, xiphoid process, and nipples → initially place chest tube on side of injury (you are going to the OR) and on contralateral side if pneumothorax / hemothorax; while in OR need **pericardial window, bronchoscopy,** and **esophagoscopy**; may also need angiogram if near Zone I neck injury
  - **Esophageal injuries** are the hardest to diagnose (consider **gastrografin swallow** before commencing diet to rule-out occult esophageal injury)
    Esophageal injuries can be hard to Dx with esophagoscopy alone
  - Penetrating **outside "box"** without pneumothorax or hemothorax → need chest tube on side of injury if patient requires intubation, otherwise follow with serial CXRs (every 4-6 hours)
  - **Pericardial window** - if you find blood, need **median sternotomy** to fix possible injury to heart or great vessels; place pericardial drains
  - Penetrating injuries **anterior-medial to midaxillary line** and **below nipples** → need **laparotomy** or **laparoscopy** to rule-out **peritoneal entry**; may also need evaluation for penetrating **"box" injury** depending on exact location
  - Some are using **FAST scan** of the pericardium instead of pericardial window for "box" injuries
- **Penetrating chest injury** and patient is ***unstable*** (SBP < 90)
  - DDx: hemorrhage, tension PTX, cardiac tamponade
  - *Place chest tube right away* (on side of injury, consider bilateral chest tubes) → diagnostic for tension pneumothorax (PTX)
  - If chest tube has **high output** (> 1000-1500 cc with insertion) → go to OR for **anterolateral thoracotomy** on the bleeding side (keep the patient supine)
    Clamshell incision if you need to see whole heart or contra-lateral side
    Clamp **hilum** if severe **lung injury** (then repair)
    Clamp **aorta** if **aortic injury** (then repair)
    Put finger in hole (digital compression) for **heart injury** (then repair)
    Intercostal arteries and IMA can bleed significantly
  - If **tension PTX** (SBP improves with chest tube) → just manage chest tube
  - If not much blood from chest tube(s) and no tension PTX → OR for **pericardial window**
    If window is **positive** → median sternotomy (cardiac injury)
    If window is **negative** and **high chest injury** → median sternotomy (you actually have a Zone I neck injury)
    If window is **negative** and **low chest injury** → laparotomy (you actually have a penetrating abdominal injury)
  - When patient is stable, if "box" injury need completion work-up described above
- **ED thoracotomy** (coding in the ED; **SBP < 60** or **no pulse**)
  - Consider tension PTX before thoracotomy
  - Blunt trauma - use only if pressure or pulse lost **in ED**
  - Penetrating trauma - use only if pressure or pulse lost **on way to ED** or **in ED**
  - Thoracotomy - **open pericardium** anterior to phrenic nerve (looking for hemopericardium) and **cross-clamp aorta** (avoid esophagus anterior to aorta)
  - Penetrating **right chest injury** and patient codes → still do left thoracotomy (possible clamshell if you need to get to the right chest)
  - Need pressure to rise > 70 mmHg after cross-clamping to continue (otherwise further Tx is futile)
- **Persistent hypotension** despite fluid resuscitation (other than ongoing bleeding) - tension pneumothorax, pericardial tamponade, air embolism, myocardial infarction, adrenal insufficiency, neurogenic shock

HEAD INJURY

Glasgow Coma Scale (GCS)
Motor
6 - follows commands
5 - localizes pain
4 - withdraws from pain
3 - flexion with pain (decorticate)
2 - extension with pain (decerebrate)
1 - no response
Verbal
5 - oriented
4 - confused
3 - inappropriate words
2 - incomprehensible sounds
1 - no response
Eye opening
4 - spontaneous opening
3 - opens to command
2 - opens to pain
1 - no response

GCS score:
≤ 14 → head CT
≤ 10 → intubation (prior to head CT)
≤ 8 → ICP monitor

- Most important prognostic score - **motor**
- **Penetrating** head injury has the worst survival of any head injuries
- Lowest score is **3**; intubated patients are given a verbal score of **1T**

Indications for Head CT

Suspected skull penetration by a foreign body
Discharge of cerebrospinal fluid (CSF), blood, or both from the nose
Hemotympanum or discharge of blood or CSF from the ear
Altered state of consciousness at the time of examination
Focal neurologic Sx's
Any situation precluding proper surveillance (eg going to OR)
Loss of unconsciousness at any point
Head injury plus additional trauma
Head injury with alcohol or drug intoxication
Head injury and on anticoagulation (eg warfarin, Plavix, Xarelto, Eliquis, Pradaxa)

- **Epidural hematoma** - MC arterial bleeding from **middle meningeal artery**
  - Often associated with temporal bone Fx
  - Head CT - shows a lenticular (lens-shaped) deformity adjacent the skull
  - Sx's: often have **loss of consciousness** (LOC) → then **lucid interval** (awake) → then **sudden deterioration** (HA, vomiting, restlessness, stupor, LOC)
  - **Craniotomy** indications (evacuate hematoma): GCS < 9, hematoma volume > 30 cm^3, or a midline shift **> 5 mm**
- **Subdural hematoma** - MC from torn **venous plexus (bridging veins)** that cross between the dura and arachnoid
  - Greater incidence than epidural
  - Head CT - shows a crescent-shaped deformity adjacent the skull
  - **Craniotomy** indications: hematoma thickness > 10 mm, a midline shift **> 5 mm**, worsening GCS (drops another 2 points after initial evaluation), fixed and dilated pupils, anisocoria, or ICP > 20 mmHg
  - Chronic subdural hematomas - usually in elderly after minor falls

- **Intracerebral hematoma** - usually in **frontal lobe** (typically do not require operation but if causing significant mass effect will need decompression)
- **Cerebral contusions** - can be coup or contracoup (rarely require operation)
- **Head trauma** in a patient on **anticoagulation** (eg warfarin, Plavix) → get **Head CT**
  - **Negative study** - repeat study in 8-12 hours (do <u>not</u> reverse patient)
  - **Hemorrhage**: *reverse warfarin* - **prothrombin complex** *(fastest) or* **FFP** <u>and</u> **Vit K** (IV); *Plavix Tx*- **platelets**; repeat head CT (8-12 hrs) if not going for craniotomy
- **Intraventricular hemorrhage** - need **ventriculostomy** if causing hydrocephalus
- **Diffuse axonal injury** - shows up better on **MRI** (most sensitive test) than CT scan
  - Tx: supportive; may need craniectomy if ICP elevated
  - Extremely poor prognosis
- **Cerebral perfusion pressure** (CPP = MAP - ICP); *want **CPP > 60 mmHg***
  - CPP = mean arterial pressure (MAP) *minus* intracranial pressure (ICP)
  - Signs of **elevated ICP on head CT** - decreased ventricular size, loss of sulci, loss of cisterns
  - **ICP monitors** indicated for: **GCS ≤ 8**, suspected **increased ICP**, or moderate-severe head injury and **unable to follow exam** (eg going to OR)
  - **Reduced CPP** results in **secondary traumatic brain injury**
- Tx to *increase* MAP - **volume** and **pressors** (phenylephrine)
- Tx to *decrease* ICP (normal is 10, > 20 usually requires Tx)
  - **Sedation** and **paralysis**
  - **Raise head of bed**
  - **Relative hyperventilation** for modest cerebral vasoconstriction (pCO_2 30-35); do not want to over-hyperventilate and cause cerebral ischemia from too much vasoconstriction
  - Keep **Na 140-150**, serum **osmolality 295-310** - may need to use <u>hypertonic saline</u> at times (draws fluid out of brain)
  - **Mannitol** - draws fluid from brain
  - **Barbiturate coma** - consider if above not working
  - **Ventriculostomy** with CSF drainage (want ICP < 20)
  - **Craniectomy** decompression - if refractory to all of above (decompresses ICP)
  - **Fosphenytoin** or **Keppra** - can be given prophylactically to prevent seizures in moderate to severe head injury
  - **Dilated pupil** - from **temporal lobe compression** on the same side (**CN III**, oculomotor)
- **Basal skull fractures**
  - **Raccoon eyes** (peri-orbital ecchymosis) - anterior fossa fracture
  - **Battle's sign** (mastoid ecchymosis) - middle fossa fracture; can injure **facial nerve** (CN VII)
  - Can also have **hemotympanum** and **CSF rhinorrhea / otorrhea**
  - Majority of basal skull Fx's do <u>not</u> require surgery
- **Temporal skull fractures** - can injure CN VII
  - Most common site of **facial nerve injury** (VII) - *geniculate ganglion*
  - Associated with lateral skull or orbital blows
- **Skull fracture** indications for **surgery** (majority do <u>not</u> require surgery):
  - **Significantly depressed** (> 1 cm, needs elevation) <u>or:</u>
  - **Contaminated** (dura penetration) <u>or:</u>
  - **Persistent CSF leak** not responsive to conservative Tx (up to 2 weeks; close dura with operation)
- **CSF leaks** after skull fracture - Tx: treat expectantly; can use **lumbar drain with CSF drainage** if persistent
- **Dilated pupil** (blown pupil)
  - Possible **ipsilateral temporal lobe** pressure on **cranial nerve III** (oculomotor), can progress to **temporal uncal herniation**
  - In ED, patient intubated with **blown pupil** and *stable* → get head CT (do not want to perform Burr Hole for baseline anisocoria)
  - In ED, patient intubated with **blown pupil, head injury,** and *unstable*→ address **hypotension** *before* getting head CT (eg go to OR for abdominal bleeding, go to angio for pelvic bleeding) - consider Burr hole if not going to make it to head CT for awhile (5 cm anterior and superior to external auditory canal)

- **Brain swelling** - maximum at **48-72 hours** after trauma (**peak ICP**)
  - Sx's of **elevated ICP** - *hypertension*, HR lability, slow respirations; stupor, HA
  - **Intermittent bradycardia** is a sign of severely elevated ICP and impending **herniation** (shift of brain across skull structures; usually fatal)
  - **Cushing's Triad** - HTN, bradycardia, and decreased RR (Kussmaul breathing); signals impending **herniation**
- **Diabetes insipidus / SIADH** (see Fluids and Electrolytes chapter)

SPINE TRAUMA
- **Cervical spine** *(MC spine injury)*
  - **Dens = odontoid process**
  - MC <u>location</u> for spine injury - **cervical spine**
  - MC cervical spine <u>Fx</u> - **dens Fx**
  - Screening - **Neck CT scan**
  - **C-1 burst Fx** (Jefferson) - caused by axial loading; Tx: rigid collar
  - **C-2 Fx** (hangman) - caused by distraction / extension; Tx: traction-halo
  - **C-2 odontoid process (dens) Fx**
    - Type I - above base, stable
    - Type II - at base, unstable (Tx: cervical fusion or halo brace)
    - Type III - extends into vertebral body (Tx: fusion or halo brace)
  - **Facet** fractures or dislocations - can cause cord injury; usually associated with hyperextension and rotation with ligamentous disruption
- **Thoracolumbar spine**
  - Screening for Fx - **CT scan**
  - 3 columns of the thoracolumbar spine (anterior, middle, posterior)
  - If more than 1 column is disrupted, the spine is considered unstable:
    - **Compression fractures** (wedge) usually involve the anterior column only and are considered stable (Tx: **TSLO brace** [thoraco-lumbar sacral orthosis])
    - **Burst fractures** are considered unstable (2 or more columns - usually anterior and middle); Tx - **spinal fusion**
- **Upright fall** - at risk for calcaneus, lumbar, and wrist/forearm Fx's
- **Neurologic deficits *without* bony injury** on CT scan - get **MRI** to check for ligamentous injury
- **Pre-vertebral soft tissue** swelling on CT scan and no bony injury - get **MRI** (high risk for occult ligamentous injury)
- **Indications for emergent spine surgery**:
  - Open fractures
  - Soft tissue or bony compression of the cord
  - Progressive neurologic dysfunction
- The higher the spine injury, the higher the morbidity and mortality
- The best indication for **<u>steroids</u>** is **worsening neurologic deficit**

MAXILLOFACIAL TRAUMA
- *Fracture of the **temporal bone** is the MCC of **facial nerve injury*** (CN VII, at **geniculate ganglion**); if severe injury → repair
  - **iatrogenic** facial nerve injury in OR → **repair** immediately
- Try to preserve skin and not trim edges with facial lacerations
- Scalp lacerations - hair removal is generally <u>not</u> necessary
- Facial trauma - at high risk for cervical spine trauma

Le Fort Classification of Maxillofacial Fractures

Type	Description
I	Maxillary fracture straight across (-)
II	Lateral to nose, underneath eyes, diagonal down to maxilla (/ \)
III	Lateral orbital walls (- -)

- **Le Fort Fx's** - most repaired with **ORIF**
- **Nasoethmoidal orbital Fx's** - 70% have a CSF leak
  - CSF has **tau protein** and **beta-transferrin**
  - Conservative Tx for up to **2 weeks**

- Can try **lumbar drain** to lower CSF pressure and help close leak
- May need surgical closure of **dura** to stop leak
- If undergoing facial reconstruction, repair at that time
■ **Nosebleeds** (epistaxis)
  - **Anterior** (MC, 90%) - Tx: pressure, Vaseline gauze packs (Kiesselbach plexus)
  - **Posterior** (associated with **HTN** and **atherosclerosis**) - can be hard to deal with
    Posterior packing
    Can try **balloon tamponade** (Foley catheter; may need to **intubate**)
    May need angio-embolization of **internal maxillary** or **ethmoidal** artery
    Some use endonasal cautery / ligation (**sphenopalatine** artery)
    Life-threatening problem (higher mortality compared to anterior bleeds)
■ **Orbital blowout fractures** - patients with <u>impaired upward gaze</u> or <u>diplopia</u> (double vision) need repair; Tx: restoration of orbital floor with bone fragments or bone graft
■ **Mandibular injury** - **malocclusion** #1 indicator of injury
  - Dx: fine-cut facial CT scans with reconstruction
  - Most repaired with **inter-maxillary fixation** (IMF; upper / lower dental arches; 6-8 weeks) or open reduction and internal fixation (ORIF)
■ **Tripod fracture** (zygomatic bone) - ORIF for cosmesis only *(not a functional problem)*
■ Patients with maxillofacial Fx's are at high risk for **cervical spine injuries**

NECK TRAUMA
■ *Asymptomatic* **blunt** - neck CT angio
■ *Asymptomatic* **penetrating** - controversial; MC method below

Penetrating Neck Injury Zones

Zone	Evaluation of Asymptomatic Patients
I	Clavicle to cricoid cartilage
	Need angiogram, bronchoscopy, esophagoscopy, and barium swallow; a pericardial window may also be indicated.
	May need **median sternotomy** to reach these injuries (*almost <u>always</u> needed for **vascular injuries** in order to obtain proximal control*)
II	Cricoid to angle of mandible
	***Neck exploration in OR** for <u>all</u> of these injuries (lateral neck incision)*
III	Angle of mandible to the base of skull
	Need angiogram and laryngoscopy
	May need **jaw subluxation** / digastric and sternocleidomastoid muscle release / mastoid sinus resection to reach **vascular** injuries here

■ *Symptomatic* neck trauma (*blunt <u>or</u> penetrating*): hypotension, pulsatile bleeding, expanding hematoma, palpable thrill, crepitus, stridor, hemoptysis, neurologic deficit (eg hemiplegia) → *all need **neck exploration in OR** (use exposure methods above)*
  - Losing or lost airway in ED (ie respiratory distress) → cricothyroidotomy in ED
  - <u>Dysphagia</u> [for 1) blunt <u>or</u>; 2) Zone I or Zone III penetrating] - most get swallow studies and EGD to rule-out an injury (not exploration)
  - Penetrating carotid injury can be repaired primarily or with interposition graft
■ **Carotid artery injury** (internal or common carotid artery)
  - **Hemorrhage, pseudoaneurysm**, or **AV fistula** (continuous bruit) - Tx: **open primary repair**
  - Can present **late** after blunt trauma and often have **normal head CT scans** (ie late neuro deficit develops after negative head CT at original trauma work-up)
  - RFs: forceful compression or hyperextension
  - Dx: head / neck CT angio
  - **Carotid dissection** (isolated; should not have aortic dissection)
    Asymptomatic - Tx: heparin or Plavix (prevents thrombosis)
    Symptomatic - Tx: endovascular covered stent *(best)* <u>unless</u> the artery is completely thrombosed (then just give heparin or Plavix)
  - **Carotid disruption** (presents with carotid thrombosis)
    Complete occlusion- Tx: heparin or Plavix (prevents thrombus extension)
    Antegrade flow present - Tx: endovascular covered stent or open repair to prevent Cx's (eg pseudoaneurysm, rupture, complete thrombosis), even if patient is asymptomatic

- Confirm no intra-cranial hemorrhage before starting heparin / Plavix
- **Internal carotid artery ligation** - stroke in 20% (*avoid* ligation)
- **Esophageal injury**
  - *Hardest neck injury to find*
  - **Esophagoscopy** and **esophagogram** (swallow study) - best combined modalities (find 95% of injuries when using both methods)
  - **Contained** injuries - treated conservatively
  - **Non-contained** injuries (*need surgery*):
    If **small** injury and **minimal contamination** → primary closure
    If **extensive** injury or severe **contamination** (ie not repairable)→
      Neck - just place drains (will heal; *no* esophagectomy)
      Chest - chest tubes to drain injury, place neck spit fistula, staple across lower esophagus (eventually need esophagectomy)
  - Always drain esophageal and hypopharyngeal repairs - 20% leak rate
  - Approach to **esophageal injuries**:
    Neck - **left side**
    Upper ⅔ thoracic esophagus - **right thoracotomy** (avoids aorta)
    Lower ⅓ thoracic esophagus - **left thoracotomy** (left sided course)
- **Laryngeal fracture** and **tracheal** (neck) injuries
  - *These can be airway emergencies*
  - If **stridor** or **respiratory compromise** → secure airway *emergently* in *ED* (possible cricothyroidotomy)
  - If **crepitus** or **bloody sputum** → intubate in *OR* (RSI can change airway status here - be in OR for emergency airway management)
  - Tx: primary repair, can use strap muscle for airway support; tracheostomy necessary for most to allow edema to subside and to check for stricture (need to convert cricothyroidotomy to tracheostomy, otherwise will have vocal cord Cx's)
- **Thyroid gland** injuries - suture ligation for bleeding; place drains (*not* thyroidectomy)
- **Recurrent laryngeal nerve** injury (can be iatrogenic injury intra-op) - can try to repair or can re-implant in cricoarytenoid muscle (Sx - hoarseness)
- **Shotgun injures** to neck - **CT angio** if asymptomatic with **esophagus** and **trachea** evaluation
- **Vertebral artery** bleeds - can embolize or ligate without sequela in majority

CHEST TRAUMA
- **Hemothorax**
  - Indications for **OR thoracotomy** (on side of injury) after **chest tube placement:**:
    > 1000-1500 cc after initial insertion
    > 250 cc/h for 3 hours
    > 2,500 cc over 24 hours
    Bleeding in an unstable patient
  - Need to drain all of the blood (in < 48 hours) to prevent fibrothorax, pulmonary entrapment, infected hemothorax, and empyema
  - **Unresolved hemothorax** despite 2 well-placed chest tubes → Tx: VATS drainage (wait until patient stable from trauma)
  - Most important RF for **empyema** in trauma - **retained hemothorax**
- **Persistent large pneumothorax after chest tube**
  - Make sure **1st chest tube** has good placement and system working
  - Place **2nd chest tube anteriorly in apex**
  - Still doesn't resolve → **bronchoscopy** to look for **tracheo-bronchial injury** or **mucus plug**
- **Sucking chest wound** (open pneumothorax)
  - Needs to be at least ⅔ the diameter of the trachea to be significant
  - Cover wound with dressing that has tape on three sides → prevents development of tension pneumothorax while allowing the lung to expand with inspiration
- **Trachea** (chest) **and bronchial injury**
  - MC with blunt trauma
  - Sx's: **worsening oxygenation** after chest tube placement (patient takes a deep breath in and it goes out chest tube), large **continuous air-leak**, extensive **pneumomediastinum, persistent pneumothorax**

- MC in <u>right</u> mainstem bronchus (not as flexible)
- May need to **mainstem intubate** patient on unaffected side (use **long single lumen** tube - *avoid double lumen tube which can cause more injury*)
- One of the few indications in which **clamping the chest tube** may be indicated (prevents chest tube from sucking air out the injury and away from the lungs)
- Dx: **bronchoscopy** (95% of these injuries are within 1 cm of carina)
- **Indications for repair**:
  1) Respiratory compromise
  2) Unable to get lung up
  3) After 1-2 weeks of persistent air leak
  4) Injuries > 1/3 the size of the tracheal or bronchial lumen
- **Right thoracotomy** - for right mainstem, trachea in chest, and proximal *left* mainstem injuries (avoids the aorta)
- *Rare* left thoracotomy for very unlikely <u>distal left mainstem injuries</u>
- Note - you rarely ever want to clamp a chest tube in trauma because of the risk of developing a tension pneumothorax
- **Esophageal injury** - see section "Neck Trauma"
- **Diaphragm rupture**
  - MC on **left side** and to result from **blunt trauma**
  - CXR - may see **air-fluid level** in chest from **stomach herniation** through ruptured diaphragm (Dx can be made on that finding); may see NG tube in chest
  - Chest CT - these injuries can be hard to find
  - Tx:
    - **Trans-abdominal** (eg laparotomy) approach if **< 1 week** since injury
    - **Chest** approach (thoracotomy) if **> 1 week** since injury (need to take down adhesions in chest)
    - Usually need **mesh** (PTFE [Gortex]) to repair hole in the diaphragm
- **Aortic transection** - usually from rapid deceleration injury (usually MVA)
  - 80% of these patients die at the scene
  - **CXR** - widened mediastinum, 1st or 2nd rib Fx's, apical capping, loss of aortopulmonary window, loss of aortic contour, left hemothorax, trachea deviation to the right
  - Mediastinal widening is usually from laceration of bridging veins and arteries in the mediastinum (*not* blood leaking from aorta itself*)
  - MC tear location - **ligamentum arteriosum** (just distal to subclavian)
  - CXR normal in 5% - need aortic evaluation in patients with significant mechanism (head on car crash > 45 mph, fall > 15 feet)
  - Dx: **chest CT angio** (to screen; **aortogram** is the gold standard)
  - *Important to* **treat other life-threatening injuries** <u>before</u> *the aortic transection* → positive FAST scan or other life-threatening injury (eg large subdural hematoma, pelvic Fx with hemorrhage) needs to be addressed <u>before</u> the aortic transection; patient should be stable before aortic repair (may take 24-48 hours)
  - Significant **intra-cranial hemorrhage** is a <u>contraindication</u> to open repair (Tx: covered stent endograft)
  - Operative approach:
    1) **Left thoracotomy** (posterolateral) and repair on partial left heart bypass with **interposition graft** <u>or</u>;
    2) Place a **covered stent endograft** (*best*, distal transections only)
- **Thoracic vascular injuries**
  - In general get **proximal** and **distal control** before open repair (bypass graft often used but primary repair possible); endovascular repair being used for some injuries (eg descending aortic transection)
  - **Median sternotomy** for injuries to:
    - Ascending aorta
    - Innominate artery (may need cervical extension)
    - Proximal right subclavian artery (cervical extension)
    - Proximal right (cervical extension) or proximal left common carotid artery
    - Proximal left subclavian artery (need **trap door incision** by dividing the left 2nd intercostal space and elevating the 1st and 2nd ribs)
    - Innominate vein
    - Superior vena cava (and intra-thoracic inferior vena cava)

- **Left thoracotomy** for injuries to:
  - Distal left subclavian artery
  - Descending aorta (eg aortic transection at ligamentum arteriosum)
- **Right mid-clavicular incision ± resection of medial clavicle**
  - Distal right subclavian artery
- Ligation of the **subclavian artery** can *generally* be performed in *emergency settings*; usually well tolerated (lots of collaterals around shoulder - issue is that 1-2% of patients have an incomplete Circle of Willis and a dominant vertebral artery, which comes off the subclavian artery [results in posterior stroke])
- **Cardiac contusion** (myocardial contusion)
  - Sx's (RFs): sternal fracture (high risk), sternal contusion, no seatbelt
  - MCC of *death* - **ventricular fibrillation** (VF; highest risk in 1st 24 hrs)
  - MC *arrhythmia* overall in these patients - **supra-ventricular tachycardia** (SVT)
  - Dx: **EKG** *(best test)* - **conduction abnormalities** most significant finding; any finding other than NSR is considered significant
  - If *both* the **EKG** *and* **troponin I** are **normal** → do *not* need telemonitoring (these patients do not have cardiac contusion - essentially 0% false negative rate)
  - If either the EKG is abnormal *or* troponin I is elevated → **telemonitoring** for 24-48 hours (EKG with anything other than normal sinus rhythm is *abnormal*)
  - Tx: **telemonitoring** for 24 hours (**amiodarone** for stable arrhythmias other than SVT; **cardioversion** for unstable arrhythmias)
- **Flail chest** - ≥ 2 consecutive ribs broken at ≥ 2 sites → results in paradoxical motion of the chest wall
  - Underlying **pulmonary contusion** is the biggest pulmonary impairment (not the flail chest itself)
  - Tx: may need **intubation** for underlying pulmonary impairment
- **Multiple rib Fx's** and patient is **splinting** → consider paravertebral block or thoracic epidural (allows pain relief; improves breathing and hypoxemia)
- **Aspiration** - may not produce CXR findings immediately
- Traumatic causes of **cardiogenic shock** - cardiac tamponade, cardiac contusion, tension pneumothorax
- **Tension pneumothorax** (one-way valve effect causes air entry into pleural space and pressure builds up)
  - Sx's: hypotension, tachycardia, tachypnea, *high* airway pressures on ventilator, *decreased* breath sounds, bulging neck veins, trachea shift away from injured side
  - Hypotension can worsen after **intubation**
  - Can see **bulging diaphragm** during laparotomy
  - Cardiac compromise from **decreased venous return** (SVC + IVC compression)
  - Tx: **chest tube** (thoracostomy tube); needle decompression an option if chest tube not available
- **Cardiac tamponade**
  - Sx's: hypotension, distended neck veins, and muffled heart sounds (Beck's Triad)
  - Dx: **FAST scan**; If FAST scan shows **pericardial fluid** → **pericardiocentesis** or **OR pericardial window** to decompress tamponade
  - If pericardial window or pericardiocentesis shows **blood** → need **median sternotomy** to find injury
  - Patient **coding** → ED left anterior-lateral thoracotomy, open pericardium
  - Mechanism - **decreased right ventricle filling** due to compression from pericardial fluid (blood)
- **Lung injury bleeding** - perform **pulmonary tractotomy** with stapler to get to the bleeding spot; can staple bleeding site and air leaks *(not formal lobectomy)*
  - **Severe bleeding lung injury** → clamp **pulmonary hilum** for control
- **Hole in the heart** → digital compression (finger in the hole), pledgetted suture closure
- **Aortic penetrating injury** - clamp aorta proximally and distally, fix hole with pledgetted suture
- Intercostal arteries and the internal mammary artery can bleed significantly
- **Sternal Fx** - these patients are at high risk for **cardiac contusion**
- **1st and 2nd rib Fx's** - high risk for **aortic transection**

PELVIC TRAUMA (see previous blunt trauma section for acute management)

■ Pelvic fractures can be a major source of **blood loss**

■ If hemodynamically unstable with pelvic fracture and negative FAST scan, negative CXR, and no other reasons for blood loss → stabilize pelvis (C-clamp, external fixator, or sheet) and go to angio for **embolization**

■ **Anterior** pelvic fractures - more likely to have **venous** bleeding from pelvic venous plexus (MC bleeding source with pelvic Fx)

■ **Posterior** pelvic fractures - more likely to have **arterial** bleeding

■ **Pelvic fixation** (external fixator) will tamponade most pelvic venous bleeding

■ **Angio-embolization** is required for most pelvic arterial bleeding

■ **Severe pelvic fractures** - high risk for **genitourinary** and **rectal** injuries
  ● Need **proctoscopy, retrograde urethrogram** (RUG), and **cystogram**

■ May need colostomy for severe rectal or perineal lacerations

■ Pelvic Fx repair itself may need to be delayed until other associated injuries are repaired

■ **Penetrating injury** pelvic hematomas intra-op - open
  ● Vascular control at aortic bifurcation and where common iliac veins join IVC
  ● At times may need **angio-embolization** or **covered stent** for associated vascular injuries

■ Blunt injury pelvic hematomas intra-op - leave
  ● If expanding or patient unstable → stabilize pelvic fracture, pack pelvis if in OR, and go to angiography for **embolization**; if packs are placed intra-op, remove after 24-48 hours when the patient is stable

■ **Isolated anterior ring** (eg pubic rami Fx) with minimal sacro-iliac displacement → Tx: weight bearing as tolerated (WBAT)

■ MC **associated injury** with pelvic fracture → **closed head injury** (CHI)

DUODENAL TRAUMA

■ Usually from **blunt** trauma (crush or tears from deceleration)

■ MC location for *tears* - **2nd portion** of duodenum (descending, usually near ampulla of Vater) - can also get tears near ligament of Treitz

■ MC location for *hematoma* - **3rd portion** (overlying spine)

■ Up to 25% mortality with **blunt duodenal injuries** due to associated **shock**

■ **Debridement** and **primary repair** - 80% of injuries requiring surgery can be treated this way

■ *Segmental resection with **primary end-to-end anastomosis** is possible with **all segments** except the **2nd portion** of the duodenum (Ampulla of Vater and ductal system prevents resection; can do **primary repair** to most 2nd portion injuries)*

■ **Diagnosing blunt duodenal injury** - **CT scan** with contrast initially; UGI contrast study *(best test)*
  ● CT scan may show bowel wall thickening, hematoma, free air, contrast leak, or retroperitoneal fluid / air
  ● **Intra-peritoneal free air** or leak → go to OR for repair
  ● **Retro-peritoneal air** or leak → non-operative management (NGT, NPO, TPN, bowel rest, and antibiotics)
  ● If CT scan is worrisome for injury but non-diagnostic, can repeat CT in 6-8 hours to see if finding is getting worse or get an UGI study

■ **Para-duodenal hematomas** on **CT scan** (or missed on initial CT scan)
  ● Can present with high **small bowel obstruction** 12-72 hours after injury (eg N/V); MC in children
  ● Dx: **UGI study** *(best test)* will show "**stacked coins**" or "**coiled spring**" appearance (usually in **3rd portion** of duodenum; should have no extravasation of contrast)
  ● Tx: **conservative** (NPO, NG tube, and TPN) - cures 90% over 2-3 weeks (hematoma is reabsorbed); if **contrast leak** is found → need open repair

■ **Intra-op paraduodenal hematomas** (≥ 2 cm) - open (both penetrating and blunt)

■ If at laparotomy and duodenal injury suspected, perform **Kocher maneuver** and **open lesser sac** through the omentum; check for hematoma, bile, sucus, and fat necrosis → if found, need formal inspection of the entire duodenum (also need to check for pancreatic injury)

- Kocher maneuver - the peritoneum to the right of the duodenum is incised and the duodenum / pancreas are reflected towards midline (mobilize colon hepatic flexure first)
  - Inspects the 2nd and 3rd portions of duodenum, the pancreas head, and portal triad structures
  - Indications for Kocher maneuver:
    - RUQ bile staining
    - Sucus drainage
    - Fat necrosis
    - Paraduodenal hematomas discovered intra-op
- Duodenal wall compromise (eg leak or loss of integrity) - Tx:
  - Try to get primary repair *(80% of injuries requiring surgery are treated with primary repair)*
    - If it involves > 75% of the bowel wall circumference, can't use primary repair (need segmental resection and primary anastomosis)
    - If the bowel wall circumference or the luminal diameter will be reduced by > 50%, can't use primary repair (need segmental resection and primary anastomosis)
    - May also need segmental resection and primary anastomosis if extensive injury (eg significant bowel wall missing; also through and through injuries)
    - Consider diversion with pyloric exclusion (staple but do not cut across the pylorus) and gastro-jejunostomy to allow healing
    - Place a distal feeding jejunostomy and a proximal draining jejunostomy tube that threads back to duodenal injury site
    - Place drains
  - If in 2nd portion of duodenum and can't get primary repair (eg large segment of wall missing; > 75% circumferential lesion; bowel lumen or circumference would be reduced to < 50% normal) →
    - *Resection and reanastomosis is generally not an option due to the proximity of the Ampulla of Vater and ductal system*
    - Place jejunal serosal patch over hole; may need future Whipple
    - Use pyloric exclusion, gastro-jejunostomy, drains, feeding tube
    - Duodeno-jejunostomy (end to end) may be an option depending on proximity to the Ampulla of Vater (eg >75% circumferential lesion)
    - *Single stage trauma Whipple is almost never indicated (very high mortality);* always perform staged procedure with damage control surgery first followed by Whipple 24-48 hours later (also allows time for ERCP or MRCP to fully evaluate the ampulla and ductal system)
  - Drains - remove when tolerating diet without an increase in drainage
  - Fistulas (major source of morbidity with duodenal injuries) - often close with time; Tx - bowel rest, TPN, octreotide, conservative Tx for 3-4 months (be patient with these)

SMALL BOWEL TRAUMA (other than duodenum)
- Usually penetrating injury - *MC organ injured with penetrating abdominal injury* (some texts say liver)
- Can be hard to find on CT with blunt trauma
- Occult small bowel injuries
  - CT scan showing intra-abdominal fluid not associated with a solid organ injury, bowel wall thickening, or a mesenteric hematoma is suggestive of injury
  - Need close observation and possibly repeat CT scan after 6-8 hours to make sure the finding is not getting worse
  - Make sure patients with non-conclusive findings can tolerate a diet before discharge
- Repair lacerations transversely → avoids stricture
- Large lacerations that are > 50% of bowel circumference or result in a lumen diameter or bowel circumference < 50% normal → Tx: resection and anastomosis
- Multiple close large lacerations - just resect that bowel segment
- Mesenteric hematomas - open if expanding or large (≥ 2 cm)

COLON TRAUMA (sigmoid colon considered left colon here)
- Most associated with **penetrating** injury
- **Right** and **transverse colon** injuries Tx: 1) primary repair _or_ 2) resection and anastomosis (for <u>destructive injuries</u> [ie > 50% circumference or associated with significant colon devascularization]); all are essentially treated like small bowel injuries
  - _No diversion needed for right and transverse colon injuries_
- **Left colon** - perform **primary repair <u>without diversion</u>** for all injuries if < 50% circumference and not associated with colon devascularization (treats <u>majority</u>)
  - If **left sided colectomy** is performed (ie for <u>destructive</u> lesions [> 50% circumference or colon devascularization]), _diverting ileostomy_ is indicated for: **gross contamination** (eg peritonitis), ≥ **6 hours** has elapsed between injury and repair, significant **comorbidities**, _or_ ≥ **6 units** pRBCs have been given
  - If patient is in **shock** and can't perform primary repair → just bring up **end colostomy** and leave **Hartman pouch** after resection (avoids left sided anastomosis in a sick patient and diverts stool)
- **Paracolonic hematomas** - <u>open</u> both blunt and penetrating

RECTAL TRAUMA
- Most associated with **penetrating** injury
- _Intra-peritoneal injuries:_
  - _Perform primary repair <u>without diversion</u> for all injuries if non-destructive_ (< 50% circumference and <u>not</u> associated with devascularization) - _treats <u>majority</u>_
  - If **low anterior resection** (LAR) is performed (ie for destructive lesions [> 50% circumference or for rectal devascularization]), _a diverting loop colostomy is <u>always indicated</u> (different than above);_ if in **shock**, place end colostomy <u>only</u>
- _Extra-peritoneal injuries_
  - _**High** rectal_ (proximal 1/3) - **primary repair** usual (**laparotomy**, mobilize rectum); if LAR needed, place diverting loop colostomy (follow LAR pathway above)
  - _**Middle** rectal_ (middle 1/3) - often inaccessible due to location (too low for laparotomy, too high for transanal repair); if repair not easily feasible, there is extensive damage, or if you can't find it → _**place end-colostomy** <u>only</u> (<u>not</u> APR);_ this area will heal after 6-8 weeks, take down colostomy at that time
  - _**Low** rectal_ (distal 1/3) - most repaired **primarily** with **transanal approach**; if repair not easibly feasible, there is extensive damage, or if you can't find it → _**place end-colostomy** <u>only</u> (<u>not</u> APR)_
- Presacral drains and rectal washout are generally <u>not</u> recommended

LIVER TRAUMA
- MC with **blunt** trauma (some texts say liver is MC blunt trauma intra-abdominal injury)
- Lobectomy almost <u>never</u> necessary
- **Common hepatic artery** - can be ligated under _emergency_ circumstances (collaterals through the gastroduodenal artery [GDA]; confirm GDA is present first)
- **Pringle maneuver** (intermittent clamping of the **portal triad**)
  - Used for **severe hepatic bleeding**
  - Does <u>not</u> stop bleeding from **hepatic veins** or **IVC**
  - Clamp for 15 min then remove for 5 min; allows time for repair of liver injuries
  - Effective for portal venous or hepatic artery bleeding
  - **Hepatocytes most sensitive to ischemia** - central lobar (acinar zone III)
  - The portal triad structures include the **portal vein** (posterior), **common bile duct** (lateral), and the **proper hepatic artery** (medial). The portal triad enters the liver at **segments IVb and V**
- **Damage control peri-hepatic packing** - can pack severe hepatic bleeding if the patient is unstable (and possibly coagulopathic) in the OR and the injury is not easily fixed (eg retro-hepatic IVC or hepatic vein injury)
  - Consider **angio-embolization**
  - Go to ICU and get patient resuscitated and stabilized (RBCs, FFP, and platelets; warm patient; correct acidosis and hypocalcemia)
  - Remove packs the next day
- **Severe retro-hepatic venous bleeding** (from **hepatic veins** or **IVC**) and not easily repaired →

- Tx: **Place packs** *(best option)*; hard to fix these injuries; perform damage control peri-hepatic packing and see if its **controlled**:
     - a. If **bleeding controlled** → consider angio-embolization; go to ICU and follow damage control peri-hepatic packing pathway above
     - b. If **bleeding not controlled** → 1) **Atrio-caval shunt** (diverts blood and allows repair; supra-renal IVC; use 32 Fr chest tube or ET tube as shunt) or 2) **extracorporeal bypass** (infra-renal IVC to right atrium)
- Place **sterile covering** (instead of closing the abdomen primarily) to prevent abdominal compartment syndrome if its hard to get abdominal contents back in the abdomen (occurs with massive resuscitation)
- **Portal triad hematomas** - need to be explored
- **Common bile duct injury**
     - Kocher maneuver and dissect out the portal triad to find these injuries
     - < 50% circumference - **repair over stent**
     - > 50% circumference or complex injury - **choledochojejunostomy**
     - May need intra-op cholangiogram to define injury
     - 10% of duct anastomoses leak - **place drains** intra-op
     - Late Cx - **biliary stricture** at site of repair
- **Portal vein injury** (or **superior mesenteric vein**) - need to repair (50% mortality with ligation)
     - May need to **transect** the pancreas to get to portal vein injury
     - Will need to perform **distal pancreatectomy** with that maneuver
     - Tx: side biting clamp (allows blood flow with primary repair [lateral venorrhaphy])
- **Subcapsular** hepatic hematomas → *leave alone if <u>stable</u> (ie <u>no</u> contrast extravasation, <u>no</u> pseudoaneurysm)*
- **Leave drains** intra-op with liver injuries
- **Unstable patients** (SBP < 90 despite 2 L LR) with blunt liver injuries should **go to the OR** (may need angio-embolization later)
- **Non-operative management** of blunt liver injuries (only in **stable** patients)
     - If the patient becomes **unstable** (SBP < 90) or is a **transient responder** despite aggressive resuscitation including ≥ **4 units** of pRBCs or requires ≥ **4 units** of pRBCs to keep Hct > 25 → **go to OR** (if unstable) *or* angio-embolization (if transient responder)
     - **Active contrast extravasation** (ie blush) or **pseudoaneurysm** on CT scan and patient is **stable** or transient responder → **angio-embolization**
     - With non-operative management requires bed rest for **5 days**
     - The higher the injury grade, the more likely an intervention is needed (highest is **grade VI** - <u>hepatic avulsion</u>, likely not compatible with life)
- **Fluid collection** late after severe liver injury → Tx: place **percutaneous drain** <u>only</u> (likely bile leak; **95%** resolve with conservative Tx)
- **Hemobilia** after trauma
     - Sx's: **abdominal pain, jaundice,** and **hematemesis** (± melena) <u>late</u> after trauma (*classic*; mean **4 weeks** after initial event; can also occur after hepatic surgery or percutaneous intervention to liver)
     - **MCC** - <u>iatrogenic</u> (eg PTC tubes, laparoscopic liver Bx, lap choly and injury to right hepatic artery)
     - **MC situation** - hepatic artery to biliary duct fistula
     - Dx: **EGD** - will see **blood coming out of the Ampulla of Vater**
     - Tx: **angio-embolization**; surgical ligation if that is unsuccessful

SPLEEN TRAUMA

- Usually **blunt trauma** *(MC organ injured with blunt trauma)*; fully healed after **6 weeks**
- Post-splenectomy sepsis greatest risk **within 2 years** of splenectomy
- Splenic salvage is associated with increased transfusion rate
- Threshold for splenectomy in **children** is high - *unusual to have splenectomy*
- **Subcapsular** splenic hematomas → *leave alone if <u>stable</u> (ie <u>no</u> contrast extravasation, <u>no</u> pseudoaneurysm)*
- **Unstable patients** (SBP < 90 despite 2 L LR) with blunt splenic injuries → **go to OR**
- **Non-operative management** of blunt splenic injuries (only in **stable patients**)
     - If the patient becomes **unstable** (SBP < 90) or is a **transient responder** despite aggressive resuscitation including ≥ **2 units** of pRBCs or requires ≥ **2 units** of

pRBCs to keep Hct > 25 → **go to OR** (if unstable) *or* **angio-embolization** (if transient responder)

- **Active contrast extravasation** (ie blush) or **pseudoaneurysm** on CT scan and patient is **stable** or **transient responder** → angio-embolization
- With non-operative management need bed rest for **5 days**
- The higher the injury grade, the more likely an intervention will be needed (highest **grade V** - completely shattered spleen or complete hilar disruption that devascularizes spleen)

- **Fluid collection** late after splenectomy → Tx: place **percutaneous drain** *only* (likely injured the tail of the pancreas, fluid will be high in **amylase**); vast majority (> 95%) resolve with conservative Tx
  - Can also present as late fluid collection after conservative Tx for splenic trauma (fracture in tail of pancreas); same Tx as above
- *Contraindications* to intra-op splenic salvage - unstable patient, grade V injury, coagulopathy, or other serious injury (eg concomitant severe liver trauma with closed head injury → removes confounding issue)
- **Need immunizations 2 weeks** after splenectomy (pneumococcus, meningococcus, Haemophilus influenza) - see Splenectomy chapter for post-splenectomy issues

PANCREATIC TRAUMA

- Most associated with **penetrating injury** (80%)
- **Blunt injury** - can result in **pancreatic fractures** (results in duct fracture), usually perpendicular to the duct (Tx: distal pancreatectomy)
- **Kocher maneuver** - evaluates pancreatic head (also **open the lesser sac** by going through the omentum to inspect the rest of the pancreas) - need to evaluate the duodenum with pancreas injuries
- Edema or necrosis of peri-pancreatic fat usually indicative of injury
- **Pancreatic contusion** - leave if stable, place drains if in OR
- **Intra-op pancreatic hematoma** - open (both penetrating and blunt)
- 80% of injuries found **intra-op** are treated with **drains only** (ie the pancreatic duct is not involved)
- The **primary concern** for pancreatic injuries is to figure out whether or not the **pancreatic duct** is injured
- **Distal pancreatic duct injury** - Tx: distal pancreatectomy, can take up to 80% of the gland (leave drains)
  - **Splenic vein** is directly posterior to pancreas
  - **Splenic artery** is superior and posterior
- **Pancreatic head duct injury that is not reparable** - place **drains** initially and damage control surgery first *(mortality too high with single stage trauma Whipple → 50%)*
  - Damage control surgery *first* with delayed Whipple (after 24-48 hours) improves survival (staged Whipple)
- Whipple vs. distal pancreatectomy based on duct injury in relation to the **SMV** (superior mesenteric vein)
- Persistent / rising **amylase** or **abdominal pain** *late* after blunt trauma or *late* after distal pancreatectomy → may indicate missed pancreatic injury or suture line leak
  - Dx: **CT scan** (will show fluid collection near pancreas)
  - Tx: **percutaneous drain** *only* as initial step (95% resolve; fluid will be high in **amylase**), may need ERCP with stent if it fails to resolve
- CT scans can be poor at diagnosing pancreatic injuries initially
  - Delayed signs - fluid, edema, necrosis
- **ERCP** good at finding duct injuries; may be able to treat with sphincterotomy and temporary stent

ORTHOPEDIC TRAUMA (also see Orthopedic chapter)

- Can have **> 2 L blood** loss from a **femur fracture** (hypotensive patient)
- Orthopedic emergencies - pelvic Fx in unstable patients, spine injury with deficit, open fractures, dislocations or fractures with vascular compromise, compartment syndrome
- Femoral neck fractures and hip dislocations - are at high risk for **avascular necrosis** (should be repaired within 24 hours)
- **Long bone fracture** or **dislocation** with **loss of pulse** (or weak pulse) → Tx: immediate reduction and reassessment of pulse / ABI:

- If pulse does not return → **go to OR** for vascular bypass or repair (may need angiography in OR to define injury)
- If pulse is weak (ABI < 0.9) → **CT angio**
- All **posterior knee dislocations** need a **formal angiogram** after reduction, unless pulse is absent, in which case you would just go to OR (25% risk of popliteal artery injury); return of pulses after reduction does not rule-out arterial injury after posterior knee dislocations
- Concomitant major arterial, venous, and nerve injuries increase risk of amputation

Fracture / Dislocation	Concomitant Injury
Upper Extremity	
Anterior shoulder (humerus) dislocation	Axillary nerve
Posterior shoulder (humerus) dislocation	Axillary artery
Proximal humerus Fx	Axillary nerve
Mid-shaft humerus Fx (or spiral Fx)	Radial nerve
Distal (supracondylar) humerus Fx	Brachial artery
Elbow (ulnar) dislocation	Brachial artery
Distal radius Fx	Median nerve
Lower Extremity	
Anterior hip (femur) dislocation	Femoral artery
Posterior hip (femur) dislocation	Sciatic nerve
Distal (supracondylar) femur Fx	Popliteal artery
Posterior knee dislocation	Popliteal artery
Fibula neck Fx	Common peroneal nerve
Other	
Temporal bone Fx	Epidural hematoma, facial nerve
Parietal bone Fx	Epidural hematoma
Maxillofacial Fx	Cervical spine Fx
Sternal Fx	Cardiac contusion
First or Second rib Fx	Aortic transection
Scapula Fx	Aortic transection
Rib Fx's (left, 8-12)	Spleen laceration
Rib Fx's (right, 8-12)	Liver laceration
Pelvic Fx	Bladder, urethral, rectal injuries

VASCULAR TRAUMA

- **Vascular repair** (or vascular shunt) performed _before_ **orthopedic repair**
- Pulse deficit or distal ischemia with orthopedic injury → reduce fracture or dislocation 1st, then re-assess pulse / ABIs (ankle brachial index)
- **Major signs** of extremity vascular injury (hard signs):
  - Active hemorrhage
  - Pulse deficit
  - Expanding or pulsatile hematoma
  - Distal ischemia
  - Bruit or thrill
  → go to **OR for exploration** for any of above (may need angio in OR to define injury)
- **Minor signs** of extremity vascular injury (soft signs):
  - History of hemorrhage
  - Large stable / non-pulsatile hematoma
  - ABI < 0.9
  - Unequal pulses
  → get **CT angio** for any of above (formal angiogram if vascular injury found)
- Proximity of injury to a major artery and injury to an anatomically related major nerve are **not** indications for CT angio
- ABI ≥ 0.9, no major/minor signs, and no fracture → Tx: **observation** (no further work-up, discharge from ED; _exception_ - posterior knee dislocations)
  - _All_ posterior knee dislocations require formal angiogram
- Injuries with **flow limitation** → Tx: need primary repair, interposition graft, or place a covered stent
- **Exposure for lower leg:**

1) **Above knee** popliteal - posterolateral retraction of **sartorius**
2) **Below knee** popliteal - posterolateral retraction of **gastrocnemius** (medial head)
■ **Saphenous vein interposition graft** - needed if artery segment **> 2 cm** is missing
  ● Use vein from the **contralateral leg** when fixing lower extremity arterial injuries (*avoid* PTFE)
■ Cover site of anastomosis with viable tissue and muscle
■ Consider *prophylactic* **fasciotomy** if ischemia **> 4-6 hours** (prevents compartment syndrome)
■ **Compartment syndrome** - consider if compartment pressures are **> 20 - 25 mmHg** or if clinical exam suggests elevated pressures (see also Vascular chapter)
  ● **Classic scenario**: injury with loss of blood flow → repair (> 4-6 hours later) → **pain** and **swelling** *soon* post-op
  ● Sx's: **pain with passive motion** *(1st finding)* and a **swollen tender extremity** (loss of pulse is a late finding)
  ● High risk injuries - supracondylar humeral fractures (Volkman contracture), tibial plateau fractures, crush injuries (especially lower extremities), or other injuries that result in a disruption and then restoration of blood flow after 4-6 hours
  ● Can occur in *any* muscle compartment (compartment pressure exceeds capillary filling pressure; ischemia / **rhabdomyolysis** occurs)
  ● In the lower extremity, the **anterior compartment** is most likely to be affected (get foot drop from dead muscle)
  ● Is a **reperfusion injury** mediated by **PMNs** (neutrophils); tissues in the compartment **swell**, leading to increased **pressure** in the compartment, which eventually *exceeds* capillary filling pressure, and results in **ischemia**
  ● Dx: *based on **clinical suspicion** (if suspected → fasciotomy)*
  ● Tx: **fasciotomy** (medial and lateral incisions for four compartment fasciotomy in the leg)
      With fasciotomy, you are through the fascia when the **muscle bulges**
      Incise the **total length** of the compartment (eg length of the leg)
      Remove all dead tissue (myoglobinemia if you don't resect)
      After 5-10 days place skin grafts
  ● The **superficial peroneal nerve** can be injured with the **lateral fasciotomy incision** for the lower extremity (decreased foot eversion)
  ● The **soleus muscle** must be detached from the proximal tibia to reach the deep muscle compartment with medial fasciotomy incision for the lower extremity
  ● Undiagnosed compartment syndrome can present as **renal failure** (dark urine from myoglobinuria; myoglobin release from injured / dead muscle)
  ● **Myoglobinuria Tx**: aggressive **normal saline hydration** *(best)*, **alkalinize urine** with HCO_3^- (prevents precipitation to ferrihemate - the toxic metabolite)
■ **Rhabdomyolysis** - can occur with compartment syndrome, severe extremity trauma, crush injuries, and burns
  ● Results in **myoglobin** release as well as **hyperkalemia, acidemia,** and **hyperphosphatemia;** have significant release of **creatine kinase** (> 5000 U/L)
  ● Always check for **compartment syndrome** if rhabdomyolysis occurs
■ **IVC injury** (infra-hepatic, Cattell for exposure) - primary repair if residual diameter is > 50% the normal IVC; otherwise place saphenous vein or synthetic patch
  ● Bleeding from IVC is best controlled with proximal and distal pressure, not clamps → can tear it
  ● Repair posterior wall injury through the anterior wall (may need to cut through the anterior IVC to get to posterior IVC injuries)
■ **Celiac** or **SMA** with **pseudoaneurysm, blush**, or large **hemo-retroperitoneum** - Tx: OR for repair *or* angiography for covered stent (*do not embolize these injuries*)
■ **Vein injuries** that need **repair** - vena cavae; portal vein; superior mesenteric, femoral, popliteal, innominate, subclavian, and axillary veins (primary repair or vein patch)
■ **Arterial injuries** that can *generally* be **ligated** in the *emergency* setting (should always attempt **repair** for following as ligation has a 1-2% risk of severe ischemia) →
  ● Either **subclavian artery** (lots of collaterals around shoulder)
  ● Either the **radial** *or* **ulnar artery** (need a pulse in other vessel)
  ● Either the **anterior tibial artery** *or* **posterior tibial artery** (need a pulse in other vessel [ie dorsalis pedis or posterior tibialis])

URETER TRAUMA
- MCC - **penetrating** trauma
- *Hematuria is not a reliable indicator*
- **Multi-shot IVP** *(best test,* good for penetrating wounds to lower quadrants or if worried about ureteral injury; identifies injury and presence of 2 functional kidneys)
  - other tests - retrograde cysto-urethrogram, CT scan with contrast
- **Cattell or Mattox** maneuver for exposure
- If *large* (≥ **2 cm**) ureteral segment is missing → you can not perform primary anastomosis (ends will not reach):
  - **Upper** and middle ⅓ **injuries will not reach bladder** (ie above the pelvic brim) Tx: temporize with percutaneous nephrostomy (tie off both ends of the ureter) or externalized drainage catheter (connect to ureter); eventual trans-ureteroureterostomy (connects to other ureter) or ileal conduit
  - **Lower** ⅓ injuries Tx: implant in the bladder (ureterocystostomy); may need bladder psoas hitch procedure so that the ureter can reach
- If *small* (< 2 cm) ureteral segment is missing:
  - **Upper** and middle ⅓ **injuries** Tx: mobilize both ends of ureter and perform primary anastomosis over stent (absorbable suture, 6-0 PDS)
  - **Lower** ⅓ **injuries** - Tx: still implant in the bladder (easier anastomosis than primary repair)
- **Partial transections** can be repaired over stent
- Avoid stripping the ureters (devascularization) - blood supply is **medial** to upper 2/3 of ureter and **lateral** to lower 1/3 of ureter
- **Leave drains** for all ureteral injuries
- These injuries can also occur with LAR, APR, and pelvic gynecologic / sarcoma resections *(95% involve the **lower** ⅓ of the ureter with repair using ureterocystostomy)*

RENAL TRAUMA
- MCC - **blunt** trauma
- 95% of renal injuries are treated non-operatively (eg **cortical lacerations**, collecting system disruptions, urine extravasation)
- **Hematuria** is the best indicator of renal trauma
- All patients with hematuria need an abdominal CT scan
- IVP (intravenous pyelogram) can be useful in the OR for patients without a CT scan → will identify the **injury** and presence of a functional **contralateral kidney**, which can affect intra-op decision making
- Anatomy
  - **Gerota's Fascia** covers kidney
  - **Anterior to posterior renal hilum** structures (VAP) - renal vein, renal artery, renal pelvis
    - **Right renal artery** is **posterior to IVC** (MC)
    - **Left renal vein** is **anterior to aorta** (MC) - need to watch for retro-aortic left renal vein when placing aortic clamp for open AAA repair
  - **Left renal vein**
    - Can be **ligated near IVC** in emergency situation (has **adrenal vein** and **gonadal vein** collaterals)
    - Right renal vein does not have these collaterals (plugs directly into IVC) - need repair or nephrectomy *(only if life saving)*
- **Urine extravasation** on **CT scan** - *vast majority do not require operation*
- Vascular pseudoaneuryms and active contrast extravasation - *majority* treated with angio interventions (eg stents, embolization)
- **Indications for operation:**
  - *Acutely* - ongoing renal hemorrhage in an unstable patient
  - *After acute phase (any):*
    - Major collecting system disruption
    - Unresolving urine extravasation
    - Severe hematuria
- With exploration, get control of **vascular hilum 1st** (aorta at base of transverse mesocolon to control origins of renal arteries [high at level of left renal vein])
  - *Unstable patients* - control aorta at diaphragm (intra-abdominal)

- Intra-op findings:
  - **Blunt** renal injury with **stable hematoma** → leave unless IVP or pre-op CT shows no blood flow or significant blood extravasation
  - **Penetrating** renal injury with **stable hematoma** → open unless IVP or pre-op CT shows good function without significant blood extravasation
  - **Expanding peri-renal hematoma** or **active hemorrhage** → explore
- Kidney exploration
  - **Left** side → Mattox maneuver
  - **Right** side → Cattell maneuver
  - Can use SVG (saphenous vein graft) if not enough length for primary renal artery or renal vein repair
- Intra-op and find a **kidney cortical laceration** - Tx: primary repair (although uncomplicated kidney cortical lacerations are *not* an indication for laparotomy - see above indications for operation)
- Place **drains** intra-op after repair, especially if collecting system is injured
- *Intra-venous* **methylene blue dye** can be used to check for urine leaks
- **Trauma to flank** and CT scan (or IVP) shows **no renal contrast uptake** (ie no blood flow to kidney) in a stable patient - Dx and Tx: **angiogram**; can stent if flap is present
- **Persistent shock** with severe vascular kidney injury and other concomitant life-threatening injuries - Tx: **nephrectomy** (feel for a kidney on contralateral side 1st)

BLADDER TRAUMA
- MCC - **blunt** trauma (> 95% associated with **pelvic fractures** - *MC associated injury*)
- **Hematuria** - best indicator of bladder trauma (although not specific)
- Sx's: meatal blood; sacral or scrotal hematoma
- Dx: **retrograde cystourethrogram** (*best test*)
- **Extra-peritoneal** bladder rupture - cystogram shows starbursts
  - Tx: **urinary catheter** (Foley) for 7-14 days (*no surgery*)
- **Intra-peritoneal** bladder rupture - often in kids, cystogram shows **leak**
  - Tx: laparotomy and **primary repair** of defect

URETHRA TRAUMA
- MCC - **blunt** trauma (> 95% associated with **pelvic fractures**)
- Increased incidence in **males**
- Sx's: **hematuria, blood at meatus, scrotal hematoma**; free floating prostate
- *No* **urinary catheter** *if urethral injury suspected* (membranous portion of urethra at risk for dissection / false passage / disruption)
- Dx: **retrograde urethrogram** (RUG, *best test*) shows contrast extravasation
- **Significant tears** - Tx: percutaneous **suprapubic cystostomy tube**, delayed repair in 2-3 months (*safest method* - high stricture / impotence rate if repaired early)
- **Small, partial tears** - Tx: may get away with bridging urethral catheter across tear area (leave for 2-3 weeks → is definitive Tx)
- **Genital trauma** - can get fracture in erectile bodies from vigorous sex
  - Tx: repair tunica albuginea / Buck's fascia if damaged (enclose erectile bodies)
- **Testicular trauma** - get U/S to see if tunica albuginea violated, repair if necessary

PEDIATRIC TRAUMA
- MCC of childhood death
- Trauma bolus - **LR** 20 cc/kg × 2, then give **blood** 10 cc/kg
- Increased risk of **hypothermia** (high BSA compared with weight) and **head injury**
- **Tachycardia** - *best indicator of shock in children*
  - Others - tachypnea, mental status changes (eg lethargy)
  - BP is not a good indicator of blood loss in children - *last thing to go*

Normal Vital Signs by Age

Age Group	Heart Rate (beats/min)	Respiratory Rate (breaths/min)
Infant (< 1 yr)	140	40
Preschool (1 - 5 yr)	120	30
Adolescent (5 - 12 yr)	100	20
Teen (≥ 13 yrs)	80	15

TRAUMA DURING PREGNANCY

- There should be an emphasis on **maternal stabilization** *(shock is the MCC of placental abruption)*
- Blood volume increases with normal pregnancy and **Hct decreases** (3rd trimester Hct is normally **27-33**)
- Pregnancy should not lead to "underdiagnosis" or "undertreatment" due to unfounded fears of fetal effects (rads < 5-10 have not been shown to have a negative impact on the fetus, especially after the 1st trimester)
- Fetal radiation risk is highest in the <u>1st trimester</u>
- Estimate pregnancy based on **fundal height** (20 cm = 20 wk = umbilicus)
- Place **fetal monitor** and **uterine tocodynamometer**
  - Indications for *__continuous__* fetal monitoring (<u>*any*</u> below; leave for 4-24 hours) - vaginal bleeding, abnormal trauma labs (eg lactate, AST, amylase), ≥ 4 contractions per hour
  - *Normal* fetal HR: **120-160**
- Check for vaginal discharge (blood, amnion)
- Check for effacement, dilation, and fetal station
- Roll **patient to the left** to decrease compression on IVC *(prevents* **hypotension**)
- **Significant trauma** and **stable** patient (eg abdominal pain, closed head injury, pelvic fracture, significant extremity injury, hematuria, paraplegia)
  - Get work-up - **CXR**; **head / neck CT**, and **abdomen / pelvic CT** (total rads 3.5)
- **Significant trauma** and **unstable** patient - use **FAST scan** as initial assessment
- Significant <u>mechanism</u> (eg high speed MVA), **stable** patient, and **no physical signs of injury** - use **FAST screening** (CT scan of the abdomen and pelvis if positive); admit patient for 24 hour observation
- **Minor** trauma (eg ground level fall, minor injury) - directed work-up, use uterine shielding
- Fetus needs to be at least **24 weeks** to survive outside mother
- Signs of **placental abruption** - uterine tenderness, contractions ≥ 4 per hour, fetal HR < 120, vaginal bleeding
  - Can be caused by **shock** (#1) or **mechanical forces** (#2)
  - Placental lining separates from the uterus (50% fetal demise)
- Indications for **C-section** in a **stable mother** (> 24 weeks) <u>*any*</u> below;
  - Prsistent fetal bradycardia
  - Late decelerations despite adequate fluid resuscitation
  - Placental abruption
- Indications for **C-section** at **laparotomy** or in a **critically ill mother** (<u>*any*</u> below):
  - Persistent maternal shock or severe injuries and pregnancy near term (> 34 weeks)
  - Pregnancy a threat to the mother's life (eg hemorrhage, DIC)
  - Mechanical limitation to a life-threatening vessel injury
  - Risk of fetal distress exceeds risk of immaturity
  - Direct intra-uterine trauma

HEMATOMAS

Intra-op Hematoma Management

Hematoma ($\geq$ 2 cm)	Penetrating	Blunt
Pelvic	Open	Leave
Paraduodenal	Open	Open
Portal triad	Open	Open
Retrohepatic	Leave if stable	Leave
Midline supramesocolic	Open	Open
Midline inframesocolic	Open	Open
Pericolonic	Open	Open
Perirenal	Open[a]	Leave[b]
[a]Unless pre-op CT scan or IVP shows no significant injury		
[b]Unless pre-op CT scan or IVP shows no blood flow or major blood extravasation		

Retroperitoneal Hematoma Management

Zone	Location	Potential Injuries
1	**Central** (medial to psoas)	Pancreas, duodenum, aorta and its proximal branches, IVC - **explore** for *both* blunt and penetrating injury Divided into **Supramesocolic** and **Inframesocolic** (see below for exposure and proximal vascular control)
2	**Flank** (lateral to psoas)	Kidney, ureter, or colon - **explore** for penetrating; **leave** for blunt (unless expanding / pulsatile perirenal hematoma or a colon injury) Need Mattox / Cattell for exposure **Aortic** control (if needed) at **diaphragmatic hiatus** (best in acute situations) **IVC** control (if needed) after **Cattell** *Retrohepatic hematoma* - **leave** for both blunt and penetrating unless ruptured, expanding, or pulsatile *(hard to fix)*
3	**Pelvis**	Penetrating injury - generally **explore** although angio-intervention may be indicated; vascular control at **aortic bifurcation** and junction of **iliac veins with IVC** Pelvic fractures (blunt) - **leave** hematomas alone; pelvic stabilization and angio-embolization may be needed

Supramesocolic Zone I - at or above the root of the transverse mesocolon (supra-renal aorta, celiac axis, renal vessels, and proximal SMA)
*Proximal **aortic control** - at abdominal **diaphragmatic hiatus** (need left thoracotomy if hematoma is at the level of the **diaphragm**); then Mattox maneuver for exposure (not Cattell - liver is in the way)*

Inframesocolic Zone I - below the root of the transverse mesocolon (infra-renal aorta, infra-hepatic IVC)
*Proximal **aortic control** (if needed) - infra-renal aorta just **below the left renal vein** (same exposure as AAA repair) at the **base of the transverse mesocolon** (transverse mesocolon pulled towards head, small bowel to the right)*
*Proximal **IVC control** (if needed) - just **below renal vein insertions** (use compression, not clamp); **Cattell maneuver** for exposure*

- In general, **penetrating** retroperitoneal hematomas are **explored** (except retro-hepatic)
- Management of **blunt** retroperitoneal hematomas is variable (see above table)
- **Mattox maneuver** - spleen, pancreas, and left colon are medially rotated (good for aortic, left renal, and left iliac structures)
- **Cattell maneuver** - duodenum and right colon are medially rotated (good for infra-hepatic IVC, right renal, and right iliac structures)

SHOCK
- **Respiratory rate** progressively ↑s with shock
- *Shock* = inadequate tissue perfusion
- **1st response** to hemorrhagic shock - ↑ed diastolic pressure (vasoconstriction)

TRAUMA STATISTICS
- **Trauma deaths**
  - **1st peak** (0 to 30 min) - most deaths due to **hemorrhage** (MC, lacerations of heart, aorta) and brain; can't save these patients
  - **2nd peak** (30 min to 4 hrs) - deaths due to **head injury** (MC) and **hemorrhage**; patients you can save with rapid assessment (golden hour)
  - **3rd peak** (days to weeks) - deaths due to **MSOF** and **sepsis**

1) **Hemorrhage** - MCC of death in 1st hour
2) **Head injury** - MCC death after reaching the ED alive
3) **Infection** - MCC death long term

OTHER

- **Blunt injury** - 80% of all trauma
- **Penetrating injury** - **small bowel** MC injured
- **Blunt Injury** - **spleen** MC injured (some say liver)
- **Tongue** - MCC of upper airway obstruction → perform jaw thrust
- **Seat belts** - small bowel perforations, lumbar spine Fx, sternal Fx
- **Catecholamines** - peak 24-48 hours after injury
- **ADH, ACTH,** and **glucagon** - all ↑ after trauma (fight or flight response)
- **Thyroid hormone** - _not involved in flight or flight_
- **Serum lactate** (< 2.5) - best measure of adequate resuscitation in trauma patients (or patients in hemorrhagic shock for other reasons)
- **Drains** - leave drains intra-op for pancreatic, liver, biliary system, urinary, and duodenal injuries
- **Snakebites** (Sx's depend on species) - shock, bradycardia, and arrhythmias can result; Tx: stabilize patient, anti-venin, tetanus shot
- **Hypothermia** (< 35 C; bradycardia, reduced cardiac output, and arrhythmias develop as temp drops)
  - Best initial Tx: **warm air conduction** (Bair hugger)
  - Extreme (< 27 C) Tx: **cardiopulmonary bypass** (highest rate of heat transfer)
  - Do not stop CPR until warm and dead
- **Electrical Injuries**
  - At high risk for **rhabdomyolysis** and **compartment syndrome**
  - All extremities susceptible
  - Do not put IVs into affected limbs
  - All need volume resuscitation (cell necrosis inside body)
  - **EKG** and **telemetry** for 24-48 hours if having arrhythmias
  - Concomitant injuries - solid organ fracture, intestinal or gallbladder rupture, quadriplegia, cataracts
  - MCC of death - _cardiac arrest from **ventricular fibrillation**_
  - **Electrical burns to mouth in children** (electrical cord) – wait 6-9 months before repair unless child cannot eat
  - **Highest resistance** bone
- **Lightning strike** MCC death - cardiac arrest

Critical Care

387. Which of the following is the correct equation for systemic vascular resistance (SVR):
     a.   80 x [(wedge – CVP) / C.O.]
     b.   80 x [(MAP – wedge) / C.O.]
     c.   80 x [(MAP – CVP) / C.O.]
     d.   80 x [(CVP – wedge) / C.O.]

     Answer c. 80 x [(MAP – CVP) / C.O.]

388. Early sepsis is associated with all of the following except:
     a.   Respiratory alkalosis
     b.   Hyperglycemia
     c.   Confusion and irritability
     d.   Hyperkalemia

     Answer d. Early sepsis is not associated with hyperkalemia.

389. Following massive pulmonary embolism, wedge pressure is likely to be:
     a.   3 x normal
     b.   2 x normal
     c.   Normal
     d.   Below normal

     Answer d. Below normal. Massive PE will cause elevated PA pressures, right ventricular pressures, and central venous pressure. Wedge pressure will be low as blood cannot traverse the lungs to the left atrium. This results in hypotension.

390. All of the following are true except:
     a.   Pulmonary wedge pressure reflects mean left atrial pressure
     b.   The most basic definition of shock is low blood pressure
     c.   PEEP improves oxygenation by increasing functional residual capacity
     d.   Mixed venous saturation measurements are taken from the pulmonary artery
     e.   The best sign of appropriate fluid resuscitation in hemorrhagic shock is lactate level

     Answer b. The most basic definition of shock is **inadequate tissue perfusion**.

391. While performing a difficult left hepatectomy for hepatocellular CA in a patient with Child's A cirrhosis you encounter diffuse bloody oozing and bile leakage from the liver bed. Despite numerous blood products and argon beam coagulation you are not able to stop the oozing. After 12 hours in the OR, he has the following values: pH 7.30, UOP 30 cc/8 hours, BP 85/50, and HR 110. The most appropriate next step is:
     a.   Pack the liver, admit to ICU, and aggressive fluid resuscitation
     b.   Give DDAVP
     c.   Pringle maneuver
     d.   Palliative care only

     Answer a. Damage control surgery / resuscitation is appropriate here. Packing the area will help control bleeding and allow time for blood product resuscitation. Take the patient back to the OR the next day to remove the packs and provide definitive control of the bleeding. DDAVP could help with the bleeding, however, at this stage damage control surgery is appropriate.

392. During a difficult distal gastrectomy and gastro-jejunostomy for gastric CA, you test your anastomosis with dye through an NG tube. Dye freely flows out your anastomosis and onto the operative field. The case has taken 8 hours and you spend another 4 hours trying to repair the area. She has the following values: pH 7.30, UOP 10 cc/4 hours, BP 90/50, and HR 120. The most appropriate next step is:
     a.   Redo the anastomosis this time using a stapler

b.   Take down the anastomosis
c.   Total gastrectomy
d.   Place drains, admit to ICU, and aggressive fluid resuscitation
e.   Palliative care only

Answer d. Place drains, admit to ICU, and aggressive fluid resuscitation. Again, damage control surgery / resuscitation is appropriate here. Definitive repair should be performed when the patient is stable.

393. All of the following are true except:
    a.   Coronary sinus blood has the lowest venous oxygen tension
    b.   Renal vein blood has the highest venous oxygen tension in the body
    c.   The most important determinant of myocardial oxygen consumption and energy expenditure is wall tension
    d.   Arterial pressure is equal to heart rate x systemic vascular resistance

Answer d. Arterial pressure is equal to cardiac output x systemic vascular resistance.

394. All of the following are most often associated with a decrease in SVO$_2$ (mixed venous oxygen saturation) except:
    a.   Myocardial infarction
    b.   Cardiac tamponade
    c.   Hemorrhagic shock
    d.   Septic shock

Answer d. A **decrease in SVO$_2$** is caused by either decreased delivery of oxygen to the periphery or increased consumption. Delivery problems can result from a low cardiac output (eg MI, cardiac tamponade, hypovolemia), decreased oxygen carrying capacity (eg low Hct, hemorrhage), or a low oxygen saturation.

An **increase in SVO$_2$** can occur with anything that causes shunting of blood or causes a decreased oxygen consumption in the periphery. Cirrhosis and septic shock cause shunting and an increased SVO$_2$. Cyanide toxicity would result in decreased peripheral oxygen consumption and an elevated SVO$_2$.

395. All of following cause a left shift in the oxygen dissociation curve except:
    a.   Decreased CO$_2$
    b.   Low temperature
    c.   High pH
    d.   2-3 DPG

Answer d. Left shift (oxygen becomes more bound to hemoglobin) is caused by decreased CO$_2$, decreased temp, and high pH. **Right shift** is caused by low pH, increased CO$_2$, 2-3 DPG (diphosphoglycerate), and ATP.

396. Which of the following equations determines oxygen delivery:
    a.   C.O. x [(Hgb x 1.34 x mixed venous saturation) + (pO$_2$ x 0.003)] x 10
    b.   Wedge x [(Hgb x 1.34 x O$_2$ saturation) + (pO$_2$ x 0.003)] x 10
    c.   C.O. x [(Hgb x 1.34 x O$_2$ saturation) + (pO$_2$ x 0.003)] x 10
    d.   Wedge x [(Hgb x 1.34 x mixed venous saturation)+(pO$_2$ x 0.003)] x 10

Answer c. C.O. x [(Hgb x 1.34 x O$_2$ saturation) + (pO$_2$ x 0.003)] x 10

397. Which of the following equations determines myocardial oxygen consumption (CaO$_2$ = arterial O$_2$ content, CvO$_2$ = venous O$_2$ content):
    a.   = C.O. x (CaO$_2$ – CvO$_2$)
    b.   = C.O. x (CvO$_2$ – CaO$_2$)
    c.   = C.O. - (CaO$_2$ – CvO$_2$)
    d.   = C.O. - (CvO$_2$ – CaO$_2$)

Answer a. O_2 consumption (VO_2; **Fick equation**) = C.O. x ($CaO_2 - CvO_2$)

O_2 **content** = (Hgb x 1.34 x O_2 saturation) + (pO_2 x 0.003)

398. A critical care patient has the following pulmonary artery catheter values: BP 80/50, cardiac index 5.0, systemic vascular resistance 500, and CVP 5. This is most consistent with:
    a.   Septic shock
    b.   Hypovolemic shock
    c.   Cardiogenic shock
    d.   Neurogenic shock

    Answer a. An elevated cardiac index of 5, a low SVR of 500, and a low CVP of 5 suggests **septic shock** (is associated with a high cardiac output).

399. The most appropriate next step in the above patient is:
    a.   IV fluid
    b.   Inotrope
    c.   Vasopressin
    d.   Norepinephrine
    e.   Blood products

    Answer a. IV fluid resuscitation is the first step in the treatment of septic shock. Persistent hypotension despite adequate fluid resuscitation is then an indication for pressors.

400. A 67 yo woman develops urosepsis following a low anterior resection (LAR) for adenocarcinoma. She has been started on broad spectrum antibiotics and given volume resuscitation. She is intubated, has a wedge pressure of 18, a HR of 120, a blood pressure of 70/50, and a C.O. of 8. The most appropriate next step is:
    a.   Norepinephrine
    b.   Dobutamine
    c.   Dopamine
    d.   Epinephrine

    Answer a. Levophed (norepinephrine) is primarily an alpha agent and decreases vasodilatation associated with septic shock. This is the initial **pressor of choice** for septic shock despite fluid resuscitation. The 2nd agent to give for persistent septic shock is **vasopressin**.

401. A 50 yo ICU patient has a C.O. of 3.0 with a wedge pressure of 20 and a systemic pressure of 85/50. His HR is 90 and his SVR is 2400. The most appropriate initial step for this patient is:
    a.   Phenylephrine
    b.   ACE inhibitor
    c.   Nitroglycerin
    d.   Dobutamine

    Answer d. Poor cardiac output associated with high filling pressures, low blood pressure, and a high SVR is consistent with **cardiogenic shock**. Initial Tx is an **inotrope** (eg dobutamine).

402. You place a swan ganz catheter in a 70 kg man through the left subclavian vein and get a wedge pressure. The approximate swan distance into the patient should be:
    a.   45 cm
    b.   50 cm
    c.   55 cm
    d.   60 cm

    Answer c. The approximate swan distance to wedge from the left subclavian vein is 55 cm. If you place a swan-ganz catheter and wedge it but the distance is significantly longer than expected (8 cm or greater), you likely have a loop or your catheter is in the wrong place.

403. All of the following concerning pulmonary artery catheters are true except:
   a. If possible, they should be avoided in patients with left bundle branch blocks
   b. Excessive PEEP can artificially decrease wedge pressure
   c. Zone III of the lung is the optimal site of placement
   d. Pulmonary vascular resistance (PVR) can only be measured using a PA catheter (ECHO does not measure PVR)

   Answer b. Excessive PEEP can artificially increase wedge pressures. The optimal site of placement of the PA catheter is in **lung zone III** (bases usually) to avoid the effects of airway pressures on wedge pressures. Wedge pressure measurement is taken at **end expiration**.

404. A critical care patient following a thoracoabdominal aortic aneurysm repair has the following pulmonary artery catheter values: cardiac index 1.8, systemic vascular resistance 3000, BP 80/40, and wedge pressure of 5. This patient needs
   a. Levophed (norepinephrine)
   b. Dobutamine
   c. Volume
   d. Phenylephrine

   Answer c. Poor cardiac index, poor filling pressures and a high SVR suggests **hypovolemic shock**. This patient needs volume

405. A critical care patient has the following pulmonary artery catheter values: cardiac output 2.0, systemic vascular resistance 500, and wedge pressure of 5. This is most consistent with:
   a. Septic shock (early)
   b. Hypovolemic shock
   c. Cardiogenic shock
   d. Neurogenic shock

   Answer d. A low cardiac output, low filling pressures (wedge pressure), and a low SVR is most consistent with **neurogenic shock**. (note that late, end stage septic shock could present like this as the heart starts to give out but the answer above states *early* septic shock). Early stage septic shock would be associated with a high cardiac output.

406. After fluid resuscitation, the most appropriate next step in the above patient is:
   a. Dobutamine
   b. Milrinone
   c. Nitric oxide
   d. Phenylephrine

   Answer d. Phenylephrine is appropriate for neurogenic shock *after* appropriate **fluid resuscitation**. This usually occurs in trauma scenarios and patients usually have associated paraplegia.

407. A 35 yo woman is hypotensive despite fluid resuscitation (CVP 18) and pressors (Neosynephrine and Levophed) following thymectomy for Myasthenia Gravis. She has had a persistent hyperpyrexia (fever). The most appropriate next step is:
   a. Dexamethasone
   b. Add another pressor
   c. Calcium
   d. Blood transfusion

   Answer a. This patient is likely suffering from **acute adrenal insufficiency** based on the clinical scenario. **Dexamethasone** is indicated.

408. Which of the following are the most likely electrolyte values in the above patient:
   a.   Na 130 and K 5.3
   b.   Na 150 and K 5.3
   c.   Na 130 and K 3.3
   d.   Na 150 and K 3.3

   Answer a. Na 130 and K 5.3. **Hyponatremia** and **hyperkalemia** occur with adrenal insufficiency. Decreased aldosterone in primary adrenal insufficiency causes **hyperkalemia** (decreased excretion). Aldosterone deficiency and compensatory hypersecretion of ADH (anti-diuretic hormone) result in **hyponatremia**.

409. The most sensitive test for adrenal insufficiency is:
   a.   ACTH stimulation test
   b.   24 urine cortisol
   c.   Random serum cortisol
   d.   Serum ACTH level

   Answer a. The most sensitive test for adrenal insufficiency is the **corticotropin (ACTH) stimulation test.**

410. Each of the following drugs causes stimulation of adenylate cyclase except:
   a.   Dopamine
   b.   Dobutamine
   c.   Epinephrine
   d.   Milrinone

   Answer d. Milrinone works by inhibiting **cAMP phosphodiesterase** (which increases cAMP). Milrinone is not subject to receptor down-regulation with prolonged use. Dopamine, epinephrine, and dobutamine are all beta-agonists, stimulate **adenylate cyclase** to increase cAMP, and are subject to receptor down-regulation.

411. All of the following are true of nitric oxide except:
   a.   Increases cAMP
   b.   The precursor is arginine
   c.   It is primarily released from vascular endothelium
   d.   Inducible nitric oxide synthetase is involved in hypotension with sepsis

   Answer a. **Arginine** is the precursor to **nitric oxide** (NO). NO acts on soluble **guanylate cyclase** to increase **cGMP** and cause **vasodilatation**.

412. All of the following are true of intra-aortic balloon pumps (IABPs) except:
   a.   The tip should be placed 2-3 cm below the aortic arch
   b.   Inflation occurs with T wave and deflation on P wave
   c.   Improvement in coronary blood flow is primarily due to diastolic augmentation
   d.   The IABP is inflated during systole
   e.   It improves cardiac output

   Answer d. The IABP is *deflated* during systole to help reduce afterload.

413. Which of the following is a contraindication to IABP:
   a.   Aortic valve insufficiency
   b.   Ventricular septal rupture
   c.   Acute mitral insufficiency
   d.   Large MI with cardiac failure

   Answer a. Aortic valve insufficiency is a contraindication to IABP.

414. Which of the following is most renal protective for patients with renal insufficiency receiving a dye load:
   a. ASA
   b. Pre-dye hydration
   c. HCO3-
   d. N-acetylcysteine

   Answer b. Pre-dye **hydration** has been shown to be the most renal protective measure in patients with an elevated creatinine receiving a dye load. HCO_3^- and **N-acetylcysteine** are also protective agents.

415. All of the following are true except::
   a. The MCC of acute renal failure (or oliguria refractory to fluid challenge) post-op is hypotension intra-op
   b. Renin converts angiotensinogen to angiotensin I
   c. Angiotensin converting enzyme (ACE) converts angiotensin I to angiotensin II
   d. The highest concentration of ACE is in the liver
   e. Bilateral renal artery stenosis is likely to raise renin levels and cause HTN

   Answer d. The highest concentration of ACE is in the **lung.**

416. All of the following are true of aldosterone except:
   a. Causes reabsorption of Na
   b. Causes excretion of H and K ions
   c. Acts at the distal convoluted tubule
   d. Primarily acts on protein kinase C

   Answer d. Aldosterone is a steroid hormone that causes the resorption of Na and excretion of H and K at the distal convoluted tubule by stimulating **transcription** of Na/K ATPase and Na/H ATPase (causes **water reabsorption**).

417. A patient stops making urine after surgery. All of the following values are consistent with pre-renal renal failure except:
   a. Urine Na < 20
   b. BUN/Cr ratio 45
   c. FeNa = 0.1%
   d. Urine osmolality 200 mOsm

   Answer d. Urine osmolality > 500 mOsm is consistent with pre-renal azotemia. **FeNa** is the *most sensitive test* for **acute renal failure**. Urine Na is low because the kidney is reabsorbing it, increasing the Na gradient for water reabsorption.

418. FeNa is:
   a. [(Urine creatnine/Plasma creatnine) / (Urine sodium/Plasma sodium)]
   b. [(Urine sodium/Plasma sodium) / (Urine creatnine/Plasma creatnine)]
   c. [(Plasma sodium/Urine sodium) / (Urine creatnine/Plasma creatnine)]
   d. [(Urine sodium/Plasma sodium) / (Plasma creatnine/Urine creatnine)]

   Answer b. This is the formula for FeNa.

419. An 85 yo man POD 3 from aortic valve replacement has not had any urine output since his urinary catheter was removed 12 hours earlier. His BUN is 50 and creatinine is 1.8. You suspect his benign prostatic hyperplasia (BPH) is contributing to the problem The most appropriate test in this patient is:
   a. FeNa
   b. PET scan
   c. U/S
   d. Uroscopy
   e. IVP

Answer c. U/S is the best test for obstructive uropathy (post-renal obstruction; eg transected ureter, BPH, nephrolithiasis). Bladder scanning can be done at the bedside.

420. You are performing a difficult open thoracoabdominal aortic replacement with re-implantation of the celiac, SMA, and renal vessels. He has the following values: BP 90/60, HR 100, PA 50/30, pH 7.25, potassium 5.0, creatinine 5.5. He is on high amounts of norepinephrine, vasopressin, neosynephrine. You try several rounds of diuretics however he has not made urine in 8 hours. The most appropriate next step is:
   a.   Peritoneal dialysis
   b.   Continued management
   c.   Hemodialysis (HD)
   d.   More diuretics
   e.   Continuous veno-venous hemofiltration (CVVH)

   Answer e. CVVH has much less blood pressure fluctuation and hemodynamic compromise compared to HD. The other answers are not appropriate.

421. All of the following are true of peritoneal dialysis except:
   a.   An uncorrected inguinal hernia is considered an absolute contraindication to placement
   b.   The MCC of flow obstruction is omentum
   c.   The catheter should be placed under the diaphragm
   d.   The catheter should be placed through the rectus
   e.   The exit site should be above the beltline

   Answer c. The catheter should be placed in the deep pelvis (not under diaphragm).

422. While trying to treat a patient with severe ARDS, you increase the PEEP to improve oxygenation. After doing this, you notice a decrease in urine output. The mechanism of decreased urine output with increased PEEP is:
   a.   Compartment syndrome
   b.   Decreased cardiac output (C.O.)
   c.   Reduced oxygenation
   d.   Retained CO2

   Answer b. Progressively increasing **PEEP** (beyond 10-15 cm H_2O) will compress the SVC and IVC, leading to decreased right atrial filling and **decreased C.O.**

423. PEEP improves oxygenation by:
   a.   Increasing functional residual capacity
   b.   Increasing tidal volumes
   c.   Increasing respiratory rate
   d.   Increasing residual volume

   Answer a. Positive end expiratory pressure **(PEEP)** improves oxygenation by improving **functional residual capacity** (FRC). This effectively keeps alveoli open at the end of the breath so oxygen exchange can continue.

424. All of the following are true of lung dead space except:
   a.   Refers mostly to the conductance portion of the airway
   b.   Is about 150 ml in most adults
   c.   Refers to areas that are ventilated and not perfused
   d.   Refers to areas that are perfused but not ventilated

   Answer d. Dead space is the area of lung that is ventilated but not perfused. In normal individuals, this is about 150 cc and refers mostly to the conduction portion of the airways (everything proximal to the respiratory bronchioles). Pathology which can increase dead space includes excessive PEEP (collapses the alveolar capillaries), PE, ARDS, and pulmonary hypertension. Increased dead space can lead to CO_2 **build-up.**

425. All of the following are true except:
   a. Vital capacity is the maximal amount of air exhaled after a normal inhalation.
   b. Residual volume is the volume of air left in the lung after maximal exhalation.
   c. Tidal volume is the volume of air exhaled with normal inspiration and exhalation.
   d. Functional residual capacity is the volume of air left in the lung after a normal exhalation

   Answer a. Vital capacity is the maximal amount of air exhaled after a maximal inhalation.

426. All of the following are within normal extubation parameters except:
   a. NIF (negative inspiratory force): – 35
   b. PO_2 of 92 on 40% FiO_2
   c. Minute ventilation 25
   d. PCO_2 35
   e. Awake and alert

   Answer c. Normal minute ventilation should be 10-15 L/min.

427. Post-op day 1 after a right upper lobectomy, your patient has a fever to 102.0. The most likely source of the fever is:
   a. PMNs
   b. Platelets
   c. Macrophages
   d. Lymphocytes

   Answer c. Alveolar macrophages are activated with **atelectasis** and release of **IL-1**, which acts on the hypothalamus to cause **fever**.

428. A patient with severe pancreatitis develops diffuse pulmonary infiltrates, hypoxemia, and eventually requires intubation. All of the following are true of the patients condition except:
   a. High plateau pressures improve patient outcome.
   b. Diffuse bilateral pulmonary infiltrates versus uni-lateral infiltrate suggests ARDS over pneumonia
   c. Diffuse bilateral pulmonary infiltrates with low filling pressures suggests ARDS over cardiogenic pulmonary edema
   d. Reducing barotrauma by lowering tidal volumes and allowing permissive hypercapnea has improved the outcome for ARDS

   Answer a. Acute Respiratory Distress Syndrome **(ARDS)** can result from various issues (eg pancreatitis, shock, sepsis, etc.). ARDS is characterized by impaired gas exchange leading to hypoxemia and diffuse infiltrates on CXR. **Maintaining low plateau pressures** with **permissive hypercapnia** is a key principle for ARDS Tx.

429. A 35 yo woman undergoing routine laparoscopic bilateral tubal ligation develops severe hypotension, tachycardia, and a drop in end-tidal CO_2. The patient still has bilateral breath sounds. The most likely Dx is:
   a. A disconnection between the patient and the ventilator
   b. The patient has developed atelectasis
   c. Myocardial infarction
   d. CO_2 embolus

Answer d. End tidal CO2 specifically reflects the exchange of CO_2 from blood to the alveolus. A gradual *rise* in ET-CO_2 usually reflects impaired exchange from lung collapse or atelectasis.

A *drop* in ET-CO_2 can be from something simple like disconnection from the ventilator or something more serious such as an embolus (eg **air embolus** through a central line, **CO_2 embolus** with laparscopic procedures, or **thromboemboli**). The abrupt drop in ET-CO_2 following an embolus is from interruption of CO_2 exchange at the alveolar level.

Because of the hypotension associated with the drop in ET-CO_2 in the above patient, the most likely Dx is CO_2 embolus.

430. Tx of the above problem involves removing the abdominal insufflation and:
        a.   Emergent TPA therapy
        b.   Coronary catheterization
        c.   Bilateral chest tubes
        d.   Trendelenburg, left side down, and 100% oxygen

Answer d. Tx of a CO_2 embolus involves **stopping insufflation** (1st step), placing the patient in **trendelenburg** (head down) position with the **left side down** (prevents any more propagation of CO_2 into lungs), and then **ventilating with 100% oxygen** (CO_2 is reabsorbed faster as it comes into equilibrium).

431. A 50 yo woman undergoing laparoscopic tubal ligation has a sudden drop in her ET-CO_2. The anesthesiologist states he cannot hear any breath sounds. Her blood pressure is 120/60 and her HR is 70. The most likely diagnosis is:
        a.   A disconnection between the patient and the ventilator
        b.   The patient has developed atelectasis
        c.   Myocardial infarction
        d. CO_2 embolus

Answer a. Because this patient is totally stable, the most likely cause of the decreased ET-CO_2 is **disconnection from the ventilator**.

432. A 35 yo woman undergoing routine laparoscopic bilateral tubal ligation has a sudden rise in ET-CO_2. The anesthesiologist states that the patients breath sounds are present but are decreased in both the bases. Her blood pressure is 120/60 and her HR is 70. The most likely diagnosis is:
        a.   A disconnection between the patient and the ventilator
        b.   Atelectasis
        c.   Myocardial infarction
        d. CO_2 embolus

Answer b. The most likely cause of the rise in ET-CO_2 is **atelectasis**. The patient needs larger tidal volumes.

433. All of the following are true except:
        a.   Presence of deep tendon reflexes precludes diagnosis of brain death
        b.   A positive test for apnea is consistent with brain death
        c.   An absent oculocephalic reflex is consistent with brain death
        d.   Fixed and dilated pupils are consistent with brain death

Answer a. You can still have **brain death** with intact deep tendon reflexes.

434. A 27 yo man is in the ICU 6 hours after splenectomy following a MVA. The patient had a prolonged transport time and received 10 units of blood prior to arrival and 5 liters of crystalloid. You are having trouble ventilating the patient. Currently, his peak airway pressures are 70 (plateaus 50), his abdomen is distended, he is not making any urine, and his bladder pressure is 40. His CVP is 15 and his BP is 85/40. The most appropriate maneuver in this patient is:

a. Increase PEEP
b. Volume resuscitation
c. Decompressive laparotomy
d. CT scan

Answer c. This patient has classic signs of **abdominal compartment syndrome**. A bladder pressure > 20-25 is usually seen in this syndrome. Tx - **decompressive laparotomy**

435. A 25 yo woman involved in a MVA has a severe posterior hepatic laceration that you are trying to treat with damage control. You pack the area off and head to the ICU. She has received 20 units of blood, 10 FFP, and 10 platelets but remains hypotensive (BP 80/40). Her hematocrit is stable at 30. The most likely cause of her persistent hypotension is:
    a. Cardiac tamponade
    b. Sepsis
    c. Low calcium
    d. Low magnesium

Answer c. **Low calcium** can occur after massive transfusion. This in turn can cause hypotension. Calcium should be replaced with massive transfusion.

436. All of the following are true except:
    a. High PEEP will increase renin production
    b. Respiratory acidosis with laparoscopy can be reduced by decreasing pneumoperitoneum pressure and by increasing minute ventilation
    c. Pneumoperitoneum will increase renin production
    d. Reperfusion injury is mediated primarily by lymphocytes

Answer d. Reperfusion injury is mediated primarily by **PMNs**.

Pneumoperitoneum compresses the IVC, decreases venous return to the heart, lowers C.O. and BP which is sensed by the kidney, and results in increased **renin** production.

437. All of the following are true except:
    a. Tx for nipride toxicity is amyl nitrate, then sodium nitrite
    b. Tx for methemoglobinemia is methylene blue
    c. Tx for carbon monoxide (CO) poisoning is primarily amyl nitrate
    d. Methemoglobinemia results in a right shift on the oxygen-hemoglobin dissociation curve

Answer c. The primary Tx for **CO poisoning** is **intubation with 100% oxygen**

CARDIOVASCULAR SYSTEM

Normal Values

Parameter	Value
Systemic blood pressure (mmHg; average)	120/80
Pulmonary artery pressure (mmHg)	25/10 (15)
Cardiac output (C.O., L/min)	4 - 6
Cardiac index (C.I., L/min)	2.5 - 4
Systemic vascular resistance (SVR)	**1100** (800-1400)
Pulmonary capillary wedge pressure (wedge pressure)	**11** ± 4
Central venous pressure (CVP)	**7** ± 2
Mixed venous oxygen saturation (SvO_2)	**75** ± 5

- **Hemodynamics**
  - **Mean arterial pressure** = C.O. x SVR
  - **Cardiac output** (C.O.) = HR x stroke volume
  - **Cardiac index** (C.I.) = C.O. / BSA
  - **Systemic vascular resistance** (SVR) = 80 x [(MAP – CVP) / C.O.]
  - **Cardiac Output** - Kidney gets 25%, Brain gets 15%, Heart gets 5%
  - **Left ventricular performance** - determined by pre-load, afterload, contractility, and heart rate
  - **Preload** - pressure stretching the ventricle of the heart
    - Linearly related to left ventricular end-diastolic **volume** (LVEDV)
    - **Wedge pressure** - used as a measurement of preload
    - **Starling's Law** - the greater volume of blood entering the heart (LVEDV), the greater the ejection (stroke volume or ejection fraction); termed **right shift along curve**; at some point along the curve, increased volume no longer increases ejection and can worsen it (over-distension → **extreme right shift on Starling curve**)
  - **Afterload** - tension produced by the heart in order to contract
    - Related to the resistance (ie SVR) against the ventricle contracting
    - **High SVR** - hard for the ventricle to contract
    - **Low SVR** - easier for the ventricle to contract
    - **Diabetics** - have increased SVR from arteriopathy
  - **Contractility** - force of contraction
  - **Stroke volume** = LVEDV – LVESV
    - Is determined by LVEDV, contractility, and afterload
    - **LVEDV** - determined by preload and distensibility of ventricle
    - **LVESV** (LV end-systolic volume) - determined by contractility and afterload
  - **Ejection fraction** = stroke volume / LVEDV

OXYGEN DELIVERY / CONSUMPTION
- **Arterial O_2 content** (CaO_2) = (Hgb x 1.34 x O_2 saturation) + (pO_2 x 0.003)
- **O_2 delivery** = C.O. x [(Hgb x 1.34 x O_2 saturation) + (pO_2 x 0.003)] x 10
- **O_2 consumption** (VO_2; Fick equation) = C.O. x (CaO_2 - CvO_2)
  - CvO_2 = venous O_2 content (mmHg)
- Normal O_2 delivery to O_2 consumption ratio is 4:1 (25% utilized; **SvO_2 = 75%**)
  - Thus there is 4 x more oxygen delivered then used
  - C.O. will increase to keep ratio constant
  - O_2 consumption is normally **supply independent**
- Most important determinant of **myocardial O_2 consumption** (energy expenditure) - **wall tension** (followed by heart rate, contractility)
- **Oxygen-Hemoglobin dissociation curve**
  - 1) **Right Shift** (decreased O_2 affinity, p50 increases) occurs with: ↑ CO_2 (Bohr effect), ↑ temp, ATP, 2,3-DPG, ↓ pH, and methemoglobinemia
  - 2) **Left shift** (increased O_2 affinity, p50 decreases) occurs with: opposite above, fetal Hgb, carbon monoxide poisoning
  - **Normal p50** (O_2 tension with 50% of the O_2 receptors saturated) = 27 mmHg
- **Mixed venous saturation** (SvO_2, pulmonary artery catheter)
  - Oxygen saturation of mixed venous blood (normal: 75% ± 5), measurements taken from **pulmonary artery** (allows mixing), assesses tissue oxygenation
  - **Elevated SvO_2** occurs with:
    - **Shunting of blood** (eg septic shock, cirrhosis, L→R cardiac shunt) or;
    - **Decreased O_2 extraction** (eg hypothermia, paralysis, coma, cyanide)
  - **Decreased SvO_2** occurs with:
    - **Decreased O_2 delivery** (eg low C.O., hypoxia, low Hct) or;
    - **Increased O_2 extraction** (eg malignant hyperthermia)
- **Bronchial blood flow** becomes unsaturated after delivery to bronchus and lung tissue, then empties into pulmonary veins; thus, left ventricle blood pO_2 is 5 mmHg lower than pulmonary capillaries
- **Coronary sinus blood** (ie coronary venous blood) - has lowest venous oxygen saturation in body (**30%**); heart consumes a lot of oxygen

- **Renal veins** - have highest venous oxygen saturation in body (**80%**); kidneys receive 25% of the C.O. but do not have a high oxygen expenditure
- **Pulse oximeter** - reads Hgb-O_2 as **red** and unbound Hgb as **infrared**
  - (**Red / Red + Infrared**) x 100 = % sat
  - Pulse oximeter **miss-reads** - dark skin, low C.O., ambient light, low hematocrit, hypothermia, carbon monoxide
- During **hypoxia**, blood is _shunted_ to the **heart** and **brain**
- **Shock** = inadequate tissue perfusion (most basic definition)
- **Tachypnea** and **mental status changes** occur with progressive shock

PULMONARY ARTERY CATHETERS (PA catheter)
- **Inaccurate measurements** can be caused by:
  1) PA catheter <u>not</u> **in lung zone III** (lower lobes)
  2) **Wedge pressure > LA pressure** (mediastinal fibrosis, pulmonary vein obstruction, pulmonary HTN, high PEEP [compresses pulmonary veins])
  3) **LA pressure > LV end diastolic pressure** (mitral regurgitation, mitral stenosis)
- **Wedge pressure** measurement reflects **mean left atrial pressure** (or pre-load)
- **PA catheter distances to wedge** (apx):

Right subclavian	45 cm
Right internal jugular	50 cm
Left subclavian	55 cm
Left internal jugular	60 cm

  - If distance much longer/shorter than expected (ie 8 cm) → in wrong place or have loop
- **Optimal lung placement** for PA catheter - **zone III** (lower lobes)
  - Has **less respiratory influence** on measurements
  - Measurements should be taken at **end-expiration**
- **Contraindications**
  - **Absolute** - right sided endocarditis or thrombus, right mechanical heart valve
  - **Relative** - coagulopathy (reverse), recent pacemaker (use fluoroscopy), left bundle branch block (can cause complete heart block)
- **High PEEP:**
  - Can artificially increase wedge pressure measurements
    Subtract ½ the PEEP from the wedge value if PEEP > 10
  - Can cause **decreased C.O.** from **decreased <u>right atrium</u> filling** (<u>main mechanism</u>); **high PEEP** causes **poor urine output** (UOP) due to **decreased C.O.** (will also increase **renin**)
- **Pulmonary vascular resistance** (PVR) can be measured <u>only</u> using a PA catheter (<u>not</u> measured with ECHO); **PVR** = [(PA pressure – wedge) /cardiac output] x 80

SHOCK

Types of Shock

Shock	CVP / wedge	C.O.	SVR	SvO_2
Hemorrhagic	↓	↓	↑	↓
Septic	↓	↑	↓	↑
Cardiogenic (eg MI, cardiac tamponade)	↑	↓	↑	↓
Neurogenic (eg head, spinal cord injury)	↓	↓	↓	↑
Adrenal Insufficiency (acute)	↓	↓	↓	↓
PE (or air / CO_2 embolism)	↑	↓	↑	↓

- **Shock** = inadequate tissue perfusion (most basic definition)
- **Tachypnea** (↑ RR) and **mental status changes** occur as shock progresses
- **Hemorrhagic shock** - <u>initial response</u> is an **increase** in diastolic pressure
  - Tx: volume (LR, then blood in trauma patients)
- **Septic shock** - hyperventilation (respiratory alkalosis), mental status changes (eg confusion), and hypotension (early sepsis triad)
  - **Hyperglycemia** - often occurs just before clinical sepsis and can occur throughout course

171

Early sepsis - ↓ insulin, ↑ glucose (impaired utilization)
Late sepsis - ↑ insulin, ↑ glucose (insulin resistance)
- Tx: *volume resuscitation 1st and antibiotics*; then **norepinephrine** for continued hypotension; **vasopressin** if still refractory
- **Optimal glucose** level in sepsis: **80 - 120** (insulin drip)
- Consider testing for **adrenal insufficiency** if refractory to volume and pressors
- Inducible nitric oxide synthetase is involved in **hypotension** with sepsis

- **Cardiogenic shock** (eg myocardial infarction, CHF exacerbation)
  - Sx's: dyspnea, pulmonary edema, low C.O., poor urine output
  - Heart can't contract effectively → **pulmonary congestion**
  - Heart also becomes **over-distended** → worsens contractility
  - Tx: **dobutamine** (inotrope); **intra-aortic balloon pump** may be necessary to stabilize *(see below)*; diuretics if pulmonary edema

- **Cardiac tamponade** (causes cardiogenic shock)
  - Mechanism of hypotension is decreased **right ventricular filling** due to fluid in the pericardial sac around the heart
  - Sx's (Beck's triad): hypotension, jugular venous distention, and muffled heart sounds
  - Dx: **1st ECHO sign** of early cardiac tamponade → **impaired diastolic filling of right atrium** (from compression)
  - Tx: **pericardial window** or **pericardiocentesis** to drain fluid; fluid resuscitation to temporize; pericardiocentesis blood does not form clot

- **Neurogenic shock** - loss of sympathetic tone; usually spine or head injury
  - Sx's: low HR, low BP, and warm skin; low SVR
  - Tx: **volume resuscitation 1st**; **phenylephrine** for continued low BP (raises SVR)

- **Adrenal insufficiency** (Acute)
  - MCC - **withdrawal of exogenous steroids**; others - bilateral adrenal hemorrhage (MC related to sepsis, eg Waterhouse-Friderichsen syndrome), adrenalectomy
  - Sx's: N/V, abdominal pain, fever (hyperpyrexia), hypotension (unresponsive to fluids / pressors), lethargy; ↓ glucose, ↓ Na, and ↑ K
    - **Relative adrenal insufficiency** can occur in severely ill critical care patients (hypotension refractory to fluid and pressors)
  - Dx: increased **ACTH** and decreased **cortisol**
    - **Corticotropin stimulation test** (*best test*, ACTH given, cortisol in blood then measured)
      - **Baseline cortisol < 15** or **change < 9** ug/dl after stimulation test = adrenal insufficiency
  - Tx: **Dexamethasone** (2 mg IV q6) - give prior to corticotropin stimulation test (dexamethasone does NOT interfere with test)

EMBOLI
- **Pulmonary embolism** (PE)
  - Sx's: dyspnea; tachycardia and tachypnea; hypoxia and hypocarbia; chest pain
  - Hypotension and shock can occur if **massive** (*high* pulmonary artery pressures, *low* wedge pressure)
  - ABG - ↓ pO_2 and ↓ pCO_2, respiratory alkalosis (from hyperventilation)
  - MC EKG finding - **sinus tachycardia**
  - Intubated patients can present with a **sudden drop in ET-CO_2** and **hypotension**
    - Blood can't get to left side of heart due to PE
  - Most arise from **ilio-femoral region DVT**
  - Dx: **CT angio** (99% sensitive); elevated **D-dimer**; 1/3 have negative LE duplex
  - Tx: **heparin** (*Do not wait on chest CT to give heparin if PE suspected*)
    - Suspicion of PE = give heparin
    - Volume, inotropes, and pressors if hypotensive
  - Consider open (on cardiopulmonary bypass) or percutaneous (suction catheter) **embolectomy** if patient is in shock despite massive pressors and inotropes *(thrombolytics have not shown survival improvement)*

- **Fat emboli** - petechiae, hypoxia, and confusion (can also be similar to PE)
  - **Sudan red stain** may show fat in sputum and urine
  - MCC - lower extremity fractures / orthopedic procedures (eg hip, femur)

- **Air emboli** (CO_2 embolus similar)
  - MCC - sucking air through **central line** or central line site
  - **CO_2 embolus** can occur with **laparoscopic** procedures (eg laparoscopic cholecystectomy)
  - Sx's: **hypotension** and **tachycardia**, 'mill wheel' murmur
    - **Air** and **CO_2 embolus** will have a sudden drop in ET-CO_2 *(usual 1st sign)*
    - If CO_2 embolus, there is a *transient* rise in ET-CO_2, followed quickly by a *precipitous drop* in ET-CO_2
  - Air (or CO_2) can lodge in right sided heart chambers and/or pulmonary arteries, causing an **air lock** which prevents blood from going to the **left heart**
  - Tx: 1st step - **stop insufflation** if laparoscopic procedure
    - **Trendelenburg** (head down)
    - **Left lateral decubitus** position (keeps air in right heart)
    - Give **100% oxygen** (equilibrates with embolus and is reabsorbed faster) - *stop nitrous oxide (doesn't diffuse quickly)*
    - **Hyperventilation** (increase minute ventilation, RR x TV)
      - ↓s blood pCO_2, which ↑s gradient for CO_2 or air to diffuse
      - Reabsorbs embolus faster
    - **Aspirate central line** if present (gets embolus out of RA)
    - **Intubate** if not already; fluids, pressors, and inotropes to maintain BP
    - **Prolonged CPR** if needed to allow embolus to be absorbed

CARDIOVASCULAR DRUGS
- **Receptors**
  - Inotropes that **directly ↑ cAMP** - Dopamine, Dobutamine, Epinephrine (mostly an inotrope, some pressor activity), Isoproterenol
  - Inotropes that **inhibit cAMP phosphodiesterase** (indirectly ↑ cAMP) – Milrinone
  - Inotropes that **inhibit Na/K transporter** - Digoxin
- **Inotropes** (↑ cardiac output)
  - **Dopamine** (1-20 µg/kg/min)
    - **Low** (1-5)   **Renal dopamine receptors** (renal perfusion)
    - **Medium** (6-10)   **Beta-1 + Beta-2** (↑ contractility + ↑ HR)
    - **High** (>10)   **Alpha-1** (vasoconstriction, ↑ MAP)
  - **Dobutamine** (1-20 µg/kg/min) - **Beta-1** (contractility)
    - Some beta-2 (vasodilation) at higher doses (> 15)
  - **Milrinone**
    - **cAMP phosphodiesterase inhibitor** (results in ↑ed cAMP)
    - Ca^{++} influx ↑s myocardial **contractility**
    - Also a **pulmonary vasodilator** (relaxes vascular smooth muscle)
    - **Not subject to beta-receptor down-regulation like other inotropes** (good for long-term use; eg patients awaiting heart TXP); other drugs lose potency with time
  - **Isoproterenol**
    - **Beta-1** (↑ HR and contractility) and **Beta-2** (vasodilates)
    - **Side-effects**: arrhythmogenic; increases heart metabolic demand (rarely used); may actually ↓ BP (beta-2)
  - **Epinephrine** (Epi, 1-20 µg/min)
    - **Low Dose** (1-5)   **Beta-1** and **Beta-2**
    - **High Dose** (> 5)   **Alpha-1** and **Alpha-2**
    - Can *lower* blood pressure at low doses (Beta-2 > Beta-1)
- **Pressors** (↑SVR and ↑MAP; NE also inotropic)
  - **Phenylephrine** - **Alpha-1** (vasoconstriction)
  - **Norepinephrine** (NE, Levophed; 1-40 µg/min)
    - Predominantly **Alpha-1 + Alpha-2** (vasoconstriction); some Beta-1 (contractility)
    - Acts as a potent **splanchnic vasoconstrictor**
  - **Vasopressin** (0.01 - 0.1 U/min); **V-1** receptor (different mechanism than above pressors); arterial **vasoconstriction**

- **Vasodilators**
  - **Nipride** - arterial vasodilator (NO mediated)
    - **Cyanide toxicity** occurs at doses > 3 mcg/kg/min for 72 hours; can check **thiocyanate levels** and signs of **metabolic acidosis**
    - Cyanide binds to cytochrome c in mitochondria and **disrupts electron transport chain**; cell cannot use O_2 so you get a **left to right shunt** (↑s SvO_2)
    - Tx for <u>cyanide toxicity</u> - **amyl nitrite**, then sodium nitrite; can also use **hydroxocobalamin**
  - **Nitroglycerin** - NO mediated; predominantly venodilation, decreases **ventricle wall tension** by decreasing pre-load; also a coronary artery vasodilator
  - **ACE inhibitors** - **decrease angiotensin II** (predominantly results in vasodilation and *decreased* aldosterone)
    - 1) reduce mortality post-MI *and;* 2) prevent CHF post-MI
    - *Absolute contraindications* - previous angioedema, renal artery stenosis
    - *Relative contraindications* - impaired renal function, hypovolemia, aortic stenosis
    - S/Es - cough, angioedema
  - **Nitric Oxide** - vasodilator (binds soluble guanylate cyclase receptor)
    - Also called **endothelium-derived relaxing factor** (EDRF)
    - **Arginine** is the precursor to **nitric oxide** (nitric oxide synthetase is located in the endothelium)
    - Nitric oxide then acts on **soluble guanylate cyclase** to increase **cGMP** which causes **vasodilation**
    - **Inhaled Nitric Oxide** is a selective pulmonary artery vasodilator
  - **Sildenafil** (Viagra) - is a pulmonary artery vasodilator (NO mediated)

INTRA-AORTIC BALLOON PUMP (IABP)
- **Sequence:**
  - **Inflation** - on **T wave** (diastole)
  - **Deflation** - on **P wave or start of Q wave** (systole)
- Tip should be just distal to left subclavian (2 cm below top of arch)
- Effects:
  - *Improves* **MAP** (inflation with ventricular diastole)
  - *Improves* **diastolic coronary perfusion** (coronaries fill in diastole; ↑ed diastolic MAP improves coronary perfusion)
  - *Decreases* **afterload** (deflation with ventricular systole)
  - Decreases preload (allows more forward flow; unloads heart)
- **IABP indications:**
  - 1) **Cardiogenic shock** post-MI
  - 2) **Ventricular septal rupture** (VSR) post-MI
  - 3) **Acute mitral regurgitation** (MR, eg ruptured papillary muscle either spontaneously or post-MI)
  - 4) **Unstable angina** (improves coronary flow)
  - 5) Pre-op before high risk cardiac surgery (eg patients with low EF)
- Increases survival following 1) VSR or 2) acute MR
- *Absolute contraindications* - aortic regurgitation (insufficiency), aortic dissection, severe aortoiliac occlusive disease
- *Relative contraindications* - vascular grafts in aorta; aortic aneurysms

OTHER CARDIOVASCULAR
- **Atrial fibrillation** is the MCC of **delayed discharge** after cardiac surgery
- **Magnesium** is used to Tx **torsades de pointes** (a type of ventricular tachycardia)
- **Prolonged QT interval**
  - Occurs with certain **drugs** (amiodarone, fluoroquinolones) or **hypomagnesemia**
  - An **early after de-polarization** (ie premature ventricular complex) can occur within the QT interval precipitating ventricular tachycardia (torsades de pointes)
  - Stopping the precipitating drugs or correcting hypomagnesemia shortens QT interval and lessens the likelihood of this happening
  - **Magnesium** can be used to treat torsades de pointes

PULMONARY FUNCTION TESTS (PFTs)

- **Total lung capacity** (TLC)
  - Lung volume after maximal inspiration
  - TLC = VC + RV
- **Vital capacity** (VC)
  - Volume of air with maximal exhalation after maximal inhalation
- **Residual volume** (RV)
  - Lung volume after maximal expiration (comprises 20% of TLC)
- **Tidal volume** (TV)
  - Volume of air with a normal inspiration and expiration
- **Functional residual capacity** (FRC)
  - Lung volume after normal exhalation
  - FRC = ERV + RV
  - Surgery (atelectasis), sepsis (ARDS), and trauma (contusion, atelectasis, ARDS) – all ↓ FRC
  - *PEEP increases FRC*
- **Expiratory reserve volume** (ERV)
  - Volume of air forcefully expired after normal expiration
- **Inspiratory capacity**
  - Maximum amount of air breathed in after normal exhalation
- **FEV_1** - forced expiratory volume in 1 sec (after maximal inhalation)
- **Minute ventilation** = tidal volume x respiratory rate
- **Compliance** = (change in lung volume) / (change in lung pressure)
  - **High compliance** - lungs easy to ventilate (eg COPD)
  - **Low compliance** - lungs hard to ventilate (eg ARDS, fibrotic lung diseases, reperfusion injury, pulmonary edema)

VENTILATOR

- Improving **Oxygenation** →
  - ↑ **PEEP** - improves **functional residual capacity** (FRC; *best initial method to increase pO_2*); causes **alveolar recruitment** and keeps alveoli open at end-expiration so oxygen exchange continues
  - ↑ **FIO_2** - not as effective as ↑ed PEEP; *avoid* FIO_2 > 60% for > 24 hrs (causes **O_2 radical** induced **lung injury**)
- Improving **Ventilation** (removing CO_2) →
  - ↑ **respiratory rate**
  - ↑ **tidal volume**
- **Pressure support** - decreases work of breathing (inspiratory pressure held constant until minimum TV is achieved)
- *Excessive PEEP Cx's:*
  - Decreases **right atrial filling** → **decreases C.O.** → decreases renal blood flow → **decreases UOP** *(main mechanism of decreased UOP with increased PEEP is low C.O.);* also results in **increased renin**
  - ↑s **pulmonary vascular resistance** (pulmonary capillary compression)
  - ↑s **wedge pressure** measurement
  - **Hypercapnia** (elevated CO_2) from increased dead space ventilation due to pulmonary capillary compression
- **Barotrauma** - prevent by keeping **plateau pressure < 30** (most important) and peak pressure < 50
  - **Decrease TV** if pressures are elevated; consider pressure control ventilation (see below)
- **Excessive increase in inspiratory time** (inverse ratio ventilation) can result in significant **auto-PEEP** because lungs are not given enough time to exhale (stacking breaths, results in barotrauma or decreased C.O. from decreased right atrial filling)
- Normal inspiration to expiration time ratio (I:E ratio) is **1 : 3**
- **Mechanical inspiration** increases airway pressure, decreases **right atrial filling**, decreases blood flow across the lungs, reduces C.O., and reduces BP
- **Intermittent mechanical ventilation** (IMV) - uses a preset volume
- **Pressure control ventilation** (PCV) - uses a preset pressure limit (often used as a permissive hypercapnia strategy with ARDS)

- **Normal extubation parameters:**
  - $FiO_2 \leq 40\%$
  - PEEP 5 (physiologic)
  - Pressure support 10
  - RR < 24
  - Minute ventilation 5-10 L/min (TV x RR)
  - Negative inspiratory force (NIF): - 20 or less (meaning more negative)
  - HR < 120
  - $PO_2 > 60$
  - $PCO_2 < 50$
  - pH 7.35-7.45
  - Saturations > 93%
  - Off pressors, follows commands, can protect airway
  - Often have **CPAP trial** before extubation in the ICU

ATELECTASIS (alveolar hypoventilation)
- MCC of **hypoxia** early post-op (abdominal and thoracic surgery)
- MCC of **fever** in first 48 hours after surgery
  - **Fever** is caused by release of **IL-1** from **alveolar macrophages** (IL-1 acts at the hypothalamus to cause fever)
- Collapse of alveoli causes **hypoxia** (increased pulmonary shunt)
- Sx's: fever, tachycardia, hypoxia (is caused by poor inspiration, mucus plugging)
- RFs: COPD, upper abdominal surgery, obesity
- Tx: incentive spirometer, ambulation, pain control

LUNG INJURY

Types of Lung Injury

Acute Respiratory Distress Syndrome (ARDS)
  Acute onset
  Bilateral pulmonary infiltrates
  $PaO_2/FiO_2 \leq 300$
  Absence of CHF (ie low filling pressures, wedge $\leq$ 18)
Ventilator Associated Pneumonia (VAP)
  New _unilateral_ infiltrate
  Fever
  Purulent sputum (consider bronchoalveolar lavage)
  > 48 hours on ventilator
Pulmonary Embolus (PE)
  Normal CXR (possible wedge shaped infarct)
  Hypoxia _and_ hypocarbia
  Sudden onset
  Predisposing condition (eg gastric bypass patient)
Congestive Heart Failure (CHF)
  Bilateral pulmonary edema
  Cardiomegaly
  Elevated filling pressures (wedge > 18)

- **ARDS** (acute respiratory distress syndrome) - **hypoxia** primary problem; impaired gas exchange overall; can lead to systemic inflammatory response syndrome (SIRS), shock, and multi-system organ dysfunction (failure)
  - **Criteria** *(see table above)*
  - **PMNs** have a prominent role in ARDS with **inflammation** of lung parenchyma
  - MCC - **pneumonia** (40%); others - sepsis, multi-trauma, severe burns, pancreatitis, aspiration, shock
  - Tx: regardless of ventilator mode (IMV vs. PCV) the goal is to **reduce barotrauma,** allow **permissive hypercapnia**, and **improve oxygenation**
    If IMV is used, want tidal volumes 5-7 cc/kg
    If PCV is used, want plateau pressure < 30 and peak pressure < 50
    Increasing RR can help reduce CO_2
    pH should be kept above 7.25 (Tx: sodium bicarbonate [HCO_3^-])

- **Permissive hypercapnia** - increases **inspiratory time** (to improve oxygenation) at the expense of expiratory time (causes pCO2 to rise); **correct pH to > 7.30** (give **HCO3⁻**, may be able to ↑ RR)
- **Aspiration** - chemical pneumonitis from aspiration of gastric secretions
  - MC site - **superior segment of the right lower lobe**

VENTILATION TO PERFUSION RATIO (V/Q ratio)
- Normally highest in upper lobes, lowest in lower lobes
- **Dead space**
  - Part of lung that is ventilated but <u>not</u> perfused
  - Normally, dead space is the airway to level of the bronchiole (comprises 150 ml; conductive airways)
  - **MCC of increased dead space** (high V/Q ratio) - **excessive PEEP** (due to capillary compression); others - ↓ed C.O. (capillary collapse), PE, pulmonary hypertension
  - *Increased* dead space leads to *increased* pCO₂
- **Shunt** (poor ventilation but good perfusion)
  - **MCC of increased shunt** (low V/Q ratio) – **atelectasis** *(alveolar hypoventilation)*; others - mucus plug, ARDS (alveoli filled with edema)
  - **Shunt** causes **hypoxia** *(decreased pO₂)*
- **Pulmonary vasodilators** - inhaled nitric oxide, prostacyclin
- **Pulmonary vasoconstrictors** - **hypoxia** (very potent), acidosis
- **Pulmonary shunting** can be caused by nipride, nitroglycerin and nifedipine; manifests as **hypoxia**

RENAL SYSTEM
- **Renin-Angiotensin System**
  - Glomerular filtration rate (GFR) is controlled by the **efferent limb**
  - **Renin** (released from **kidney** juxta-glomerular apparatus)
    Release caused by:
      ↓ed **pressure** sensed by **juxta-glomerular apparatus**
      ↑ed **sodium** concentration sensed by **macula densa**
      Additional releasing factors: **Beta-1 receptor, high K⁺**
    Inhibition of release - low K⁺
    Renin converts **angiotensinogen** (synthesized in **liver**) to **angiotensin I**
  - **Angiotensin converting enzyme** (ACE, located in **lung**)
    Converts angiotensin I to angiotensin II
    ACE inhibitors work here (eg captopril)
    ACE also breaks down **bradykinin**
  - **Angiotensin II** effects (binds AG II receptor):
    *Primary effect - release of **aldosterone** from **adrenal cortex***
    Secondary effects:
      1) <u>Vasoconstrictor</u> (potent, reduces renal blood flow), increases BP
      2) ↑ed <u>sympathetic tone</u> (↑ed HR and contractility)
      3) Release of <u>ADH</u> (vasopressin, posterior pituitary)
  - **Aldosterone** (steroid hormone)
    Up-regulates **Na⁺/K⁺ ATPase** in **distal convoluted tubule** (cell membrane) → causes **Na⁺** and **water reabsorption; K⁺ excretion**
    Also up-regulates **Na⁺/H⁺ exchanger** → causes H⁺ excretion (can get metabolic alkalosis)
    Hyperkalemia can also stimulate aldosterone release
- **Anti-diuretic hormone** (ADH; vasopressin)
  - Released by posterior pituitary gland when **osmolality** is high
  - Acts on *collecting ducts* for **water resorption**
  - Also a **vasoconstrictor**
- **Renal Toxic Drugs**
  - **NSAIDs** - *inhibit* **prostaglandin synthesis** which causes renal arteriole vasoconstriction
  - **Aminoglycosides, contrast dyes** and **myoglobin** - direct injury to renal tubules

POOR URINE OUTPUT POST-OP (or azotemia post-op)
- MCC of poor urine output post-op - **hypovolemia**
- Azotemia = elevated **BUN** and **Cr**
- **Oliguria** (poor urine output) or **azotemia post-op**
  - 1st - check urinary catheter; make sure **volume loaded** (CVP 11-15) and consider volume challenge (1-2 L LR or NS); send urine electrolytes and consider renal U/S
  - 2nd - try **diuretic trial** → furosemide (Lasix)
  - 3rd - dialysis if needed
- FE_{Na} (fractional excretion of sodium) = (urine Na/Cr) / (plasma Na/Cr)
  - *Best test for **acute azotemia** or **poor urine output** not responsive to volume*
  - Determines pre-renal vs. intrinsic renal cause
- **Renal U/S** - *best test for **acute obstructive nephropathy / uropathy*** (azotemia or poor urine output due to obstruction)
  - Etiologies - kidney stone, iatrogenic ligation of ureter, BPH
  - **U/S** - shows **hydronephrosis**
- **Tx:**
  - **Pre-renal** oliguria / azotemia
    - Tx: **optimize volume**
  - **Renal** oliguria / azotemia (intrinsic; parenchymal)
    - Intrinsic renal failure is usually from **acute tubular necrosis** (ATN)
    - MCC of renal ATN - **hypotension** intra-op
    - Tx: **diuretic trial** (eg furosemide); try to make **non-oliguric**
  - **Post-renal** oliguria / azotemia (ie obstructive nephropathy / uropathy)
    - Tx: **relieve obstruction**
- MCC of post-op acute renal failure (ie ATN) - **hypotension** intra-op (eg s/p open AAA repair now with oliguria despite fluid resuscitation)

Diagnostic Values for Azotemia or Poor Urine Output

Parameter	Pre-renal	Renal (intrinsic, parenchymal)
FE_{Na}	< 1%	> 3%
Urine sodium	< 20	> 40
Urine osmolality	> 500	< 350
BUN / Cr ratio	> 40	< 20

- **Indications for dialysis** - high K (*most immediate, life-threatening issue*), fluid overload, metabolic acidosis, uremic encephalopathy, uremic coagulopathy, poisoning
- **Hemodialysis** – rapid; can cause large volume shifts and instability (**hypotension**) in sick patients
  - Hct increases by 5-8 for each liter taken off with dialysis
- **CVVH** - slower; good for ill patients who can not tolerate hemodynamic instability (eg cardiogenic shock, septic shock)
- **Contrast dyes** - direct tubular injury; Tx: **pre-hydration** before contrast exposure *(best)*; HCO_3^-, N-acetylcysteine
  - Note - **gadolinium** for MRI can cause **contrast nephropathy** and **nephrogenic systemic fibrosis** in patients with **renal insufficiency**
  - Can use CO_2 **angiogram** (contrast not as good, less renal toxic)
- **Myoglobinuria**
  - Released from muscle after trauma (eg crush injury) or compartment syndrome
  - Myoglobin converted to **ferrihemate** in acid environment (renal toxic)
  - Urine shows presence of heme (positive for blood) *without* RBCs
  - Tx: fluids *(best)* + $HCO3^-$ to alkalinize urine (prevents conversion to ferrihemate)

SIRS (Systemic Inflammatory Response Syndrome)
- Causes - **infection** (MCC; eg bacteremia, pneumonia), any form of shock, burns, multi-trauma, pancreatitis, ARDS, severe inflammatory responses
- **Sepsis** = SIRS + infection
- SIRS → shock → multisystem organ failure → death
- All mediated by massive **TNF-alpha** and **IL-1** cytokine release

- *Most potent <u>stimulant</u> for **SIRS** (and **TNF-alpha** release) - **gram negative rod endotoxin** (lipopolysaccharide; lipid A portion)*
- Criteria for SIRS (need $\geq$ 2):
  - **Temp**   > 38°C or < 36°C
  - **HR**   > 90 (or on pressors)
  - **RR**   > 20 (or requiring intubation)
  - **pCO$_2$**   < 32 mmHg
  - **WBC**   > 12 or < 4
- Goals are to **stop the cause of SIRS** and **supportive care**

SEPSIS (SIRS + infection)
- **Hyperglycemia** - often occurs *<u>just before</u>* clinical sepsis
- **Optimal glucose level in septic patients**: 80 - 120
- Sepsis + hypotension = **septic shock**
- **Hypotension** with septic shock is related to up-regulation of **inducible nitric oxide synthetase** (iNOS)

BRAIN DEATH
- **Precludes diagnosis** - temperature < 32 C, SBP < 90, drugs (eg ETOH, phenobarbital, pentobarbital), metabolic derangements (eg hyperglycemia, uremia), desaturation with apnea test
- **Following must exist for 6-12 hours** - unresponsive to pain, absent cold caloric oculovestibular reflexes, absent oculocephalic reflex (patient doesn't track), no spontaneous respirations, no corneal reflex, no gag reflex, fixed and dilated pupils, positive apnea test
- **EEG** - shows electrical silence; **MRA** - will show no blood flow to brain
- **Apnea test** - the patient is pre-oxygenated, a catheter delivering O$_2$ at 8 L/min is placed at the carina through the ET-tube; CO$_2$ should be normal before starting the test
  - The patient is disconnected from the ventilator for **10 minutes**
  - A **CO$_2$ > 60 mm Hg** or *increase* in CO$_2$ by 20 mmHg at the end of the test is a **positive test for apnea** (meets brain death criteria)
  - If <u>SBP</u> drops (< 90), the patient <u>desaturates</u> (< 85% on pulse oximeter), or <u>spontaneous breathing</u> occurs the test is terminated (<u>negative test for apnea</u>) → place back on the ventilator (cannot declare brain death)
- Can still have **deep tendon reflexes** with brain death

TOXICITIES AND OTHER CONDITIONS
- **Carbon monoxide poisoning**
  - **MCC fatal poisoning** (from suicide) - carbon monoxide
  - Can also occur with **fires** and **smoke inhalation**
  - Sx's: HA, N/V, confusion (mental status changes), coma, death
  - Binds hemoglobin (Hgb) directly (creates **carboxyhemoglobin**) → O$_2$ can't bind anymore (all the binding sites are filled)
  - **Carbon monoxide** has as a **greater affinity** for Hgb than oxygen (250 x)
  - Also results in a **left shift** on the Hgb-oxygen dissociation curve
    - Hgb will not let go of bound O$_2$
  - Dx: **Falsely elevates oxygen saturation reading** on pulse oximeter
  - Abnormal carboxyhemoglobin levels:
    - **Non-smokers** > 10%
    - **Smokers**   > 20%
    - **Coma**   > 50%
    - **Death**   > 70%
  - Tx: **100% oxygen on ventilator** (*best* Tx, displaces carbon monoxide); rarely need hyperbaric O$_2$
- **Methemoglobinemia** (eg Hurricaine spray, fertilizers; nitrites act as oxidizers)
  - Sx's: tachypnea (↑ RR), dyspnea, metabolic lactic acidosis
  - Oxygen carrying **ferrous ion** (Fe2+) of heme group is oxidized to ferric ion (Fe3+) → forming **methemoglobin** which *cannot* bind oxygen
  - Results in a **right shift** on the Hgb-oxygen dissociation curve
  - Oxygen saturation reads 85% on pulse oximeter

- Tx: **methylene blue** and oxygen
- **Nipride toxicity** (cyanide toxicity)
  - Sx's: N/V, confusion, metabolic acidosis, elevated SvO_2
  - Tx: **amyl nitrite**, followed by **sodium nitrite** and **sodium thiosulfate**; hydroxocobalamin (IV Vit B12)
- **Critical illness polyneuropathy** - motor > sensory neuropathy; occurs with sepsis; can lead to failure to wean from ventilator
- **ETOH withdrawal Sx's**: HTN, tachycardia, delirium, seizures after 48 hours
  - Tx: thiamine, folate, B_{12}, Mg, K, PRN lorazepam (Ativan)
- **ICU psychosis** - generally occurs on 3rd post-op day and is frequently preceded by lucid interval
  - Need to rule-out metabolic (eg hypoglycemia, DKA, hypoxia, hypercarbia, electrolyte imbalances) and organic (eg MI, CVA) causes
- **Damage control** - at times during major elective surgeries (eg major liver resection, complicated gastrectomy, leak following gastric bypass) patients will become cold, acidotic, hypotensive and oliguric; the approach here is to come to a logical stopping point in the operation, take the patient to the ICU for resuscitation, and bring the patient back to the OR to finish the procedure when they are stabilized (after 24-48 hours)
- **Reperfusion injury** – critical role of **PMNs**

CHRONIC RENAL FAILURE CHANGES
- **Anemia** (low erythropoietin)
- $\uparrow$ **K,** $\uparrow$ **BUN,** $\uparrow$ **Cr,** $\uparrow$ **Mg** and $\uparrow$ **PO$_4^-$**
- $\downarrow$ **Na,** $\downarrow$ **Ca** and $\downarrow$ **pH**
- **Volume overload** (can't make urine)
- Hemodialysis can remove fluid, K, BUN, Cr, Ca, Mg, PO_4^-, and H^+
- *Avoid* Mg-containing laxatives

PERITONEAL DIALYSIS
- *Absolute contraindications* - extensive adhesions, physical / mental condition making them incapable of performing PD, uncorrected mechanical defects (eg inguinal hernia)
- *Relative contraindications* - recent intra-abdominal foreign material (eg aortic tube graft, recent ventricular-peritoneal shunt), peritoneal leaks, body size limitations, inflammatory bowel disease, severe malnutrition, frequent diverticulitis
- Catheter should be placed in the **deep pelvis**
- The catheter should be directed downward after exiting the skin (exit site should be above the beltline)
- Catheter is placed through the **rectus muscle**
- Early Cx's - bowel perforation (1%), outflow failure (catheter placement in omentum [MCC], catheter tip migration, fibrin clot, kinking)
- Late Cx's - exit-site infection, tunnel infection, peritonitis, cuff protrusion, outflow failure (obstruction by omental wrapping [MCC], constipation - stool in rectum presses on catheter, kinking), dialysate leaks, hernias

ABDOMINAL COMPARTMENT SYNDROME
- Sx's:
  1) **Hypotension**
  2) **Distended abdomen**
  3) **Low urine output** (**decreased C.O.** from **IVC compression** biggest factor; also renal vein compression)
  4) **High airway pressures** (upward displacement of diaphragm)
- Occurs with **hypotension** and **massive blood / fluid resuscitation** due to trauma (especially with prolonged transport time) or prolonged, extensive abdominal surgery
- Abdominal contents become **swollen** and **compress IVC**, leading to *decreased* C.O. (visceral / renal malperfusion; low urine output)
- **IVC compression** (leading to decreased venous return) is the final common pathway for **decreased C.O.**
- Dx: **bladder pressure > 20 - 25** (hook bladder catheter up to CVP monitor to measure)
- Cx's: gut malperfusion, poor ventilation

- Tx: **decompressive laparotomy**, sterile cover for abdominal contents
- **Can't get abdomen closed because of swollen bowel** → cut sterile IV bag and sew to skin; loban drape over that; bring back in 48 hours and close abdomen when visceral swelling goes down

CO_2 PNEUMOPERITONEUM (normal pressure 10-15 mmHg)
- Cardiopulmonary dysfunction can occur with intra-abdominal pressure > 20 (try to keep insufflation pressure **10-15 mmHg**)
  - High initial insufflation pressure → malpositioned insufflation needle
  - Zero initial insufflation pressure → stopcock is closed
- Are *increased* with pneumoperitoneum: mean arterial pressure, pulmonary artery pressure, HR, systemic vascular resistance, central venous pressure, mean airway pressure, peak inspiratory pressure, and CO_2
- Are *decreased* with pneumoperitoneum: pH, venous return (IVC compression), cardiac output, renal flow secondary to decreased cardiac output (renin will increase)
- **Hypovolemia** lowers pressure necessary to cause compromise
- **PEEP** worsens effects of pneumoperitoneum
- CO_2 can cause some decrease in myocardial contractility
- Can minimize **respiratory acidosis** from CO_2 pneumoperitoneum by *decreasing* pneumoperitoneum pressure and *increasing* minute ventilation (RR or TV)

SURGICAL TECHNOLOGIES
- **Harmonic scalpel**
  - Cost-effective for **medium vessels** (short gastric arteries)
  - Disrupts **protein hydrogen bonds** and causes **coagulation** of vessels
- **Ultrasound**
  - **B-mode** (MC used, B = brightness; assesses relative density of structures); forms 2 dimensional structure
    - **Shadowing** - dark area posterior to object indicates solid mass (eg gallstone)
    - **Enhancement** - brighter area posterior to object, indicates fluid-filled cyst or structure (eg gallbladder)
  - **Lower frequencies** - good for deep structures, less resolution
  - **Higher frequencies** - good for superficial structures, more resolution
- **Duplex ultrasound** combines **B mode** (above) with **doppler**; looks at how sound waves bounce off moving objects like blood; gives colored visual description of blood flow (can see velocity, stenosis, and direction)

ACUTE GOUT FLARE
- Due to **uric acid** buildup (end product of purine metabolism)
- Sx's: painful arthritis, especially the MTP of great toe (podagra); warm, tense joint
- Dx: needle shaped ***negatively birefringent crystals***; ↑ WBCs in joint
- Tx: **Acute attacks** - **indomethacin** (NSAID), **colchicine** (microtubule inhibitor, prevents WBC migration), steroids if severe
  - **Allopurinol** (xanthine oxidase inhibitor) - inhibits uric acid synthesis
  - **Probenecid** - inhibits renal reabsorption of uric acid

Burns

438. Each of the following are true of 1st and superficial 2nd degree burns except:
  - a. Epithelialization occurs primarily from hair follicles
  - b. Epithelialization can occur from the edges of the wound
  - c. Superficial 2nd degree burns usually require skin grafts
  - d. A sunburn is an example of a 1st degree burn
  - e. Scald burns are the MC type of burn

  Answer c. Superficial 2nd degree burns do not require skin grafts.

439. The primary fuel used in burn wounds is:
  - a. Protein
  - b. Fatty acids
  - c. Glucose
  - d. Glutamine

  Answer c. WBCs use glucose in an obligatory fashion (primary cell in burn wounds) although this does not require modification of TPN components.

440. The most important nutritional component for healing severe burns is:
  - a. Protein
  - b. Fatty acids
  - c. Glucose
  - d. Glutamine

  Answer a. Burn wounds require a significant amount of protein to heal the area (1.5 mg/kg x % BSA burn).

441. All of the following patients require referral to a burn center except:
  - a. A 25 yo woman with a 4% BSA second degree burn to the back of hand
  - b. A 25 yo man with a 15% BSA second degree burn to her back
  - c. A 25 yo man with a 4% BSA second burn to his elbow
  - d. An 80 yo man with a 11% BSA second degree burn to his back
  - e. A 25 yo man with a 6% BSA third degree burn to his back

  Answer b. This patient would not require referral.

442. Second degree burns involving the entire left leg and entire left arm would be considered:
  - a. 20% BSA
  - b. 27% BSA
  - c. 34% BSA
  - d. 41% BSA

  Answer b. 27% BSA (leg - 18%; arm - 9%)

443. A 54 yo man involved in a house fire was trapped in an enclosed space. As you evaluate him, he spits up carbonaceous sputum. You notice upper airway stridor and his throat feels tight. All the following are true except:
  - a. This patient should be intubated
  - b. Lung and tracheal injury primarily result from carbon products, not heat
  - c. Burn wound infection is the MC infection with severe burns (>30% BSA)
  - d. ETOH is a risk factor for inhalational injury

  Answer c. Pneumonia is the MC infection in patients with significant burn wounds. In some series, 70% of all patients with large burns get pneumonia.

444. A 28 yo man suffers severe 2nd and 3rd degree burns (60% BSA). He is intubated and currently undergoing appropriate fluid resuscitation. The patient has 3rd degree burns across his entire chest extending to his back and is hard to ventilate. The patient also

has a circumferential burn to his right arm and hand with decreased perfusion to his digits. The next appropriate step is:

    a.   Escharotomy
    b.   Arm elevation
    c.   Thrombectomy of the right brachial artery
    d.   TPA

Answer a. Patients with circumferential 2nd and 3rd degree burns and poor distal perfusion should undergo **escharotomy** to that extremity. Occasionally for deep burns, escharotomy is not enough because the muscle compartment is involved in the burn and <u>fasciotomy</u> is required. For the arm, opening the dorsal and ventral compartments is required. Patients with severe burns **across the chest** can have trouble with ventilation due to decreased chest wall compliance (from both the burn and from edema with subsequent fluid resuscitation; Tx - chest escharotomy). Patients with severe burns to the **fingers** and decreased perfusion require **mid-axial incisions** (*not* lateral – the nerves travel here).

445. All of the following are true of fluid resuscitation for burn patients except:

    a.   Lactated ringers is the fluid of choice
    b.   Aggressive fluid resuscitation is indicated for $\geq$ 2 degree burns over $\geq$ 15% BSA
    c.   CVP is the best measure of fluid resuscitation
    d.   ½ the volume should be give in the 1st 8 hours

Answer c. **Urine output** is the best measure of fluid resuscitation in burns patients.

In trauma patients with **hemorrhage** or other conditions resulting in hemorrhage, **serum lacatate** is the best indicator of resuscitation.

446. A 70 kg man has 15% BSA 2nd degree burns and 10% BSA 3rd degree burns. Appropriate total volume resuscitation should be:

    a.   5000 cc
    b.   6000 cc
    c.   7000 cc
    d.   8000 cc
    e.   9000 cc

Answer c. 7000 cc. Give 4 cc/kg × % burn in first 24 hours (4 cc x 70 kg x 25% BSA burn). Give half that volume in the first 8 hours.

447. Treatment of patients with severe burn injuries and myoglobinuria consists of:

    a.   Broad spectrum antibiotics
    b.   Aggressive inotropic support
    c.   Fluid resuscitation and HCO_3^- drip
    d.   CVVH to clear the myoglobin

Answer c. The best Tx for patients with burn injuries and myoglobinuria is fluid resuscitation and sodium bicarbonate (HCO_3^-) to prevent precipitation of myoglobin.

448. The best way to diagnose burn wound sepsis is:

    a.   Culture swab of the wound
    b.   Biopsy of the wound
    c.   Blood cultures
    d.   Examination

Answer b. The best way to Dx burn wound infection is wound biopsy.

449. You are getting ready to place a skin graft on a burn area. A burn wound biopsy shows 10^4 staph epidermidis/gram of tissue. The next appropriate step in management is:
   a. Nothing
   b. Broad spectrum antibiotics
   c. Vancomycin
   d. Proceed with auto-grafting

   Answer d. The diagnosis of a burn wound infection requires $> 10^5$ organisms/gram of tissue, otherwise it is considered colonization. The best way to diagnose a burn wound infection is with a burn wound biopsy (avoids contaminates from just swabbing it)

   If there was an **infection** present in the burn wound, in addition to starting antibiotics, going ahead with excising the burn wound (and the infection) and placing a temporary porcine allograft is a reasonable option. *You would not want to place an autograft in this situation.*

450. The most common organism involved in burn wound infection is:
   a. Staph epidermidis
   b. Pseudomonas
   c. Strep viridans
   d. Klebsiella

   Answer b. Pseudomonas is the MC organism in burn wound infection (some studies state staph aureus is the MC organism, but pseudomonas is the classic answer; often times it just depends on the institution reporting the data)

451. All of the following are true of topical burn agents except:
   a. Silvadene can result in neutropenia and thrombocytopenia
   b. Silver nitrate can result in methemoglobinemia
   c. Mafenide acetate can result in metabolic alkalosis
   d. Topical antibiotics result in decreased burn wound infections
   e. Mupirocin can be effective for MRSA infections

   Answer c. Sulfamylon (**mafenide acetate**) can result in **metabolic acidosis** (not metabolic alkalosis) through inhibition of carbonic anhydrase.

452. Skin grafts survive in the 1st 48 hours primarily by:
   a. Neovascularization
   b. Reliance on stored glycogen
   c. Gluconeogenesis
   d. Imbibition

   Answer d. Skin grafts survive by **imbibition** (osmotic exchange of nutrients) for the 1st 48 hours. After that, neovascularization takes over.

453. In comparison of split thickness skin grafts (STSG) to full thickness skin grafts (FTSG), all of the following are true except:
   a. STSG are more likely to survive
   b. FTSG have less wound contraction
   c. FTSG are good for palmar burns
   d. The most common reason for skin graft loss is infection

   Answer d. The MCC of **skin graft loss** is **seroma** (or hematoma) formation underneath skin graft, which raises it, and prevents neovascularization. Make sure the skin graft is compressed down with xeroform gauze to prevent this.

454. You bring an intubated 30 yo man with a 60% BSA burn back to the OR for his 3rd debridement in 3 days and the anesthesiologist gives him succinylcholine. Shortly after this, his EKG shows T wave abnormalities, then a widened QRS, and then

asystole. You cannot feel a pulse so you start CPR. The 1st drug you should give for this problem is:

   a.   Dantrolene
   b.   Calcium gluconate
   c.   Methylene blue
   d.   Atropine

Answer b. Burn patients are at increased risk for **hyperkalemia** because of myonecrosis and leaking of potassium into the blood stream. This, combined with succinylcholine which causes potassium release when it depolarizes the cell membrane, results in hyperkalemia. The 1st Tx of choice for **hyperkalemia** with arrhythmias is **calcium gluconate** (stabilizes myocardial membranes).

Given general ACLS guidelines, epinephrine or vasopressin could have been given but these were not options. If you know the problem is **hyperkalemia**, give **calcium gluconate**.

455. All of the following are true of frostbite except:
   a.   Tetanus prophylaxis is indicated
   b.   Early aggressive debridement for gangrene is indicated
   c.   Topical antibiotics are indicated
   d.   Rapid re-warming is indicated

Answer b. Early debridement should be _avoided_ for early gangrene. One should wait up to 3-4 months so that viable and necrotic areas are clearly demarcated to avoid removing viable tissue.

456. All of the following are true of carbon monoxide poisoning except:
   a.   CO results in a left shift on the oxygen-hemoglobin dissociation curve
   b.   CO binds heme molecules with 200 times more affinity than oxygen
   c.   CO falsely elevates the pulse oximetry reading
   d.   The primary treatment is hyperbaric oxygen

Answer d. The primary treatment is **intubation** with 100% oxygen

457. All of the following are true except:
   a.   Seizures following burn wounds are MC due to stroke
   b.   Ectopia is best treated with surgical release
   c.   Hydrofluoric acid burns are best treated with calcium (topical, intra-arterial)
   d.   Steroids are contraindicated in Toxic Epidermal Necrolysis
   e.   The MC burn type is accidental scald burn

Answer a. Seizures following burn wounds are MC due to **hyponatremia** related to fluid resuscitation

Burn Classification

Degree	Description
1st degree	Sunburn (epidermis)
2nd degree	
Superficial dermis (papillary)	Painful to touch; blebs and blisters; hair follicles intact; blanches _Do not need skin grafts - heals in 2 weeks_
Deep dermis (reticular)	Decreased sensation; **loss of hair follicles**, slow to blanch (need **skin grafts**)
3rd degree	Leathery (charred parchment); down to subcutaneous fat (sub-dermal)
4th degree	Down to bone, adipose, tendon, or muscle tissue

- Burn Injury RFs: alcohol or drug use, age (very young or old), smoking, low socioeconomic status, violence, epilepsy
- Highest deaths - **children** and **elderly** (can't get away)
- 1st and superficial 2nd degree burns heal by **epithelialization** - epithelial cells come from **hair follicles** (primary site) and edges of wound

ADMISSION CRITERIA
- 2nd and 3rd degree burns > 10% BSA in patients aged < 10 or > 50 years
- 2nd and 3rd degree burns > 20% BSA in all other patients
- 2nd and 3rd degree burns to significant portions of hands, face, feet, genitalia, perineum, or skin overlying major joints
- 3rd degree burns > 5% in any age group
- Electrical and chemical burns
- Concomitant inhalational injury, mechanical trauma, or preexisting medical conditions
- Patients with special social, emotional, or long-term rehabilitation needs
- Suspected child abuse or neglect

CHILD ABUSE
- Accounts for 15% of burn injuries in children

History and Exam findings that suggest abuse

Delayed care	Lack of splash marks
Conflicting histories	Stocking or glove pattern
Previous burns or injuries	Flexor area sparing
Sharp demarcation	Dorsal area of hands
Uniform depth of burn	Deep and localized contact

BURN ASSESSMENT AND INITIAL MANAGEMENT
- **Scald** burns (heated fluids, eg hot water bath) - MC type of burn (usually accidental)
- **Flame** burns (ie fire) - more likely to come to hospital and be admitted
- **Contact** burns (ie hot stove)
- % burn with 50% mortality (LD_{50}) - **65% BSA**
- SIRS occurs at 15-20% BSA burn
- Assessing **percentage of body surface area** burned (rule of 9s)
  - Head = 9, arms = 18, chest = 18, back = 18, legs = 36, perineum = 1
  - Can also use patient's palm to estimate injury (palm = 1%)
- **Parkland formula**
  - Use only for $\geq$ **2nd degree burns** that are ≥ **15% BSA**
  - Give 4 cc/kg × % BSA burn in first 24 hours:
    - Give ½ of that volume within the first 8 hours
    - Give the next ½ over the next 16 hours
  - Use **Lactated Ringer's** solution (LR) in first 24 hours
    - Switch to D5 1/2 NS after 24 hrs
  - Parkland formula can grossly underestimate volume requirements with inhalational injury, ETOH, electrical injury, or post-escharotomy
  - **Children** need **glucose** (D5) in the first 24 hours as well; also need <u>maintenance</u> IVFs in addition to resuscitation fluids
    - Parkland underestimates fluid requirement in children by about 30%
    - Children should have aggressive fluid resuscitation started $\geq$ **2nd degree burns** that are ≥ **10% BSA**
  - *Avoid* colloid (albumin) in the first 24 hours (causes *increased* **respiratory Cx's**)
- **Escharotomy indications** (usually **circumferential** burns):
  - Cold extremity, weak pulse, ↓ capillary refill, ↓ pain sensation, or ↓ motor / neuro function in extremity
  - Problems ventilating patient with significant chest torso burns
  - May also need **fasciotomy** if compartment syndrome suspected
- **Escharotomy incisions** - perform within **4-6 hours** to prevent **myonecrosis**
  - **Forearms** - <u>dorsal</u> longitudinal incision, <u>ventral</u> S-shaped incision (relieves compression for both median and ulnar nerves)
  - **Hands** - incisions on the dorsum of hand (avoid palmar surface)

- **Fingers** - mid-axial incisions on ventral surface (avoid lateral incisions - the nerves are there)
- **Chest** (ie trouble ventilating patient) - lateral chest wall, subcostal, and subclavicular incisions
- **Legs** and **feet** - medial and lateral incisions
- **Extremely deep** and **electrical burns** can cause **compartment syndrome** and **rhabdomyolysis** (myoglobinuria, hyperkalemia, acidemia, and hyperphosphatemia)

INHALATIONAL INJURY
- Primarily caused by **carbonaceous materials** and **smoke,** not heat
- Important prognostic factor for **mortality** after burn
- Sx's of possible injury: stridor, facial burn, wheezing, carbonaceous sputum
- RFs: ETOH, trauma, closed space, rapid combustion, extremes of age (age < 10 <u>or</u> > 50), delayed extrication
- **Indications for intubation** - upper airway stridor or obstruction; worsening hypoxemia
- Massive volume resuscitation can worsen Sx's (pulmonary edema)
- Dx: **fiberoptic bronchoscopy** (see soot, erythema, edema)
- Keep intubated until patient has a **cuff leak** with the balloon down on the ET tube (ie swelling has decreased) and has a **normal ABG**
- **Cx's of inhalational injury**: pneumonia, airway obstruction, atelectasis, carbon monoxide poisoning, ARDS
- **Pneumonia** - MC infection in patients with > 30% BSA burns
  - MCC of <u>death</u> after significant burn - **pneumonia**
  - Pneumonia RFs: #1 **inhalational injury**, #2 massive fluid resuscitation with pulmonary edema

FIRST WEEK
- Goals for the 1st week: 1) **start nutrition** *and* 2) **excise burned areas**
- **Caloric need**: 25 calories/kg/day + (30 calories × % burn) - *don't exceed* 3000 kcal/d
- **Protein need**: 1 g/kg/day + (3 g × % burn) - *protein nutrition is a major concern for burn wound healing*
- Excise burn wounds **48-72 hours** after burn, but not until <u>after</u> appropriate fluid resuscitation and the patient is stable
  - Use **dermatome** to remove burn wound and **place skin graft**
  - Dermatome used for **deep 2nd, 3rd,** and some **4th degree** burns
  - Skin / tissue viability after dermatome excision is based on **punctate bleeding** (#1), color, and texture after eschar removal (if not viable, go deeper)
- Wounds to **face, palms, soles,** and **genitals** are *deferred* for the 1st week
- **For each burn wound excision session**:
  - Want < 1 L blood loss
  - < 20% of skin excised
  - < 2 hours in OR
  - *Blood loss is to be expected*
  - *Patients can get extremely sick if too much time is spent in OR*
- Autografts are *contraindicated* if wound Bx is positive for **beta-hemolytic strep** or **bacteria > 10^5**
- **Autografts** (split-thickness [STSG] or full-thickness [FTSG]) - *best*
  - Have decreased infection, desiccation, protein loss, pain, water loss, heat loss, and RBC loss compared to dermal substitutes
  - Donor skin site for STSGs undergoes re-epithelialization from **hair follicles** *(primary site)* and **skin edges**
    Takes **3 weeks** for donor site to heal (healing time *inversely* proportional to thickness of graft harvested)
    Can use a **donor site again** (re-epithelializes)
  - **Imbibition** (osmotic absorption of nutrients and oxygen) - blood supply to skin graft in days 0-3
  - **Neovascularization** (new blood vessel growth to graft) - starts around day 3
  - **Poorly vascularized beds** <u>unlikely</u> to support skin grafting:
    Tendon
    Bone without periosteum
    XRT areas (radiated skin)

- - **Unusual areas** that <u>can</u> support skin grafts - omentum, bone with periosteum, bowel wall
  - **STSG** - includes epidermis and part of dermis
  - **FTSG** - includes epidermis and all of the dermis
  - Skin grafts need to be **compressed** with xeroform gauze / cotton balls to inhibit **seroma** or **hematoma** formation which prevents the graft from attaching *(MCC of skin graft failure)*
- **Homografts** (allografts - human cadaveric skin; xenografts - usually porcine)
  - Good **temporizing material**; last **4 weeks**
  - Good for infected burn wounds
  - Allografts **vascularize** and are eventually **rejected** at which time they must be excised and replaced with autograft
- **Skin grafting:**
  - **Reasons to delay autografting:**
    - Infection
    - Not enough skin donor sites
    - Patient septic or unstable
    - Avoidance of more donor sites with concomitant blood loss
  - MCC of skin graft loss - **seroma** or **hematoma** formation under graft (lifts the graft and it won't neovascularize); apply gauze pressure dressing to the graft to prevent this
  - STSGs are more likely to **survive** compared to FTSG
    - Graft not as thick so easier for **imbibition** and subsequent revascularization to occur
    - **STSG** - 0.015 cm, includes **epidermis** and **part of dermis**
    - **Meshed** grafts - use for back, flank, trunk, arms, and legs
  - FTSGs have **less wound contraction** compared to STSG
    - Good for small areas such as the palms and back of hands
    - Not as many donor sites
    - Not good for large areas
    - Can get better skin color match
    - FTSG **donor site** must be **closed primarily**
    - Good FTSG donor sites - behind ear, above clavicle, groin (loose skin)
  - **STSG donor site**
    - **Hemostasis** with **epinephrine soaked gauzes**
    - Cover with Op-site (**semi-occlusive dressing**)
    - Donor site heals in **3 weeks**
    - Can use as a **STSG donor site again** (epithelium migrates primarily from **hair follicles**, also from wound edges; these are termed **epithelial appendages**)
    - Donor site **healing time** *inversely* proportional to **thickness of graft** harvested
  - **FTSG donor site** - need primary closure
- **Hands** and **fingers** - splint in extension prior to FTSG

WEEKS 2-4 (specialized areas addressed and allograft replaced with autograft)
- **Face** - topical antibiotics 1ˢᵗ week, **FTSG** for unhealed areas (non-meshed)
- **Hands**
  - **Superficial** - topical antibiotics, range of motion exercises; splint with fingers extended if edematous
  - **Deep**
    - Topical antibiotics and immobilize in extension for 1ˢᵗ week
    - May need wire fixation of joints if unstable or open
    - Immobilize in extension for 7 days after skin graft (need **FTSG**)
    - Physical therapy after that
  - **Palms** - try to preserve palmar attachments (palmar aponeurosis)
    - <u>Avoid</u> palmar fasciotomy or escharotomy - go on dorsal surface
- **Genitals** - topical antibiotics for 1 week; can use **STSG** (meshed)

BURN WOUND INFECTIONS

- Apply **topical antibiotics** (eg Silvadene, bacitracin, Neosporin, sulfamylon) immediately after burns (decreases incidence of burn wound infections)
- <u>No</u> role for prophylactic IV antibiotics
- **Silvadene** (silver sulfadiazine)
  - Can cause **neutropenia** and **thrombocytopenia**
  - *Contraindicated* in patients with sulfa allergy
  - Limited eschar penetration (bacteriostatic); can inhibit epithelialization
  - Ineffective against some *Pseudomonas*; effective for *Candida*
- **Silver nitrate**
  - Can cause **methemoglobinemia** - contraindicated in patients with G6PD deficiency (causes hemolysis)
  - Can cause **electrolyte imbalances** (hyponatremia, hypochloremia, hypocalcemia, and hypokalemia)
  - Discoloration
  - Limited eschar penetration
  - Ineffective against some *Pseudomonas* species and GPCs
- **Sulfamylon** (mafenide acetate) - <u>painful</u> application
  - Can cause **metabolic acidosis** due to carbonic anhydrase inhibition (decreased renal conversion of $H_2CO_3 \rightarrow H_2O + CO_2$)
  - Good eschar penetration; good for burns overlying <u>cartilage</u>
  - Broadest spectrum against *Pseudomonas* and GNRs
- **Mupirocin** (Bactroban) - good topical agent for MRSA
- **> 30% BSA burns** are at high risk for infection (larger burn = greater risk)
  - **Cell mediated immunity** is decreased in burn wound due to decreased granulocyte chemotaxis
- MC organisms in burn wound infection - **pseudomonas** and *Staph aureus*
- MC fungal infection - **Candida**
- **Sx's** (burn wound infection):
  - Peripheral edema
  - 2nd to 3rd degree burn conversion
  - Hemorrhage into scar
  - Ecthyma gangrenosum (pseudomonas); green fat, focal discoloration
  - Black skin around wound
  - Rapid eschar separation
  - Pseudomonas smell
- **Burn wound sepsis** - usually due to pseudomonas *or S. aureus*
- Best method to **diagnose burn wound infection** (and differentiate from colonization) – biopsy (Bx) of burn wound
  - $< 10^5$ organisms on Bx - <u>not</u> a burn wound infection (just colonization)
- **Tx** (burn wound infection):
  - **Burn wound excision** with <u>allograft</u> replacement
    Do <u>not</u> use autograft when excising infected burn wounds
  - **Systemic antibiotics**
  - Excise allograft and place autograft after the infection clears
  - If just cellulitis around burn wound → systemic and topical antibiotics

UNUSUAL BURNS

- **Acid** and **alkali burns** - copious water irrigation (30-60 min)
  - Alkalis produce deeper burns than acid due to **liquefaction** necrosis
  - Acid burns cause **coagulation** necrosis
- **Hydrofluoric acid** burns - intra-arterial **calcium**; spread calcium on wound (neutralizes burn)
- **Powder** burns - wipe away before irrigation
- **Tar** burns - cool, then wipe away with a **lipophilic solvent** (glycerol, eg adhesive remover)
- **Phenol** burns - are not water soluble; use lipophilic solvent (eg glycerol)
- **Electrical** burns - need cardiac monitoring
  - Can cause rhabdomyolysis and compartment syndrome

- • Other Cx's - polyneuritis, quadriplegia, transverse myelitis, cataracts, liver necrosis, hollow viscous perforation, pancreatic necrosis
- ■ **Lightning** - cardiac arrest secondary to ventricular fibrillation

COMPLICATIONS AFTER BURNS
- ■ **Seizures** - MC iatrogenic (related to **Na^+ concentration** and resuscitation)
- ■ **Hyperkalemia** - can occur with large burns from myonecrosis
  - • *Avoid **succinylcholine*** - releases potassium (can cause a lethal arrhythmia or asystole → Tx: **calcium gluconate**)
- ■ **Myoglobinuria** (from dead muscle); Tx: **fluid resuscitation** *(best Tx)* + HCO3⁻ to alkalinize urine and prevent precipitation of myoglobin
- ■ **Renal failure** (from volume loss, myoglobinuria)
- ■ **Ectopia** - contraction of burned adnexae and can't see out of eye
  - • Tx: surgical eyelid release
- ■ **Eyes** - fluorescein staining to Dx injury; Tx: fluoroquinolone ointment
- ■ **Corneal abrasion** - Tx: topical fluoroquinolone ointment
- ■ **Symblepharon** - eyelid stuck to underlying conjunctiva
  - • Tx: release with glass rod and amniotic tissue transplantation
- ■ **Curling's ulcer** - duodenal ulcer that occurs with burns
- ■ **Marjolin's ulcer** - highly malignant, ulcerative **squamous cell CA** in **chronic non-healing burn wounds** or in chronic healing unstable scars (osteomyelitis, venous ulcers, post-XRT); latency period is up to 30 years
- ■ **Acalculous cholecystitis**
- ■ **Peripheral neuropathy** - from small vessel injury and demyelination
- ■ **Heterotopic tendon ossification** - Tx: physical therapy; may need surgery
- ■ **Fractures** - Tx: often need external fixation to allow for treatment of burns
- ■ **Hypertrophic scar**
  - • Does <u>not</u> go beyond original border of scar like keloids
  - • Usually occurs 3 - 4 months after injury
  - • Secondary to increased **neovascularization**
  - • MC with **deep** thermal injuries, take > 3 weeks to heal, heal by contraction and epithelial spread, or heal across flexor surfaces
  - • Tx: **steroid injection** into lesion *(best)*, silicone injection, compression
  - • Wait at least 1 year before scar modification surgery (scar excision, primary closure, then steroid injections)

FROSTBITE
- ■ Need rapid re-warming (40-42 C in circulating water; want sensation to return)
- ■ Tetanus prophylaxis, topical antibiotic, pain control
- ■ *Avoid early surgery (even if gangrene is present)* → *may take 3-4 months to differentiate between viable and necrotic tissue*
- ■ Allow time for the necrotic tissue to autoamputate
- ■ Avoid pressure on the area and use non-abrasive cleaning

ERYTHEMA MULTIFORME (and variants)
- ■ **Erythema Multiforme** - least severe form (self-limited; target lesions)
- ■ **Stevens-Johnson Syndrome** - more serious (< 10% BSA)
- ■ **Toxic Epidermal Necrolysis** (TEN) - most severe form (> 30% BSA)
- ■ **Staph Scalded Skin Syndrome** - caused by **staph aureus** (can be associated with toxic shock syndrome; Sx's - fever, N/V/D, diffuse erythema, hypotension, desquamation)
- ■ All have *skin epidermal detachment from the dermis (<u>desquamation</u>)*
- ■ Mouth, lungs, and GI tract can also be involved
- ■ Caused by a variety of **drugs** [**penicillin** (MC), Dilantin, Bactrim] and **viruses**
- ■ Tx: fluid resuscitation (weeping wounds); apply topical antibiotics; prevent wound desiccation with Telfa gauze wraps (non-stick); IV antibiotics if due to *Staph*; may need future skin grafts
- ■ *<u>No steroids</u>*
- ■ <u>No</u> silvadene if thought to be sulfa related

Head and Neck

458. All of the following are true except:
   a. Torus palatine is generally resected
   b. The inferior thyroid artery is a branch of the thyrocervical trunk
   c. The facial nerve provides motor function to the face
   d. The phrenic nerve is located along the anterior scalene muscle

   Answer a. Torus palatine (benign congenital bony mass on upper palate of mouth) should be left alone.

459. Patients with head and neck squamous cell CA are at high risk for:
   a. Esophageal CA
   b. Melanoma
   c. Lung CA
   d. Brain CA
   e. Nasopharyngeal CA

   Answer c. Around 5% of all patients with head and neck CA will have either a synchronous or metachronous lung CA. Screening for lung CA in these patients is appropriate (these are often diagnosed at an earlier stage for this population).

460. A 55 yo man presents to your office with an asymptomatic left sided 2 cm neck mass on the anterior border of the sternocleidomastoid muscle near the clavicle. The mass has been present for about 3 months. He denies fevers or other Sx's. The mass is not tender. On exam, the mass is mobile and you do not feel any adenopathy. Physical exam is otherwise normal. The most appropriate next step for this patient is:
   a. Perform excisional biopsy
   b. FNA in the office
   c. I-131
   d. Antibiotics

   Answer b. FNA (with U/S if possible) is the next appropriate step. FNA can make a definitive Dx 90% of the time.

461. Which of the following is the most likely diagnosis in the above patient:
   a. Squamous cell CA
   b. Adenocarcinoma
   c. Lymphoma
   d. Thyroid CA
   e. Parathyroid CA

   Answer a. Squamous cell CA

462. If the above patient was age 35, which of the following would be most likely:
   a. Squamous cell CA
   b. Adenocarcinoma
   c. Lymphoma
   d. Thyroid CA
   e. Parathyroid CA

   Answer c. Lymphoma (squamous cell CA if $\geq$ 50, lymphoma if < 50)

463. FNA in the above patient shows squamous cell CA in a lymph node. In addition to physical exam, the test most likely to identify this patient's primary lesion is:
   a. MRI
   b. Pan endoscopy with random biopsies
   c. CT scan
   d. PET scan

Answer b. You are trying to find the primary tumor here. It would be premature to go with just excisional biopsy. Although CT scan will be needed in the work-up, **physical exam** and **pan-endoscopy** detects 80% of head and neck tumors.

464. Instead of the above, FNA is negative despite 3 attempts. Pan-endoscopy with random biopsies and neck/chest/abdominal CT are negative except for the 2 cm lesion. The lesion is non-cystic and does not appear to be invading any other structures. The most appropriate next step in this patients management is:
    a. Excisional Biopsy
    b. Modified radical neck dissection
    c. Radiation therapy
    d. I-131

Answer a. Perform excisional biopsy is the most appropriate next step. You have performed an appropriate work-up to find the primary tumor and the patient does not have diffuse adenopathy suggestive of lymphoma. One should always be prepared to perform a modified radical neck dissection (MRND) when biopsying an anterior neck mass in case multiple nodes are found but this should not be the initial step.

465. The excisional biopsy for the above patient comes back as a lymph node with squamous cell carcinoma. The most likely source for the primary tumor is:
    a. Palate
    b. Tonsil
    c. Tongue
    d. Pharynx

Answer b. The MC location for a head / neck CA of unknown origin is **tonsils**.

466. For the above, which of the following is the most appropriate next step:
    a. Selective neck dissection
    b. Induction chemo with 5-FU and cisplatin
    c. XRT only
    d. Modified radical neck dissection and ipsilateral tonsilectomy

Answer d. Metastatic squamous cell CA with **occult primary** is treated with **ipsilateral MRND**, **ipsilateral tonsillectomy** and post-op **bilateral neck XRT**.

467. Instead of the above, the excisional biopsy shows thyroid tissue (pathology reports it as lateral aberrant thyroid tissue). All of the following are true _except_:
    a. The patient should undergo total thyroidectomy
    b. The patient should undergo MRND
    c. The patient should receive post-op XRT
    d. The patient should be treated with I-131

Answer c. Occult papillary thyroid CA can present in this fashion (the papillary CA has spread to a cervical node). Tx - total thyroidectomy, MRND, and I-131. Post op XRT is indicated for papillary (and follicular) CA only if it is not responsive to I-131.

468. A 50 yo man with a long history of chewing tobacco presents with a 2 cm ulcer on his inner cheek. You get a core needle biopsy which shows a verrucous (buccal squamous cell) CA. The most appropriate management of this patient is:
    a. Pre-op chemo-XRT followed by resection
    b. Chemo-XRT only
    c. Full cheek resection with flap
    d. Full cheek resection with modified radical neck dissection

Answer c. Verrucous ulcer CA (buccal squamous cell CA) is not aggressive and can undergo full cheek resection with 0.5 cm margins +/- a flap. No chemo or XRT is indicated. Lymph node dissection is <u>not</u> indicated either.

469. All of the following are true of oral cavity squamous cell CA except:
   a.   The lower lip is more commonly involved than the upper lip
   b.   Nasopharyngeal SCCA is associated with human papilloma virus
   c.   Nasopharyngeal SCCA is treated primarily with chemo-XRT
   d.   Flaps are needed if more than 1/3 of the lip is removed

   Answer b. Nasopharyngeal CA is associated with **Epstein Barr Virus**
   and is treated primarily with **chemo-XRT** (_very_ sensitive to XRT; stage I
   nasopharyngeal CA gets XRT only).

470. A 50 yo man has a mass just anterior to the ear. The mass causes him pain and he
   has a facial droop. CT of the head shows the tumor is involved in both the deep and
   superficial portions of the gland. This most likely represents:
   a.   Mucoepidermoid carcinoma
   b.   Adenoid cystic carcinoma
   c.   Pleomorphic adenoma
   d.   Warthin's Tumor

   Answer a. There are 2 features of this presentation that make the parotid tumor
   almost certainly malignant. The first is that it invades both the superficial and
   deep glands (unusual for benign tumors) and the second is that the **facial nerve**
   is affected (facial droop). Given that this tumor is almost certainly malignant, you
   have to go with the MC malignant tumor of the parotid, which is mucoepidermoid
   carcinoma. The **facial nerve** courses through the **parotid gland** and controls
   motor function to face.

471. The nerve most likely injured with submandibular resection is:
   a.   Vagus
   b.   Hypoglossal
   c.   Auriculo-temporal
   d.   Marginal mandibular

   Answer d. The nerve most commonly injured with resection of the
   submandibular gland is the **marginal mandibular nerve** (branch of the facial
   nerve). The marginal mandibular nerve has fibers that go to the mental nerve
   which provides sensation and motor to the corner of the mouth and chin (the
   inferior alveolar nerve, off the trigeminal nerve, also gives fibers to the mental
   nerve)

472. A 55 yo man with a pre-auricular mass undergoes head, neck and chest CT which
   shows a parotid tumor involving both lobes with no additional lesions or adenopathy.
   EGD and bronchoscopy are also negative. The patient has a normal neurologic exam.
   At resection, a mucoepidermoid carcinoma is completely encasing the facial nerve.
   Which of the following is the appropriate next step:
   a.   Superficial parotidectomy
   b.   Total parotidectomy and stripping the tumor off the facial nerve
   c.   Total parotidectomy and resection of the facial nerve
   d.   Close and give XRT

   Answer b. Due to the morbidity associated with resection of the facial nerve, an
   attempt should be made to preserve it, even if you have to peal the tumor off.
   This area should receive post-op XRT after surgery. If the neuro exam revealed
   the nerve was already non-functional (an uncommon scenario), it could then be
   sacrificed.

473. A 55 yo woman with a pre-auricular mass undergoes head, neck, and chest MRI which
   show a diffusely infiltrative parotid tumor extending to and encasing the carotid sheath
   and vagus nerve. The external carotid artery is narrowed from compression. Bx
   shows adenoid cystic CA. The most appropriate next step is:
   a.   Total parotidectomy with carotid reconstruction

        b.   Total parotidectomy and stripping the tumor off the carotid artery
        c.   XRT
        d.   chemo

Answer c. Adenoid cystic CA can be extensively infiltrative, with a propensity to invade nerve roots. Additionally, it is very sensitive to XRT and typically has a long indolent course. Given the diffuse disease in this patient, **XRT** is indicated as sole therapy.

474. All of the following are true except:
        a.   The MC benign parotid tumor is pleomorphic adenoma
        b.   The tumor most likely to involve bilateral parotid glands at time of Dx is Warthin's Tumor
        c.   Tx of most benign parotid tumors involves enucleation
        d.   Following a parotidectomy, gustatory sweating is most likely caused by cross-innervation of the auriculotemporal nerve with sympathetic nerves to the skin
        e.   Most parotid tumors are benign, although pleomorphic adenomas can undergo malignant degeneration

Answer c. Tx of most **benign parotid tumors** involves **superficial parotidectomy**. *Enucleation is contra-indicated due to high recurrence rate.*

475. A mass in which of the following areas has the highest malignancy risk:
        a.   Parotid gland
        b.   Submandibular gland
        c.   Sublingual gland
        d.   Minor salivary gland

Answer d. Although the parotid gland is the MC location for malignant tumors, minor salivary gland tumors are more likely to be malignant compared to all the others. **Risk of tumor being malignant:** minor salivary > submandibular / sublingual > parotid

476. A 35 yo woman presents with unsteadiness, tinnitus and hearing loss. You order a head MRI and there is a tumor at the cerebello-pontine angle. The most likely diagnosis is:
        a.   Glioma
        b.   Glioma multiforme
        c.   Neuroma
        d.   Meduloblastoma

Answer c. Unsteadiness, tinnitus, and hearing loss are the classic symptoms of an **acoustic neuroma**. A tumor at the cerebello-pontine angle almost ensures the diagnosis.

477. A 10 yo boy presents with a cyst and a cyst tract near the angle of his mandible. This cyst has had recurrent infections in it. This cyst most likely connects to the:
        a.   External auditory canal
        b.   The tonsillar pillar
        c.   The nasal septum
        d.   Thoracic duct

Answer a. Type I branchial cleft cysts can extend from the angle of the mandible to the **external auditory canal**.
Type II (MC Type) can go from anterior SCM muscle to the **tonsillar pillar**
Type III can go from the deep SCM muscle to the **pyriform sinus**
Tx for all of these cysts is resection

478. A 5 yo girl presents with a midline anterior neck mass that moves up and down with tongue protrusion and swallowing. This most likely represents:

a.   Thyroid cancer
b.   Branchial cleft cyst Type I
c.   Branchial cleft cyst Type II
d.   Thyroglossal duct cyst

Answer d. A midline anterior neck mass in a child that moves with tongue protrusion and swallowing is classic for a **thyroglossal duct cyst**. Thyroid CA would appear more lateral as would branchial cleft cysts.

479. Treatment for the above lesion is:
    a.   Cyst resection only
    b.   XRT
    c.   Chemo
    d.   Includes removal of the central portion of the hyoid bone

Answer d. Tx for a thyroglossal duct cyst is excision of the entire **cyst, tract, and central portion of hyoid bone** (midportion) through lateral neck incision (Sistrunk procedure).

480. A 1 yo girl has a fluctuant multi-loculated mass on the lower lateral neck (posterior to the sternocleidomastoid [SCM] muscle) that has repeated infections. This most likely represents a:
    a.   Branchial cleft cyst Type I
    b.   Branchial cleft cyst Type II
    c.   Thyroglossal duct cyst
    d.   Cystic hygroma

Answer d. Given the lesion is posterior to the SCM muscle (posterior neck triangle), this most likely represents a **cystic hygroma** (_benign_ lymphatic malformation). Tx - simple **resection**

481. All of the following are true except:
    a.   The MC childhood aural CA is rhabdomyosarcoma
    b.   Pinna lacerations should be repaired with full thickness sutures including cartilage
    c.   The most effective surgery for obstructive sleep apnea is uvulopalatopharyngoplasty
    d.   Sepsis from suppurative parotitis despite antibiotics requires parotidectomy
    e.   Suppurative parotitis can be caused by dehydration or salivary calculi

Answer d. **Sepsis** (MC from staph aureus) from **suppurative parotitis** despite antibiotics requires **incision and drainage**

NERVES
- **Accessory nerve** (spinal accessory nerve) - innervates trapezius, sternocleidomastoid muscle (SCM), and platysma
  - Injury - _trouble with head turning, shoulder droop, poor shoulder shrug_
  - MC nerve injury with **posterior neck triangle** dissection (eg lymph node dissection or tumor removal)
- **Vagus nerve** - runs between internal jugular vein and carotid artery; gives off the **recurrent laryngeal nerve** (innervates larynx)
  - Injury - _hoarseness_
  - MCC of vagus nerve injury - **carotid endarterectomy**
- **Phrenic nerve** - runs on top of anterior scalene muscle; **diaphragm** innervation
  - Injury - _shortness of breath_
- **Long thoracic nerve** - runs posterior to middle scalene muscle; innervates **serratus anterior**
  - Injury - _winged scapula (can't raise hands above head)_
- **Trigeminal nerve** - ophthalmic, maxillary, and mandibular branches; **sensation** to face; muscles of **mastication**

- Injury - *chewing difficulties; facial numbness*
- **Facial nerve** - temporal, zygomatic, buccal, marginal mandibular, and cervical branches; **motor** function to face; runs through the **parotid gland**
  - Injury - *facial droop*
- **Glossopharyngeal nerve** - taste to posterior 1/3 tongue; motor to pharynx
  - Injury - *swallowing difficulties*
- **Hypoglossal nerve** - motor to tongue; tongue deviates to **same side** of hypoglossal nerve injury
  - Injury - *slurred speech, swallowing difficulties*
- **Lingual nerve** - located under tongue; taste to anterior 2/3 tongue and floor of mouth; comes off mandibular branch of trigeminal nerve (has facial nerve fibers as well)
  - Injury - *poor taste sensation*
- **Inferior alveolar nerve** - travels inside the mandible and provides sensation to teeth; is a branch of trigeminal nerve; gives off **mental nerve**
  - Injury - *jaw numbness, droop at corner of mouth (mental nerve)*
- **Mental nerve** (fibers from both inferior alveolar nerve [Trigeminal] and marginal mandibular nerve [Facial]) - comes out of the mental foramen and innervates the corner of the mouth and chin (motor and sensation)
  - Injury - *droop at the corner of the mouth, chin numbness*

THYROCERVICAL TRUNK - "STAT":
- **S**uprascapular artery
- **T**ransverse cervical artery
- **A**scending cervical artery
- Inferior **T**hyroid artery

FLAPS
- **Trapezius muscle flap** - based on **transverse cervical artery**, spinal accessory nerve
- **Pectoralis major muscle flap** - based on thoracoacromial artery or internal mammary artery
- **Latissimus dorsi flap** - **thoracodorsal artery**, thoracodorsal nerve
- **Serratus anterior flap** - **lateral thoracic artery**, long thoracic nerve

HEAD AND NECK DISSECTIONS
- **Anterior neck triangle** dissection - SCM, sternal notch, inferior border of digastric muscle; contains **carotid sheath**; risk injury to **thoracic duct** (if left sided dissection) and **vagus nerve**
- **Posterior neck triangle** dissection (usually for suspicious node) - posterior border of SCM, trapezius muscle, and clavicle; risk injury to **accessory nerve** and **brachial plexus**
- **Parotid gland** dissection
  - MC nerve injury - **greater auricular nerve** (*numbness over lower ear*)
  - **Facial nerve** also at risk
- **Frey's syndrome** - occurs after **parotidectomy**
  - Injury of **auriculotemporal nerve** that then cross-innervates with **sympathetic fibers** to sweat glands of skin
  - Sx's: **gustatory sweating** (sweating while eating)
  - Tx: if severe, allograft skin graft between nerve and skin
- **Submandibular gland dissection**
  - MC nerve injury - **marginal mandibular nerve** (mental nerve comes off this)
  - Sx's: **droop at corner of mouth,** chin numbness
- **Modified radical neck dissection** (MRND) takes **cervical nodes** *and*:
  - Omohyoid
  - Sensory nerves C2-C5
  - Cervical branch of facial nerve
  - Submandibular gland
  - *No mortality difference compared with RND*
- **Radical neck dissection** (RND, *rarely used*) - same as MRND *plus*:
  - Accessory nerve (CN XII)

- Sternocleidomastoid
- Internal jugular resection
- *Most morbidity occurs from* **accessory nerve resection** *(muscles of neck including sternocleidomastoid and trapezius)*
■ **Jaw fractures** can injure the **inferior alveolar nerve** (gives branches to mental nerve); Sx's - droop at corner of the mouth

ASYMPTOMATIC HEAD AND NECK MASSES (often an enlarged lymph node)
■ **MC etiology** of asymptomatic neck mass (eg neck lymph node)
- Age < 50 - **lymphoma**
- Age > 50 - **squamous cell CA**
■ **Neck mass workup** (or enlarged lymph node)
- **1st** - H and P, laryngoscopy and **FNA** *(best test for Dx)*
  FNA is definitive 90% of the time (if it shows CA, base work-up on type of cells)
  Can consider antibiotics for 2 weeks with re-evaluation if thought to be inflammatory (tender, upper respiratory infection Sx's) – should get smaller, if not getting smaller need FNA and follow below
- **2nd** - if above non-diagnostic → EGD and bronchoscopy to look for primary; multiple random Bx's if no primary found; neck / chest CT if still not found
- **3rd** - if still cannot find a primary tumor → perform excisional biopsy and send frozen section; need to be prepared for MRND
  Neck mass with negative work-up, Dx at time of excisional Bx → **squamous cell CA** (90%)
■ **Epidermoid CA** (or other squamous cell CA variant) found in **cervical node** *without* **known primary** →
- **1st** - EGD and bronchoscopy to look for primary; get random Bx's
- **2nd** - neck / chest CT
- **3rd** - if still cannot find primary →
  Ipsilateral **MRND**
  Ipsilateral **tonsillectomy** (MC area for occult head/neck tumor - **tonsils**)
  Bilateral **XRT** (to nodal regions + potential primary sites)
■ **Thyroid tissue in a cervical node** (**lateral aberrant thyroid tissue**, ie thyroid CA with lymph node metastases)
- Tx: **total thyroidectomy, MRND, and post-op** ^{131}I
■ **Preauricular masses** (or lumps)
- All lumps in front of the ear are parotid tumors until proved otherwise
- Dx usually made after superficial lobectomy

SALIVARY GLAND TUMORS
■ **Parotid** (80% benign), **submandibular** (50% benign), **sublingual** (50% benign), and **minor** (20% benign) salivary gland tumors
■ **Mass in large salivary gland→** MC benign
■ **Mass in minor salivary gland→** MC malignant (smaller gland = more likely malignant)
- Although parotid gland is MC site for a malignant tumor
■ **MC salivary gland tumor in children** - hemangiomas
■ MC injured nerve with submandibular gland resection - **marginal mandibular nerve** (inferior alveolar nerve branch; motor function to lower lip and chin)

PAROTID GLAND TUMORS
■ Preauricular masses (just above mandible, anterior to ear)
- All are **parotid tumors** until proved otherwise
■ Sx's: usually a painless mass; **pain or facial nerve paralysis** suggests CA
■ Pre-op work-up - **head, neck** and **chest CT** (looking for invasion or if it represents a metastasis from another primary)
■ Dx is usually made by **superficial parotidectomy** (*do not shell out - high recurrence rate for both benign and malignant lesions with enucleation*)
- *No* FNA unless deep in the parotid on CT scan, it is felt to be a metastasis, or if the patient is a poor surgical risk
■ 80% of all salivary gland tumors are in the **parotid**
■ 80% of parotid tumors are **benign** (60% are pleomorphic adenomas)

- **Facial nerve** - courses through parotid gland and controls motor function to face
- MC injured nerve with parotid surgery - **greater auricular nerve** (numbness over lower portion of ear auricle)
- **Deep parotid tumors** can extend to **parapharyngeal space**
  - Can deviate the tonsil towards the midline
  - Tx: median mandibulotomy for exposure (mandibulectomy if bone involved)
- **Malignant tumors**
  - Often present as a painful mass but can also present with facial nerve paralysis or lymphadenopathy
  - Lymphatic drainage - intra-parotid and anterior cervical chain nodes
  - MC metastatic site - **lung**
  - **Mucoepidermoid CA** - #1 malignant tumor of parotid
    Wide range of aggressiveness
  - **Adenoid cystic CA** - #2 malignant tumor of parotid
    Long, indolent course
    Propensity to invade **nerve roots**
    Very sensitive to XRT (just give XRT if extensive non-resectable tumor)
  - Tx for both:
    Total parotidectomy (superficial and deep lobes)
    Prophylactic **MRND**
    Post-op **XRT**
  - Try to **preserve facial nerve** branches, even if you have to peel tumor off (unless nerve already out on pre-op exam) - **XRT** to that area post-op
  - **Low grade mucoepidermoid** - consider total parotidectomy *without* MRND or XRT
  - **Deeply invasive adenoid cystic CA** - do *not* resect, just give **XRT** (can have a long indolent course)
  - Melanoma and SCCA skin CA can metastasize to parotid gland (see Skin and Soft Tissue chapter)
- **Benign tumors**
  - Often present as a painless mass
  - **Pleomorphic adenoma** (mixed tumor) - #1 benign tumor of parotid
    <u>Malignant degeneration</u> in 5%
    If malignant degeneration, need total parotidectomy
  - **Warthin's tumor** (papillary cystadenoma lymphomatosum) - #2 benign tumor of parotid
    Males, **smoking** *(strong RF)*
    Bilateral in 10%
  - Tx for both: **superficial parotidectomy** (total parotidectomy if deep gland involved); <u>No</u> enucleation *(high recurrence rate for benign tumors)*

PAROTID - OTHER CONDITIONS
- **Stensen's duct** (ie parotid duct) - opens into vestibule of mouth opposite upper 2nd molar
- **Parotitis** - acute inflammation of parotid gland usually due to obstruction by a **duct stone** (salivary calculi); most calculi near orifice
  - Recurrent parotitis is due to ascending infection from oral cavity
  - Tx: **incise duct** and **remove stone**
  - Gland excision may eventually be necessary for recurrent disease
- **Post-op parotitis** (can be **suppurative**, MC POD 4-12) - usually elderly men
  - RFs: **dehydration** (decreased saliva), poor oral hygiene, decreased oral intake
  - Can be caused by **salivary calculi**
  - MC organism - *staph aureus*
  - Sx's: pain, swelling, erythema over parotid gland (near cheek), fever, high WBCs
  - Tx: fluids, stimulate salivation (eg give candy sucker), and antibiotics
    If due to a **stone** → incise duct and remove it
  - Need open **surgical drainage** if **abscess** develops or if patient does not improve in **48 hours**
  - Can be **life-threatening**
- **Stensen's duct laceration** - repair over catheter stent
  - Ligation can cause painful parotid atrophy and facial asymmetry

- **Sialoadenitis** (acute inflammation of salivary gland usually related to **stone** in duct)
    - Most salivary calculi are near the orifice of the duct
    - Tx: **incise duct and remove stone**

ABSCESSES
- **Peritonsillar** abscess - older kids (usually > 10 years; called **quinsy**)
    - Sx's: trismus (reduced opening of jaw), odynophagia
    - Usually does <u>not</u> obstruct airway
    - Tx: needle aspiration 1st, then drainage through <u>tonsil bed</u> if no relief in 24 hours (may need to intubate to drain; will self-drain with swallowing once opened)
- **Retropharyngeal** abscess - younger kids (usually < 10 years)
    - Sx's: fever, odynophagia, drool; is an **airway emergency**
    - Can occur in elderly with Pott's disease
    - Tx: intubate in a calm setting; drainage through <u>posterior pharyngeal wall</u>; will self-drain with swallowing once opened
- **Parapharyngeal** abscess - all age groups; occurs with dental infections, tonsillitis, and pharyngitis
    - Morbidity comes from vascular invasion and **mediastinal spread** via prevertebral and retropharyngeal spaces
    - Tx: drain through <u>lateral neck</u>; leave drains
- **Ludwig's angina** - acute mouth floor infection; involves **mylohyoid muscle**
    - MCC - **dental infection** of the mandibular teeth
    - May rapidly spread to deeper structures and cause airway obstruction
    - Tx: airway control, surgical drainage, antibiotics

EAR DISORDERS (ear = pinna)
- **Cauliflower ear** (ie boxers ear, UFC fighters) - un-drained hematomas that organize and calcify; Tx: drain hematomas to avoid this
- **Pinna lacerations** - need full thickness sutures through involved cartilage
- **Ear infections** need to be treated promptly to avoid **cartilage necrosis**
- **Cholesteatoma** - epidermal inclusion cyst of ear
    - Slow growing but erode as they grow - damage middle ear bones (malleus, incus, and stapes) and/or mastoid
    - Sx's: hearing loss and brown/yellow/bloody drainage from ear
    - Tx: **surgical excision** ± mastoidectomy
- **MC childhood aural CA** - rhabdomyosarcoma of middle or external ear

ORAL AND PHARYNGEAL CAVITY CANCER (above larynx)
- RFs: **ETOH** and **tobacco**
- *These patients are also at high risk for **lung CA** (all need **CXR**)*
- MC type - vast majority **squamous cell CA** (ie epidermoid)
- CA risk - **erythroplakia** worse than leukoplakia
- Division **oral cavity** and **pharynx** marked by:
    - Tonsillar pillars
    - Junction between the hard and soft palates
    - Tongue papilla
- **Oral cavity** includes mouth floor, anterior 1/3 tongue, gingival, hard palate, anterior tonsillar pillars, and lips
- MC site for **oral cavity CA** - lower lip (needs to involve mucosa)
- **Tonsillar CA** considered an oral cavity CA
- **Oral cavity CA** → <u>submental</u> + <u>submandibular</u> nodes 1st
    - *Exception* - **tongue CA** goes to cervical chain nodes (early)
- **Pharyngeal CA** → <u>cervical</u> chain nodes 1st
    - **Nasopharyngeal CA**: Sx's - epistaxis or obstruction; EBV associated; Chinese; *very responsive to XRT (do <u>not</u> resect these tumors)*
    - **Oropharyngeal CA**; Sx's - neck mass, sore throat
    - **Hypopharyngeal CA**; Sx's - hoarseness (**early LN spread**)
- **Location with lowest survival rate** - hard palate (hard to resect)
- Need **1 cm margin** for all *except* tongue (2 cm margin required)
- Tx:

- Stage I + II *oral cavity* (< 4 cm, no nodal or bone invasion) → *Resection*
- Stage I + II *pharyngeal* (< 4 cm, no nodal or bone invasion) → *XRT only*
  Include neck nodes with XRT; hard to resect these tumors
  ***Note - nasopharyngeal SCCA is very sensitive to XRT (Stage I – XRT;
  Stage II – chemo-XRT)**
- Stage III *oral cavity* or *pharyngeal* tumors (> 4 cm _or_ nodal or bone invasion)
  All get:1) *Resection*, 2) *MRND*, and 3) post-op *chemo-XRT*
  Exception – **nasopharyngeal CA** → get **chemo-XRT** only (no resection;
  include neck nodes in XRT field)
- Stage IV (metastases) - palliative chemo-XRT (5-FU + cisplatin)

SPECIAL ISSUES
- **Verrucous ulcer**
  - Very **low grade,** well-differentiated squamous cell CA
  - Often occurs on **inner cheek** (**buccal** squamous cell CA) but can occur anywhere in mouth
  - Often presents as **leukoplakia**
  - Associated with **chewing tobacco**
  - Not aggressive, rare metastasis
  - Tx: **Full cheek resection** (0.5 cm margins) ± flap
    No lymph node dissection
    No chemo or XRT
- **Lip CA**
  - **Lower lip** CA (95%) more common than upper due to sun exposure
  - RFs: men, ETOH, tobacco, sun exposure
  - Lesions at **commissure** (angle of mouth) are **most aggressive**
  - Majority are **squamous cell CA**, some melanoma
  - Needs to involve **mucosa** or its *not* lip CA (would then Tx like skin CA [MC basal cell CA]); usually presents as ulcerated lesion
  - **High cure rate** and **low risk** of nodal or systemic metastases
  - Tx: **MOHS surgery** for most (if squamous cell CA, not melanoma); **flaps needed** if more than 1/3 of lip is removed; _no prophylactic neck dissection_
- **Tongue CA** - jaw invasion still operable; **early nodal invasion** (cervical chain)
  - Commando procedure - removes portion of the mandible
- **Maxillary sinus CA Tx**: maxillectomy
- **Tonsil CA**: Sx's - asymptomatic until large; RFs - ETOH, tobacco
  - MC type - squamous cell CA
  - Considered **oral cavity** CA
  - 80% have **lymph node spread** at time of Dx
  - Tx: **tonsillectomy** (best way to get Dx + Tx lesion); therapy then same as above for oral cavity tumors
- **Other nasopharynx tumors**
  - **MC benign tumor of nasopharynx** - papilloma
  - **MC malignant tumor of nasopharynx in children** - lymphoma (Tx: chemo)
  - **Nasopharyngeal angiofibroma** - benign; **extremely vascular**
    Males < 20 years (obstruction or epistaxis)
    Tx: **angio-embolization** (MC internal maxillary artery), then resection
    XRT for inaccessible tumors

LARYNGEAL CANCER
- Includes vocal cord and surrounding structures
- MC type - vast majority **squamous cell CA** (ie epidermoid)
- Sx's: hoarseness, aspiration, dyspnea, dysphagia
- Tx: **XRT** (if vocal cord only) or **chemo-XRT** (if beyond vocal cord)
  - *Surgery is not the primary Tx; want to preserve larynx*
  - **XRT** - spread field to get **ipsilateral neck nodes** (cervical chain)
    If tumor **crosses midline** → bilateral neck XRT
  - **Stage III** (positive nodes) → need above + MRND (take **ipsilateral thyroid**)
- MC benign tumor of larynx - **papilloma**

ACOUSTIC NEUROMA (vestibular schwannoma, CN VIII, vestibulocochlear)
- Benign, slow growth
- Associated with neurofibromatosis (von Recklinghausen's DZ)
- Sx's: tinnitus, hearing loss, unsteadiness, vertigo
- Dx: **MRI** *(best test)* - classically at the **cerebello-pontine angle**
- Tx: Craniotomy and resection including superior/inferior vestibular nerves
    - **Facial nerve** at risk with surgery
    - XRT is an alternative

PARAGANGLIOMA
- **MC ENT site** - carotid body (ie **carotid body tumor**, at bifurcation)
- Can secrete **norepinephrine** (↑ HR + HTN; palpations, headaches)
- Sx's: **neck mass** with **bruit**
- Dx: CT angiography - highly vascular
- Tx: surgical excision (see Vascular chapter)

OTHER CONDITIONS
- **Nasal fractures** - set after swelling decreases
- **Septal hematoma** - Tx: drain to avoid infection and necrosis of septum
- **TMJ dislocations** (temporomandibular joint) - Tx: closed reduction
- **Tracheostomy** - consider in patients who will require intubation for > 7-14 days; decreases secretions and pneumonia risk; provides easier ventilation
- **Mastoiditis** - infection of mastoid cells; can destroy bone; rare
    - Results from untreated **acute supportive otitis media**
    - Ear is pushed forward
    - MC organism - *strep pneumoniae*
    - Tx: **tympanostomy tube** and **antibiotics**, may need emergency **mastoidectomy** if those fail
- **Esophageal foreign body**
    - Sx's: dysphagia; most just below the cricopharyngeus (95%)
    - Dx and Tx: **rigid EGD** under anesthesia
    - Perforation risk increases with <u>length of time</u> in the esophagus
- **Fever** and **pain** after EGD removal of foreign body → Dx: gastrografin followed by barium swallow to rule-out perforation
- **Laryngeal foreign body** - coughing; emergent cricothyroidotomy as a last resort may be needed to secure airway
- **Torus palatini** - benign congenital bony mass on upper palate of mouth; Tx: nothing
- **Torus mandibular** - as above but on anterior lingual surface of mandible
- **Sleep apnea**
    - Patient rarely aware of problem (spouse brings them in)
    - Pauses in breathing with sleep
    - Cx's: cor pulmonale, myocardial infarction (MI), arrhythmias, death
    - Tx: **CPAP** (continuous positive airway pressure at night *(best Tx)* **Uvulopalatopharyngoplasty** (UPP, best surgical option)
- **Prolonged oral intubation** - can lead to **sub-glottic stenosis**
    - Tx: tracheal resection and reconstruction *(best Tx)*; can dilate temporarily
- **Median rhomboid glossitis** - failure of fusion of the tongue; Tx: <u>none</u> required
- **Cleft lip** (primary palate)
    - **Highest prevalence** – Native Americans
    - Failure of fusion of **maxillary** and **medial nasal processes**
    - Involves lip, alveolus, or both structures; may have poor feeding
    - *Repair at* **10 weeks** *of age,* **10 pounds,** *and a* **Hgb 10**
    - Tx: **Millard procedure** (Z plasty); repair nasal deformities at same time
- **Cleft palate** (secondary palate)
    - Two plates of hard palate are not completely joined; also involves soft palate
    - **Hole in roof of mouth** connects directly with **nasal cavity**
    - Affects **speech** and **swallowing** if not closed soon enough; can affect maxillofacial growth if closed too early → *repair at* **12 months**
    - **Palatal obturator** used to temporarily close hole before surgery
- **Hemangioma** - MC benign head and neck tumor in adults
    - **MC tumor overall of childhood**

Adrenal

482. All of the following are true except:
    a. The right adrenal vein drains into the right renal vein
    b. Cortisol level generally peaks between 4-6 am
    c. Adult excess androgen or estrogen secretion from an adrenal source is almost always CA
    d. Glucocorticoid and mineralocorticoid Tx after adrenalectomy prevents Addison's Disease and Nelson's Syndrome
    e. The MCC of primary adrenal insufficiency is autoimmune disease

    Answer a. The right renal vein drains into the inferior vena cava. Careful ligation here during adrenalectomy (can get massive bleeding from the IVC).

483. During a negative trauma workup, you discover an adrenal tumor. All of the following are appropriate in this patient's management except:
    a. Urine catecholamines and metabolites should be checked
    b. > 4-6 cm is an indication for resection
    c. A functioning tumor requires resection
    d. Angiomyolipomas require adrenalectomy
    e. A high attenuation tumor is an indication for FNA

    Answer d. Angiomyolipomas are benign and can be observed.

484. A 65 yo woman with previous bladder CA has an asymptomatic 3 cm left adrenal mass on CT scan. Work-up including serum ACTH, serum cortisol, serum aldosterone, and urine catecholamines are all negative. What is the most appropriate next step:
    a. Tagged RBC scan
    b. CT guided Bx
    c. Tagged WBC scan
    d. U/S
    e. Observation

    Answer b. CT guided Bx is indicated for an adrenal mass in a patient with previous CA history.

485. All of the following are true of pheochromocytomas except:
    a. The MC location for an extra-adrenal pheochromocytoma is the aortic bifurcation
    b. Alpha blockers should be given before beta-blockers to avoid hypertensive crisis
    c. The most sensitive test for pheochromocytoma localization is MIBG
    d. Adrenal venous sampling is the best method for localizing adrenal pheochromocytomas
    e. Volume replacement is indicated before surgery

    Answer d. Adrenal venous sampling should be _avoided_ to prevent hypertensive crisis. An open approach should be used for <u>malignant</u> pheochromocytomas.

486. All of the following are true of pheochromocytoma except:
    a. The MC sign is episodic hypertension
    b. The MC extra-adrenal site is the Organ of Zuckerkandl
    c. Malignant tumors should be removed with open surgery
    d. They are associated with the MEN1 gene (menin protein)

    Answer d. Pheochromocytomas are associated with the **RET proto-oncogene**.

487. The most sensitive test for pheochromocytoma is:
    a. Plasma metanephrines
    b. Plasma VMA
    c. Urine VMA

d.   Urine metanephrines

Answer d. Urine metanephrines (<u>not</u> plasma concentration)

488. A 25 yo women presents to the hospital with HTN, polydipsia, and polyuria. She has a serum sodium of 150 and a serum potassium of 2.9. She has been off diuretics for some time. All of the following are true except:
    a.   This patient likely has a plasma aldosterone to renin ratio > 20
    b.   A 24 urine aldosterone > 14 mcg after a 3 day salt loading (salt suppression test) helps confirm the diagnosis
    c.   Metabolic alkalosis is consistent with the disease
    d.   The MC primary cause of this syndrome is adrenal hyperplasia.
    e.   Renin level is likely low

Answer d. The MCC of **hyperaldosteronism** is **aldosterone adenoma**.

489. What is the best initial study for localizing the above lesion:
    a.   MRI
    b.   CT scan
    c.   Venous sampling
    d.   MIBG scan

Answer b. CT scan (high resolution)

490. All of the following are true except:
    a.   Weight gain is the MC symptom of Cushing's Syndrome
    b.   High ACTH and a high dose dexamethasone test that does not suppress cortisol production suggests an ectopic ACTH producer and CT scan is indicated
    c.   Mitotane is used for unresectable adrenocortical CA
    d.   The best initial test for the diagnosis of Cushing's Syndrome is a 24 hour urine free cortisol
    e.   Adrenal adenoma is the MC non-exogenous cause of primary Cushing's Syndrome

Answer e. Pituitary adenoma is the MC non-exogenous cause of Cushing's Syndrome.

ADRENAL BLOOD SUPPLY
- **Superior adrenal artery** - off inferior phrenic artery
- **Middle adrenal artery** - off aorta
- **Inferior adrenal artery** - off renal artery

- **Left adrenal vein** - goes to **left renal vein**
- **Right adrenal vein** - goes directly into **IVC** (*careful* ligating this during adrenalectomy - can get massive hemorrhage from the IVC)
- **Lymphatics** - drain to sub-diaphragmatic and renal lymph nodes

HYPOTHALAMIC-PITUITARY-ADRENAL AXIS
- **Hypothalamus** releases **CRH** (corticotrophin releasing hormone), which goes to anterior pituitary gland
- **Anterior pituitary gland** then releases **ACTH** which goes to adrenal cortex
- **Adrenal cortex** then releases **cortisol**
  - Diurnal (high am, low pm) peak at 4-6 a.m.
  - Also increased with **stress**
- **Cortisol effects** - proteolysis, lipolysis, gluconeogenesis, hyperglycemia (partly from insulin resistance), inotropic, increases vascular tone
- **After bilateral adrenalectomy → need glucocorticoids + mineralocorticoids**
  - Prevents **Addison's Disease** (adrenal insufficiency)
  - Prevents **Nelson's Syndrome** (pituitary enlargement compresses optic nerve); from chronic CRH stimulation of pituitary adenoma

ADRENAL MEDULLA

- Produces **catecholamines** (norepinephrine and epinephrine)
- **Tyrosine hydroxylase** - rate-limiting step for catecholamines
- **Phenylethanolamine N-methyltransferase** (PNMT), converts norepinephrine (NE) → epinephrine (EPI), enzyme _only_ found in **adrenal medulla** (exclusive producer of endogenous EPI)
- _Only_ _adrenal_ pheochromocytomas produce **EPI**
- **Monoamine oxidase** (MAO) - breaks down NE and EPI to normetanephrine and metanephrine; **Vanillylmandelic acid** (VMA) produced from these

ASYMPTOMATIC ADRENAL MASS

- 1% of **CT scans** show adrenal **incidentaloma** (> 1 cm; 5% are metastases)
- Increase with age
- **MC adrenal tumor** (also MC malignant adrenal tumor) - **metastasis** from another primary (MC - lung; breast, melanoma); adrenals are common sites for metastases
- **MC adrenal tumor** _without_ **previous history of CA** (also MC primary adrenal tumor) – **non-functional adrenal adenoma** (50%)
- Dx: _Rule-out a_ **functional tumor 1st** _before_ **any** _biopsy_ - need to send:
  - Urine metanephrines
  - 24-hour urine cortisol and ACTH (adrenocorticotropic hormone)
  - Serum potassium, renin, and aldosterone levels
- **CA history** with asymptomatic adrenal mass - need **CT guided Bx**
- **Adrenocortical CA** - CT/MRI findings generally suggests diagnosis
- **FNA** indications (_any_ below):
  - > 10 hounsfield units (**high attenuation**)
  - **Poor contrast washout** (< 50%)
  - **Previous CA** or you think it's a **metastasis** from a separate primary
- **Surgery** indications (_any_ below):
  - **Ominous characteristics** (non-homogenous or complex)
  - **> 4-6 cm**
  - **Functioning** tumor
  - **Enlarging** tumor
  - **Significant FNA finding** (eg adrenocortical CA)
- Some **isolated** metastases to adrenal can be resected with adrenalectomy
- Anterior approach for adrenal CA resection
- If going to follow an incidentaloma, need repeat imaging every 3 months for 1 year, then yearly
- **Angiomyolipoma** (on Bx) - benign, leave alone

ADRENAL CORTEX

- **GFR** (salt, sugar, sex; outer to inner zones) - zone **granulosa** (aldosterone), zona **fasciculate** (cortisol), zona **reticularis** (androgens)
- **Aldosterone** - stimulates **water reabsorption** (absorbs Na, secretes K)
- **Cortisol** - gluconeogenesis and glycogenolysis (increases **blood glucose**) and increases vascular tone _(part of fight or flight response)_
- Excess estrogens and androgens by adrenals - almost always CA
- **Hyperaldosteronism** (Conn's syndrome)
  - Sx's: **HTN** (sodium retention _without_ edema) and **hypokalemia**
    Weakness, polydipsia, polyuria
    Check for hyperaldosteronism in patients with **HTN** _and_ either 1) low K$^+$, 2) an **adrenal mass**, or 3) who are **refractory to medical Tx**
  - **Primary** disease (renin is <u>low</u>) - **adenoma** (MC, 85%), hyperplasia (15%), ovarian tumors (rare), cancer (rare)
  - **Secondary** disease (renin is high) - more common than primary disease; **CHF** (MCC), renal artery stenosis, Bartter syndrome (renin-secreting tumor)
  - Dx for **primary hyperaldosteronism** (need both 1 _and_ 2 below):
    1) **Salt-load suppression test** (_best test_) - urine aldosterone <u>stays high</u> after salt-load (24 hr **urine aldosterone > 14 mcg**)
    2) **Aldosterone : renin ratio > 20**
    Labs - ↓ **K** (usually < 3), ↑ **Na, metabolic alkalosis**

Plasma renin will be low

- **CT scan** (high resolution) - *best initial test* to localize a suspected aldosteronoma (tumor is generally 0.5-2 cm); if tumor is not found or if <u>bilateral</u> adrenals look either normal or abnormal → get adrenal venous sampling
- **Adrenal venous sampling** - *most accurate test* to localize an adenoma and to differentiate adenoma vs. hyperplasia but is *invasive* (1% adrenal vein rupture rate)
- Pre-op need **control of HTN** and **potassium replacement**
- **Adenoma Tx** - adrenalectomy
- **Hyperplasia Tx** - high morbidity with bilateral resection
    - Medical Tx 1st for hyperplasia using **spironolactone** (inhibits aldosterone), **calcium channel blockers**, and **potassium** *(treats the majority of patients)*
    - If **bilateral resection** is performed (usually done for **refractory hypokalemia**), patient will need **fludrocortisone** (mineralocorticoid) and **hydrocortisone** post-op

- **Hypercortisolism** (Cushing's syndrome)
  - Sx's: **weight gain** (MC), acne, abdominal striae, moon face, obesity, depression
  - MCC - **iatrogenic** (exogenous steroids)
  - **1st** - get **24-hour urine cortisol** *(best initial test for Dx)* and **serum ACTH**
      - If ACTH is **low** (and cortisol is high), patient has a cortisol secreting lesion (eg adrenal adenoma, adrenal hyperplasia) → get Adrenal CT scan
      - If ACTH is **high** (and cortisol is high), patient has a pituitary adenoma or an ectopic source of ACTH (eg small cell lung CA) → go to 2nd below
  - **2nd** - if **ACTH** is **high**, give **high dose dexamethasone suppression test** (suppresses pituitary adenoma) and measure **urine cortisol**:
      - If cortisol is suppressed → **pituitary adenoma**
      - If cortisol is not suppressed → **ectopic producer of ACTH** (eg small cell lung CA)
  - **Pituitary adenoma** (Cushing's disease)
      - **MC non-iatrogenic cause of Cushing's syndrome** (80% of cases)
      - Cortisol is suppressed with dexamethasone suppression test
      - Mostly **microadenomas**
      - **Brain MRI** - *initial test to localize*
      - **Petrosal sampling** - *best test to localize (but is invasive)*
      - Tx: most tumors removed with **trans-sphenoidal** approach; unresectable or residual tumors treated with XRT
  - **Ectopic ACTH**
      - **#2 non-iatrogenic** cause of Cushing's syndrome
      - MCC - **small cell lung CA**
      - Cortisol is <u>not</u> suppressed with dexamethasone suppression test
      - **Chest (#1)** and **abdominal CT** - *best test to localize* source of ACTH (MC – small cell lung CA)
      - Tx: resection of primary if possible; medical suppression if inoperable
  - **Adrenal adenoma**
      - **#3 non-iatrogenic** cause of Cushing's syndrome
      - Low ACTH and high cortisol (unregulated production)
      - **Adrenal CT** - *best initial test to localize* a suspected adenoma (high resolution, compares non-contrast to delayed contrasted images)
      - Tx: adrenalectomy
  - **Adrenal hyperplasia** (macro or micro)
      - **NP-59 scintigraphy** - *best test for 1) equivocal adrenal CT or; 2) suspected hyperplasia;* figures out adenoma vs. hyperplasia
      - Tx: **metyrapone** and **aminoglutethimide**; (inhibit steroid production); bilateral adrenalectomy if medical Tx fails
      - If bilateral adrenalectomy is performed, need to give both **hydrocortisone** and **fludrocortisone** (mineralocorticoid) post-op
  - **Adrenocortical CA** - rare cause of Cushing's syndrome (see below)
  - **Bilateral adrenalectomy** - consider in patients with ectopic ACTH from tumor that is unresectable (would need to be a slow growing tumor - rare) or ACTH from a pituitary adenoma that cannot be found

- Give **hydrocortisone** post-op when operating for Cushing's Syndrome
- Need **hydrocortisone** and **fludrocortisone** post-op when performing bilateral adrenalectomy
- **Adrenocortical carcinoma** (rare)
  - Bimodal distribution (before age 5 and in the 5th decade)
  - Usually **large** (> 6 cm) and usually **advanced** at Dx (ie metastases)
  - Sx's: abdominal pain, weight loss, weakness, HTN
    - 60% are **functional** - cortisol (MC; Cushing's), aldosterone (HTN, hypokalemia), sex steroids (virilization, feminization, masculinization)
  - **Adrenal CT** - *best test to localize*; differentiates adenoma vs CA; can usually make Dx based on CT scan findings (eg necrosis, hemorrhage, local invasion)
  - Tx: **radical adrenalectomy** (include **kidney**) - open anterior approach
    - Debulking helps Sx's and prolongs survival
    - **Mitotane** (adrenolytic) for residual, recurrent, or metastatic disease - prolongs disease-free survival
  - 5-year survival (all patients) - 20%
- **Hypocortisolism** (adrenal insufficiency; Addison's disease)
  - MCC - **withdrawal of exogenous steroids** (is a secondary cause)
  - Other secondary causes - pituitary disease, bilateral adrenalectomy
  - MC primary cause - adrenal **autoimmune disease;** others - <u>bilateral</u> adrenal infection, hemorrhage, metastasis, or fibrosis
  - Sx's of **acute adrenal insufficiency** (Addisonian Crisis) - hypotension (not responsive to fluids / pressors), fever (hyperpyrexia), lethargy, abdominal pain, N/V
    - Labs: ↓ glucose, ↑ K, ↓ Na
    - Dx: high **ACTH** and low **cortisol**
      - **Cosyntropin test** (*best test*, ACTH given and cortisol measured)
      - **Baseline cortisol < 15** or **change < 9** ug/dl after stimulation test = adrenal insufficiency
    - Tx: **dexamethasone**; fluids to temporize, cosyntropin test
      - (dexamethasone does <u>not</u> interfere with test)
  - **Chronic adrenal insufficiency** - hyperpigmentation, weakness, weight loss, abdominal pain Tx: **hydrocortisone + fludrocortisone**
    - Adrenal insufficiency causes *decreased* **cortisol** (ACTH will be high unless pituitary disease) and *decreased* **aldosterone**
  - **Fever, N/V, abdominal pain,** and **hypotension** after thymectomy for myasthenia gravis or splenectomy for ITP → **Addisonian Crisis** (Tx: **dexamethasone**)

ADRENAL MEDULLA
- **Pheochromocytoma** (chromaffin cells)
  - Rare; usually slow growing; Chromaffin cells that arise from adrenal medulla, sympathetic ganglia, or ectopic neural crest cells
  - **10% rule** - malignant, bilateral, in children, familial, extra-adrenal
  - Can be associated with MEN IIa, MEN IIb, von Recklinghausen's disease, tuberous sclerosis, Sturge-Weber disease, von Hippel-Lindau
  - MC location - **adrenal** (right-sided predominance)
    - **Extra-adrenal** tumors are more likely **malignant** (25%) and do <u>not</u> produce epinephrine *(do <u>not</u> have **PNMT enzyme**)*
    - Malignancy based on invasion / metastases (not histology)
  - Sx's: **HTN** (MC; can be **episodic,** eg weight lifting), headache, diaphoresis, palpitations
  - Dx:
    - 24 hour **urine metanephrines** *(<u>best test for Dx</u> - most accurate)* + VMA
    - **CT scan** (or MRI) to localize tumors
    - **MIBG scan** (norepinephrine analogue) - *<u>best test to localize tumor</u>*
    - Clonidine suppression test - tumor does <u>not</u> respond, catecholamines will remain high
    - <u>*No* adrenal venous sampling</u> → *can cause **hypertensive crisis***
  - <u>Pre-op</u>: oral **volume replacement** (should gain weight) and start an **α-blocker** (phenoxybenzamine)

Need to be careful with β-blockers and give only *after* α-blocker → β-blockers can precipitate **hypertensive crisis** (unopposed alpha stimulation, can lead to **stroke**, **CHF,** or **MI**)

Consider β-blocker only for persistent tachycardia or arrhythmias

- Tx: **adrenalectomy** (or resection of ectopic tumor) - many removed *laparoscopically*

  Open approach if malignant tumor

  Ligate adrenal veins 1st to avoid spilling catecholamines during tumor manipulation

  Debulking helps Sx's in patients with unresectable disease

  Persistent **hypertension** after removal → check other sites below

  Hypotension after removal → give **fluids** to restore normal volume status

  Should have nipride, phenylephrine, and anti-arrhythmic agents (eg amiodarone) ready during the time of surgery

  Metyrosine - inhibits tyrosine hydroxylase and *decreases* catecholamines (given pre-op or for metastatic disease)

- **Post-op Cx's** - persistent hypertension, hypotension, hypoglycemia, bronchospasm, arrhythmias, intracerebral hemorrhage, CHF, MI
- Other sites for pheochromocytomas - **aortic bifurcation** (called **Organ of Zuckerkandl**; *MC extra-adrenal location*), vertebral bodies, opposite adrenal, bladder
- **Falsely elevated VMA** - coffee, tea, fruits, vanilla, iodine contrast, labetalol, α- and β-blockers
- **Extra-medullary tissue** - responsible for **medullary CA of thyroid** and **extra-adrenal pheochromocytoma**

■ **MIBG** - metaiodobenzylguanidine (NE analogue)

Thyroid

491. All of the following are true except:
    a. T3 is the most active form of thyroid hormone
    b. Thyroid hormone is <u>not</u> involved in the fight or flight response
    c. Albumin carries the majority of thyroid hormone in circulation
    d. TSH is the most sensitive and accurate indicator of thyroid function (best test for either hyperthyroidism or hypothyroidism)
    e. A non-recurrent laryngeal nerve is more common on the right

    Answer c. Thyroxin-binding globulin (TBG) carries majority of T3 and T4.

492. A 50 yo woman presents to your clinic with a thyroid nodule. After H and P, the most appropriate next step in management is:
    a. Thyroid lobectomy
    b. Total thyroidectomy
    c. FNA
    d. Neck MRI

    Answer c. FNA (with U/S) is the best initial Dx test for a thyroid nodule.

493. Ultrasound on the above patient reveals a 1.2 cm mass. Pathology from the FNA shows follicular cells. The most appropriate next step in management is:
    a. Thyroid lobectomy
    b. Nothing
    c. Neck CT
    d. Neck MRI

    Answer a. Follicular cells on FNA results in **follicular cell CA** in 5-10% of patients. Thyroid lobectomy is required for definitive Dx.

494. You take the above patient to the operating room and perform a thyroid lobectomy. Pathology shows this is a 1.5 cm follicular cell carcinoma. The most appropriate next step is:
    a. Completion total thyroidectomy
    b. Close
    c. Post op chemotherapy
    d. Post-op XRT

    Answer a. Follicular cell or papillary thyroid CA > 1 cm requires total thyroidectomy.

495. The above patient also had palpable lymph nodes in her neck on physical exam prior to surgery. The most appropriate management is:
    a. Cherry pick the lymph nodes out of the neck
    b. Radical neck dissection
    c. Modified radical neck dissection (MRND)
    d. Post op XRT

    Answer c. Patients with thyroid CA and clinically positive lymph nodes should undergo total thyroidectomy and MRND.

496. After total thyroidectomy and MRND above, post-op this patient should also undergo:
    a. I-131 therapy
    b. XRT
    c. Chemotherapy (5-FU)
    d. Tamoxifen therapy

    Answer a. I-131 is indicated for either papillary and follicular thyroid CA > 1 cm.

Do not give thyroid replacement until after Tx with ^{131}I to avoid suppressing ^{131}I uptake (want TSH level high before Tx with ^{131}I)

497. Post-operatively the above opera singer has a loss of voice pitch and voice fatigue. This is most likely due to injury of the:
   a. Superior laryngeal nerve
   b. Recurrent laryngeal nerve
   c. Vagus nerve
   d. Glossopharyngeal nerve

   Answer a. Loss of pitch is most consistent with **superior laryngeal nerve** injury. Careful ligation of the **superior thyroid artery** branches at the level of the thyroid capsule can help avoid this complication.

498. Instead of the above, the patient has a hoarse voice, most likely due to injury of the:
   a. Superior laryngeal nerve
   b. Recurrent laryngeal nerve
   c. Vagus nerve
   d. Glossopharyngeal nerve

   Answer b. Hoarseness is most consistent with **recurrent laryngeal nerve** injury and abduction of the vocal cord. This nerve often tracks with the **inferior thyroid artery** inferiorly. The hoarseness may get better (wait 6-8 weeks); if that fails, medialize the vocal cord with a silicone wedge or silicone injection *(not re-op repair of nerve)*.

   The **right RLN** normally loops around the **innominate artery** and the **left RLN** loops around the **aorta**.

499. Post-op, a patient undergoing a difficult total thyroidectomy has severe respiratory stridor and impending respiratory arrest immediately after extubation in the post-anesthesia care unit. She does not have any signs of hematoma. The most effective way of airway access is:
   a. Re-intubation
   b. Open the wound and place emergent tracheostomy
   c. Take her back to the OR for re-exploration
   d. Racemic epinephrine

   Answer b. Given the clinical scenario, this patient likely suffered **bilateral RLN injury**. Trying to intubate a patient with bilateral RLN injury and medialization of both vocal cords (ie both cords are in a *paramedian* location) is very difficult. The best option is emergent tracheostomy through the collar incision (which you performed for the thyroidectomy).

   At times both vocal cords may be *abducted*, resulting in severe **hoarseness** and **aspiration**. Tracheostomy is needed in these patients as well.

500. A 50 yo woman presents with a thyroid lump. You perform an U/S and it appears to be a 1.5 cm cyst. The most appropriate next step is:
   a. Percutaneous cyst drainage
   b. I-131
   c. Observation
   d. Thyroid lobectomy
   e. Thyroxine

   Answer a. Percutaneous cyst drainage

501. You completely drain the cyst in the above patient and send the fluid to pathology which shows serous fluid. One month later she returns to clinic with the same complaint and the cyst has returned on U/S. You drain it again and again one month later the cyst reappears. The most appropriate next step is:

a. I-131
b. Thyroxine
c. XRT
d. Thyroid lobectomy
e. Methimazole

Answer d. Thyroid lobectomy. Repeated occurrence of thyroid cyst is an indication for surgery (cyst size > 3-3.5, previous neck XRT, incomplete resolution, or bloody fluid are all indications for **thyroid lobectomy** [*not* cyst *excision*]). Cystic papillary thyroid CA can present with a recurrent cyst.

502. Following I-131, the most effective way of suppressing the growth of any residual follicular or papillary thyroid CA is:
a. Thyroid hormone replacement
b. Daily calcium
c. Daily phosphate replacement
d. Daily potassium

Answer a. Thyroid hormone replacement following resection for thyroid CA is a very effective tumor suppressor adjunct. By giving thyroid hormone, you effectively suppress TSH production and inhibit tumor growth.

503. A 50 yo woman with previous radiation therapy as a child has a 0.8 cm papillary thyroid CA. You do not feel any adenopathy. The most appropriate treatment is:
a. Thyroid lobectomy
b. Total thyroidectomy
c. Total thyroidectomy and MRND
d. Observation

Answer b. History of **XRT** is an indication for **total thyroidectomy.**

504. All of the following are risk factors for metastatic spread and recurrence of papillary and follicular thyroid CA except:
a. Males
b. Previous XRT
c. Age 20-50
d. Extra-capsular invasion

Answer c. RFs for thyroid CA **metastases** or **recurrence**: grade (poorly differentiated), age (< 20 or > 50), male gender, extra-thyroidal disease, size > 1 cm, previous XRT

505. All of the following are true of medullary thyroid carcinoma (MTC) except:
a. Amyloid is found in the tissue
b. Flushing and diarrhea occur
c. Family members of patients with MEN IIb should be screened for the RET proto-oncogene
d. MEN IIa patients have the worst prognosis

Answer d. MEN IIb and sporadic forms have the worst prognosis. *Family members of patients with MEN IIb should be screened for the **RET proto-oncogene.***

Screening using calcitonin is not recommended as these patients already have medullary thyroid CA.

506. Which of the following is true of MTC:
a. It is less aggressive than papillary or follicular thyroid CA
b. Chemo is effective
c. I-131 is effective

d. Total thyroidectomy, central node dissection, and ipsilateral MRND is indicated for patients who present with a palpable mass.

Answer d. Total thyroidectomy, central node dissection, and ipsilateral MRND is indicated for patients who present with a palpable mass. Chemo and I^{131} are <u>not</u> effective for MTC. MTC is more aggressive than papillary or follicular thyroid CA.

507. All of the following are true of Hurthle cell thyroid tumors except:
    a. 80% are malignant
    b. MC occurs in elderly
    c. Pathology shows oncocytic or oxyphilic cells
    d. Diagnosis is usually made with lobectomy

Answer a. 80% of **Hurthle cell thyroid tumors** are _benign_.

508. All of the following are true of anaplastic thyroid CA except:
    a. Is usually resectable
    b. Usually presents in elderly patients with long-standing goiters
    c. Has a propensity to invade other structures
    d. Is the most aggressive thyroid CA

Answer a. **Anaplastic thyroid CA** is the most aggressive thyroid CA and is usually beyond surgical management at the time of Dx (5-YS - 5%).

509. A 5 yo presents with a mid-line cervical mass that has had recurrent infections. The mass seems to move upward with swallowing. It also moves when the tongue is protruded. Which of the following is the most appropriate next step:
    a. Continued antibiotics
    b. Observation
    c. Resection of the cyst only
    d. Resection of the cyst and total thyroidectomy
    e. Resection of the cyst and the central portion of the hyoid bone

Answer e. Tx for a thyroglossal duct cyst is resection of the cyst and the central portion of the hyoid bone.

510. A 31 yo woman is 21 weeks pregnant and has severe tremors, tachycardia, and sweating. Her endocrinologist makes the diagnosis of hyperthyroidism and starts her on propylthiouracil (PTU), however, she continues to have Sx's. You advise the physician that the most appropriate next step is:
    a. Propranolol
    b. I-131
    c. Thyroidectomy
    d. Switch to methimazole

Answer c. The problem in this patient is that you <u>cannot</u> use either I-131 or methimazole because of their teratogenic effects. I-131 will ablate the fetal thyroid. Methimazole causes cretinism (stunted physical and mental growth due to hypothyroidism). Propylthiouracil (PTU) is safe because it does not cross the placenta.

You could use a beta-blocker, but you would still have hyperthyroidism (albeit with a lower heart rate) and an increased risk of stillbirth. Also, beta-blockers are contraindicated in the 3rd trimester of pregnancy as they have been associated with fetal growth retardation.

511. All of the following are true except:
    a. The Wolff Chaikoff effect is iodide inhibition of T3 and T4 release
    b. The mechanism of propylthiouracil is inhibition of peroxidases and iodide binding
    c. The most appropriate initial Tx for thyroid storm is I-131

d. Serum thyroglobulin is the best lab value for detecting thyroid papillary or follicular cell CA recurrence
e. Serum calcitonin is the best lab value for detecting recurrent medullary thyroid CA (MTC)

Answer c. The most appropriate initial Tx for thyroid storm is a **beta-blocker** (eg propranolol). High doses of **iodine** (Lugol's solution, potassium iodide) inhibit TSH action on the thyroid and inhibits organic coupling of iodide to tyrosine, resulting in less T3 and T4 release (**Wolff-Chaikoff effect**).

512. All of the following are true except:
a. Follicular cell CA MC spreads hematogenously
b. The MC thyroid CA in children is papillary thyroid CA
c. Hashimoto's disease is a risk factor for thyroid lymphoma
d. Psammoma bodies (calcium deposits) are most consistent with follicular cell thyroid CA
e. The majority of substernal goiters can be removed with a cervical collar incision

Answer d. Psammoma bodies (calcium) are found in **papillary thyroid CA**.

THYROID ANATOMY AND FUNCTION

- **Hypothalamus** - releases **thyrotropin-releasing hormone** (TRH) → goes to anterior pituitary gland
- **Anterior pituitary gland** - releases **thyroid-stimulating hormone** (TSH) → goes to thyroid gland
- **Thyroid Gland** – releases T4 and T3 (thyroid hormones)
  - TRH and **TSH** release controlled by a T4 + T3 negative feedback loop
  - **Peroxidases** links tyrosine and iodine to form T4 and T3
  - **Thyroglobulin** - stores T4 and T3 in **colloid**
  - Only **free T4** and T3 are **active** (protein bound <u>not</u> active) - free hormone represents < 1% of total serum T4 and T3
  - T4 : T3 serum ratio is **20:1**
  - Most T3 comes from T4 to T3 conversion in periphery (**deiodinases** - remove iodine ions)
  - T3 is the **more active form** (4x more potent than T4)
  - **Thyroid binding globulin** - transports the majority of T4 and T3 in bloodstream
- T4 and **T3** bind the **thyroid hormone receptor** in the <u>**nucleus**</u>
- **Thyroid hormone function** - ↑s C.O., HR, and basal metabolic rate; potentates effects of catecholamines
  - Is <u>not</u> involved in flight or fight stress response
- *TSH (nl. 0.3 - 3) - best test for thyroid function (hyperthyroidism or hypothyroidism)*
- **Thyroxine treatment** - TSH levels should fall 50%; **osteoporosis** long-term S/E
- **Thyroid gland** is derived from the **1st and 2nd pharyngeal pouches**
- **Vascular supply**
  - **Superior thyroid artery** - 1st branch off *external carotid artery*
    At superior pole of thyroid
  - **Inferior thyroid artery** - off **thyrocervical trunk** (inferior)
    Supplies **both inferior** and **superior parathyroids**
    With thyroidectomy, need ligation of the inferior thyroid arteries close to thyroid gland to avoid injury to parathyroid glands
  - **Ima artery** (3%) - off aorta or innominate artery; goes to thyroid gland
  - **Superior** and **middle thyroid veins** - *internal jugular vein* drainage
  - **Inferior thyroid vein** - *innominate vein* drainage
- **Superior laryngeal nerve** (external branch)
  - *MC injured nerve with thyroidectomy*
  - Motor to **cricothyroid muscle**
  - Runs superior and lateral to thyroid lobes
  - Usually tracks close to <u>superior thyroid artery</u> at the upper pole of the thyroid
  - Injury results in **loss of projection** and **easy voice fatigability** (opera singers)
  - Ligate the superior thyroid arteries close to the gland to avoid injury

- **Recurrent laryngeal nerve** (RLN)
  - Motor to all of the **larynx** (controls vocal cords) except cricothyroid
  - Runs posterior and medial to thyroid lobes in the tracheoesophageal groove
  - Can track with <u>inferior thyroid artery</u> but variable
  - **Left** RLN loops around **aorta**; the **right** RLN loops around **innominate artery**
  - **Non-recurrent laryngeal nerve** - in 2%; more common on the **right**
    - Intra-op injury risk is higher for a non-recurrent laryngeal nerve
  - *Unilateral* injury can result in **hoarseness** (if vocal cord *abducts*) or can be **asymptomatic** (if vocal cord adducts, *termed paramedian location*)
    - **Hoarseness** - may get better (wait 6 months), **medialize vocal cord** with silicone wedge or injection if persistent Sx's *(not re-op repair of nerve)*
    - **Asymptomatic** - leave alone
    - **Intra-op RLN injury** - repair at that time
  - *Bilateral* injury
    - Can **obstruct airway acutely** (vocal cords adducted, both in *paramedian* location); Sx's - severe stridor, respiratory distress → *need* **emergency tracheostomy** (can't intubate - *vocal cords block airway*)
    - Can cause **profound aspiration** (both vocal cords *abducted*) → will usually need **tracheostomy**
- Post-thyroidectomy **stridor**
  - If due to **hematoma** → <u>*emergently*</u> **re-open neck incision** and remove hematoma (can result in airway compromise)
  - If due to **bilateral RLN injury** → would need <u>*emergent*</u> **tracheostomy**
- Post-thyroidectomy **oral paresthesias**
  - Due to **hypocalcemia** from <u>devascularized parathyroid glands</u>
  - Tx: **calcium**
  - Avoid this by ligating inferior thyroid arteries <u>close</u> to the thyroid gland

THYROID STORM
- Sx's: tachycardia, fever, irritability, N/V, diarrhea, diaphoresis, high-output cardiac failure *(MCC of death in thyroid storm)*
- MC after surgery in a patient with undiagnosed **Graves' disease**
- Also precipitated by anxiety, excessive gland palpation, adrenergic stimulants
- Tx: **beta-blockers** *(1st drug to give)*, **Lugol's solution** (potassium iodide; *most effective drug but takes awhile*, give 1 hr after methimazole), **methimazole**, cooling blankets, oxygen, glucose
- Emergent thyroidectomy <u>*rarely*</u> indicated
- **Wolff-Chaikoff effect** - very effective for thyroid storm; patient given high doses of **iodine** (Lugol's solution, potassium iodide), which inhibits TSH action on thyroid and inhibits organic coupling of iodide, resulting in less T3 and T4 release

ASYMPTOMATIC THYROID NODULE
- 90% of thyroid nodules are benign; female predominance
- Check for **attachment** to trachea and cervical **adenopathy**
- Get **FNA** *(best initial test)*, **U/S**, and **thyroid function tests** (TSH, T3, and T4)
- **FNA** is determinant in 80%, follow appropriate Tx →
  - Shows **follicular cells** → Tx: lobectomy (10% CA risk; see Thyroid CA section)
  - Shows **thyroid CA** → Tx: thyroidectomy or lobectomy and appropriate Tx (see Thyroid CA section)
  - Shows **cyst fluid** → Tx: drain fluid
    - If it <u>recurs</u>, is <u>bloody</u>, size > <u>3-3.5</u>, previous neck <u>XRT</u>, *or* <u>incomplete resolution</u> → Tx: lobectomy
  - Shows **colloid tissue** → most likely **colloid goiter**
    - Low chance of malignancy (< 1%)
    - Tx: thyroxine; lobectomy if it continues to enlarge
  - Shows normal **thyroid tissue** and **T3 / T4 are elevated** → likely **solitary toxic nodule**
    - Asymptomatic - Tx: <u>*observation*</u>
    - Symptomatic - Tx: methimazole and ^{131}I
- **FNA** is <u>indeterminant</u> in 20% → get radionuclide study (technetium 99)

- **Hot** nodule → Tx:
  - Asymptomatic - *observation*
  - Symptomatic - methimazole and ^{131}I (lobectomy if that fails)
- **Cold** nodule → lobectomy (more likely malignant than hot nodule)
- **Thyroid adenomas** - need to differentiate from CA → *requires lobectomy*
- Thyroid CA is the MC **endocrine malignancy** in the U.S.

GOITER
- Refers to any abnormal enlargement
- Most identifiable cause is iodine deficiency; Tx - iodine replacement
- **Non-toxic multinodular goiter** (colloid goiter) - diffuse enlargement without evidence of functional abnormality (from low grade stimulation of TSH receptor or iodine deficiency)
  - Operative indications - **airway compression** (eg stridor, dyspnea on exertion), **suspicious nodule**, or **cosmesis**
  - Pathology - shows **colloid tissue**
  - **Tracheomalacia** can occur from compression
  - Tx: **thyroxine**
  - **Subtotal** or **total thyroidectomy** if indicated; subtotal has a decreased risk of RLN injury
- **Mediastinal thyroid tissue** (substernal goiter)
  - Almost all cases are from acquired disease with *inferior extensions of a normally placed thyroid gland* (usually multinodular goiter)
  - Considered substernal when > 50% of the thyroid gland is below thoracic inlet
  - Blood supply is from normal vessels in the neck (*not* intra-thoracic vessels)
  - Tx: 95% of these can be removed through a **neck collar incision** (cervical incision) alone (ie *without* median sternotomy)

ABNORMALITIES OF THYROID DESCENT
- **Pyramidal lobe** - occurs in 10%; extends from the isthmus to thymus
- **Lingual thyroid**
  - Thyroid tissue that persists in foramen cecum at **tongue base**
  - Represents complete failure of thyroid migration
  - Sx's: dysphagia, dyspnea, dysphonia ("strawberry lump" at tongue base)
  - 2% malignancy risk (MC - papillary thyroid CA)
  - Tx: **thyroxine** suppression; abolish with ^{131}I if that fails
    - Resection if worried about CA or if it does not shrink after medical Tx
  - Is the only thyroid tissue in 70% of the patients who have it (get U/S to check for the presence of thyroid gland)
- **Thyroglossal duct cyst**
  - Midline cervical mass; goes through the **hyoid bone**
  - Thyroglossal tract arises from **foramen cecum** (tongue base); thyroglossal duct cysts can arise anywhere from tongue to thyroid pyramidal lobe (thyroid descent path)
  - Most are located between the **hyoid bone** and **thyroid isthmus**
  - Classically moves **upward** with swallowing or tongue protrusion
  - Sx's: usually asymptomatic; susceptible to **infection** *(MC issue)*, dysphagia, dysphonia, dyspnea, fistula; may be **premalignant** (MC - papillary thyroid CA)
  - May be all the thyroid tissue the patient has
  - Surgical indications: **infection** *(MC indication)*, CA, increasing size
  - Tx: resection → take mid-portion of **hyoid bone** along with the **thyroglossal duct cyst** all the way to the **tongue base** (Sistrunk procedure); use a lateral neck incision

HYPERTHYROIDISM TREATMENT
- **Thionamide drugs** - includes propylthiouracil (PTU) and methimazole
  - Inhibit thyroid hormone (T3 and T4) formation (**inhibit peroxidases**)
- **Methimazole** - *1st line therapy*; *not used in pregnancy*
  - Side effects: **cretinism** in newborns (crosses placenta), aplastic anemia, agranulocytosis (rare)
- **PTU** - safe with pregnancy; not 1st line therapy due to **hepatotoxicity**

- Side effects - **hepatotoxicity** (especially <u>children</u>), aplastic anemia, agranulocytosis (rare)
■ **Radioactive iodine** (^{131}I)
  - Good for poor surgical risk patients or those unresponsive to thionamides
  - **Children** - there is general concern for the development of CA in young children treated with ^{131}I so it is *not used*
  - ^{131}I should <u>not</u> be used in **children** (malignancy risk), during **pregnancy** (cretinism, can traverse placenta), or in **lactating mothers** (in milk)
  - **Toxic multinodular goiter** - ^{131}I is much <u>less effective</u> for toxic multi-nodular goiter than for Grave's Disease and toxic adenoma due to non-homogenous uptake
■ **Thyroidectomy** indications for hyperthyroidism:
  - **Cold nodules**
  - **Grave's** or **toxic adenomas** not responsive to thionamides and ^{131}I
  - **Pregnant patients** or **children** not controlled with thionamides
  - **Toxic multi-nodular goiters** (thyroidectomy is considered 1st line here as medical Tx is generally ineffective, but a trial of medical Tx should be considered, *especially in the frail and elderly*)
■ Best time to operate during pregnancy is early **2nd trimester** (lowest overall risk of teratogenic events and premature labor)
■ Subtotal thyroidectomy can leave patient euthyroid

CAUSES OF HYPERTHYROIDISM
■ Sx's of hyperthyroidism - atrial fibrillation, heat intolerance, thirst, increased appetite, weight loss, sweating, palpitations; usually in women
■ Sx's can worsen with **contrast dyes**
■ *Unusual* to have to operate for hyperthyroidism *except* for toxic multinodular goiter
■ **Graves' disease** (toxic diffuse goiter; often in older women)
  - MCC of hyperthyroidism (80%)
  - Sx's only found in Grave's - **exophthalmos, pre-tibial edema**
  - Caused by **antibodies** (IgG) to **TSH receptor** (activate the receptor)
    IgG antibodies - long acting thyroid stimulator (LATS) and thyroid stimulating immunoglobulin (TSI)
  - Dx: low TSH, high T3/T4; ^{123}I scan shows diffuse homogenous uptake
  - Medical Tx usually manages hyperthyroidism (effective in > 95%)
  - Tx: **thionamides** (50% recurrence), ^{131}I (5% recurrence), or **thyroidectomy** if medical Tx fails; **beta-blocker** (helps with Sx's only)
  - **Unusual to have to operate** on these patients:
    Pre-op preparation: <u>methimazole</u> until euthyroid, <u>beta-blocker</u>, <u>Lugol's solution</u> for 14 days to decrease friability and vascularity (operate <u>only</u> after euthyroid)
    Operation: bilateral subtotal (5% recurrence) or total thyroidectomy (need lifetime thyroxine replacement)
  - **Indications for surgery**:
    Concomitant suspicious thyroid nodule *(MC indication)*
    Non-compliant patient
    Recurrence after medical Tx
    Children and pregnant women not controlled with thionamides *(^{131}I contraindicated)*
■ **Toxic multinodular goiter**
  - Older women usual; are usually non-toxic 1st
  - Sx's: tachycardia, weight loss, insomnia, airway compromise
  - Caused by hyperplasia secondary to chronic low-grade TSH stimulation
  - Pathology shows **colloid tissue**
  - Thyroid scan shows diffuse <u>non-homogenous</u> uptake
  - ^{131}I is <u>less</u> *effective for toxic multinodular goiter* (has non-homogenous uptake)
  - Tx: **surgery** (subtotal or total thyroidectomy) is the **preferred initial Tx** for toxic multinodular goiter but a **trial of ^{131}I** should be considered, especially if the patient is **elderly** and **frail**
    If compression or a suspicious nodule is present - Tx: **surgery**
■ **Single toxic nodule**

- Younger women usual; usually ≥ 3 cm to have Sx's; function autonomously
- Dx: **thyroid scan** (shows localized hot nodule)
  U/S - may show adenoma
- 20% of hot nodules eventually cause Sx's
- Tx: **thionamides** and ^{131}I (95% effective); lobectomy if medical Tx fails
- Rare causes of hyperthyroidism - trophoblastic tumors, TSH-secreting pituitary tumors
- **Pregnancy** and hyperthyroidism (usually Grave's disease)
  - If **PTU** is working, they do not need surgery
  - If **PTU** has not effectively treated the problem (eg still requiring beta-blocker to control Sx's) → Tx: **total** or **sub-total thyroidectomy**
  - Control of Sx's with beta-blocker can help but the patient is still hyperthyroid and at increased risk of **stillbirth** → will need surgery in the 2nd trimester
  - Can not use ^{131}I in pregnancy (cretinism)
  - Best time for thyroidectomy in pregnancy - early 2nd trimester (lowest overall risk of teratogenic events and premature labor); need total thyroidectomy or sub-total thyroidectomy
  - *Methimazole should not be used during pregnancy (cretinism)*

CAUSES OF THYROIDITIS
- **Hashimoto's disease**
  - *MCC of hypothyroidism in adults*
  - *MCC of thyroiditis*
  - Sx's: painless **enlarged gland**; chronic thyroiditis
  - Women; history of childhood XRT
  - Is an **autoimmune disease** (anti-microsomal and anti-thyroglobulin antibodies)
  - Erythrocyte sedimentation rate (ESR) is normal
  - Goiter due to lack of organification of **trapped iodide** inside gland
  - Pathology shows a **lymphocytic infiltrate**
  - Unusual to have to operate unless there is a suspicious nodule
  - These patients are at risk for **thyroid lymphoma** (Tx: chemo-XRT)
  - Tx: **thyroxine** *(1st line - treats vast majority)*
  - **Thyroidectomy** indicated if gland continues to grow despite thyroxine, if suspicious nodules appear, or if compression Sx's occur
- **Bacterial thyroiditis** (rare)
  - Usually secondary to **contiguous spread**
  - **Bacterial** upper respiratory tract infection (URI) usual precursor (staph and strep)
  - Sx's: fever, dysphagia, tenderness; normal thyroid function tests
  - Tx: **antibiotics**
  - May need **lobectomy** to rule-out CA with unilateral Sx's or if not responsive to antibiotics
  - May need total thyroidectomy for persistent inflammation
- **De Quervain's thyroiditis**
  - **Viral** URI precursor; tenderness, sore throat, weakness, fatigue; women
  - **ESR** is elevated
  - Tx: **steroids** and **ASA**
  - May need **lobectomy** to rule-out CA if unresponsive to medical Tx
  - May need total thyroidectomy for persistent inflammation
- **Riedel's fibrous struma** (rare)
  - **Woody** and **fibrous** component that can involve adjacent strap muscles and carotid sheath
  - Can resemble thyroid CA or lymphoma (need **Bx**)
  - Disease frequently results in **hypothyroidism** and **compression**
  - RFs: sclerosing cholangitis, fibrotic diseases, retroperitoneal fibrosis
  - Tx: **steroids** and **thyroxine**
  - Possible **isthmectomy** (resect thyroid isthmus) or **tracheostomy** for airway Sx's
  - If resection needed, watch for RLNs

THYROID CANCER

- *MC endocrine CA in the U.S.*
- Sx's: asymptomatic nodule; voice changes (dysphonia), dysphagia
- **Follicular cells** on FNA → 5-10% chance of CA (can <u>not</u> differentiate between follicular cell adenoma, follicular cell hyperplasia, and follicular cell CA on FNA)
- Worrisome for **malignancy** - solid, solitary, cold, slow growing, or hard nodule
  - Males; age > 50; previous neck XRT; MEN IIa or IIb
- **Sudden growth** - could be hemorrhage into previously undetected nodule or represent CA
- **Follicular adenomas** (colloid, embryonal, fetal subtypes) → <u>no increase in CA risk</u>, although still need **lobectomy** to prove it is an adenoma
- **Papillary thyroid carcinoma**
  - MC type of thyroid CA (85%)
  - Least aggressive and slow growing (best prognosis thyroid CA)
  - Often occurs in **women** and **children**
    - Large and firm nodules in children are worrisome
    - Older age (> 50) predicts a worse prognosis
  - RFs: **childhood XRT** (very high risk; MC tumor following neck XRT [usually given for previous lymphoma]); **long-standing goiter** (> 5 years)
  - Pathology - **psammoma bodies** (calcium deposits) and **Orphan Annie nuclei**
    - Many are **multicentric**
    - Can present as a **cyst** (a **complex cyst** or **bloody cyst fluid** *worrisome*)
    - **Lymphatic** spread 1st but is <u>not</u> prognostic
    - Prognosis based on **local invasion** *(MCC of death)*
  - **Children** are more likely to be **node positive** (75%) compared to adults (15%)
  - <u>Rare</u> metastases (**lung**)
  - 5-year survival rate - **95%**; death secondary to local invasion (usually airway)
- **Follicular thyroid carcinoma**
  - More aggressive than papillary thyroid CA
  - **Women** and **older adults** (50-60s); low iodine diet
  - Pathology - if FNA shows just **follicular cells** → have 5-10% chance of malignancy; Tx: **lobectomy**
    - **Hematogenous** spread (MC - **bone**) → 50% have metastatic disease at the time of presentation
  - **Lobectomy** on pathology shows **adenoma** or **follicular cell hyperplasia** → nothing else needed
  - 5-year survival rate - **70%**; prognosis based on hematogenous spread (stage)
- **Surgery** for **papillary** and **follicular** thyroid CA → start with lobectomy
  - Indications for <u>total</u> **thyroidectomy**:
    - Tumor **> 1 cm**
    - **Extra-thyroidal disease** (beyond thyroid capsule, clinically positive nodes, metastases)
    - **Multi-centric** or **bilateral** lesions
    - **Previous XRT**
  - Indications for **MRND**:
    - **Extra-thyroidal disease**
  - Indications for **post-op** ^{131}I (6 weeks after surgery, want TSH high for maximum uptake):
    - Tumor **> 1 cm**
    - **Extra-thyroidal disease**
    - *Need <u>total thyroidectomy</u> for ^{131}I to be effective*
  - Enlarged lateral neck lymph node that shows **thyroid tissue** (**lateral aberrant thyroid tissue**; ie papillary thyroid CA with lymphatic spread) → Tx: **total thyroidectomy, MRND**, and ^{131}I
- **Medullary thyroid carcinoma** (MTC)
  - Can be MEN IIa, MEN IIb, familial MTC only, and sporadic MTC (80%)
  - Associated with the **RET proto-oncogene**
  - **Worse prognosis** - MEN IIb and sporadic
  - More *aggressive* than follicular and papillary CA
  - Usually the 1st manifestation of MEN IIa and IIb (Sx - **diarrhea**)
  - Pathology - tumor arises from **parafollicular C cells**

> C-cell hyperplasia considered <u>premalignant</u>
> Amyloid deposition in thyroid gland
> Secrete calcitonin - can cause diarrhea and flushing
> Majority (90%) have multicentric disease

- Need to screen for hyperparathyroidism and pheochromocytoma
- Lymphatic spread - most have involved nodes at time of diagnosis of palpable disease (70%)
- Often early metastases (lung, liver, bone; prevents attempt at cure)
- Prophylactic Tx (thyroidectomy and central node dissection) - indicated for patients with a family history of MTC who have the RET proto-oncogene:
  > MEN IIa - at age 6 years
  > MEN IIb - at age 2 years
  > Not done earlier due to difficulty in finding recurrent laryngeal nerves in children (too small); high risk of injury (including bilateral injury and need for permanent tracheostomy)
- MTC Tx (presenting as a mass): need total thyroidectomy, central node dissection, <u>and</u> ipsilateral MRND
  > Bilateral MRND if both lobes have tumor or if extrathyroidal disease present
  > XRT may be useful for unresectable local or metastatic disease
  > Chemo of little benefit (I^{131} does <u>not</u> work)
- Monitor calcitonin level to detect disease recurrence
- 5-year survival for patients who present with palpable MTC:
  > MEN IIa - 50% (prognosis based on distant metastases)
  > MEN IIb - 10%
- Patients with a family history of MEN IIa, MEN IIb, or Familial MTC should undergo genetic testing for the RET proto-oncogene
  > *Calcitonin elevation is <u>not</u> a good screening tool as most of those patients have already developed MTC if calcitonin is elevated.*

■ Hürthle cell carcinoma
- Most are benign (80%; Hürthle cell adenoma); usually older patients
- Metastases go to bone and lung if malignant
- Pathology - Askenazy cells (oncocytic or oxyphilic cells)
- *Can <u>not</u> make Dx of benign vs malignant based on FNA (need lobectomy to make Dx)*
- Tx: thyroid lobectomy, total thyroidectomy if malignant
  > MRND for clinically positive nodes

■ Anaplastic thyroid cancer
- *Most aggressive thyroid CA (<u>all</u> are malignant)*
- Elderly patients with long-standing goiters
- Rapidly lethal (5-year survival: 0-5%) - propensity to invade other structures (eg trachea)
- Usually beyond surgical management at time of Dx
- Pathology - vesicular appearance of nuclei
- Tx: total thyroidectomy for the rare lesion that can be resected (possible tracheal resection)
- Can perform palliative thyroidectomy for compressive Sx's or give palliative chemo-XRT

ADJUVANT THERAPY AND FOLLOW-UP FOR THYROID CANCER
■ ^{131}I effective for papillary and follicular thyroid CA <u>only</u>
- Can cure bone and lung metastases
- Given 4-6 weeks after surgery when TSH levels are highest (want TSH 3 x normal)
- Do <u>not</u> give thyroid replacement until <u>after</u> treatment with ^{131}I → would suppress TSH and uptake of ^{131}I
- Indications for ^{131}I Tx:
  > Tumors that are > 1 cm or have extrathyroidal disease (beyond thyroid capsular, nodal spread, or metastases)
  > Primary inoperable tumors due to local invasion
  > Recurrent CA

- Need _**total** thyroidectomy_ for ^{131}I to be effective (otherwise it just gets taken up by the gland)
- ^{131}**I side-effects** (rare): sialoadenitis, GI Sx's, infertility, bone marrow suppression, parathyroid dysfunction, leukemia
- **Not** used in **children** (CA risk), **during pregnancy** (cretinism, can traverse the placenta), or in **lactating mothers** (cretinism, in milk)

■ After Tx with ^{131}I, give **thyroxin** to keep TSH levels low:
- Want TSH $\leq$ 0.03 and patient mildly thyrotoxic
- This is very effective for suppressing metastatic disease

■ ^{123}I can be used to look for recurrence late after total thyroidectomy for papillary and follicular thyroid CA

■ **XRT** is used in papillary and follicular thyroid CA _only_ for unresectable disease not responsive to ^{131}I

■ **XRT** can be used for medullary, Hürthle, and anaplastic thyroid CA

■ **Thyroglobulin** level is used to detect recurrence of **papillary** and **follicular** cell thyroid CA after total thyroidectomy _(must have had a total thyroidectomy to use this as a screen)_

■ **Calcitonin** level is used to detect recurrence of **medullary thyroid CA** after thyroidectomy

■ RFs for thyroid CA **metastases** or **recurrence** : X-GAMES (previous XRT, tumor grade, age < 20 or > 50, males, extra-thyroidal disease, size > 1 cm)

Parathyroid

513. All of the following are true except:
    a. Superior parathyroid glands are derived from the 3rd pharyngeal pouch
    b. Parathyroid hormone (PTH) increases renal reabsorption of Ca and increases bone resorption (release of Ca and PO_4^- into the blood)
    c. PTH level should drop to 50% or less of the pre-op level within 10 minutes after successfully removing a parathyroid adenoma
    d. Active Vit D increases gut Ca absorption by increasing calcium binding protein
    e. PTH stimulates 1-hydroxylation of Vit D in the kidney

Answer a. The **superior parathyroid glands** are derived from the **4th pouch**.

514. All of the following are true except:
    a. The MC location for a missed parathyroid gland at re-exploration is normal anatomic position
    b. The MC location for an ectopic parathyroid gland is the thymus
    c. The superior thyroid artery goes to the superior glands and the inferior thyroid artery for the inferior glands
    d. The MCC of hypo-parathyroidism is previous thyroid surgery
    e. The inferior glands are more likely to be found in an ectopic position compared to the superior glands

Answer c. The blood supply to both the superior and inferior parathyroid glands is the **inferior thyroid arteries**.

515. All of the following are true except:
    a. The MCC of hypercalcemia is hyper-parathyroidism
    b. Malignant hypercalcemia is most commonly from tumor osteolysis
    c. Parathyroid CA is the malignancy with the highest risk of hypercalcemia
    d. PTH related peptide (PTH-rp) causes an increase in urine cAMP
    e. MEN 2B is not associated with hypercalcemia

Answer b. Malignant hypercalcemia is most commonly from PTH-rp release.

516. All of the following are true except
    a. Tertiary hyperparathyroidism most commonly occurs after kidney TXP
    b. Calcitonin stimulates bone resorption by osteoclasts
    c. Age < 50 is a relative indication for parathyroidectomy in asymptomatic patients with hyperparathyroidsim
    d. Vit D undergoes 1-hydroxylation in the kidney
    e. Pregnant patients with primary hyperparathyroidsim should undergo parathyroidectomy in the 2nd trimester

Answer b. Calcitonin *inhibits* bone resorption by osteoclasts

517. Which of the following is most consistent with primary hyperparathyroidism?
    a. Ca 11, PTH 200, elevated urine Ca
    b. Ca 8, PTH 200, elevated urine Ca, serum creatnine 7
    c. Ca 11, PTH 40, low urine calcium
    d. Ca 8, PTH 35, normal urine calcium

Answer a. Ca 11, PTH 200, elevated urine Ca

518. Which of the following lab values are most consistent with primary hyperparathyroidism?
    a. Cl 105, phosphate 4 and elevated renal cAMP
    b. Cl 107, phosphate 3 and decreased renal cAMP
    c. Cl 106, phosphate 4 and decreased renal cAMP
    d. Cl 105, phosphate 3 and elevated renal cAMP

Answer d. Primary hyperparathyroidism is associated with an elevated PTH, elevated Ca, elevated renal cAMP (effect of PTH on the PTH receptor in the kidney), and a Cl:PO4 ratio > 33.

519. Which of the following is most consistent with secondary hyperparathyroidism:
   a. Ca 11, PTH 200, elevated urine Ca
   b. Ca 8, PTH 200, elevated urine Ca, serum creatnine 7
   c. Ca 11, PTH 40, low urine calcium
   d. Ca 8, PTH 45, normal urine calcium

   Answer b. Secondary hyperparathyroidism occurs primarily in dialysis patients who have chronic loss of Ca.

520. A 50 yo man on chronic dialysis complains of severe and refractory bone pain despite aggressive treatment with sevelamer chloride, Ca, and cinacalcet. PTH level in this patient is most likely:
   a. 0.35
   b. 3.5
   c. 35
   d. 305

   Answer d. The PTH level is elevated in secondary hyperparathyroidism.

521. The most appropriate next step in the above patient is:
   a. Total parathyroidectomy and autoimplantation
   b. More frequent dialysis
   c. Alendronic acid
   d. Mithramycin

   Answer a. Total parathyroidectomy and autoimplantation

522. Which of the following is most consistent with familial hypercalcemic, hypocalciuria (FHH)?
   a. Ca 11, PTH 200, elevated urine Ca
   b. Ca 8, PTH 200, elevated urine Ca, serum creatnine 7
   c. Ca 11, PTH 40, low urine calcium
   d. Ca 8, PTH 35, normal urine calcium

   Answer c. Ca 11, PTH 40, low urine Ca. FHH is due to a defect in kidney PTH receptor that results in increased Ca resorption. Urine Ca will be low. *Tx for FHH – nothing (leave alone, Ca level never gets that high).*

   Patients with primary hyperparathyroidism have elevated urine Ca.

523. You are performing a parathyroidectomy for primary hyperparathyroidism and find 3 normal sized glands. All of the following are true *except*:
   a. The tail of the thymus should be resected
   b. You should resect 2 and 1/2 glands
   c. If you can't find an adenoma - close and get a sestamibi scan
   d. Median sternotomy should be *avoided* at this stage

   Answer b. *You should not resect normal glands.* If you cannot find the missing gland, you should close and get a post-op sestamibi scan.

524. You are performing a parathyroidectomy for primary hyperparathyroidism and find 3 abnormally large glands. Which of the following is true:
   a. You should resect 1 gland
   b. You should resect 3 glands
   c. You should resect 2 and 1/2 glands
   d. You should close and get a sestamibi scan

 e. You should resect 1 gland and biopsy the rest

Answer c. If the glands are abnormally large, resect 2 and ½ glands. You should then follow Ca and PTH levels - if they remain high, obtain a sestamibi scan post-op to find the missing gland.

You should <u>avoid</u> biopsy of parathyroid glands – can cause hemorrhage and devascularization (resulting in hypoparathyroidism).

525. You are performing a minimally invasive parathyroidectomy and you resect a large parathyroid gland. PTH falls from 200 to 150 after 30 min. The most appropriate next step is:
  a. Investigate the other 3 glands
  b. Close and check post-op PTH and Ca levels
  c. Ipsilateral thyroid lobectomy
  d. I-131 post-op
  e. Close and give Cinacalcet

Answer a. Investigate the other 3 glands. This patient has either parathyroid hyperplasia or a missing 2nd adenoma. PTH should go to < 50% of the pre-op value within 10 minutes.

526. All of the following are true of parathyroid CA except:
  a. The MCC of mortality is airway invasion
  b. The MC site of metastases is lung
  c. PTH is elevated
  d. Surgery should include en bloc parathyroidectomy and ipsilateral thyroidectomy

Answer a. The MCC of mortality with parathyroid CA is **hypercalcemia** - these patients can have extremely high Ca levels (> 15). Surgery should include **en bloc parathyroidectomy** and **ipsilateral thyroidectomy**.

527. A 30 yo woman recently diagnosed with MEN I syndrome develops confusion, somnolence, and a shortened QT on EKG. The next appropriate step is:
  a. Alpha-blockade
  b. Beta-blockade
  c. Calcium
  d. Intravenous fluids and lasix

Answer d. MEN I includes parathyroid hyperplasia, pancreatic tumors, and pituitary tumors. Of these, only **hypercalcemia** from hyperparathyroidism is associated with confusion, somnolence, and short QT. *Tx -* ***rapid normal saline bolus (200-300 cc/hr) and Lasix***

528. Which of the following is characteristic of MEN I:
  a. Parathyroid hyperplasia, medullary carcinoma of the thyroid, and pheochromocytoma
  b. Medullary carcinoma of the thyroid, pheochromocytoma, marfanoid habitus, mucosal neuroma
  c. Parathyroid hyperplasia, pancreatic tumors (MC - gastrinoma), pituitary tumors
  d. Von Recklinghausen's Disease

Answer c. MEN I consists of parathyroid hyperplasia, pancreatic tumors (gastrinoma is MC for this syndrome), and pituitary tumors (MC - prolactinoma).

Gastrinoma is the MC MEN I tumor overall. (Note insulinoma is the MC endocrine pancreatic tumor in the general population but not in MEN I).

529. All of the following are true except:
- a. Urine catecholamines should be checked in MEN IIa and IIb patients before elective surgery
- b. MEN1 inactivation is associated with MEN IIa
- c. Ca levels should be checked in MEN I and MEN IIa patients before elective surgery
- d. Ret proto-oncogene is associated with MEN IIa and IIb

Answer b. MEN1 inactivation is associated with MEN I. **Ret proto-oncogene** is associated with MEN IIa and IIb.

530. All of the following are true except:
- a. Parathyroid hyperplasia with hypercalcemia is usually the first part of MEN I to become symptomatic
- b. The MC pituitary neoplasm in MEN I is prolactinoma
- c. MEN IIb patients are likely to have a marfanoid habitus
- d. Medullary thyroid CA occurs in 50% of patients with MEN IIa or IIb

Answer d. Medullary thyroid CA occurs in nearly all (almost 100%) of patients with MEN IIa or IIb.

531. All of the following are true except:
- a. MEN I patients with simultaneous tumors should have the hyperparathyroidism corrected 1st
- b. MEN IIa patients with simultaneous tumors should have the pheochromocytoma corrected 1st
- c. MEN IIb patients with simultaneous tumors should have the medullary thyroid CA corrected 1st
- d. Gastrinoma is the MC pancreatic tumor in MEN I patients

Answer c. MEN IIb patients with simultaneous tumors should have the **pheochromocytoma** corrected 1st.

ANATOMY AND FUNCTION

- **Superior parathyroids** - found <u>lateral</u> to recurrent laryngeal nerves (RLNs), <u>above</u> inferior thyroid artery, posterior surface of superior portion of thyroid gland
  - Derived from **4th pouch** (associated with the **thyroid complex**)
  - Can migrate to the **posterior** mediastinum
- **Inferior parathyroids** - found <u>medial</u> to RLNs, <u>below</u> inferior thyroid artery
  - More anterior
  - Derived from **3rd pouch** (associated with **thymus**)
  - Inferior parathyroids have a more **variable location** and are more likely to be **ectopic**
  - Occasionally are found in the **tail of the thymus** (MC ectopic site) and can migrate to the anterior mediastinum
  - Other ectopic sites - intra-thyroid, mediastinal, near tracheoesophageal groove
- 85% of patients have all 4 glands (10% have 5 or more glands; 5% have 3 glands)
- **Inferior thyroid artery** - blood supply to <u>both</u> **superior** and **inferior parathyroid glands**
- PTH - *increases* serum Ca by:
  - **Kidney Ca reabsorption** in distal tubules
    Also ↓s kidney PO_4^- and HCO_3^- absorption (all mediated by **cAMP**)
  - Stimulates **bone resorption** (stimulates **osteoclasts**; **releases Ca** and PO_4^-)
  - Increases **Vitamin D production in kidney** (↑s 1-hydroxylation of Vit D)
  - Net serum PO_4 *decreases* due to PTH
- Calcitonin - *decreases* serum Ca by:
  - **Inhibits resorption of Ca from bone** (osteoclast inhibition)
  - **Increases kidney Ca and PO_4 excretion**
  - Net serum PO_4 *decreases* due to calcitonin

- **Vit D** (1,25-dihydroxy-cholecalciferol)
  - **Synthesis**: 7-dehydrocholesterol → **UV light** → Vit D3 → **liver** (**25-hydroxylation**) → Vit D3-25OH → **kidney** (**1-hydroxylation**) → Vit D
  - **Active Vit D** _increases_ intestinal Ca and PO_4 absorption by increasing synthesis of **calcium binding protein**
- *The MCC of hypo-parathyroidism is* **previous thyroid surgery** *(disrupted vascular supply to the parathyroids during thyroid surgery)*
- **Normal Values**
  - **Normal Ca**:   8.5-10.5 mg/dL
  - **Normal Ionized Ca**:   1.1 - 1.5 mmol/L
  - **Normal PTH**:   10 - 60 (pg/ml)
  - **Normal PO_4**:   2.5 - 5.0
  - **Normal Cl⁻**:   98 - 107
  - **Parathyroid gland weight**   60 - 80 gm

PRIMARY HYPERPARATHYROIDISM

- **PRAD-1** oncogene increases risk for parathyroid adenomas
- **Genetic Syndromes** - MEN I and IIA, familial hyperparathyroidism
- Often in older women
- Most patients are **asymptomatic** - high Ca found on routine lab work
- Sx's (from **hypercalcemia**): weakness, myalgias, nephrolithiasis, pancreatitis, peptic ulcers, bone pain, fractures, depression, bone loss (densitometry), HTN (renal impairment), cholelithiasis
- **Osteitis fibrosa cystica** (brown tumors, osteoclastomas) - bone lesions from Ca resorption; characteristic of hyperparathyroidism
- Dx: **high PTH** and **high Ca** (autonomously secreted PTH)
  - Other values:
    - Low PO_4^-
    - Cl⁻ to PO_4^- ratio > 33
    - Hyperchloremic metabolic _acidosis_
    - ↑ cAMP in urine (action on PTH receptor in kidney)
  - Urine Ca is **elevated** (unlike FHH - see below)
- Indications for **surgery**:
  - Symptomatic disease
  - Asymptomatic disease with (_any_ below):
    - Ca > 11.6
    - Decreased creatinine clearance (< 60 ml/min; from Ca overload)
    - Kidney stones
    - Substantial bone loss (densitometry t-score < −2.5, any site)
    - Age < 50 (relative indication; lowers lifetime risk of Cx's)
- **Single adenoma** - 80% of patients
- **Diffuse hyperplasia** - 15%; MEN I and IIa have 4-gland hyperplasia
- **Multiple adenomas** - 5%
- **Parathyroid adenocarcinoma** - very rare; can get very high Ca levels
- Tx:
  - **Adenoma** - resection; consider inspection of other glands to rule out hyperplasia or multiple adenomas (ie if PTH fails to drop)
  - **Parathyroid hyperplasia**
    - Do _not_ Bx all glands → hemorrhage and hypo-parathyroidism risk
    - Tx: resect 3½ glands (subtotal parathyroidectomy, form the ½ gland 1ˢᵗ) or total parathyroidectomy and auto-implantation (parathyroid graft tissue placed in strap muscles or forearm; forearm used in MEN so you don't have to go back into neck for recurrence)
  - **Parathyroid CA** → radical parathyroidectomy (take **ipsilateral thyroid lobe**)
  - Remember to **give calcium** post-op (bone hunger will use up Ca)
  - **Pregnancy** - surgery in 2ⁿᵈ trimester; high risk of **stillbirth** if not resected
- **Intra-op frozen section** → confirms tissue taken was indeed parathyroid
- **Intra-op PTH levels** → determines if the causative gland is removed (PTH should go to < **50%** of the pre-op value within **10 minutes**; peripheral vein draw)
  - *If PTH does not fall appropriately, you need to* **check all of the other glands** *(ie you have multiple adenomas or parathyroid hyperplasia)*

- Trouble finding adenoma → check missing gland locations below
- **Missing gland locations - thymus tissue** (*MC ectopic location*; can remove thymus tail from the neck and see if PTH drops [possible *transcervical* thymectomy, *but not median sternotomy*]), near carotid bifurcation, anterior to vertebral bodies, superior to pharynx, tracheo-esophageal groove, intra-thyroid (use U/S to find it), mediastinum
- **Still cannot find adenoma** despite checking missing gland locations → close and follow PTH; if PTH is still high, get **sestamibi scan** to localize
- If you find 3 <u>large</u> glands (ie you have **hyperplasia** and are missing a gland or you have hyperplasia and the patient was born with 3 glands)
  - Check missing gland locations above
  - Take **2 ½ glands** (or 3 glands with auto-implantation)
  - Check **intra-op PTH**:
    1) If decreased > 50% in 10 min → you're done
    2) If still high PTH → take **tail of thymus** (or transcervical thymectomy) → if PTH still high, close and get post-op sestamibi scan to localize missing gland
- If you find 3 <u>normal</u> sized glands (ie you can't find the adenoma)
  - Check missing gland locations and **take tail of thymus** (or transcervical thymectomy)
  - Still not found → close and get post-op sestamibi scan
  - *Do <u>not</u> resect normal glands*
  - *Also do <u>not</u> biopsy normal glands → can cause hemorrhage and devascularization, resulting in <u>hypo-parathyroidism</u>*
- **Follow Ca post-op** (remember to give Ca post-op)
  - Post-op **hypocalcemia** etiologies:
    Bone hunger (early) - normal PTH, decreased HCO_3^-
    Graft / Remnant failure (late) - low PTH, normal HCO_3^-
- **Persistent hyperparathyroidism** (1%) - MC from missed adenoma remaining in neck
  - **Sestamibi scan** to localize missing gland and re-operate
  - At reoperation for a missing gland, the MC location for the gland is **normal anatomic position**
  - **Reoperation** is associated with increased risk of <u>RLN injury</u> and permanent <u>hypoparathyroidism</u>
- **Recurrent hyperparathyroidism** - occurs after a period of hypocalcemia or normocalcemia
  - Can be due to new adenoma formation
  - Can be due to tumor implants at original operation that have grown
  - Consider recurrent parathyroid CA
- **Sestamibi scan** - some use this for all patients with hyperparathyroidism
  - Will have preferential uptake by the overactive parathyroid gland (adenoma)
  - Good for picking up adenomas but not 4-gland hyperplasia
  - Best for trying to pick up ectopic glands

SECONDARY HYPERPARATHYROIDISM
- MCC - **chronic renal failure**
- Dx: **high PTH** in response to **low Ca** (Ca may be low normal)
- Ca is lost with dialysis
- Serum PO_4 is high
- Sx's: pruritus, bone pain, fractures
- *Most do <u>not</u> need surgery (medical Tx effective in 95%)*
- Tx: **Ca supplement** and **sevelamer chloride** (Renagel - binds phosphate), **calcitriol** (Vit D), control diet PO_4 (low dairy products)
  - **Cinacalcet** - mimics Ca; inhibits PTH release from parathyroids *(very effective)*
- Surgery indications (refractory to medical Tx and any of the following):
  - Refractory **bone pain** *(MC indication)*
  - **Fractures**
  - **Pruritus** (itching)
- 85% get relief with surgery
- Surgery involves **total parathyroidectomy** with auto-transplantation or **subtotal parathyroidectomy**

TERTIARY HYPERPARATHYROIDISM
- Renal disease now corrected with kidney transplant but still overproduces PTH
- Has similar lab values as primary hyperparathyroidism (high PTH, high Ca)
- Surgical indications same as primary hyperparathyroidism
- Tx: **subtotal** (3½ glands) or **total parathyroidectomy** with autoimplantation

FAMILIAL HYPERCALCEMIC HYPOCALCIURIA (FHH)
- Patients have mildly **high serum Ca** and **_low_** urine Ca *(urine Ca would be increased if it was primary hyperparathyroidism)*
- Caused by a defect in the PTH receptor at the kidney distal convoluted tubule that causes *increased* resorption of Ca
- These patients are never symptomatic
- Dx: Ca 9-11, have normal PTH (10-60), **_low_ urine Ca** *(key finding, opposite that of primary hyperparathyroidism)*
- Tx: nothing (Ca not that high in these patients); *no* parathyroidectomy

PARATHYROID CANCER
- Rare cause of hypercalcemia
- Dx: ↑ Ca, ↑ PTH, and ↑ alkaline phosphatase (can have extremely high Ca)
- MC metastatic site - **lung**
- Tx: wide en bloc excision (total parathyroidectomy and ipsilateral thyroidectomy)
- 5-year survival rate - 50%
- Mortality is due to **hypercalcemia** (can have extremely high Ca levels)

CALCIPHYLAXIS (calcific uremic arteriopathy)
- Associated with **chronic renal failure** and secondary hyperparathyroidism
- Get **calcification + thrombosis** of small-medium **blood vessels**; occurs in any tissue
- Has a very **poor prognosis**
- 1st sign - painful **skin ischemia** and **necrosis**
- Dx: **skin Bx** (shows calcium deposits)
- Tx: **dialysis** to keep Ca low; **Cinacalcet**; wound care
  - Want Ca x PO_4^- product to be low

HYPERCALCEMIA
- 90% due to either **primary hyperparathyroidism** (#1) or **malignancy**
- MC mechanism of **malignant hypercalcemia** - PTH-rp (*not tumor destruction of bone*)
- **Non-hematologic malignancies** - can release **PTH-rp** (rp = related peptide); causes **hypercalcemia**
  - MC CA causing malignant hypercalcemia - **breast CA**
  - CA with high risk of malignant hypercalcemia - **squamous cell lung CA**
  - *Highest* risk CA - **parathyroid CA**
  - Elevated Ca is not due to bone destruction
  - PTH-rp is not detected by the lab PTH assay test
  - Get high **urine cAMP** with PTH-rp (acts on kidney PTH receptor)
- **Hematologic malignancies** - can cause bone destruction (osteolysis) with increased Ca; MC - **multiple myeloma**; can also get excess Vit D precursors

MULTIPLE ENDOCRINE NEOPLASIA SYNDROMES
- Neoplasms can develop synchronously or metachronously
- Autosomal dominant; () = % of patients who develop each part
- **MEN I** (MEN1 gene, menin protein)
  - **Parathyroid hyperplasia** (90%)
    - Usually 1st part to become symptomatic (hypercalcemia, **kidney stones**)
    - Tx: 4-gland resection with autotransplantation
    - Don't leave gland in neck - hard re-op if recurrence
  - **Pancreatic islet cell tumors** (70%)
    - Gastrinoma #1 - 50% multiple, 50% malignant
    - MCC of **mortality** in these patients
  - **Pituitary adenoma** (70%)
    - Prolactinoma #1
  - Need to correct hyperparathyroidism 1st if simultaneous tumors

- **MEN IIa** (RET proto-oncogene)
  - **Parathyroid hyperplasia** (50%) - same as above
  - **Medullary CA of thyroid** (>99%)
    - *Nearly **all patients** get this (hallmark of MEN IIa and IIb)*; often bilateral
    - Usually **1st part** to be symptomatic (MC Sx - **diarrhea**)
    - MCC of **mortality** in these patients
  - **Pheochromocytoma** (50%)
    - Often bilateral, nearly always benign
  - Need to correct <u>pheochromocytoma</u> 1st if simultaneous tumors
- **MEN IIb** (RET proto-oncogene)
  - **Medullary CA of thyroid** (>99%)
    - Same as above except <u>MEN IIb</u> is ***more aggressive*** than MEN IIa
  - **Pheochromocytoma** (50%) - same as above
  - **Mucosal neuromas** (anywhere in GI tract)
  - **Marfan's habitus** and **musculoskeletal** abnormalities
  - Need to correct <u>pheochromocytoma</u> 1st if simultaneous tumors
- Always check **Ca** on MEN I and IIa patients before operating on them
- Always check **urine metanephrines** on MEN IIa and IIb patients before operating on them

Pituitary Gland

532. All of the following are true except
    a. A calcified cyst near the sella turcica in a 5 yo boy is most consistent with meningioma
    b. Trouble lactating following peri-partum hypotension is consistent with Sheehan's syndrome
    c. Most prolactinomas can be treated with bromocriptine
    d. ADH is released primarily in response to high plasma osmolarity

    Answer a. A calcified cyst near the sella turcica is most consistent with **craniopharyngioma.** Tx – resection if symptomatic (benign cyst)

HYPOTHALAMUS
- Releases **TRH, CRH, GnRH, GHRH,** and **dopamine** into median eminence
- Hormones then pass through the posterior pituitary (neurohypophysis) on their way to the anterior pituitary (adenohypophysis)
- **Dopamine** - inhibits prolactin secretion (constitutive inhibitor)

POSTERIOR PITUITARY GLAND (neurohypophysis)
- Consists of axons extending from **supraoptic** and **paraventricular nuclei** of **hypothalamus** into the posterior pituitary gland
- Secretes **2 hormones** into capillaries of the hypophyseal circulation:
    1) **ADH** (anti-diuretic hormone; ie vasopressin)
        Release controlled by **supraoptic nuclei** mostly
        Primarily regulated by **osmolar receptors** in hypothalamus; released in response to **high plasma osmolarity**
        Causes increased **water absorption** in **kidney collecting ducts**
    2) **Oxytocin** - release controlled by **paraventricular nuclei** mostly
- *Posterior pituitary does not contain cell bodies*

ANTERIOR PITUITARY GLAND (adenohypophysis; 80% of the pituitary gland)
- **ACTH, TSH, GH, LH, FSH,** and **prolactin** released
- *No direct blood supply*; has **portal system** with blood passing through neurohypophysis 1st
- Pituitary gland found in **sella turcica**
- **Bi-temporal hemianopia** (visual problems with pituitary mass) - from a pituitary mass compressing optic nerve (CN II) at the chiasm
- *Contraindications* to trans-sphenoid resection of tumors - supra-cellar extension (dumbbell-shaped tumor), massive lateral extension
- **Bromocriptine** - can be used reduce all endocrine secreting pituitary tumors *except* ACTH secreting

PROLACTINOMA
- *MC pituitary tumor; MC are **micro-**adenomas*
- Sx's: amenorrhea, galactorrhea, infertility, poor libido, visual problems
- Dx: ↑ **prolactin** (> 150 usual); MRI and visual field testing
- Tx: *most prolactinomas do not need surgery*
    1) **Asymptomatic** and **micro-adenoma** (≤ 10 mm) - follow with MRI
    2) **Symptomatic** or **macro-adenoma** (> 10 mm):
        Bromocriptine or **cabergoline** (dopamine agonist) - 85% success (safe with pregnancy)
        Trans-sphenoid surgery (for failed medical Tx, hemorrhage, visual loss, wants pregnancy, or CSF leak) - 85% successful (15% recurrence)

ACROMEGALY (excessive growth hormone, GH)
- GH stimulates secretion of **insulin-like growth factor-1** (IGF-1)
- MC are *macro-adenomas*
- Sx's: jaw enlargement (macroglossia), HA, ↑ soft tissue, HTN, amenorrhea, DM, giganticism; visual problems related to size
  - Can have **life-threatening cardiac issues** (valves, cardiomyopathy)
- Dx: ↑ **IGF-1 level** (*best test, random GH level* <u>*not*</u> *useful*)
  - **MRI** to look for tumor
- Tx:
  - *Surgery 1st choice if not invading surrounding tissues* (→ trans-sphenoid resection)
  - **Octreotide** and **bromocriptine** can shrink tumor and relieve Sx's
  - **Pegvisomant** (GH receptor antagonist)

OTHER
- **Sheehan's syndrome**
  - Pituitary insufficiency in mother after childbirth
  - From hypovolemia or shock following childbirth causing **pituitary ischemia**
  - *1st sign* - postpartum **trouble lactating**; can also have amenorrhea, adrenal insufficiency, hypothyroidism
  - Affects **anterior pituitary** (portal venous blood supply), posterior pituitary usually not affected (direct arterial blood supply)
  - Tx: **replace deficiencies**
- Craniopharyngioma
  - **Benign**
  - MC children aged 5-10 years
  - *Calcified cyst* near anterior pituitary, remnants of **Rathke's pouch**
  - Sx's: headaches, growth failure, bi-temporal hemianopia, endocrine abnormalities, hydrocephalus
  - Tx: surgery if symptomatic
  - **Diabetes insipidus** - frequent Cx post-op
- **Bilateral pituitary masses** - if non-endocrine producing → probably metastases

Breast

533. All of the following are true except:
   a. Laceration of the long thoracic nerve will result in a winged scapula
   b. Laceration of the thoracodorsal nerve will result in weak arm adduction and internal rotation
   c. Batson's plexus is a venous plexus that allows direct metastases to the spine (bone)
   d. The MCC of malignant axillary adenopathy is metastatic breast CA
   e. The MC injured nerve with MRM or ALND is the intercostobrachial nerve which results in axillary numbness and is generally well tolerated

   Answer d. The MCC of malignant axillary adenopathy is **lymphoma.**

534. All of the following are true of mastodynia except:
   a. < 1% represents breast CA
   b. The MCC of cyclic mastodynia is fibrocystic disease
   c. Continuous mastodynia is more refractory to treat than cyclic mastodynia
   d. The MCC of continuous mastodynia is DCIS

   Answer d. The MCC of continuous mastodynia is **infection**.

535. All of the following are treatments for mastodynia except:
   a. Bromocriptine
   b. Avoidance of tobacco (nicotine) and caffeine
   c. Evening primrose oil
   d. OCP's
   e. Tamoxifen

   Answer e. All are treatments for mastodynia except Tamoxifen.

536. A 27 yo breastfeeding woman develops pain, erythema, and tenderness adjacent the nipple-areolar complex. U/S shows an associated abscess which you drain percutaneously. This patient most likely has:
   a. Mondor's Disease
   b. Fibrocystic disease
   c. Fibroadenoma
   d. Periductal mastitis
   e. Galactocoele

   Answer d. Periductal mastitis

537. All of the following are true in the above patient's condition except:
   a. There is usually an associated infection
   b. Incisional biopsy should be performed if it fails to improve after 2 weeks
   c. Initial treatment should be antibiotics and continued breast feeding
   d. Klebsiella is frequently found in the excreted milk
   e. Dilated mammary ducts are usually present

   Answer d. Staph is the MC organism associated with peri-ductal mastitis.

538. All of the following are true of non-breast feeding periductal mastitis except:
   a. It is associated with a bloody discharge
   b. Nipple piercings and tobacco are risk factors
   c. Erythema is often present
   d. Non-cyclical mastodynia is a common clinical feature
   e. Initial Tx should be antibiotics and follow-up

   Answer a. Non-breast feeding periductal mastitis is associated with a creamy (not bloody) discharge.

539. A 25 woman has pain in the left breast with a palpable cord, surrounding erythema, and tenderness. This most likely represents:
   a. Inflammatory breast CA
   b. Breast abscess
   c. Periductal mastitis
   d. Fibroadenoma
   e. Mondor's disease

   Answer e. Mondor's Disease (superficial thrombophlebitis of the breast)

540. All of the following are true of the above condition except:
   a. It is associated with trauma and strenuous exercise
   b. Surgery is generally required after the acute process resolves
   c. It is often painful
   d. NSAIDs and warm compresses are appropriate initial Tx
   e. It usually occurs in the breast in women

   Answer b. Surgery is not required. Tx is NSAIDs and warm compresses.

   Superficial thrombophlebitis can also occur in the limbs, axilla, and trunk.

541. A 45 yo woman undergoes breast CNBx and the pathology shows phyllodes tumor. You find no metastatic disease. The most appropriate management is:
   a. Modified radical mastectomy
   b. Lumpectomy and axillary lymph node dissection
   c. Radical mastectomy
   d. Wide local excision and no axillary node dissection

   Answer d. Phyllodes tumors consist of stromal cells (mesenchymal origin, not epithelial) and can be hard to differentiate from fibroadenomas. Unlike fibroadenomas, a margin must be obtained with resection. *Tx – WLE with 1 cm margin and no ALND*

   Only 15% are malignant (cystosarcoma phyllodes) and behave like sarcomas *(nodal disease is extremely rare). Tx - WLE with 1 cm margin, no ALND*

   Malignancy is determined by mitoses per high powered field *(not cytology).*

542. A girl in her mid-teens has a quickly enlarging breast mass. U/S shows a 7 cm diameter hypoechoic mass. Given the most likely diagnosis, the most appropriate next step is:
   a. Serial U/S follow-up only
   b. Excisional biopsy and SLNB
   c. Mass excision only
   d. Chemo-XRT
   e. Lumpectomy and ALND

   Answer c. Mass resection. This likely represents a giant juvenile fibroadenoma and should be resected to avoid permanent breast damage.

543. A 80 yo man is in you clinic for a large right breast. He has a right 2.0 cm mass and normal exam on the left side. The most appropriate next step is:
   a. Local resection of the right mass
   b. Observation with follow-up in 6 months
   c. Send off hormonal studies and follow-up in 6 months
   d. Core needle biopsy (CNBx)
   e. XRT

   Answer d. CNBx. This is worrisome for **male breast CA**. Senescence gynecomastia is bilateral, not unilateral.

544. All of the following are true of adolescent gynecomastia except:
   a. Pathologic work-up is _rarely_ required other than a breast and testicular exam
   b. This condition is often unilateral
   c. Reassurance and follow-up is the standard of care
   d. These patients generally require surgery in their late teens
   e. There is no breast CA risk

   Answer d. These patients do <u>not</u> require surgery. The condition generally resolves after adolescence.

545. A 50 yo woman presents with bloody nipple discharge. All of the following are true except:
   a. This patient needs bilateral mammograms
   b. This MC occurs with invasive ductal CA
   c. This patient likely requires a ductogram and directed excision
   d. This patient should have a breast U/S
   e. Any expressed bloody fluid should be sent to cytology

   Answer b. The MCC of bloody nipple discharge is **intra-ductal papilloma.**

546. A 50 yo woman presents with serous nipple discharge. On exam you express fluid from a duct. The immediate next step is:
   a. Breast MRI
   b. Collect the expressed fluid for examination
   c. Nothing
   d. Mammogram

   Answer b. Around 5% of patients with suspicious nipple discharge have malignant or suspicious cells on cytology. Around 90% of those patients will have CA on excision.

547. A 50 yo woman presents with bloody nipple discharge. You send the fluid off to cytology and it is negative for malignant or suspicious cells. Mammogram and U/S do not reveal any lesions. The most appropriate next step is:
   a. Breast MRI
   b. Ductogram
   c. Subareolar resection
   d. Breast biopsy

   Answer b. Ductogram. **Intraductal papilloma** is the MCC of bloody nipple discharge. This is best diagnosed with a ductogram.

548. A 50 yo woman presents to you with breast pain and lumpy breast tissue that seems to vary with her hormonal cycle. She thinks she feels a dominant area that she hadn't felt before. All of the following are true except:
   a. She needs bilateral mammograms
   b. She needs an U/S
   c. She needs a core needle biopsy of the dominant area
   d. Observation is indicated

   Answer d. A breast CA work-up is indicated in this patient.

549. Mammogram shows suspicious calcifications (BIRADS IV) and CNBx shows atypical ductal hyperplasia in the above patient. The most appropriate next step is:
   a. Subcutaneous mastectomy
   b. Chemotherapy
   c. Excisional biopsy
   d. Lumpectomy and XRT
   e. Observation and repeat mammography in 6 months

Answer c. Excisional biopsy These lesions do <u>not</u> require negative margins although you do need to get all of the lesion that appears on mammogram (ie you need to get all of the suspicious calcifications).

550. A 50 yo woman presents with a palpable mass in her left breast. You do not feel any axillary adenopathy. The mass feels firm and mobile. U/S shows a 1.75 cm mass with no associated findings. A BIRADS II lesion (benign finding) is demonstrated on mammography. The most appropriate next step is:
   a. Observation only
   b. Repeat mammography in 3-6 months
   c. Excisional biopsy
   d. CNBx
   e. Lumpectomy and XRT

   Answer d. CNBx (or FNA) is indicated for all suspicious **palpable breast masses**, even if mammography and/or U/S demonstrate a benign lesion.

   CNBx <u>without</u> excisional biopsy allows **appropriate staging with SLNB** (mass is still present) and **one-step surgery** (avoids 2 surgeries) for patients diagnosed with breast CA.

   CNBx <u>prior</u> to any excision is appropriate for both: 1) suspicious palpable masses <u>and</u> 2) patients with appropriate BIRAD or U/S indications.

551. Which of the following benign breast diseases has a significant risk of breast CA:
   a. Complex fibroadenoma
   b. Papilloma
   c. Sclerosing adenosis
   d. Florid hyperplasia without atypia
   e. Atypical lobular hyperplasia

   Answer e. Atypical lobular hyperplasia has a relative risk (RR) of 5 and excisional biopsy is indicated.

552. A 50 yo woman undergoes CNBx for a BiRADS IV lesion and it shows radial scar. The most appropriate next step is:
   a. Observation and repeat mammography in 6 months
   b. XRT
   c. Simple mastectomy
   d. Excisional biopsy
   e. Lumpectomy and XRT

   Answer d. Excisional Bx. Patients with a **radial scar** have a **10%** risk of underlying breast CA. Radial scars can be seen on mammogram and are confirmed by histology. CNBx is often used before excicional biopsy.

553. A 50 yo woman undergoes CNBx for a BiRADS V lesion and it shows normal tissue. The most appropriate next step is:
   a. Observation and repeat mammography in 6 months
   b. XRT
   c. Simple mastectomy
   d. Excisional biopsy
   e. Lumpectomy and XRT

   Answer d. Excisional Bx. A BiRADS V lesion has a **95%** breast CA risk. At some point the lesion needs excision. XRT, simple mastectomy, and lumpectomy + XRT are not appropriate at this stage.

554. A 50 yo woman undergoes a CNBx for a BiRAD IV lesion (suspicious linear calcifications) and it shows ductal carcinoma in situ (DCIS). All of the following are true except:

a. Comedo type DCIS is an indication for subcutaneous mastectomy
b. Males with DCIS should undergo simple mastectomy
c. SLNB is indicated if mastectomy is performed
d. DCIS does not require negative margins
e. Lumpectomy with XRT is an option for most DCIS lesions

Answer d. Negative margins are required for DCIS.

555. A 2nd CNBx in a separate quadrant in the above patient also shows DCIS. What is the most appropriate next step:
a. Lumpectomy x 2 and SLNB
b. Lumpectomy and PET scan
c. Simple mastectomy and PET scan
d. Simple mastectomy and SLNB
e. Simple mastectomy only

Answer d. Simple mastectomy and **SLNB**. Can't go with lumpectomy x 2 as she has 2 separate primary DCIS lesions in separate quadrants (multi-centric / multi-focal disease). You need SLNB when performing mastectomy for DCIS (last chance to sample the sentinel lymph node).

Around 10% of patients with DCIS undergoing mastectomy will actually have invasive ductal CA at final pathology. Around 2% of patients with DCIS undergoing mastectomy will have a positive SLNB showing ductal CA.

556. A 40 yo woman undergoes a stereotactic excisional biopsy for a suspicious lesion on mammogram. The suspicious area is completely resected however the pathology comes back lobular carcinoma in situ (LCIS) with positive margins. Her mother had breast CA at age 60. All of the following are true except:
a. Re-excision for negative margins is required
b. Observation with repeat mammography and examination in 6 months can be performed
c. Tamoxifen can be used to treat this patient
d. Ductal CA is the most likely breast CA to occur in this patient
e. Bilateral simple mastectomy may be an option in this patient if she has a strong family history of breast CA

Answer a. LCIS does not require negative margins.

557. All of the following are true for LCIS except:
a. Is usually not palpable
b. Is not associated with calcifications
c. It is considered a pre-malignant lesion
d. The risk of cancer is the same for both breasts

Answer c. LCIS is considered a **marker** for breast CA and is not a premalignant lesion.

558. All of the following are true for DCIS except:
a. Comedo type indicates central necrosis
b. Papillary type has the worst prognosis
c. It is often associated the calcifications
d. XRT should be given after lumpectomy

Answer b. Comedo type has the **worst prognosis.**

559. All of the following are true of the BRCA gene except:
a. Total abdominal hysterectomy and bilateral salpingo-oophrectomy decreases breast CA risk by 70%
b. BRCA I gene equates with an ovarian cancer risk of 40% (lifetime)

c. BRCA gene confers a worse prognosis in comparable staged non-BRCA breast CA
d. BRCA II gene equates with a male breast cancer risk of 10% (lifetime)
e. Bilateral mastectomy decreases breast CA risk by 90%

Answer c. Women with **BRCA** and breast CA have the same prognosis as comparable-stage breast CA in patients not having BRCA. The **HER receptor** confers a worse prognosis for comparable-stage breast CA.

560. All of the following are true of BRCA except:
   a. BRCA I breast tends to present with poorly differentiated and receptor negative breast CA
   b. BRCA II tends to present with well differentiated and hormonal receptor positive breast CA
   c. Men with BRCA and breast CA tend to present with more advanced tumors
   d. BRCA accounts for 25% of all breast CA cases

Answer d. BRCA accounts for 5% of all breast CA cases.

561. All of the following are true except:
   a. Ovarian CA risk is higher with BRCA I
   b. Breast CA risk is relatively the same for BRCA I and BRCA II
   c. Male breast CA risk is higher with BRCA I
   d. BRCA increases the risk of melanoma, pancreatic, and other CA's

Answer c. Male breast CA risk is higher with BRCA II.

562. All of the following are recommended screening for women with BRCA except:
   a. Yearly mammogram starting at age 25
   b. Yearly breast MRI starting at age 25
   c. Yearly pelvic exam starting at age 25
   d. Year brain MRI starting at age 25

Answer d. Brain MRI is not a recommendation.

563. All of the following are true of males with breast CA except:
   a. 80% are hormonal receptor positive and < 5% are HER2 positive
   b. They have the same prognosis stage for stage compared to females
   c. The 2nd highest risk CA in males with BRCA is prostate CA
   d. Most have pectoral muscle and nipple-areola involvement at time of diagnosis
   e. They are more likely to get lobular CA

Answer e. Males are more likely to get ductal CA.

564. All of the following are true of males with breast CA except:
   a. Lumpectomy is generally indicated
   b. If hormonal receptors are positive, the patient should get tamoxifen
   c. 20% of patients have pre-existing gynecomastia
   d. Klinefelter's Disease is a RF
   e. Prognosis is generally poorer compared to women due to late diagnosis and advanced stage

Answer a. Mastectomy is generally indicated due to advanced local disease (nodal assessment is also indicated). DCIS is uncommonly diagnosed in males as the disease has already advanced to CA.

565. A 60 yo woman presents with a 6 cm infiltrating ductal CA along with palpable but moveable axillary adenopathy. She has no signs of metastatic disease. All of the following are true in this patient except:
   a. This patient is a candidate for primary (neoadjuvant) chemotherapy

b. She will ultimately require a modified radical mastectomy regardless of her response to chemotherapy
c. She needs a chest/abdomen/pelvic CT scan for systemic work-up
d. She is a candidate for lumpectomy and axillary lymph node dissection if the tumor shrinks with chemotherapy
e. The most important predictor of survival in this patient is the number of positive nodes

Answer b. This patient has **Stage III-a** disease (T3, N1, M0) and initial therapy can be surgery or chemo. If the patient wishes to have breast conserving therapy (BCT), primary chemo can be given in an attempt to shrink the tumor, followed by lumpectomy and ALND. The other option is MRM with post-op chemo-XRT *(the tumor is > 5 cm so you need XRT after MRM)*.

For **Stage III-b**, neoadjuvant chemo, followed by surgery (usually MRM), then post-op chemo-XRT is standard Tx.

566. A 50 yo woman comes to clinic and has a left sided 4 cm ductal carcinoma on mammography. Exam demonstrates the lymph nodes in her axilla are fixed and matted. Work up for metastatic disease is negative. This patients clinical stage is:
    a. Stage IB
    b. Stage IIA
    c. Stage IIB
    d. Stage IIIA

Answer d. A 4 cm CA is T2 and fixed nodes is N2a; T2,N2,M0 - stage IIIa.

567. All of the following are surgical options in the above patient except:
    a. Lumpectomy and axillary lymph node dissection
    b. Modified radical mastectomy
    c. Lumpectomy and sentinel lymph node biopsy
    d. Quadrectomy and axillary lymph node dissection

Answer c. Patients with **clinically positive nodes** are <u>not</u> candidates for SLNB.

568. The above patient undergoes BCT (lumpectomy + ALND) and post-op XRT. Two years later she has a suspicious mammogram on the same breast that shows abnormal calcifications in the right lower quadrant. The most appropriate next step is:
    a. CNBx
    b. Subcutaneous mastectomy
    c. Observation
    d. Chemo-XRT

Answer a. CNBx

569. In the above patient, CNBx shows DCIS. The most appropriate next step is:
    a. Lumpectomy
    b. Subcutaneous mastectomy
    c. MRM
    d. Chemo-XRT
    e. Observation

Answer b. Subcutaneous mastectomy (simple mastectomy) is indicated since the nodes were already taken (MRM is not necessary).

Lumpectomy would <u>not</u> be appropriate as the breast has already received **XRT** (need to give XRT after lumpectomy for DCIS which is contraindicated in this patient because she has already has XRT).

570. All of the following are contraindications to breast conserving therapy (BCT) except:
    a. Pregnancy (1st or early 2nd trimester)

b. Clinically palpable axillary nodes
c. Previous XRT that would result in excessive XRT dose
d. Multi-focal disease

Answer b. Clinically palpable axillary nodes are not a contraindication to BCT (eg lumpectomy and ALND is possible).

571. A 50 yo woman presents with erythema and edema in her left breast. She was treated with antibiotics for 2 weeks but the area persists. The most appropriate next step is:
    a. XRT
    b. Biopsy including skin
    c. MRM
    d. Change antibiotics
    e. Chemo

    Answer b. (see below)

572. Skin biopsy in the above patient shows ductal CA in the dermal lymphatics. The most appropriate next step is:
    a. MRM
    b. Chemo
    c. XRT
    d. Central lumpectomy
    e. Simple mastectomy

    Answer b. This patient has **inflammatory breast CA**. Initial Tx is **chemo**, followed by **MRM**, and then **chemo-XRT**.

573. A 50 yo woman has a 2 cm ductal carcinoma on CNBx and negative nodes on exam. You decide to perform SLNB using lymphazurin blue dye and technetium labeled sulfur colloid . All of the following are true except:
    a. If you do not find blue or radio-labeled nodes, ALND is indicated
    b. If 3 blue nodes are found, they should all be taken
    c. Resection of the highest count node and any nodes 10% or greater than that node is indicated
    d. A supraclavicular node with a high gamma count should be left alone

    Answer d. This node should be sampled. Unusually, you find a node that is hot which is outside the area you were expecting. You need to go after that node for staging purposes.

574. SLNB in the above patient shows a lymph node with a small (5 mm) area of CA. The most appropriate next step is:
    a. No further treatment
    b. ALND
    c. PET scan
    d. MRI

    Answer b. ALND (still the standard of care)

575. All of the following are true of sentinel lymph node biopsy (SLNB) except:
    a. The major concern is the false negative rate
    b. Inflammatory breast CA is a contraindication to SLNB
    c. The risk of lymphedema is lower with SLNB
    d. Lymphazurin blue dye has been associated with type II hypersensitivity reaction
    e. Breast CA is multiple quadrants is not a contraindication

    Answer d. Type I hypersensitivity reaction occurs in 1% of patients receiving lymphazurin blue dye.

Although previously a contraindication, patients with breast CA (or DCIS) in multiple quadrants can undergo SLNB. You just need to inject at all the breast CA (or DCIS) sites *(although these patients still need **mastectomy**, not multiple lumpectomies)*

Similarly, **pregnant patients** can undergo **SLNB** (previously contraindicated, now felt to be **safe**).

576. All the following are true of ALND for breast CA except:
    a.   Nodes beneath and lateral to pectoralis minor should be taken (level I and II nodes)
    b.   Grossly positive level II nodes is an indication for dissection of level III nodes
    c.   The superior border for dissection is the axillary vein
    d.   The posterior border is the scapula
    e.   The anterior border is the pectoralis muscle

    Answer d. The posterior border is the **latissimus dorsi muscle**.

577. A 63 yo woman undergoes lumpectomy and SLNB for a T3,N0,M0 ductal CA. Six months later, she feels a nodule underneath the lumpectomy suture line. FNA comes back ductal carcinoma. The most appropriate next step is:
    a.   Repeat lumpectomy including the lump
    b.   Sentinel lymph node biopsy
    c.   XRT
    d.   Modified radical mastectomy (MRM)

    Answer d. Tx for breast CA recurrence after lumpectomy is **MRM**. There is a 2-3% chance of recurrence after appropriate lumpectomy.

578. All of the following are true of (Herceptin) and the HER receptor except:
    a.   The major S/E of Herceptin is neurotoxicity
    b.   HER receptor is associated with a worse prognosis for breast CA
    c.   Herceptin Tx results in a 50% reduction in breast CA recurrence when combined with chemo
    d.   Herceptin is given after chemotherapy if both are indicated

    Answer a. Trastuzumab major S/E is **cardiac toxiity** (CHF). **Taxol** major S/E is **neurotoxicity.**

579. After a MRM, pathology shows a tumor that is 4 cm and 6 lymph nodes are positive. Estrogen receptors are positive but progesterone receptors are negative. The most appropriate post-op management is:
    a.   Chemo, XRT, and hormonal therapy
    b.   Tamoxifen only
    c.   XRT only
    d.   Chemotherapy followed by Tamoxifen

    Answer a. *≥ 4 positive nodes is an indication for **XRT after MRM**. Node positive tumors get chemo. Hormone receptor positive tumors get hormonal Tx.

580. All of the following are correct nodal designations except:
    a.   Ipsilateral infra-clavicular nodes are N3a
    b.   Ipsilateral supra-clavicular nodes are N3c
    c.   Both ipsilateral axillary and internal mammary nodes is considered N3b
    d.   Positive internal mammary nodes in absence of axillary nodes is N3a

    Answer d. Positive internal mammary nodes in absence of axillary nodes is N2b

581. All of the following are true of each breast CA type except:

a. Metaplastic breast CA is more likely to be triple receptor negative compared to other types of breast CA
b. Inflammatory breast CA has a better prognosis compared to most other types breast CA
c. Tubular breast CA has the most favorable prognosis (behaves less aggressively; usually small and low grade)
d. Ductal CA is the most common type of breast

Answer b. Inflammatory breast CA has the *worst prognosis* compared to other breast CA types.

582. A 60 yo woman has a palpable node in her axilla. You get a bilateral mammogram and CXR which are both negative. You excise the node and find adenocarcinoma that is positive for estrogen receptors. The most appropriate next step is:
    a. Chemotherapy (Adriamycin and cyclophosphamide)
    b. XRT
    c. Modified radical mastectomy
    d. Sentinel lymph node biopsy

Answer c. Occult breast CA can present as an enlarged lymph node in the axilla. With the finding of breast CA in the axillary node, you should perform MRM on the same side. In 70%, you will find breast CA in the breast. Instead of excisional Bx above, **core needle biopsy** could have been performed.

583. A 55 yo woman with no PMHx presents to your office with a weepy, scaly lesion on her right nipple. Mammogram and U/S do not show any mass. You get a wedge biopsy of the skin and breast tissue which shows Paget cells and DCIS. The appropriate next step is:
    a. Modified radical mastectomy
    b. Simple mastectomy (including the nipple areolar complex) and SLNB
    c. Lumpectomy and ALND
    d. XRT
    e. Simple mastectomy alone

Answer b. Paget's disease of the breast is considered a **breast CA**. In **> 95%** of patients, an additional underlying **DCIS** or **breast CA** (MC ductal CA) is present. All patients at a minimum need:1) removal of the nipple areolar complex including the underlying breast tissue *and* 2) some form of node sampling.

DCIS with Paget's → **simple mastectomy** and **SLNB** (including nipple areolar complex resection; *classic answer*). *ALND is not indicated for Paget's with DCIS.*

Breast CA with Paget's → 1) **simple mastectomy** (including nipple areolar complex resection) and **ALND** or **SLNB** *or*, 2) **MRM**

Paget's with no DCIS or other underlying breast CA *(rare)* → 1) **simple mastectomy** and **SLNB** (including nipple areolar complex resection) *or*, 2) **central lumpectomy** (including the nipple areolar complex) and **SLNB**.

584. All the following are true of a DIEP flap except:
    a. It has replaced the TRAM flap at some institutions
    b. It relies on the inferior epigastric arteries
    c. CABG with left IMA is a contraindication to left sided DIEP
    d. Laparoscopic cholecystectomy is a contraindication

Answer d. A lap choly is *not* a contraindication to DIEP flap (deep inferior epigastric perforators). DIEP removes the fat and skin but *not* the muscle. It is anastomosed to the internal mammary artery and vein.

585. A 55 yo woman undergoes MRM for breast CA and develops chronic lymphedema. Five years later she comes to your office with a dark purple raised lesion underneath her arm. Which of the following is true of this likely condition:
    a. This represents a breast cancer recurrence
    b. This is a sarcoma
    c. This is melanoma
    d. The patient has contra-lateral breast CA

    Answer b. This is classic for **lymphangiosarcoma** following axillary dissection and chronic lymphedema (Stewart Treves Syndrome).

586. All of the following are true of breast CA in pregnancy except:
    a. Stage for stage, the prognosis is the same as non-pregnant women
    b. Breast CA in pregnancy tends to present with advanced nodal disease, leading to a worse prognosis
    c. SLNB can be used in pregnancy
    d. Chemotherapy should never be used in pregnancy
    e. XRT should never be used in pregnancy

    Answer d. Chemotherapy can be used the 2nd and 3rd trimesters (no evidence of teratogenicity).

587. A 27 yo woman is 23 weeks pregnant and presents with a firm breast lesion. You do not feel any axillary adenopathy. All of the following are true except
    a. Mammography should be the first diagnostic step
    b. If it is a cyst, it should be drained with the fluid sent to cytology
    c. If it is solid, CNBx or FNA should be performed
    d. U/S is useful in this age group

    Answer a. Mammography does not work well in these patients due to dense breast tissue. It also exposes the fetus to radiation. U/S is the best diagnostic step in this patient and also avoids fetal radiation.

588. A 27 yo woman is 9 weeks pregnant and presents with a ductal CA on CNBx. Which of the following is true
    a. SLNB is contraindicated
    b. If chemo is indicated, it should be given after delivery
    c. BCS is acceptable therapy in the first trimester
    d. Therapeutic abortion is the only option in this patient
    e. Mastectomy and assessment of the lymph nodes is the best option is this patient

    Answer e. Mastectomy and assessment of the lymph nodes (eg MRM or mastectomy and SLNB) is the best option for patients with breast CA in the 1st or early 2nd trimester.

    SLNB can be used in pregnancy. Chemo can be given in the 2nd and 3rd trimeseters without risk of teratogenic events. BCS cannot be used in the 1st or early 2nd trimesters due to the contraindication to XRT. BCS can be used in the late 2nd or 3rd trimesters, possibly followed with chemo during pregnancy, and XRT given post-partum.

589. Which region has the lowest breast CA incidence per 100,00 people:
    a. North America
    b. South America
    c. Eastern Europe
    d. Eastern Asia

    Answer d. Eastern Asia (Japan specifically) has the lowest incidence of breast CA.

BREAST

NERVES AND ANATOMY
- **Long thoracic nerve** - innervates **serratus anterior**
  - Injury results in winged scapula, trouble lifting arm above head
  - **Lateral thoracic artery** supplies serratus anterior
- **Thoracodorsal nerve** - innervates **latissimus dorsi**
  - Injury results in weak arm pull-ups and adduction
  - **Thoracodorsal artery** supplies latissimus dorsi
- **Medial pectoral nerve** - innervates pectoralis major and pectoralis minor
- **Lateral pectoral nerve** - pectoralis major only (runs near pectoralis minor; can be injured when level III axillary nodes are taken)
- **Intercostobrachial nerve** - lateral cutaneous branch of 2nd intercostal nerve; found just below axillary vein when performing axillary lymph node dissection
  - *Most commonly injured nerve with axillary dissection*
  - Injury causes numbness to medial arm and axilla
  - Can transect without serious consequences
- **Batson's plexus** - valveless vein plexus that allows direct hematogenous metastasis of breast CA to spine (bone)
- **Lymphatic drainage**
  - 97% - axillary nodes
  - 2% - internal mammary nodes
  - Any quadrant can drain to the internal mammary nodes
  - Supraclavicular nodes - considered **N3c disease**
  - MCC of primary axillary adenopathy - **lymphoma**
- **Cooper's ligaments** - suspensory ligaments; divide breast into segments
  - Breast CA involving these strands can dimple skin

BENIGN BREAST DISEASE
- **Breast Abscess**
  - MCC - **breast-feeding**
  - MC organism - ***staph aureus***
  - Tx for **lactation** associated:
    - Repeated aspiration or incision and drainage (send drainage to cytology), **antibiotics**
    - **Continue breast feeding** or breast pump to facilitate drainage of engorged area
    - **Failure to resolve** after 2 weeks (especially if older) - excisional Bx (including skin) to rule-out necrotic CA
  - Tx for **non-lactation** associated (send drainage for cytology):
    - **Periareolar** - can get pus in nipple discharge (duct fistula)
      - Tx: aspiration; antibiotics; terminal duct excision if that fails
    - **Lateral** - aspiration or incision and drainage, antibiotics
    - **Failure to resolve** (2 weeks; especially if older) - excisional Bx (including skin) to rule-out necrotic CA
- **Periductal mastitis**
  - Sx's: non-cyclical **mastodynia** (pain), **tender** mass behind nipple areolar complex, **erythema**, warmth, swelling, nipple retraction, discharge; can have sterile or infected subareolar **abscess**
  - RFs: **breast feeding**, smoking (tobacco), nipple piercings
  - Pathology - dilated mammary ducts, inspissated secretions, marked periductal inflammation; usually associated with an **infection**
  - Dx: **FNA** (send for cytology and culture)
  - **Non-breastfeeding** associated Tx: if typical creamy discharge that is non-bloody and not associated with nipple retraction, give **antibiotics** and **reassure**; if **criteria not met**, or if it **recurs**, or if it **persists** beyond 2 weeks, need to rule-out inflammatory CA (incisional Bx including the skin)
  - **Breastfeeding** associated Tx: **antibiotics** and **continue breast feeding** (facilitates drainage of ducts); failure to improve after 2 weeks → incisional Bx including the skin to rule-out inflammatory CA

- **Galactocele** - breast cysts filled with milk; occurs with breast-feeding
  - Tx: ranges from aspiration to incision and drainage
- **Gynecomastia** (breast enlargement in male, > 2 cm pinch)
  - Is a <u>normal</u> physiologic response in <u>neonates</u> (maternal hormones - will regress), <u>adolescence</u>, and <u>senescence</u>
  - Can also be associated with many drugs and hormonal imbalances
  - **Adolescence** (12-15 yrs) - frequently unilateral *(no breast CA risk)*
    - Pathologic work-up is *rarely* required other than breast and testicular exam
    - Tx: reassurance *only* (standard of care) and follow-up
  - **Senescence** (elderly) - usually bilateral (if not, suspect male breast CA)
    - Tx: <u>nothing</u> if bilateral; if unilateral need a Bx
- **Accessory breast tissue** - can present in axilla (MC location)
- **Accessory nipples** (polythelia, MC breast anomaly) - can be found from axilla (MC site) to groin
- **Breast asymmetry** - common finding
- **Breast reduction** - ability to lactate frequently compromised
- **Mastodynia** - pain in breast; *rarely represents breast CA (< 1%)*
  - Dx: history and breast exam; bilateral mammogram, and U/S
  - **Cyclic** mastodynia - pain before menstrual period; MCC - **fibrocystic disease**
  - **Continuous** mastodynia - continuous pain; MCC - **infection** *(although in many no infection is present)*; continuous mastodynia is **more refractory** to Tx than cyclic mastodynia
  - Tx: danazol, OCPs, NSAIDs, evening primrose oil, bromocriptine
  - *Avoid* nicotine and caffeine (methylxanthines)
  - Antibiotics if infection associated
- **Mondor's disease** - sclerosing superficial vein thrombophlebitis of breast
  - Sx's: feels **cordlike**, can be **painful** with surrounding erythema
  - Associated with trauma and strenuous exercise
  - MC location - lower outer quadrant of breast; can also occur in non-breast sites (eg upper extremity or lower extremity)
  - Tx: **NSAIDs** and **warm compresses** *(not surgery)*
- **Fibrocystic disease**
  - Lots of types: fibromatosis, sclerosing adenosis, apocrine metaplasia, epithelial / ductal / lobular hyperplasia
  - Sx's: breast pain, nipple discharge (usually yellow to brown), lumpy breast tissue that varies with hormonal cycle
  - Dx: Breast exam, bilateral mammogram, and U/S
  - Tx: **reassurance** (repeat studies in 3 months) *unless* **atypical hyperplasia** is present
  - Only **CA risk** is <u>atypical</u> hyperplasia (can be ductal, lobular, or columnar; relative risk 4-5) → **need to resect these lesions** (wire guided excisional biopsy); do <u>not</u> need negative margins with atypical hyperplasia, but <u>do need</u> to remove all the suspicious area that appears on mammogram (eg calcifications, asymmetrical area)
- **Intraductal papilloma** (benign)
  - *MCC of **bloody nipple discharge***
  - Are usually small, non-palpable, and close to the nipple
  - **Benign** (are <u>not</u> premalignant) → get **contrast ductogram** to find papilloma, then leave wire in the responsible duct
  - Tx: wire-guided subareolar excisional Bx (take involved duct and papilloma) → excision required to rule-out ductal CA
- **Fibroadenoma**
  - MC breast lesion in **adolescents** and **young women**; 10% multiple
  - Sx's: usually painless, slow growing, well circumscribed, firm, rubbery
  - Often grows to several cm in size and then stops
  - Can change in size with menstrual cycle and can enlarge in pregnancy
  - Pathology - prominent **fibrous tissue** compressing epithelial cells
  - Mammography - can have large, coarse calcifications (popcorn lesions) from degeneration

- In patients **< 40 years old**:
  1) Mass needs to **feel clinically benign** (firm, rubbery, rolls, not fixed)
  2) **U/S** needs to be consistent with fibroadenoma (distinct borders, homogenous, width greater than height, **hypoechoic**)
  3) Need **FNA** or **core needle biopsy** that shows fibroadenoma
     Need all 3 of the above to be able to observe, otherwise need excisional biopsy
     If the fibroadenoma continues to **enlarge** - need **excisional biopsy**
     Avoid resection of breast tissue in teenagers and younger children → can affect breast development and very rare breast CA in this group
- In patients **> 40 years old** → excisional biopsy to ensure diagnosis (or core needle Bx as a 1st step before resection); these patients need bilateral mammogram and U/S before surgery
- **Juvenile giant fibroadenoma** (> 5 cm, teenagers) - can enlarge very quickly, with compression and damage to adjacent breast tissue; can affect subsequent breast development; Tx - **resection**

NIPPLE DISCHARGE
- Most nipple discharge is **benign**
- All need a history, **breast exam, U/S,** and **bilateral mammogram**
- Try to find a **trigger point** or **mass** on exam
- _Send_ discharge for cytology (**5%** have malignant or suspicious cells)
  - > 90% of patients with **malignant** or **suspicious** cytology have CA on excision
  - Nipple discharge cytology is fairly specific in Dx of CA and can help direct Tx
- Dx: **ductogram**
- **Yellow-green-brown** discharge - usually due to **fibrocystic disease**; should have **lumpy** breast tissue consistent with fibrocystic disease
  - Tx: if **cyclical** and **non-spontaneous** - *reassure patient*
  - If there is any **doubt** → ductogram and wire-guided excisional Bx
  - Any **other type of discharge** (spontaneous or another color) → need ductogram and wire-guided excisional Bx
- **Bloody** discharge
  - MCC - intraductal papilloma; occasionally ductal CA
  - Tx: need **ductogram** and wire-guided **excision** of that ductal area
- **Serous** discharge - worrisome for CA, especially if coming from only 1 duct or is spontaneous
  - Tx: need **ductogram** and wire-guided **excision** of that ductal area
- **Spontaneous** discharge - no matter what the color or consistency is, this is worrisome for CA → all of these patients need **ductogram** and **excisional biopsy** of that ductal area
- **Non-spontaneous** discharge (occurs only with pressure, tight fitting garments, exercise, etc.) - not as worrisome but may still need excisional Bx (eg if bloody or serous)
- May have to do a complete subareolar resection if the culprit ductal area cannot be properly localized (no trigger point, no mass felt, no obvious lesion on ductogram)

DUCTAL CARCINOMA IN SITU (DCIS)
- Malignant cells of ductal epithelium _without_ basement membrane invasion
- Usually <u>not</u> palpable
- Usually presents as a <u>cluster</u> of **calcifications** (often linear or branching) on mammography
- 50% get **CA** if not resected *(ipsilateral breast is at risk)*
- Considered a **premalignant** lesion
- Can have solid, cribriform, papillary, and comedo types
- **Comedo** pattern - *most aggressive (**worst prognosis** subtype)* has **necrotic areas**
  - High risk for multicentricity, microinvasion, and recurrence
  - Tx: **simple mastectomy** and **SLNB**
- There is a <u>high</u> **recurrence risk** for **comedo** subtype and lesions **> 2.5 cm**
- **DCIS Tx options**:
  - **Lumpectomy** (≥ 1 mm margin) and **XRT**; _No_ ALND or SLNB
    Usually removed with wire-guided excision

Need to get all of the **calcifications** on mammography
Need **negative margins** for DCIS (can go for re-excision x 1)
XRT decreases the risk of local recurrence
Possible **tamoxifen / raloxifene** post-op
- **Simple mastectomy** with **SLNB** (see below for indications)
- Patients undergoing mastectomy for DCIS need **SLNB** (last chance to sample sentinel node; **10%** have invasive ductal CA and **2%** have nodal metastases on final pathology)
- Indications for **simple mastectomy** and **SLNB** in DCIS:
  - Patient **preference**
  - **Males**
  - **Comedo** (necrosis)
  - **High grade**
  - **Multi-centric** or **multi-focal** disease
  - Inability to get **margins** _despite_ re-resection
  - DCIS recurrence
  - Diffuse **malignant appearing calcifications** (hard to follow)
  - **Large tumor** not amenable to lumpectomy (inability to get good cosmetic result)
  - **Previous XRT** that would result in excessive total XRT dose
- **Tamoxifen** (if pre-menopausal) / **Raloxifene** (if post-menopausal) - for **5 years** after resected DCIS (optional)
  - Decrease risk of breast CA in DCIS patients by **50%**
  - Only for ER or PR positive lesions

LOBULAR CARCINOMA IN SITU (LCIS)
- 30% lifetime risk of breast CA (_**both breasts at risk**_; 1% per year)
- Considered a **marker** for the development of breast CA, _is not premalignant itself_
- Is not associated with calcifications, is not palpable, and is not seen on mammogram
- Usually an **incidental finding**; multifocal disease is common
- Should not have basement membrane invasion otherwise it is lobular CA
- Primarily found in **premenopausal** women
- Patients who develop breast CA are more likely to develop a **ductal CA** (70%)
- 5% have synchronous breast CA at time of Dx (most likely ductal CA)
- _Do not need negative margins_, although need excisional biopsy of all of the suspicious area if found on mammogram and core needle Bx → rules-out sampling error (ie a ductal CA next to the area of LCIS)
- **Tx options:** 1) nothing and careful follow-up, 2) tamoxifen / raloxifene, or 3) prophylactic bilateral subcutaneous mastectomy (consider if strong family history or BRCA; _no ALND or SLNB_)

Indications for Excisional Biopsy after Core Needle Biopsy

Atypical ductal hyperplasia
Atypical lobular hyperplasia
Columnar cell hyperplasia with atypia
Radial scar (need to resect to exclude breast CA; 10% have underlying malignancy)
Lobular carcinoma in situ (LCIS)
Phyllodes tumor
Papillary lesions
Lack of concordance between mammogram and histologic diagnosis
Non-diagnostic specimen (eg lack of calcifications when Bx was performed for calcifications)

BREAST CANCER
- Breast CA _decreased_ in economically poor areas and Japan
- U.S. Breast CA risk - **1 in 8 women** (12%); 5% if no risk factors
- **Screening** decreases mortality by 25%
- 10% of breast CA's have negative mammogram and negative ultrasound
- **Clinical features** - distortion of normal architecture; skin/nipple distortion or retraction; hard, tethered, indistinct borders
- **Nodal status** (number of positive nodes) is the single most important **prognostic factor** in patients devoid of systemic metastases

- **Palpable breast mass** workup:
  - **< 40 years old** - all need **U/S** and **core needle Bx** (CNBx)
    - Need mammogram in addition to above if clinical exam or U/S is indeterminate or suspicious for CA although in general want to avoid excess radiation in this group
    - Usually fibroadenomas in this group (see previous section for Tx)
  - **> 40 years old** - all need **bilateral mammograms, U/S,** and **CNBx**
  - If **CNBx** or **FNA** is indeterminate, non-diagnostic, or non-concordant with exam findings / imaging studies → will need **excisional biopsy**
  - Clinically indeterminate or suspect solid masses (on exam, U/S, or mammogram) will eventually need **excisional biopsy** unless a CA diagnosis is made prior to that
  - If **> 40**, push for **excisional biopsy**
  - If U/S shows **cyst fluid,** aspirate it
- **Cyst fluid**
  - If **bloody,** need cyst excisional biopsy
  - If **clear** _and_ **recurs,** need cyst excisional biopsy
  - If **complex cyst,** need cyst excisional biopsy

Management of Breast Masses Based on FNA or CNBx Findings

FNA / CNBx	Treatment
Malignancy	Definitive therapy
Suspicious	Excisional biopsy
Atypia	Excisional biopsy
Non-diagnostic	Repeat FNA/CNBx _or_ excisional biopsy
Benign	Possible observation - exam and imaging studies need to concordant with benign disease, otherwise need excisional biopsy (lean towards excisional Bx if > 40)

- **Core needle biopsy** (CNBx) - gives architecture
- **Fine needle aspiration** (FNA) - gives cytology (just cells)
- **Mammography**
  - Screening mammography has a 90% sensitivity / specificity
    - **7% false positive** and **10% false negative** rate
  - Sensitivity increases with age - dense parenchymal is replaced with fat
  - Mass needs to be **≥ 5 mm** to be detected
  - **Suggestive of CA** - irregular borders; spiculated; multiple clustered, small, thin, linear, crushed-like and/or branching calcifications; ductal asymmetry, distortion of architecture

BI-RADS Classification of Mammographic Abnormalities

Category	Assessment	Recommendation
1	Normal exam	Routine screening
2	Benign finding	Routine screening
3	Probably benign finding	Short-interval (3-6 months) follow-up mammogram
4	Suspicious abnormality (eg indeterminate calcifications or architecture)	Definite CA probability, _get **CNBx**_ CA risk: 4a - 15% 4b - 35% 4c - 80%
5	Highly suggestive of CA (eg suspicious calcifications or architecture)	High probability of CA; _get **CNBx**_ 95% CA risk

- **BI-RADS 4** lesion and stereotactic CNBx shows:
  - **Malignancy** → follow appropriate Tx
  - **Benign** and **concordant** with mammogram lesion (**4a** lesion _only_) → 3-6 month follow-up mammogram
  - **Non-diagnostic, indeterminate,** or **benign** and **non-concordant** with mammogram lesion (**4b** and **4c** lesions) → need needle localization **excisional biopsy**

- **BI-RADS 5** lesion and stereotactic CNBx shows:
  - **Malignancy** → follow appropriate Tx
  - ***Any other finding*** (non-diagnostic, indeterminate, or benign) → all need needle localization **excisional biopsy**
- CNBx *without* excisional biopsy allows **appropriate staging with SLNB** (mass is still present) and **one-step surgery** (avoids 2 surgeries) for patients diagnosed with breast CA

- ■ **Screening**
  - **Mammogram** every **2-3 years after age 40**, then **yearly after 50**
  - **High-risk screening** - mammogram 10 years before the youngest age of diagnosis of breast CA in first-degree relative
  - ***No mammography in patients < 40*** *unless* high risk → hard to interpret because of **dense parenchyma**; also want to **decrease radiation dose** in young patients
- ■ **BRCA I and II** (+ family history of breast CA) and **CA risk** (autosomal dominant)
  - **BRCA I** (chromosome 17):

Female breast CA	**60%** lifetime risk
Ovarian CA	**40%** lifetime risk
Male Breast CA	**1%** lifetime risk

  - **BRCA II** (chromosome 13):

Female breast CA	**60%** lifetime risk
Ovarian CA	**20%** lifetime risk
Male Breast CA	**10%** lifetime risk

  - ***BRCA is the*** *strongest* *RF for breast CA*
  - BRCA is found in **5%** of all breast CA
  - 50% of females will get CA in the other breast after CA in the 1st breast
  - Women with BRCA breast CA have the **same prognosis** stage for stage as patients with non-BRCA breast CA
  - Women with BRCA tend to present with breast CA at a **younger age** and is more likely to be **bilateral**
  - **BRCA I** - tends to be poorly differentiated and triple receptor negative
  - **BRCA II** - tends to be well differentiated and hormone receptor positive
  - BRCA increases risk for **other CA's** (eg melanoma, pancreatic, stomach, biliary)
  - **BRCA screening**:
    - Yearly **mammogram** and breast **MRI** starting at age 25
    - Yearly **pelvic exam**, pelvic **U/S**, and **CA-125** starting at age 25
  - Bilateral mastectomy with BRCA - decreases breast CA risk **90%**
  - Prophylactic total abdominal hysterectomy (TAH) + bilateral salpingo-oophorectomy (BSO) with BRCA - decreases breast CA risk **70%**
  - Bilateral mastectomy + TAH-BSO with BRCA - decreases breast CA risk **95%**
  - Highest risk CA in **males** with BRCA (aside from breast CA) - **prostate CA**
  - Men with BRCA tend to present with **more advanced** breast CA compared to women with BRCA
- ■ Consider **prophylactic bilateral mastectomy** as opposed to careful follow-up (+/- tamoxifen / raloxifene) for →
  - 1) **BRCA gene** *or;*
  - 2) **LCIS** and strong **family history** of breast CA
  - ***Also need one of the following***: high patient anxiety, poor patient access for follow-up, difficult lesion to follow on exam or with mammograms, or patient preference for mastectomy
  - There is no urgency for the above so the patient has time to consider options
- ■ **Breast CA TNM Staging**
  - **Tis** - LCIS, DCIS, Paget's disease of nipple without tumor
  - **T1**: < 2 cm, **T2**: 2-5 cm, **T3**: > 5 cm
  - **T4**: **4a** - chest wall involvement *(does not include pectoral muscles)*
    - **4b** - skin (edema, ulceration, or satellitosis), peau d'orange
    - **4c** - both above
    - **4d** - inflammatory breast CA (erythema)
  - **N1**: ipsilateral movable axillary nodes

N2: **2a** - fixed ipsilateral axillary nodes
    2b - clinically positive internal mammary nodes in absence of axillary nodes
N3: **3a** - ipsilateral infraclavicular nodes
    3b - *both* ipsilateral axillary and internal mammary nodes
    3c - ipsilateral supraclavicular nodes (considered inoperable)
M1: distant metastasis (inoperable)
Stages

Stage I	T1, N0, M0
Stage IIa	T0-1, N1, M0 or T2, N0, M0
Stage IIb	T2, N1, M0 or T3, N0, M0
Stage IIIa	T0-3, N2, M0 or T3, N1, M0
Stage IIIb	T4, N0-2, M0
Stage IIIc	N3
Stage IV	M1

5-YS:
    Stage I - 90%
    Stage II - 75%
    Stage III - 50%
    Stage IV - 15%

- **Treatment by Stage**
  - **Stage I, II, IIIa, and IIIc** (*only* N3a *or* N3b)
    - **1st Surgery** (usually)
      - **Stage I** and **II** – BCT or MRM; *exception* is T3N0M0 and patient wants BCT, can undergo primary (neoadjuvant) chemo 1st to shrink tumor, then BCT
      - **Stage IIIa** – MRM usual, *exception* is T3N1M0 and patient wants BCT, then give *primary chemo 1st* to shrink tumor, then BCT with ALND
      - **Stage IIIc** (*only* N3a or N3b) – MRM
    - **2nd Adjuvant chemo** (TAC, see below) – indicated for tumors > 1 cm, positive nodes, or ER/PR negative tumors
    - **Trastuzumab** – if HER2 positive and tumor > 1 cm or positive nodes
    - **Hormonal Tx** – for ER or PR positive tumor (or unknown status)
      - **Pre-menopausal** – *Tamoxifen*
      - **Post-menopausal** – *Aromatase inhibitor (eg anastrozole)*
    - **XRT** *follows* chemo (eg with lumpectomy *or* if indicated after MRM)
  - **Stage IIIb** (T4 tumor)
    - **1st Neoadjuvant chemo** → then **surgery** (usually MRM)** → then **adjuvant chemo-XRT** (MC scenario)
    - **Trastuzumab** – if HER2 positive
    - **Hormonal therapy** – for ER or PR positive tumor (or unknown status)
      - **Pre-menopausal** – *Tamoxifen*
      - **Post-menopausal** – *Aromatase inhibitor*
    - **MRM <u>not</u> always required after neoadjuvant chemo for T4 tumor** – if tumor shrinks can go with BCT (*except* for inflammatory CA which always requires MRM)
  - **Stage IIIc** (*only* N3c) and **Stage IV** (metastases)
    - Both non-operable disease; Tx - chemo + hormonal therapy
    - **Bony metastases Tx:** <u>calcitonin</u> and bisphosphonates (eg <u>alendronate</u>) to decrease skeletal Cx's (eg fractures)
    - Can consider MRM for **palliation** (eg ulcerative, fungating lesion)
- MC site for distant metastasis - **bone** (axial skeleton)
- **Central** and **subareolar tumors** have increased risk of <u>multicentricity</u>
- **Node levels**
  - **I** - lateral to pectoralis minor muscle
  - **II** - beneath pectoralis minor muscle
  - **III** - medial to pectoralis minor muscle (extends to thoracic inlet, ie **infraclavicular** nodes)
  - Rotter's nodes - between pectoralis major and pectoralis minor muscle
  - Need to take **level I** and **II nodes** en bloc with **ALND** for breast CA (*only take level III nodes if level II nodes are <u>grossly involved</u>*)

- **Lymphedema** and other Cx's are increased with level III dissection
- Node dissection does <u>not</u> improve survival for breast CA
- **Nodes** are the single most important **prognostic factor** in patients devoid of systemic metastases (survival directly related to number of positive nodes)
- Other factors - hormone receptor status, tumor size, tumor grade

■ Hormone receptors (estrogen and progesterone)
  - **Positive receptors** - better response to hormones, chemotherapy, and surgery; better overall prognosis
  - Receptor-positive tumors are more common in **post-menopausal** women
  - **Progesterone** receptor positive tumors have better prognosis than estrogen receptor positive tumors
  - Tumors that are both progesterone receptor and estrogen receptor positive have the *best prognosis*
  - 10% of breast CA is negative for both receptors

■ HER2/neu receptor - <u>worse</u> prognosis than same staged non-HER2 breast CA; is a receptor tyrosine kinase
  - Trastuzumab (Herceptin) blocks this receptor

■ Male breast cancer
  - < 1% of all breast CA; usually **ductal CA** (85%)
  - Poorer prognosis because of <u>late presentation</u> (**advanced stage** at Dx)
    - A DCIS Dx is uncommon in males (has already advanced to CA)
    - Stage for stage has the same prognosis as female breast CA
  - Most have **pectoral muscle** and **nipple-areola** involvement at Dx
  - 20% have pre-existing **gynecomastia**
  - **BRCA** I and II (1% and 10% male breast CA risk, respectively)
    - Also at increased risk for other CA (MC - **prostate CA**)
  - RFs: steroid use, previous XRT, family history, Klinefelter's syndrome (XXY), testicular feminization syndrome, obesity, gynecomastia, liver disease, ETOH abuse, advanced age, Jewish decent, and African Americans
  - Tx: **modified radical mastectomy** (MRM; possible SLNB vs ALND)
    - 80% are **hormone receptor positive** - Tx: **tamoxifen**
    - <u>Not</u> usually HER2 positive (< 5%)
    - Chemotherapy indicated for hormone receptor negative tumors, large primary tumors, positive nodes, or advanced tumors

■ Ductal cancer
  - *MC type of breast CA (85%)*
  - Subtypes:
    - **Ductal CA NST** (No Special Type) - *MC ductal CA (55%)*
    - **Tubular** - forms small **tubules**, *best* prognosis of all subtypes
    - **Medullary** - smooth borders, increased **lymphocytes**, bizarre cells
    - **Mucinous** (colloid) - produces an abundance of **mucin**
    - **Papillary**
    - **Sarcomatoid** - *worst* prognosis of all subtypes
  - Tx: **MRM** or **BCT with post-op XRT**

■ Lobular cancer
  - 10% of all breast CA
  - Usually does not form calcifications; extensively infiltrative
  - Has increased bilateral, multi-focal, and multi-centric disease
  - **Signet ring cells** confer worse prognosis
  - Tx: **MRM** or **BCT** with **post-op XRT**

■ Inflammatory breast CA
  - T4d disease
  - **Very aggressive** → median survival of 36 months (worse than other breast CA)
  - Represents **dermal lymphatic invasion,** which causes <u>peau d'orange</u> **lymphedema** appearance on breast; **erythematous** and warm
  - Sx's: pain, erythema, warmth
  - Dx: full thickness incisional breast Bx including the skin
  - Tx: neoadjuvant **chemo**, then **MRM**, then adjuvant **chemo-XRT** (standard method)
  - *BCT is contraindicated for inflammatory breast CA*
  - **5-YS**: 35%

- **Surgical options**
  - **Breast Conserving Therapy** (BCT = lumpectomy, quadrectomy, ect. _plus_ ALND or SLNB) and **post-op XRT**; need **> 1 mm margin**
  - **Modified Radical Mastectomy** (MRM)
    - Removes all breast tissue including the nipple areolar complex
    - Includes axillary node dissection en bloc (ALND; level I and II nodes)
    - Mastectomy with SLNB (as opposed to ALND) can be used as well in patients with clinically negative nodes who want mastectomy vs BCT
  - Simple mastectomy (subcutaneous or total mastectomy)
    - Leaves 1-2% of breast tissue
    - Preserves the nipple-areolar complex
    - _Not_ indicated for breast CA Tx
    - Used only for DCIS and LCIS
- **Neoadjuvant therapy** (primary chemo) indications:
  - **T3 tumors** (N0-1) - if trying to shrink it for BCT (chemo is given)
  - **T4 tumors** (definitely for inflammatory breast CA; can be used for skin or chest wall involvement) - chemo is given 1ˢᵗ and usually followed by MRM (definitely need MRM for inflammatory breast CA)
  - Breast CA in pregnancy (see Pregnancy section below)
- **BCT** (includes SLNB or ALND) and **post-op XRT**
  - Need **negative margins** (all ink-negative and **> 1 mm**) before XRT
  - No real difference in survival compared to MRM
  - 2% risk of **local recurrence** → Tx: **salvage MRM**
  - **Absolute** _contraindications_ to BCT
    - 1) **2 or more primaries** in separate quadrants
    - 2) **Positive margins** despite re-resection (can re-resect x 1 for negative margins)
    - 3) **Pregnancy** (if 1ˢᵗ or early 2ⁿᵈ trimester)
    - 4) **Previous XRT** that would result in excessive total XRT dose
    - 5) **Multi-focal** or **multi-centric** disease
    - 6) **Diffuse malignant appearing calcifications**
    - 7) **Inflammatory breast CA**
  - **Relative** _contraindications_ to BCT
    - 1) **Unacceptable cosmetic result** from large tumor (eg T3)
      - _If neoadjuvant Tx shrinks T3 down → can go with BCT_
    - 2) **Scleroderma** or **SLE** (lupus)
  - T4 tumors other than inflammatory can potentially undergo BCT (usually receive neoadjuvant chemo)
- **SLNB** (sentinel lymph node biopsy)
  - Fewer Cx's than ALND
  - Not indicated if clinically positive nodes → need ALND
  - Accuracy best if **primary tumor present** (gets correct lymph channels)
  - Well suited for small tumors with low risk of axillary metastases
  - Lymphazurin blue dye and technetium labeled sulfur colloid radiotracer used (injected around tumor area); need 1-4 hours for technetium uptake
  - **Type I hypersensitivity reactions** have been reported with Lymphazurin (isosulfan) blue dye (Tx: diphenhydramine [Benadryl] if just urticaria; epinephrine for anaphylaxis)
  - Usually find **1-3 nodes** (in 95% the sentinel node is found) - get permanent stains
  - Can't find blue nodes or tracer in OR → **formal ALND**
  - Tumor found in lymphatic channels → **formal ALND**
  - If SLNB is **positive** for any tumor → **formal ALND** (_still standard of care_)
  - _Contraindications_ to SLNB:
    - 1) **Neoadjuvant therapy**
    - 2) **T3** - large tumor (> 5 cm) - blocks lymphatics
    - 3) **T4** - advanced disease (eg inflammatory breast CA)
    - 4) **Palpable nodes** (clinically positive)
    - 5) **Previous axillary dissection**
    - 6) **Tumor already taken out** (relative)

- Can perform SLNB even if planning on mastectomy (eg breast CA in multiple quadrants → can inject all the sites for SLNB and still perform mastectomy)
- Take **all of the blue nodes**
- Resect the **highest count node** (radiotracer) and any nodes **10% or greater** than that node
- Node lights up in area you were not expecting (eg supra-clavicular) → **need to resect that node**

- ■ **MRM**
  - Remove drains when < 30-40 cc/day
  - **Recurrence along mastectomy scar** - Tx: <u>resection</u> (re-stage patient 1st)
  - MRM Cx's: infection, flap necrosis, seromas
- ■ **ALND** (axillary lymph node dissection)
  - For **clinically positive nodes, positive SLNB,** or **contraindication** to SLNB
  - Take **level I** and **II** nodes en bloc
    - Take level III nodes (medial to the pectoralis minor muscle) <u>only</u> for grossly positive level II nodes
  - **Superior** border - axillary vein
  - **Medial** border - chest wall (watch for long thoracic nerve)
  - **Lateral** border - skin flap
  - **Anterior** border - pectoralis minor muscle
  - **Posterior** border - latissimus dorsi (watch for thoracodorsal nerve)
  - ALND Cx's:
    - Infection, lymphedema, lymphangiosarcoma
    - **Axillary vein thrombosis** - sudden, early, post-op swelling
    - **Lymphatic fibrosis** - slow swelling over 1-2 years
    - **Intercostobrachial nerve injury** - hyperesthesia of inner arm and lateral chest wall
    - **Long thoracic nerve** or **thoracodorsal nerve injury**
    - **Drains** - leave in until drainage < 40 cc/day
- ■ Radiotherapy (XRT)
  - Usually consists of 5,000 rad for BCT
  - XRT usually *follows* chemo if both are indicated
  - **BCT with post-op XRT**
    - XRT decreases **local recurrence** after BCT
    - Need **negative margins** ($\geq$ 1 mm) before starting XRT
    - 10% chance of local recurrence, usually within 2 years
    - Need **salvage MRM** for local recurrence
  - Indications for **XRT after** <u>mastectomy</u>:
    - 1) **Advanced nodal disease (> 4 nodes, extracapsular** nodal invasion, **N2** or **N3** disease)
    - 2) **T3** or **T4** (> 5 cm; skin, chest wall, or inflammatory)
    - 3) **Positive margins**
  - *Contraindications* to XRT:
    - Pregnancy
    - Previous XRT and would exceed recommended max dose
    - Scleroderma, SLE, active rheumatoid arthritis (all relative)
  - **XRT Cx's**: edema, erythema, rib Fx, pneumonitis, ulceration, sarcoma, contralateral breast CA
- ■ Chemotherapy
  - **TAC** (Taxanes, Adriamycin, and Cyclophosphamide) for 6-12 weeks
  - **Positive nodes** - everyone gets chemo *except* <u>postmenopausal women with positive hormonal receptors</u> → they get hormonal therapy only with **aromatase inhibitor** (Anastrozole)
  - **> 1 cm** and **negative nodes** - everyone gets chemo *except* patients with <u>positive hormonal receptors</u> → they get hormonal therapy only with **Tamoxifen** if they are <u>pre-menopausal</u> or **aromatase inhibitor** (Anastrozole) if they are <u>post-menopausal</u>
  - **< 1 cm** <u>**and**</u> **negative nodes** - <u>*no chemo*</u>; hormonal therapy as above if positive hormonal receptors *(classic answers);* some give chemo if triple receptor negative (ER - , PR - , HER -); some give Herceptin for ER -, PR -, HER+

- **After chemo**, patients positive for **hormonal receptors** should receive appropriate **hormonal therapy**
- Both chemotherapy and hormonal therapy have been shown to decrease recurrence and improve survival
- Chemo is given *before* XRT
- **Taxanes** (docetaxel [Taxotere] or paclitaxel [Taxol]) side-effects - **peripheral neuropathy**
- **Adriamycin** (doxorubicin) side-effects - **cardiomyopathy** (CHF)
  - Max dose - 500 mg/cm^2 body surface area
- **Cyclophosphamide** side-effects - **hemorrhagic cystitis** (Tx: mesna)
- **Selective Estrogen Receptor Modulators** (SERMs) - hormonal therapy
  - **Tamoxifen**
    - For **pre-menopausal** breast CA, DCIS, LCIS, and high risk women
    - Breast CA - 50% decrease in **recurrence** and 35% increase in **survival**
    - DCIS, LCIS, and high risk – decreases **risk of breast CA** by about 50%
    - Need **positive hormonal receptors** for benefit
    - Mechanism - **antagonist** to progesterone and estrogen receptors
    - Side-effects: **thromboembolism** (1%; DVT, PE, stroke), **endometrial adenocarcinoma, cataracts**
    - Raloxifene not approved for breast CA Tx
    - *Contraindications* - previous thromboembolism, warfarin, pregnancy
    - Decreases osteoporosis
    - Can be used in **male** breast CA
    - Duration of therapy: 20 mg/d for **5+ years**
  - **Aromatase inhibitors** (anastrozole, letrozole)
    - For **post-menopausal** breast CA
    - 50% decrease in **recurrence** and 35% increase in **survival**
    - Need **positive hormonal receptors** for benefit
    - Mechanism - blocks peripheral conversion of testosterone to estrogen
    - Side-effects: **fractures**
    - Lower DVT, stroke, and endometrial CA compared to Tamoxifen
    - Duration of therapy: **5 years**
  - **Oophorectomy** also an option instead of oral agents
- **Trastuzumab** (Herceptin)
  - 50% decrease in **recurrence** for HER positive tumors
  - Monoclonal antibody that blocks **HER2/neu receptor** (human epidermal growth factor receptor 2; is a receptor tyrosine kinase)
  - Indicated for breast CA that is:
    - 1) HER2 positive *and*;
    - 2) Is **either > 1 cm** or has **positive nodes**
  - Side-effects: **cardiac toxicity** (heart failure)
  - *Contraindications* - previous cardiac disease
  - Duration of therapy: **1 year**
  - Can take Herceptin concomitantly with SERMs
- Almost all women with recurrence die of disease
- Increased recurrences and metastases occur with **positive nodes, large tumors, negative receptors,** and **unfavorable subtypes**
- Untreated breast CA - median survival 2-3 years
- **Metastatic flare** - pain, swelling, erythema in metastatic areas; spinal compression
  - Tx: XRT provides relief, possible steroids
- **Adenocarcinoma in axillary node** in woman with no identifiable source →
  Check for **ER** and **PR** receptors → if positive → ipsilateral MRM (70% will have ipsilateral breast CA)
- **Occult breast CA** - breast CA that presents as axillary metastases with unknown primary; Tx: **MRM** (70% will have ipsilateral breast CA)
- **Adenocarcinoma** in **axillary node** in woman with no identifiable source
  - Check for **hormonal receptors** → if positive → ipsilateral MRM (70% will have ipsilateral breast CA)
- **Paget's disease of the breast** (is considered a breast CA)
  - Scaly, weepy skin lesion on nipple (can spread to areola); may have an underlying palpable mass

- Bx shows **Paget's cells** (large, round, vacuolated cells)
- Look for an underlying mass or suspicious calcifications on **mammogram** - *majority (> 95%) of patients* have either **underlying DCIS or ductal CA**
- Dx: full thickness incisional breast biopsy including skin – shows **Paget's cells** in skin, may show DCIS or CA cells (core needle biopsy of suspicious areas)
- Tx: need MRM (ductal CA) or simple mastectomy + SLNB (ductal CA or DCIS); need to *include* the **nipple-areolar complex** with simple mastectomy in Paget's
- Some perform central lumpectomy (include nipple areolar complex) + SLNB
- ALND is indicated for clinically positive nodes

- **Phyllodes tumor**
  - 85% benign; 15% cystosarcoma phyllodes (malignant; **> 5-10 mitoses** per HPF)
  - *No nodal metastases*, hematogenous spread if any (rare)
  - Resembles giant fibroadenoma; is a stromal tumor (mesenchymal tissue)
  - Can be very <u>fast</u> growing; can increase in size in just a few weeks
  - Can often be <u>large</u> tumors
  - Considered a low grade sarcoma if malignant
  - Tx: **WLE** with 1 cm margins; *no ALND or SLNB*

- **Stewart-Treves syndrome**
  - **Lymphangiosarcoma** from **chronic lymphedema** following ALND
  - Patients present with dark purple nodules or lesions on arm or axilla 5-10 years after surgery (Dx: biopsy of lesion); very aggressive tumor
  - Tx: sarcoma work-up and resection

- **TRAM pedicle flap**
  - Transverse Rectus Abdominis Myocutaneous (TRAM) flap
  - Based off the **superior epigastric artery**
  - Avoid left sided TRAM if previous CABG with left IMA use
  - Avoid with previous incisions that have transected the upper abdominal wall
  - *Laparoscopic cholecystectomy <u>not</u> a contra-indication*
  - Consider contra-lateral rectus muscle if chest XRT for breast CA (IMA may be compromised by XRT)
  - Some use muscle-sparing TRAM to avoid abdominal wall Cx's
  - S/E's – abdominal wall weakness, bulge

- **DIEP free flap**
  - Deep Inferior Epigastric Perforator (takes fat and skin from lower abdomen 'tummy tuck')
  - Free frap with anastomosis of **inferior epigastric vessels** to the **internal mammary artery** and **vein** in chest
  - Can't use on left side if previous CABG with left IMA use
  - Has replaced TRAM at some institutions (possible fewer abdominal wall Cx's)

- **Pregnancy with mass**
  - < 25% of breast lumps developing during pregnancy are CA
  - Mammography does <u>not</u> work well in pregnancy (less sensitive due to dense breast tissue and exposes the fetus to radiation)
  - Use **U/S** and **CNBx** for work-up to avoid radiation
    - If **cyst**, drain it and send FNA for cytology
    - If **solid**, perform CNBx or FNA
  - If CNBx or FNA is <u>equivocal</u>, need **excisional biopsy**

- **Breast CA in Pregnancy**
  - Occurs in 1 : 3000 pregnancies, average age is 34
  - CA tends to present at more **advanced stage**, leading to a **worse prognosis**
  - Higher incidence of **nodal metastases** compared to non-pregnant patients - **70%** overall are **node positive** (T1 tumor → 50% risk of nodal metastases)
  - Stage for stage, have the same prognosis as non-pregnant patients
  - The main issues dictating the pathway are:
    1) the <u>contraindication to XRT</u> in pregnancy
    2) the risk of <u>teratogenic events</u> with chemo in the 1st trimester (chemo is contraindicated in the 1st trimester)
    3) the high incidence of <u>nodal metastases</u> in pregnant patients (advanced stage at Dx) - the nodes need to be assessed at some point during pregnancy

- **Breast CA Tx** by **trimester**:
    - **1st** and **early 2nd** trimester - **MRM**, chemo if indicated in 2nd trimester
        - *BCS not possible due to the contraindication to XRT in pregnancy*
        - *Chemo is contraindicated in the 1st trimester*
    - **Late 2nd** and **early 3rd** trimester (*any* option below):
        1) MRM, chemo if indicated during pregnancy
        2) BCS with SLNB, chemo if indicated during pregnancy, post-partum XRT
        3) SLNB + neoadjuvant chemo during pregnancy, post-partum local therapy (BCS and XRT)
    - If **late 3rd trimester** - BCS with SLNB only, then post-partum XRT and if indicated chemo is an option
    - No breast-feeding after delivery
    - *SLNB can be used in pregnancy*
- **Chemotherapy risks** in pregnancy
    - 1st trimester - spontaneous abortion (10%), birth defects (10%)
    - 2nd and 3rd trimesters - no evidence of teratogenicity; many consider the best Tx in the late 2nd or 3rd trimesters is neoadjuvant chemo with local breast therapy after delivery (option 3 above)

590. All of the following are true except:
    a. Right angled rigid bronchoscopy is useful for looking into the right upper lobe
    b. The thoracic duct crosses the mediastinum right to left at T4-5
    c. The greatest change in dimension with inspiration is anterior and posterior
    d. Type II pneumocytes produce surfactant
    e. Mediastinoscopy looks into the middle mediastinum

    Answer c. The greatest change in dimension with inspiration is superior and inferior (diaphragm movement).

591. All of the following are true except:
    a. The main function of surfactant is to reduce alveolar surface tension
    b. A decrease in cardiac output is likely to increase the carbon monoxide diffusion capacity (DLCO) of the lung
    c. Pre-op FEV_1 is the single best predictor of being able to wean off the ventilator following pulmonary resection
    d. The MCC of hypoxia following lung resection is alveolar hypoventilation (atelectasis)
    e. Adenocarcinoma is the MC type of lung CA

    Answer b. A decrease in C.O. is likely to decrease DLCO.

592. All of the following are true of thoracic outlet syndrome (TOS) except:
    a. Neurologic Sx's most commonly involve the ulnar nerve
    b. The phrenic nerve is located anterior to the anterior scalene muscle.
    c. The long thoracic nerve is located posterior to the middle scalene
    d. Sx's are most commonly caused by a cervical rib
    e. The subclavian vein is the MC involved structure

    Answer e. The **brachial plexus** is the MC structure involved in thoracic outlet syndrome (usually involving the ulnar distribution, C8-T1). This results in weakness and paraesthesias in the 4th and 5th digits of the hand along with pain and paraesthesias along the medial part of the forearm. Cervical rib resection risks injury to the **phrenic nerve** and **long thoracic nerve** (identify intra-op).

593. A 24 yo baseball pitcher is in the ED with acute pain and swelling in his right arm. U/S shows clot in the subclavian vein. The next appropriate step is:
    a. Catheter directed thrombolytic therapy
    b. Thrombectomy
    c. Resection of the 1st rib
    d. Resection of the subclavian vein and reconstruction with 10 mm graft

    Answer a. Paget von Schrotter's disease is acute thrombosis of the **subclavian vein**. Initial Tx is **thrombolytics** to open up the vein followed by **1st rib resection** during the **same hospital admission** (do not wait for a repeat episode). If a cervical rib is present, it should be removed.

    The subclavian artery can also be involved with thoracic outlet syndrome, which can result in injury with thrombosis (cold white hand) or an aneurysm. Emboli from the aneurysm can cause distal embolization (painful digit, dark blue necrotic area). The aneurysm can also undergo complete thrombosis.

594. Which lung CA is most likely to be associated with a paraneoplastic syndrome?
    a. Small cell lung CA
    b. Adenocarcinoma
    c. Squamous cell CA
    d. Large cell CA

Answer a. Small cell lung CA (MC - **ACTH**, also **ADH**). *Small cell lung CA is the MCC of paraneoplastic syndromes* (overall; eg compared to breast CA, renal cell CA, etc).

Squamous cell lung CA can have **PTH-rp** release.

595. A 50 yo man with a RUL lung mass presents with lethargy, vomiting, and hyponatremia. This is most likely due to:
      a.   ACTH
      b.   PTH-rp
      c.   ADH
      d.   Prolactin

    Answer c. This is most consistent with **SIADH** (syndrome of inappropriate anti-diuretic hormone), most likely related to **small cell lung CA**.

596. A 65 yo cachectic man with an apical lung CA presents with an acutely swollen face, arms, and hands. The best treatment for this patient's likely condition is:
      a.   Chemotherapy
      b.   Emergent XRT
      c.   Resection
      d.   Antibiotics

    Answer b. This patient most likely has **Superior Vena Cava (SVC) syndrome** due to CA in-growth into the SVC. *Tx requires __emergent XRT__ which will rapidly shrink the tumor and open up the SVC.*

    SVC syndrome is MC due to **CA** (MC - **lung CA**; MC type - **small cell**)

597. A 65 yo cachectic man with an apical lung CA presents with ptosis, miosis, and anhydrosis. These Sx's are most likely from:
      a.   A paraneoplastic syndrome
      b.   Invasion of the brachial plexus
      c.   Invasion of the SVC
      d.   Invasion of the sympathetic chain at T1

    Answer d.

    Pancoast Tumors (superior sulcus) may have either:
        1) Invasion of the **sympathetic chain** at T1 (stellate ganglion), which
            results in ptosis, miosis, and anhydrosis (Horner's syndrome)
        2) Invasion of the **brachial plexus** (MC - **ulnar nerve** Sx's)

598. All of the following true except:
      a.   The vast majority (> 95%) of small cell lung CA is unresectable and treated with chemo-XRT
      b.   The MCC of lung abscess is aspiration and antibiotics are the mainstay Tx
      c.   Presence of a malignant pleural effusion is considered unresectable disease for lung CA
      d.   Myasthenia gravis patients with severe refractory symptoms and a <u>normal</u> thymus should undergo thymectomy
      e.   A patient with osteogenic sarcoma resected 2 years ago, now with 2 metastases to the left lung and 2 to the right lung, should receive palliation only.

    Answer e. This patient should undergo resection (metastatectomy – use wedge resections). Sarcomas with isolated lung metastases (<u>not</u> carcinomatosis) should undergo wedge resection as long as you leave enough lung behind for survival. The primary tumor should be under control before attempting metastatectomy. The patient should also <u>not</u> have diffuse metastases.

599. Which of the following is considered an unresectable lung tumor:
   a. Ipsilateral mediastinal node
   b. Chest wall involvement
   c. Diaphragm involvement
   d. Pericardium involvement
   e. Proximal main bronchus involvement (within 2 cm of carina)

   Answer a. N2 disease is considered **unresectable**. All the rest of the answers are T3 and potentially resectable.

600. A 65 yo man with COPD has right lung CA. You get PFTs which show an FEV-1 of 1400 cc. This patient likely:
   a. Could tolerate either a pneumonectomy or lobectomy
   b. Could tolerate a lobectomy but not pneumonectomy
   c. Could tolerate wedge resection but not lobectomy
   d. Could not tolerate any surgery

   Answer b. A pneumonectomy would leave this patient with an **FEV-1** of about 700 (roughly 50% of the initial 1400). The predicted post-op FEV-1 needs to be ≥ 800 to give a reasonable chance of not being ventilator dependent. Lobectomy would leave a post-op FEV-1 of 1050.

   Due to differences in individual patient's height, weight, and lung size, a more accurate guide is to use **percent predicted FEV-1.** That is, the predicted post-operative FEV-1 should be at least 40% of the normal FEV-1 for that patient's size and age.

601. A 55 yo man has a 3 cm mass in the RLL on chest CT. Bx of the mass shows adenocarcinoma. Chest CT shows the mass and normal sized mediastinal nodes. The next appropriate step is:
   a. Bone scan
   b. V/Q scan
   c. PET scan
   d. Angiogram
   e. Head CT

   Answer c. PET scan is indicated for lung CA to rule-out metastasis.

602. PET scan in the above patient lights up in the mediastinum. You perform a mediastinoscopy and a right paratracheal lymph node is positive for CA. The most appropriate next step is:
   a. Perform right lower lobe resection only
   b. Perform RLL resection and mediastinal lymph node dissection
   c. Perform pneumonectomy and mediastinal lymph node dissection
   d. Chemo-XRT

   Answer d. Positive paratracheal nodes identified on mediastinoscopy are considered **N2 disease** and the patient is considered unresectable. Chemo-XRT *only* is indicated (unless enrolled in a specific research protocol).

   N2 disease discovered *intra-op* at time of lobectomy → **finish lobectomy** and perform lymph node dissection.

603. Three months later, the above patient presents with a bloody pleural effusion. Cytology shows malignant cells. The most appropriate next step is:
   a. Repeat chest XRT
   b. Thoracostomy tube only
   c. Observation
   d. VATS drainage and talc pleurodesis

   Answer d. VATS drainage and talc pleurodesis for malignant pleural effusion.

604. A 22 yo patient involved in a severe MVA has bright red blood around his
tracheostomy tube which was placed 2 weeks ago. The next appropriate step is:
   a. Hyperinflating the tracheostomy balloon
   b. Removing the tracheostomy tube and oral intubation
   c. Chest CT
   d. Arteriogram
   e. RBC scan

   Answer a. This is worrisome for a **tracheo-innominate artery fistula**. Hyperinflation of the tracheostomy cuff balloon should be performed as an initial
   maneuver if the site is still oozing (although this may not control the bleeding).
   The next move is to get the patient to the OR for bronchoscopy and look for the
   fistula. One should prep for median sternotomy *before* bronchoscopy.

605. A 22 yo patient involved in a severe MVA requiring tracheostomy has stridor and
dyspnea on exertion. Bronchoscopy reveals a 3 cm long subglottic stenosis with a
diameter of about 3 mm. The most appropriate next step is:
   a. Resection and reanastomosis
   b. Serial dilation
   c. Laser therapy
   d. Steroids
   e. Tracheal stent

   Answer a. The best Tx for significant **tracheal stenosis** is **resection and
   reconstruction**.

606. A 55 yo man presents to the ED with hemoptysis (150 cc while in the ED). His vital
signs are otherwise stable. CXR shows a right sided infiltrate. The next appropriate
step is:
   a. Place right side down
   b. Place left side down
   c. Go to angiography
   d. Bronchoscopy in the ED

   Answer a. This patient has significant **hemoptysis** (the strict definition of
   massive hemoptysis is > 600 cc over 24 hours). Given the **right sided infiltrate**,
   the bleeding is most likely on the **right** so that side should be placed down to
   prevent blood going into the non-bleeding lung. Once in the OR, a **double
   lumen tube** is placed to isolate the bleeding side (again, prevents blood going
   into the non-bleeding lung). **Bronchoscopy** is the first step in identifying and
   potentially treating the source.

607. The bleeding source is not controlled at the time of bronchoscopy in the above patient.
The most appropriate next step is:
   a. Pulmonary arteriography
   b. Bronchial arteriography
   c. Pulmonary venography
   d. Aortography

   Answer b. **Bronchial arteriography**. Significant (or massive) **hemoptysis** MC
   occurs from the **bronchial arteries** *(not pulmonary arteries)* and can be contolled
   with embolization.

608. The primary blood supply to the trachea is:
   a. The superior thyroid and bronchial arteries
   b. The inferior thyroid and pulmonary arteries
   c. The inferior thyroid and bronchial arteries
   d. The superior thyroid and pulmonary arteries

   Answer c. The **inferior thyroid** and **bronchial arteries**

609. The MC malignant and benign chest wall tumors are:
   a. Osteogenic sarcoma and osteoma
   b. Ewings sarcoma and osteochondroma
   c. Chondrosarcoma and osteochondroma
   d. Ewings sarcoma and osteoma

   Answer c. Chondrosarcoma and **osteochondroma**

610. All of the following are true of mediastinal tumors except:
   a. The best method for Dx of an anterior mediastinal tumor that is non-diagnostic on needle Bx is anterior thoracotomy (parasternal mediastinotomy, Chamberlain procedure)
   b. Thymomas are the MC mediastinal tumor overall
   c. Median sternotomy is generally the best operative approach for anterior mediastinal tumors
   d. The MC anterior mediastinal tumor in children is germ cell tumor
   e. The MC anterior mediastinal tumor in adults is thymoma

   Answer b. Neurogenic tumors are the MC mediastinal tumor overall (adults and children)

LUNG ANATOMY AND PHYSIOLOGY
- **Airways** (trachea to level of terminal bronchiole)
- **Conducting airways** - 150 cc of anatomic dead space
- **Blood supply**
  - <u>Upper</u> **2/3 trachea** - inferior thyroid arteries
  - <u>Lower</u> **1/3 trachea** and **lung** - bronchial arteries
  - Segmental blood supply, avoid extensive circumferential mobilization
- First complete tracheal ring - **cricoid cartilage**
- **Mediastinal structures**
  - **Azygos vein** is along right side, dumps into **superior vena cava**
  - **Thoracic duct** runs along right side of mediastinum, **crosses midline at T4-T5**, goes into *left neck*, turns around and dumps into the *left subclavian vein* at the junction with the internal jugular vein
  - **Phrenic nerve** - runs anterior to hilum
  - **Vagus nerve** - runs posterior to hilum
- **Lung**
  - **Right** lung volume   55% (3 lobes: RUL, RML, and RLL)
  - **Left** lung volume   45% (2 lobes: LUL and LLL; lingula)
  - **Right angled rigid bronchoscopy** is useful for looking into the **right upper lobe**
  - **Quiet inspiration** - diaphragm 80%, intercostals 20%
  - **Greatest change in dimension** - superior and inferior (diaphragm)
  - **Accessory muscles** - sternocleidomastoid muscle (SCM), levators, serratus posterior, scalenes
  - **Type I** pneumocytes - gas exchange (diffusion in **alveoli**)
  - **Type II** pneumocytes - surfactant production
  - **Surfactant** - **phosphatidylcholine** main agent; *decreases* **alveolar surface tension** and keeps **alveoli open**
- MC chest wall tumor (overall) - **osteochondroma**
- MC malignant chest wall tumor - **chondrosarcoma**
- **Catamenial** pneumothorax - endometrial implants in lung that cause recurrent PTX related to menstrual cycle

PULMONARY FUNCTION TESTS BEFORE PULMONARY RESECTION
- Need predicted post-op **FEV$_1$ > 0.8 L** (or at least 40% of the normal value for that patient's age / height)
  - **FEV-1** = forced expiratory volume in 1 second
  - If **FEV-1** is close → get **qualitative V/Q scan** (use the **perfusion** measurement)
    - Find the contribution of the portion of lung to be resected to overall perfusion and subtract that fraction from the FEV$_1$ to find the predicted FEV$_1$ after resection

- **FEV_1** - single best predictor of being able to **wean off ventilator** after pulmonary resection
- **FEV_1** - single best predictor for post-op **pulmonary Cx's** (_all_ surgery patients)
■ Need predicted post-op **DLCO > 10** mL/min/mmHg (or at least 40% of the normal value)
  - **DLCO > 10** = is diffusion of carbon monoxide (represents **oxygen exchange** capacity)
  - Causes of **decreased DLCO** - lowered capillary surface area, low Hgb, poor alveolar architecture, increased dead space, low C.O., pulmonary hypertension

■ No resection if pre-op pCO_2 > 50 or pO_2 < 60 at rest
■ No resection if pre-op **VO_2 max < 10-12 mL/min/kg** (maximum oxygen consumption)
■ **Pulmonary Cx's** cause **most deaths** after lung surgery (eg respiratory failure)
■ MCC post-op **hypoxemia** - atelectasis (ie alveolar hypoventilation)
■ MCC post-op **hypercarbia** - poor minute ventilation
■ **MC resection** resulting in:
  - **Persistent air leak** - segmentectomy/wedge
  - **Atelectasis** - lobectomy *(MC Cx following lung surgery)*
  - **Arrhythmias** - pneumonectomy
  - **Broncho-pleural fistula** - pneumonectomy
■ **Operative mortality** - wedge 1%, lobectomy 3%, pneumonectomy 6%

PERSISTENT AIR LEAK
1) Make sure **chest tube on suction** and **check system** → **repeat CXR**
2) **Place 2nd chest tube anteriorly**
3) **Bronchoscopy** if still having a problem with lung re-expansion [look for foreign body or bronchus problem (eg bronchopleural fistula, mucus plug)]
- Consider chest CT
- **Wait it out** if lung re-expanded and just simple air-leak (7 days)
- **Not resolved →**
  - If after **spontaneous PTX** - staple bleb, mechanical pleurodesis
  - If after **pulmonary resection** - mechanical pleurodesis

ATELECTASIS (lung collapse from alveolar hypoventilation)
■ *MC Cx following lung resection*
■ *MCC of hypoxemia following lung resection*
■ **Hypoxemia** results from **pulmonary shunting**
■ Tx: incentive spirometer, cough, pain control, walk patient, epidural
  - If refractory consider bronchoscopy to look for **mucus plugging**
  - If already on the ventilator, may need to ↑ tidal volume (TV)

LUNG CANCER
■ *MCC of CA-related death in U.S. for men / women (30% of all CA deaths)*
  - Risk proportional to **smoking** pack-years *(biggest RF)*
  - Risk ↓s after quitting smoking but not back to baseline
  - *MC type - **adenocarcinoma** (not squamous)*
  - Strongest _prognostic_ indicator - **lymph node** involvement
  - MC site of metastasis - **brain**
  - Overall 5-YS - **10%** (35% with resection for cure)
  - **Small cell lung CA** - vast majority *not* resectable; **early spread**
■ Sx's: cough, hemoptysis, atelectasis, pneumonia, pain, weight loss
  - Can be asymptomatic with finding on routine CXR
■ **Nodal involvement** has strongest influence on **survival** and **resectability**
  - N1 nodes (tumor resectable) - hilar, intra-lobar, lobar
  - N2 nodes (tumor not resectable) - ipsilateral mediastinal, subcarinal, and aorto-pulmonary (AP) window
  - N3 nodes (tumor not resectable) - contralateral mediastinal, supraclavicular
■ **T3 tumors** (all potentially resectable) – involvement of diaphragm, chest wall, pericardium, or mediastinal pleura; tumors within 2 cm of the carina
■ **Malignant pleural effusion** – _unresectable_ disease

- **Non-small cell lung carcinoma** (NSCLC)
  - 80% of all lung CA
  - **Adenocarcinoma** is the MC lung CA (*not* squamous)
  - **Adenocarcinoma** usually more peripheral (forms glands)
  - **Squamous cell CA** usually more central (keratin pearls)
  - **Bronchoalveolar** - looks like pneumonia; grows along alveolar walls
- **Small cell lung carcinoma** (is a neuroendocrine tumor, Kulchitsky cells)
  - 20% of all lung CA
  - Usually unresectable at time of Dx (< 5% candidates for surgery) - usually central with frequent metastases to mediastinum
  - Overall 5-year survival rate - **< 5%** (very poor prognosis)
  - Tx: most just get **chemo-XRT**
- **Paraneoplastic syndromes**
  - **Small cell CA** - ACTH and ADH
  - **Squamous cell CA** - PTH-related peptide (PTH-rp)
  - MC paraneoplastic syndrome - **small cell ACTH**
- **Mesothelioma**
  - *Most malignant lung CA*
  - Aggressive local invasion, nodal invasion, and distant metastases common at the time of Dx
  - Asbestos exposure (increases risk 90x)
  - Poor prognosis

- **Chest** and **abdominal CT scan** - *single best test for clinical T and N status*
- **PET scan** - indicated for patients with lung CA; *best test for clinical M status*
- **Bronchoscopy** - needed for centrally located tumors to check for airway invasion
- **Mediastinoscopy**
  - Needed for: 1) **centrally located** tumors or 2) **suspicious adenopathy** on chest CT (nodes > 0.8 cm or subcarinal nodes > 1.0 cm) or 3) **positive PET scan** (node lights up)
  - Assesses **ipsilateral** (N2) and **contralateral** (N3) **mediastinal nodes**
  - If **mediastinal nodes** are **positive**, the tumor is *unresectable*
  - Looking into **middle mediastinum** with mediastinoscopy
  - Does not assess aorto-pulmonary (AP) window nodes (left lung drainage)
  - Endobronchial ultrasound-guided transbronchial needle aspiration (EBUS-TBNA) is a possible alternative to mediastinoscopy
- **Chamberlain procedure** (anterior thoracotomy or para-sternal mediastinotomy) - assesses enlarged **AP window nodes**; go through **left 2nd rib cartilage** (unresectable tumor if positive)
- **Supra-clavicular** or **scalene** adenopathy → **FNA** (unresectable tumor if positive)
- For **formal lung CA resection** (eg lobectomy, pneumonectomy) patients need to:
  - 1) be **operable** (eg have appropriate FEV-1 and DLCO values) *and:*
  - 2) be **resectable** (eg can't have N2, N3 or M disease)
- Lung CA Tx: **formal lung resection** (lobectomy or pneumonectomy) offers best chance for survival
  - Best indication for **neoadjuvant chemo-XRT** - **T3 superior sulcus tumors** (apical tumors or Pancoast tumor); can downstage these tumors making them resectable
  - **Adjuvant chemo** - standard Tx following resection of NSCLC (all stages); improves overall 5-YS after resection by 5% (30% → 35%)
  - **XRT** - decreases local recurrence; no change in survival
- **NSCLC chemo** (stage II or higher) - carboplatin, Taxol
- **Small cell lung CA chemo** - cisplatin, etoposide
- **Superior vena cava syndrome** (SVC Syndrome)
  - MCC - **lung CA** (usually small cell lung CA; others - lymphoma); obstructs SVC
  - **Acute Sx's**: head and neck fullness and swelling, dyspnea, dizziness; brain swelling
  - Tx: *emergent XRT if CA source* (best Tx; *not* surgery or stent; dramatic effect within hours; raise head, O_2, furosemide, steroids)
  - Chronic SVC syndrome (often due to fibrosis) Tx: stent or bypass

- **Pancoast tumors** (superior sulcus)
  - Tumor invades chest wall apex
  - Usually non-small cell lung CA
  - Can get **Horner's syndrome** (invasion of T1 **sympathetic chain** [stellate ganglion] → ptosis, miosis, anhidrosis) and/or **ulnar** nerve Sx's (**brachial plexus** invasion)
- **Metastases to the lung** - if isolated and not associated with any other systemic disease, may be resected (wedge resection usual) for colon CA, renal cell CA, sarcoma, melanoma, ovarian CA, and endometrial CA; can excise multiple tumors, just need to leave enough lung to survive

PULMONARY NODULE (coin lesion)
- Overall 10% are malignant
- MC lesion - **granuloma** (histoplasmosis)
- MC tumor - **hamartoma** (benign)
- MC malignant tumor - **lung adenocarcinoma**; **#2 metastasis** (MC breast CA)
- **Age < 50 → < 5% malignant; age > 50 → > 50% malignant**
- No growth in 2 years and smooth contour suggests benign disease
- If suspicious, will need either guided Bx or wedge resection

UPPER AIRWAY TUMORS (trachea and main bronchi)
- **Children** - 90% benign
  - MC benign - **hemangioma** (usually resolves on its own)
  - MC malignant - **carcinoid**
- **Adults** - 90% malignant
  - MC benign - **papilloma** (usually resolves on its own)
  - MC malignant - **squamous cell CA** (others - bronchial gland tumors)
- **Bronchial gland** tumors - **carcinoid, adenoid cystic CA,** and **mucoepidermoid**; usually slow growing and uncommonly metastasize
- **Carcinoid** (neuroendocrine; usually central; often endobronchial)
  - Represent **90%** of all bronchial gland tumors in adults
  - 50% have Sx's (cough, hemoptysis)
  - **Typical** carcinoids (90%) - 5% metastasize; homogenous, 5-YS - **95%**
  - **Atypical** carcinoid (10%) - 50% metastasize; necrosis, disorganized, ≥ 1 mitosis/2HPF, heterogeneous, 5-YS - **50%**
  - *Strongest RF for survival* - **atypical vs. typical**
  - Recurrence increased with positive nodes or tumors > 3 cm
- **Adenoid cystic CA** (cylindroma)
  - Mucosa frequently intact, predilection to **peri-neural** invasion
  - CA spread often **well beyond endoluminal component**
  - *Very responsive to XRT*
  - **Slow growing** - can survive decades even with metastases
  - *If you can't get safe complete resection* - give post-op XRT (very sensitive to XRT) and avoid taking vital structures
- **Mucoepidermoid CA** - can be low or high grade
- Bronchial gland tumor Tx: **resection** (1 cm margin) for all if primary is resectable and no distant metastases

HAMARTOMAS
- MC **benign** adult lung tumor (75% of all benign adult lung tumors)
- Have **calcifications** and can appear as a **popcorn lesion** on chest CT
- Contain **fat, cartilage,** and **connective tissue** (eg muscle)
- Dx can be made with **CT scan** *(can be diagnostic without need for Bx)*
- *Do not require resection*
- Repeat chest CT in 3 months to confirm Dx

EFFUSIONS
- **Benign pleural effusion**
  - Tx: VATS **mechanical pleurodesis** if refractory
- **Malignant pleural effusion**
  - Tx: VATS **talc pleurodesis** (*best*; **large particle** size to avoid ARDS)

Contraindications - non-reexpansion of the lung
- *If not able to get lung up* → Tx: tunneled **indwelling pleural catheter** (PleurX catheter)
■ **Malignant pericardial effusion** Tx: pericardial window (drain into pleural or peritoneal space)
■ **Exudative effusion**: Protein > 3, Specific gravity > 1.016, LDH ratio > 0.6 (fluid:serum)

LUNG ABSCESS (intra-parenchymal)
■ **MCC** - aspiration PNA leads to necrotic area
■ RFs: ETOH
■ MC organism - ***staph aureus*** (usually polymicrobial)
■ Dx: CT scan *(best test)*
  - MC location - **superior segment of RLL**
■ Tx: ***antibiotics alone*** *(95% successful);* CT guided drainage if that fails
  - Surgery if above fails or cannot rule out CA (eg failure to resolve after 6 weeks)
■ Chest CT can help differentiate empyema from lung abscess

EMPYEMA (pleural infection)
■ MC related to **pneumonia** and subsequent **parapneumonic effusion** which becomes infected (staph, strep); also occurs after thoracic surgery (pulmonary or esophageal)
■ Sx's: pleuritic chest pain, fever, cough, SOB
■ Pleural fluid - **WBCs > 500** cells/cc, **bacteria** on Gram stain, pH < 7.4, glucose < 60
■ **3 stages**:
  - **Exudative** - swelling of pleura (low protein and cell count)
  - **Fibrinopurulent** - fibrin deposits, purulent fluid; ↑PMNs
  - **Organized** (chronic phase) - occurs after 3-4 weeks; in-growth of fibroblasts and capillaries with **lung trapping** by collagen; get frank pus and thick fibrous peel → *lung can't expand* (likely need **decortication** - removes fibrous peel)
■ Most do not require decortication
■ Tx: **chest tube** (bedside thoracostomy), **antibiotics**, and combined intra-pleural **tPA** and **DNase lytic therapy**
  - tPA + DNase improve drainage, decrease LOS, and decrease need for surgery
  - If lung does not re-expand, need **VATS deloculation** or possible open **decortication** (removes the fibrous peel)
  - **Frail, elderly**, and **refractory** to conservative Tx - consider **Eloesser flap** (open thoracic window - direct opening to external environment to allow drainage)
■ **Broncho-pleural fistula - high frequency ventilation** can assist with closure

CHYLOTHORAX
■ Associated with 2 major issues:
  1) **Respiratory Cx's** *and:*
  2) **Nutritional deficiencies**
■ Fluid - **milky white**; high in **lymphocytes** and **triglycerides** (> 110 mL/µL; TAGs)
  - Sudan red stains the TAGs
■ **Thoracic duct** crosses the mediastinum from right to left at T5-6, then goes up into the left neck and eventually dumps into the subclavian vein at the subclavian-internal jugular junction
  - Injury ***above*** T5-6 results in **left**-sided chylothorax
  - Injury ***below*** T5-6 results in **right**-sided chylothorax
■ Fluid is generally **resistant to infection** (lots of WBCs in fluid)
■ MCC - **iatrogenic** following thoracic surgery (MC - esophageal surgery)
  - MC non-iatrogenic cause - **CA** (tumor in lymphatics; MC - **lymphoma**)
  - Other causes - trauma, central venous thrombosis (from central line)
■ **Conservative Tx** (try for **1-2 weeks**):
  - **Chest tube** drainage with lung re-expansion
  - **TPN** *without* lipids (or use medium-chain fatty acids) or low fat diet
  - **Octreotide**
  - Steroids (children)
  - *If **refractory** or **> 1.5 L/day** in adults (> 100 cc/kg/day in child) after **5 days** → need surgical therapy*

- **Surgical Tx**
  - **Traumatic** or **iatrogenic** chylothorax - Tx: **ligation of thoracic duct** on **right side** low in mediastinum (80% successful)
    - If duct not found, perform mass ligation of all tissue between aorta and azygos vein just above diaphragmatic hiatus
  - **Malignant** chylothorax - Tx: **chemo** and/or **XRT**; **talc pleurodesis**

MASSIVE HEMOPTYSIS
- Technical definition is **> 600 cc / 24 hours** (a patient who suddenly coughs up 50 cc of blood in the ED has an *emergent problem*)
- Bleeding MC from high-pressure **bronchial arteries** (<u>not</u> usually pulmonary arteries [< 10%])
- MCC - **infection** (TB); others - bronchiectasis, CA
- Death is due to **asphyxiation** (<u>not</u> blood loss)
- *First step is to secure the airway*
- Tx:
  - Place bleeding side down (if known)
  - Double lumen ET tube (prevents blood going into contra-lateral lung)
  - Bronchoscopy (rigid if possible) to identify site and possibly control bleeding (Epi injection, cautery, ice saline, bronchial blockers)
  - May need lobectomy or pneumonectomy to control
  - If not suitable for surgery - **bronchial artery embolization** (majority [90%] of bleeds are from the bronchial arteries, not pulmonary arteries)

HEMOTHORAX
- **Residual hemothorax** despite 2 good chest tubes - Tx: VATS drainage
- **Clotted hemothorax** - surgical drainage if > 25% of lung, if there are air-fluid levels, or if Sx's of infection (fever, high WBCs); surgery in 1st week to avoid peel; retained hemothorax is the #1 RF for empyema after trauma

SPONTANEOUS PNEUMOTHORAX
- Tall, healthy, thin, young males; **smoking** history; MC on the right
- Recurrence risk after 1st pneumothorax 20%, after 2nd pneumothorax 60%, after 3rd pneumothorax 80%
- Results from rupture of a **bleb** usually in the **apex** of an upper lobe
- Tx: **chest tube**
- Surgery indicated for (<u>any</u> of the following):
  - Recurrence
  - Air leak > 7 days despite 2 good chest tubes
  - Non-reexpansion despite 2 good chest tubes
  - Tension PTX
  - Hemothorax
  - Bilateral PTX
  - Previous pneumonectomy
  - Large blebs
  - High-risk profession (airline pilot, diver, mountain climber)
  - Patients who live in remote areas
- Surgery - VATS **blebectomy** and **mechanical pleurodesis**

PULMONARY AVM
- Connection between pulmonary arteries and pulmonary veins
- MC site - **lower lobes**
- Sx's: **hemoptysis** and **dyspnea**
- Can occur with **Osler-Weber-Rendu Syndrome**
- Tx: **embolization** (<u>not</u> surgery)

TRACHEOSTOMY
- Want tracheostomy between the **2nd** and **3rd tracheal rings**
  - Too high - vocal cord problems
  - Too low - tracheo-innominate artery fistula

- **Tracheo-innominate artery fistula**
  - MC after **tracheostomy**
  - Sx's: usually **premonitory bleed** (oozing), followed by **no bleeding period**, then **massive hemorrhage** (very lethal problem)
  - Tx (want to **1st control airway** and **2nd stop bleeding**) → **hyperinflate tracheostomy balloon** *(best)* to try and temporize bleeding
  - Go to OR *immediately* if suspected *(bronchoscopy in OR to look for fistula, prep for median sternotomy first)*
  - After control of airway and bleeding →
    - Median sternotomy
    - **Surgical ligation** and **innominate artery _resection_** *(not reconstruction)*
      - **_No graft_** - will become infected; just tie off ends of innominate artery
      - Tracheal repair with strap muscle interposition between ligated innominate artery ends and trachea
      - Very *low* stroke rate with this method (lots of collaterals in neck)
  - This is avoided by keeping tracheostomy at **3rd tracheal ring or above**
  - Mortality - 50%

- **Tracheo-esophageal fistula** (generally in cervical portion of the trachea)
  - MC after **tracheostomy**
  - Sx's: **tracheal secretions** that look like **saliva** or **gastric distension** if intubated; coughing with swallowing if extubated
  - Dx: **Bronchoscopy** *(best test)* - pull tracheostomy tube or ETT back
    - Usually see a big posterior hole 1-2 cm below tracheal stoma (balloon site)
  - Tx: remove tracheostomy and place ET tube with balloon below fistula
    - Place decompressive PEG tube
    - Wait until extubated before repair
    - **Tracheal resection** and **re-anastomosis**
    - **Primary repair of esophagus** *(not esophageal resection)*
    - Interpose strap muscle between esophagus and trachea

TRACHEAL STENOSIS
- MC due to previous prolonged ventilation or previous tracheostomy
- Sx's: stridor, dyspnea on exertion
- Dx: upper endoscopy *(best test)*
- Small, minor irregularities may be treated conservatively (eg dilation, laser, endoscopic removal of scar tissue)
- Tx: **significant stenosis** is best treated with tracheal **resection** and **reanastomosis** (can take up to **50%** of the trachea)

THORACIC OUTLET SYNDROME (TOS)
- **Scalene triangle** - anterior scalene, middle scalene, and 1st rib
  - Subclavian vein is anterior to the anterior scalene
  - Subclavian artery and brachial plexus are between anterior and middle scalenes
- MC anatomic abnormality for TOS - **cervical rib**; others - fibrous bands, muscle hypertrophy

- **Neurogenic** *(MC type of TOS, 90%)*
  - **Pain** and **paresthesias** (present in 95%) in **medial forearm** (supinated position) and **4th - 5th fingers**
  - Usually **normal** neuro exam; Sx's worse with **manipulation**
  - **Tinsel's test** - tapping reproduces symptoms (neurogenic TOS)
  - MC nerve distribution - **ulnar** nerve (C8-T1)
  - Dx: **CXR** - look for **cervical rib**
    - **Nerve conduction velocity** < 60 m/S
  - Tx: **physiotherapy** for 3 months *(all patients)* - *don't rush to operate*
    - If above fails and **nerve conduction velocity < 60 m/S** → **1st rib resection**, cervical rib resection if present, anterior and middle scalenes divided

- **Subclavian vein thrombosis** (Paget-von Schrötter disease)
  - Usually presents as **effort-induced thrombosis** of subclavian vein (baseball pitchers, excessive use of arm)
  - Sx's: very **painful, swollen, blue limb**
  - Dx: **duplex U/S** *(best initial test)* makes Dx and quicker to get
    Venography is the gold standard but takes longer
  - 80% have associated thoracic outlet problem
  - **Venous thrombosis** much more common than arterial thrombosis
  - Tx: catheter-directed **thrombolytics** (tPA) initially; **repair at same hospital admission** (cervical rib and 1st rib resection, divide anterior scalene muscle)
- **Arterial** (Subclavian Artery, *rarest* form of TOS)
  - Arterial **damage** can occur with subsequent **thrombosis**
  - Can get **aneurysms** which can send off **distal emboli** (acute digital ischemia) *or* undergo **thrombosis**
  - **Compression** can occur from **anterior scalene hypertrophy** (eg baseball pitchers, swimmers)
  - Sx's: **pain** and **paresthesias** (due to compression of subclavian artery)
    Acute occlusion - <u>no</u> pulse, arm **cold** and **white**
    Acute digital ischemia (painful blue lesion on finger)
  - **Adson's,** hyper-abduction, costoclavicular tests - all result in loss of radial pulse (hand cold and pale)
  - Dx: **angiogram** (gold standard), **duplex U/S** if acute occlusion (faster)
  - Tx: 1st rib and cervical rib resection; usually place **interposition bypass graft** (artery usually too damaged for repair or an aneurysm is present)
  - **Acute thrombosis** - <u>open</u> balloon thrombectomy via brachial artery if threatened limb; catheter directed **intra-arterial thrombolytics** if non-threatened limb; 1st rib resection (as above) on same admission

MEDIASTINUM
- **Normal Structures**
  - **Anterior** - thymus
  - **Middle** - heart, great vessels, phrenic, vagus, trachea, main bronchi
  - **Posterior** - esophagus, descending aorta, vertebral bodies, thoracic duct, azygos vein, hemi-azygos
- **Mediastinal mass Sx's** (any location can cause Sx's)
  - Often **asymptomatic**
  - **Respiratory insufficiency** (MC Sx), chest pain, and dysphagia
- **Tumors** (majority benign)
  - MC mediastinal tumor in <u>adults</u> and <u>children</u> - **neurogenic** (MC posterior)
  - MC **location** for mediastinal tumor in <u>adults</u> and <u>children</u> - **anterior**

  Adult solitary mediastinal mass
MC mediastinal overall	neurogenic
MC anterior	*thymoma**
MC middle	cyst
MC posterior	neurogenic

  Children solitary mediastinal mass
MC mediastinal overall	neurogenic
MC anterior	*germ cell**
MC middle	cyst
MC posterior	neurogenic

  - **Anterior** (T's) - Thyroid, parathyroid, ***Thymoma** (MC adults)*, Teratoma (+ other *Germ cell*; MC children), cystic hygroma; T-cell (and other lymphomas)
  - **Middle** - *cysts* (MC; bronchogenic and pericardial), lymphoma, teratoma
  - **Posterior** - *neurogenic (MC)*, lymphoma, enteric duplication cysts
  - **Open procedure for Dx of anterior mediastinal mass** - Chamberlain (anterior thoracotomy or parasternal mediastinotomy, go through 2nd rib cartilage)
  - **Incision for removal of anterior mediastinal mass** - median sternotomy (usually)

- **Thymoma**
  - All thymomas need resection
  - Thymus too big or associated with myasthenia gravis → resection
  - 50% are **malignant** (determined by local invasion, not histology)
  - 50% are **symptomatic**
  - 50% of patients with thymomas have **myasthenia gravis**.
  - 10% of patients with myasthenia gravis have **thymomas**
  - *Children almost never get thymomas*
  - Tx: **resection** (median sternotomy)
  - *All patients* with a thymoma should undergo resection
  - Myasthenia Gravis patients with **severe refractory Sx's** and a *normal* size thymus should undergo **thymectomy** (80% get improvement)
- **Lymphoma** (MCC of mediastinal **adenopathy**) - **NHL** (MC) and **Hodgkin's**
  - May be considered the MC primary mediastinal tumor but generally does not present as solitary mass (ie presents with adenopathy)
- **Germ cell tumors**
  - **Teratoma** - MC mediastinal germ cell tumor (hair, cartilage, fat)
    - **Benign** - marker negative
    - **Malignant** - elevated AFP, beta-HCG
    - Tx: resection; chemotherapy if malignant
  - Others - Seminoma, Non-seminoma (see Urology chapter for Tx)
- **Cysts**
  - **Bronchogenic** and **Enteric Cysts** - posterior to carina, not connected to airway; can get infected and small CA risk; Tx - resection
  - **Pericardial Cyst** - MC right costophrenic angle; Tx: *leave (no CA risk)*
- **Neurogenic tumors**
  - MC in **paravertebral sulcus** (sympathetic chain or intercostal nerve); 10% have intra-spinal involvement (**MRI** if suspected)
  - Tx: **resection** (may need spinal surgery for removal if intra-spinal)
  - **Neurolemma** (MC; schwannoma, benign nerve sheath tumor)
  - **Neurofibroma** (nerve sheath) - associated with von Recklinghausen's (café-au-lait macules, freckles, optic gliomas); 5% malignant
  - Others - ganglioneuroma (benign), ganglioneuroblastoma (malignant), neuroblastoma (very malignant, children)

Cardiac

611. Three days after a large anterior myocardial infarction, a patient develops a new holo-systolic murmur and cardiogenic shock. He is intubated due to respiratory distress and is started on multiple inotropes and pressors. CVP is 20 and PA pressures are 60/30. Despite support, his pressure continues to be 80/50 with a HR of 130. The most important next step in this patients Tx is:
    a. Obtain an ECHO
    b. Fluid resuscitation
    c. Place an IABP
    d. tPA

    Answer c. A patient in persistent cardiogenic shock despite maximal support should have an IABP placed. The patient does not need fluid resuscitation as his CVP is 20.

    An **echocardiogram** (ECHO) would make the Dx (likely a **ventricular septal rupture** or possible blown papillary muscle with acute mitral regurgitation) but the patient should be stabilized first. Use of IABPs have improved survival for cardiogenic shock following MI.

612. The MCC of death following heart transplant is:
    a. Reperfusion injury
    b. Chronic allograft vasculopathy
    c. Infection
    d. Acute rejection

    Answer b. Chronic allograft vasculopathy (accelerated arteriosclerosis) is the MCC of death following **heart TXP**.

613. All of the following are true of congenital heart disease except:
    a. Tetralogy of Fallot results in decreased pulmonary perfusion and is the MC cyanotic congenital heart disease (right to left shunt)
    b. Ventricular septal defect (VSD) is the MC congenital heart defect
    c. Tet spells are often self treated by squatting
    d. Trans-esophageal ECHO is better than a swan ganz catheter at assessing pulmonary vascular resistance (PVR)
    e. Coarctation of the aorta is associated with upper extremity hypertension and lower extremity hypotension

    Answer d. ECHO cannot assess **PVR** (cannot figure out pulmonary artery and wedge pressure which is required for calculation).

    PVR = [(PA pressure – wedge) /cardiac output] x 80

614. The posterior descending artery of the heart MC arises from:
    a. The right coronary artery
    b. The left anterior descending artery
    c. The circumflex artery
    d. An obtuse marginal artery

    Answer a. The **right coronary artery** (termed right dominant system if the posterior descending artery arises from here). Around 15% of patients have a left dominant system (posterior descending artery comes off circumflex artery).

615. Stroke following CABG is most commonly due to:
    a. Air in the heart
    b. Aortic manipulation
    c. Carotid stenosis
    d. Low flow state
    e. Cerebral aneurysm

Answer b. Stroke following CABG is usually **embolic** and usually due to **aortic manipulation** (eg aortic cross-clamping).

616. The most important determinant of oxygen consumption is:
     a.   Heart rate
     b.   Wall tension
     c.   Stroke volume
     d.   Preload

     Answer b. Although both HR and wall tension are the factors involved in myocardial oxygen consumption, **wall tension** is the primary determinant.

617. Which of the following risk factors is highest for mortality after CABG surgery?
     a.   Older age
     b.   History of congestive heart failure
     c.   Prior myocardial infarction
     d.   Pre-operative cardiogenic shock

     Answer d. The highest RF for mortality after CABG is pre-op **cardiogenic shock**.

618. The patency rate of an internal mammary artery to the left anterior descending artery and saphenous vein graft to any other coronary artery are:
     a.   IMA – 90% 20 year patency, SVG – 80% 5 year patency
     b.   SVG – 90% 20 year patency, IMA – 80% 5 year patency
     c.   IMA – 50% 20 year patency, SVG – 40% 5 year patency
     d.   SVG – 50% 20 year patency, IMA – 40% 5 year patency

     Answer a. A **left internal mammary artery graft to the left anterior descending artery** has a patency of about 90% at 20 years. This has the best patency of any coronary graft. Saphenous vein grafts have patency rates of 80% at 5 years.

619. A 62 yo woman presents with tearing like chest pain radiating to her back. Her blood pressure is 190/100 in her right arm and 90/50 in her left arm. Her HR is 95. EKG shows some non-specific T wave changes and CXR looks normal. CK-MB and troponins are not back yet. All of the following are appropriate at this stage in the patient's management except:
     a.   tPA
     b.   Chest CT
     c.   BP control
     d.   Radial a-line

     Answer a. You need to check for an aortic dissection is this patient before assuming it is an MI. The tearing like chest pain radiating to her back is highly suggestive of aortic dissection. **Control of HTN** is the best initial Tx for aortic dissections (IV **beta-blocker** best, eg esmolol)

620. You obtain an emergent chest CT which shows a dissection involving only her ascending aorta. You place a radial a-line and start an esmolol drip The most appropriate next step in this patients care is:
     a.   Dissection repair
     b.   Observation
     c.   Heparin drip
     d.   Place a covered stent endograft

     Answer a. Ascending aortic dissections (Type A) <u>all</u> need repair through a **median sternotomy.**

Descending aortic dissections (Type B) require repair only 10% of the time. When intervention is required, it usually involves placement of an endograft (or endovascular intervention) and not open surgery (if open repair needed - **left posterolateral thoracotomy**).

621. Following a difficult redo mitral valve replacement and CABG, your patient's chest tube drainage has decreased from 200 cc/hr to 20 cc/ hr. BP has suddenly dropped to 75/50 despite multiple pressors. There has been no urine output over the last hour. CVP is 25, PA wedge is 25, and C.I. is 1.2. What is the most likely diagnosis:
   a.   Valve dehiscence
   b.   Aortic insufficiency
   c.   Clotted bypass graft
   d.   Cardiac tamponade

   Answer d. Cardiac tamponade. High chest tube output followed by low chest tube output, hypotension, high filling pressures, and low urine output is highly suggestive of cardiac tamponade. The high filling pressures are due to compression of the heart by hematoma.

622. Treatment for the above patient consists of:
   a.   Re-exploration
   b.   Adding dobutamine
   c.   Lasix
   d.   Temporary ventricular assist device

   Answer a. Re-exploration

623. All of the following are true except:
   a.   Significant left main disease is an indication for PTCA and stent
   b.   3 vessel disease is generally an indication for CABG
   c.   Acute ST elevation MI is an indication for PTCA with stent
   d.   Door to balloon time should be under 90 minutes for ST elevation MI
   e.   Females are at increased risk for mortality after CABG compared to males

   Answer a. Significant left main disease should be treated with CABG.

624. The MC cardiac tumor is:
   a.   Myxoma
   b.   Angiosarcoma
   c.   Rhabdomyosarcoma
   d.   Lipoma

   Answer a. Myxoma. These most frequently arise from the **left atrium**.

625. Which of the following predicts the worst survival in a patient with aortic stenosis not undergoing valve replacement:
   a.   Dyspnea on exertion
   b.   Syncope
   c.   Angina
   d.   Loud murmur

   Answer b. Of the items listed, **syncope** has the worst natural history for aortic stenosis is terms of survival (mean survival 2 years).

CONGENITAL HEART DISEASE
- **Fetal circulation** in utero
  - **Ductus arteriosus** - connection between descending aorta and left pulmonary artery (PA); blood shunted away from lungs
  - **Ductus venosum** - connection between portal vein and IVC; blood shunted away from liver
  - **Foramen Ovale** - shunts blood from right atrium to left atrium (away from lungs)

- Fetal circulation *to placenta* - 2 umbilical arteries
- Fetal circulation *from placenta* - 1 umbilical vein
- <u>High</u> **oxygen content** causes ductus arteriosus to close after birth
- <u>Lowered</u> **pulmonary vascular resistance** causes foramen ovale to close after birth
- **Ventricular septal defect** (VSD)
  - *MC congenital heart defect*
  - *80% close spontaneously* by age 1 yr
  - **L→R shunt** (high output CHF if large)
  - Timing of repair:
    - <u>Large</u> VSDs (shunt > 2.5) - at **1 year**
    - <u>Medium</u> VSDs (shunt 2-2.5) - at **5 years**
    - <u>Small</u> VSDs (shunt < 2) are usually *left alone*
  - FTT (failure to thrive) - MC reason for early repair
- **Atrial septal defect** (ASD) - repair at 1-2 years of age
- **Tetralogy of Fallot**
  - *MC cyanotic congenital heart defect*
  - **R→L shunt** (bypasses lungs; get hypoxia and cyanosis)
  - *4 anomalies* - VSD, pulmonary stenosis, overriding aorta, right ventricular (RV) hypertrophy
  - *Causes decreased pulmonary perfusion and shunting across VSD*
  - Sx's: **Tet spells** (<u>cyanosis</u> - child then squats to ↑ SVR and ↑ blood flow to lung - essentially ↓s blood flow through VSD)
  - Timing of repair: **3 - 6 months** (earlier if severe cyanosis)
- **Persistent ductus arteriosus** (PDA)
  - **L→R shunt** (high output CHF if large)
  - Tx: **Indomethacin** - closes PDA, rarely successful after neonatal period
  - Requires **surgical ligation** through left thoracotomy if it persists
- **Coarctation** - narrowing of the aorta, usually just distal to the left subclavian artery
  - Marked by *high* blood pressure in the **upper** extremities and *low* blood pressure in the **lower** extremities
  - Tx: resection of the coarctation area (some are using balloon dilatation)

CORONARY ARTERY DISEASE
- *MCC of death in US*
- RFs: smoking, HTN, males, family history, hyperlipidemia, diabetes
- Medical Tx: nitrates, smoking cessation, weight loss, statin drugs, ASA
- Anatomy: 1) **Left main coronary artery** [branches into left anterior descending (LAD) and circumflex arteries]; and 2) **right coronary artery**
- Most atherosclerotic lesions are **proximal**
- Revascularization
  - **PTCA and stent** - 90% patency at **1 year**
  - **Saphenous vein graft** - 80% **5-year** patency
  - **Left internal mammary artery** (LIMA) – off subclavian artery
  - **LIMA to the left anterior descending artery is the <u>best</u> conduit for CABG** – 90% **20-year** patency
  - **Acute ST elevation MI (STEMI) is an indication for PTCA with stent**
- CABG procedure
  - **Cold potassium** solution (cardioplegia) **arrests heart in diastole**
    - Keeps heart **protected** and **still** while grafts are placed
  - **General indications** (stenosis needs to be ≥ 70%)
    - 1) **Left main** disease
    - 2) **3-vessel** disease
    - 3) **2-vessel** disease with **proximal LAD stenosis**
- **High mortality RFs**: <u>pre-op cardiogenic shock</u> (#1), emergency surgery, age, reoperation, and low ejection fraction (EF)
- *Combined* coronary artery disease requiring CABG and carotid stenosis > 80% → treat **carotid disease 1ˢᵗ** (stent or CEA), then CABG at a *separate procedure* days later (risk of stroke / death lower with staged procedure compared to combined procedure)
- **Stroke** after CABG - MC from **embolism off aorta** and usually due to **aortic manipulation** (eg aortic cross-clamping)

CARDIAC TAMPONADE POST-OP FROM CARDIAC SURGERY

- Sx's: high chest tube drainage that suddenly stops, followed by increasing filling pressures (PA, CVP), low BP, and low UOP *(classic)*
- Dx: often clinical Dx
  - **CXR** - widened mediastinum
  - **ECHO** - tamponade
- Tx: If patient has **pulse** → emergent re-exploration in OR
  - **No pulse** → open patients chest at bedside
- **1st ECHO sign** of cardiac tamponade - right atrial diastolic compression
- <u>Mechanism</u> of tamponade - **decreased ventricular filling** due pericardial fluid (blood)

MECHANICAL COMPLICATIONS OF MYOCARDIAL INFARCTION

- MC occur **3-7 days** after myocardial infarction
- Sx's: **hypotension**; if VSR or acute MR will have a new systolic murmur
- DDx:
  1. **Ventricular septal rupture** (VSR, holo-systolic murmur heard best at right sternal border; **post-infarct heart defect**)
  2. **Papillary muscle rupture** [causes acute mitral regurgitation (MR), holo-systolic murmur heard best in axilla]
  3. **Free wall rupture** (usually quickly fatal)
- Dx: **ECHO** - best test to figure out which of the above
  - **PA catheter – step-up in oxygen content** between right atrium and pulmonary artery secondary to L→R shunt will occur with **VSR** (not with papillary muscle rupture and acute MR)
- Tx: **Intra-aortic balloon pumps** (IABP) have improved survival for VSR and acute MR (papillary muscle rupture)
  - **VSR Tx** - patch
  - **Papillary muscle rupture Tx** - replace valve
  - **Free wall rupture Tx** - patch

AORTIC STENOSIS

- ***MC valve lesion***
- **MCC** - calcification of aortic valve (RFs: age, bicuspid aortic valve)
- ****Cardinal Sx's*** (overall mean survival after onset of Sx's is **2 years**):
  - ***Dyspnea on exertion**   4 year mean survival
  - ***Angina**   3 year mean survival
  - ***Syncope**   2 year mean survival
  - Dyspnea at rest (ie heart failure)   1 year mean survival
- **Valve area < 1.0 cm^2** - considered severe
- **Indications for surgery** (only for **severe AS**; valve is replaced):
  1) **<u>Any</u> symptoms** *or*
  2) **Asymptomatic** with **valve area < 0.6 cm^2** (critical AS)

AORTIC DISSECTION

- MC <u>location</u> for intimal tear - **ascending aorta**
- Dissection occurs in **media layer** of blood vessel wall
- **Cx's of ascending aortic dissection**: aortic valve insufficiency, coronary artery or aortic branch occlusion, tamponade, aortic rupture
- Sx's: <u>tearing chest pain</u> radiating to back (knife-like); 95% have severe HTN
- RFs: **HTN**, connective tissue disease (eg Marfan's), family history, aneurysms, atherosclerosis
- Dx: chest **CT angio** *(best test)* - see dissection flap and false lumen
- **Initial medical Tx** (**control HTN** to help stabilize dissection) - **IV beta-blocker** (*best Tx*, eg esmolol)
- Tx:
  - *<u>Any</u> ascending* aortic dissection – **all need repair** (median sternotomy); graft attempts to obliterate the false lumen
  - **Descending** aortic dissection <u>*only*</u> – **intervention <u>only</u> if complications** (eg limb or organ ischemia, rupture, uncontrollable HTN or pain, extensive hemothorax); **left posterior-lateral thoracotomy** if open repair required (most now treated with **endografts** - TEVAR)

CARDIAC TUMORS
- MC <u>tumor</u> (and MC benign tumor) - **myxoma**; 80% in **left atrium**
  - Can present with distal emboli (eg stroke, leg ischemia)
- MC <u>primary malignant</u> tumor - **angiosarcoma**
- MC <u>metastatic tumor</u> to heart - **lung CA**
- MC primary pediatric cardiac tumor - **rhabdomyoma** (benign striated muscle)

MALIGNANT PERICARDIAL EFFUSION
- Can cause cardiac tamponade
- MCC - lung CA
- Tx: **pericardial window** (pericardiocentesis if unstable)

OTHER
- **Chronic allograft vasculopathy** (accelerated arteriosclerosis) is the MCC of death following **heart TXP**
- ECHO cannot assess **PVR** (cannot figure out pulmonary artery and wedge pressure which is required for calculation).
    PVR = [(PA pressure – wedge) / cardiac output] x 80

Vascular

626. All of the following are true of atherosclerosis except:
   a. The earliest identifiable lesion is fatty steak
   b. Endothelial injury is the central mechanism in the development of atherosclerosis
   c. Foam cells are macrophages filled with cholesterol deposits
   d. Smooth muscle cell regression occurs in response to atherosclerosis

   Answer d. Smooth muscle cell hypertrophy occurs in response to atherosclerosis.

627. A 50 yo man suffers a small right sided ischemic stroke on head CT scan. Carotid duplex U/S reveals a 60% ipsilateral stenosis. The most appropriate next step is
   a. Plavix only
   b. Plavix and repeat duplex U/S in 2 weeks
   c. CEA within 2 weeks
   d. CEA between 4-6 weeks

   Answer c. Assuming a patient has appropriate duplex U/S criteria for CEA (**symptomatic** > 50% stenosis, **asymptomatic** > 70% stenosis) →

   Patient with **TIAs** or **small**, non-disabling <u>ischemic</u> strokes on head CT should have CEA **within 2 weeks** (very low risk of complications)

   Patients with recent **moderate** to **large** <u>ischemic</u> strokes on head CT should **wait 4-6 weeks** (avoids *reperfusion injury* and risk of intracranial *bleeding*).

   Patients with **hemorrhagic** strokes on head CT should **wait 6-8 weeks** (avoids *intra-cranial bleeding*).

628. The above patient undergoes right CEA. In the PACU he develops left hemiplegia. Along with *immediate* heparinization, the most appropriate next step is:
   a. Re-exploration
   b. MRI
   c. CT scan
   d. Carotid duplex
   e. Angiogram

   Answer a. Emergent re-exploration to look for **thrombus** or **intimal flap** (check for pulse in ICA, if absent, re-open artery and remove thrombus). If pulse is present, use on-table U/S and intra-op angiography to figure out problem (MC - intimal flap).

   Strokes occurring **12-24 hours** after surgery should be evaluated with CT angio.

629. All of the following are indications for carotid artery stent with a cerebral protection device (as opposed to CEA) except:
   a. Previous ipsilateral CEA
   b. Previous contralateral CEA
   c. Previous ipsilateral neck XRT
   d. Previous ipsilateral neck dissection
   e. Previous damage to the contralateral recurrent laryngeal nerve

   Answer b. Previous contralateral CEA is <u>not</u> an indication for carotid stenting.

630. All of the following are true of patch closure following CEA except:
   a. Lowers peri-op stroke risk
   b. Lowers peri-op thrombosis risk
   c. Lowers long term re-stenosis risk
   d. Increases the risk of artery narrowing

Answer d. Placing a patch _decreases_ the risk of artery narrowing

631. All of the following are true except::
    a. A normal carotid artery has continuous forward flow
    b. The MC site of carotid stenosis is the carotid bulb (near the bifurcation of the internal and external carotid arteries)
    c. Cerebral hyperperfusion syndrome most commonly occurs in patients with low grade carotid stenosis
    d. Percutaneous transluminal angioplasty (PTA) is generally the best Tx for symptomatic carotid stenosis from medial fibromuscular dysplasia
    e. Patients with 100% carotid occlusions should not undergo CEA

    Answer c. Cerebral hyperperfusion syndrome most commonly occurs in patients with **high grade carotid stenosis** with peak onset on **POD 6**.

632. All of the following are true except:
    a. The vagus is the MC injured nerve with CEA and results in hoarseness
    b. The MCC of death after CEA is myocardial infarction
    c. The facial vein can be routinely ligated
    d. CEA involves removing the intima only
    e. The lower root branches of the ansa cervicalis (descendens hypoglossi) can be divided without serious consequences

    Answer d. CEA involves removing the **intima** _and_ part of the **medial** layers.

633. A 50 yo man has a painless pulsating neck mass just anterior to the left mid sternocleidomastoid (SCM) muscle. The most likely diagnosis is:
    a. SCCA
    b. Adenocarcinoma
    c. Carotid body tumor
    d. Thyroid CA
    e. Lymphoma

    Answer c. This is classic for a **carotid body tumor**.

634. The best test to confirm the above diagnosis is:
    a. WBC scan
    b. FNA
    c. CT angio
    d. RBC scan
    e. Formal angiogram

    Answer c. CT angio (shows hypervascular tumor attached to the carotid).

635. A 55 yo woman is suffering from vertigo, syncope, and frequent falls. You get a duplex U/S which shows minimal carotid stenosis bilaterally (0-49%) and reversal of flow in the left vertebral artery and antegrade flow in the right vertebral artery. Which of the following is most appropriate in this patient:
    a. Left carotid endarterectomy
    b. Left vertebral artery stent
    c. Left subclavian stent
    d. Basilar artery stent

    Answer c. The patient has **subclavian steal syndrome** from subclavian artery stenosis as evidenced by the retrograde flow through the left vertebral artery. Tx – left subclavian stent (carotid to subclavian artery bypass if that fails).

    Subclavian steal can present as **angina** (chest pain) in patients with **previous CABG** with left internal mammary to left anterior descending anastomosis (the internal mammary arteries come off the subclavian arteries). Retrograde flow through the internal mammary artery can occur, taking blood away from the heart (Sx - angina). These patients will have lower blood pressure in the left arm compared to the right. Tx: left subclavian stent.

Vascular steal in the _donor_ leg can also occur in patients with **femoral to femoral cross-over grafts** who have a **proximal stenosis** in the _donor_ artery.

636. All of the following are potential complications of left carotid to subclavian bypass except:
   a.   Vagus nerve injury
   b.   Phrenic nerve injury
   c.   Chylothorax
   d.   Hypoglossal nerve injury

   Answer d. Hypoglossal nerve injuries occur with **high** neck dissections, not low ones. The thoracic duct enters the left subclavian vein at the junction between the left subclavian vein and left internal jugular vein. Injury can result in a chylothorax (or drainage of chyle from the incision). A **right** subclavian to carotid bypass would not be at risk for thoracic duct injury.

637. The MC peripheral site for arterial embolism obstruction is the:
   a.   Common femoral artery
   b.   Aortic bifurcation
   c.   Innominate artery
   d.   Brachial artery

   Answer a. Common femoral artery

638. A 55 yo woman with presents with a cyanotic and painful left hand. You cannot feel any brachial, radial, or ulnar pulses. Cardiac exam reveals an irregular rhythm. The most appropriate next step is
   a.   tPA
   b.   Heparin _only_
   c.   Open embolectomy
   d.   Argatroban
   e.   Bivalirudin

   Answer c. Open embolectomy. This patient most likely has an **embolus** given the history and irregular rhythm. The **brachial artery** is the MC upper extremity site for an embolus to lodge. Brachial artery cut-down and open embolectomy is indicated here.

   Thrombosis of the brachial artery usually follows access procedures (eg cardiac catheterization) and usually requires an **inter-position graft** for repair due to **damage** to the vessel. Heparin and tPA are _unlikely_ to work in these situations and would take too long in a patient with a threatened hand.

639. All of the following are true except:
   a.   ASA is the Tx of choice for improving long term vascular graft patency
   b.   The best predictor of long term patency in extremity vein grafts is surgical technique
   c.   Duplex U/S is the best technique for surveillance of bypass grafts
   d.   Rest pain typically begins with an ABI < 0.5

   Answer b. The best predictor of long term patency in extremity vein bypass grafts is **vein quality**.

640. A 60 yo golfer presents with a 40-pack year smoking history and pain is his calfs after walking 150 feet. The most appropriate next step in management is:
   a.   Angiogram and PTA
   b.   Coumadin

c. Smoking cessation, exercise therapy, and ASA
d. Angiogram and bypass

Answer c. Medical Tx is the initial Tx for **claudication**.

641. Which of the following is true for claudication:
   a. The 5-year need for revascularization risk is 50%
   b. The 5-year mortality is 5%
   c. The major mortality risk is gangrene
   d. The 5-year amputation risk is 1-3%

Answer d. The 5-year amputation risk is 1-3%

5-year <u>amputation</u> risk: **1-3%**
5-year need for <u>revascularization</u> risk: **15%**
5-year <u>mortality</u>: **30%**
Mortality is mostly related to **cardiovascular events** (myocardial infarction [#1], stroke, sudden death)

642. All of the following are true except:
   a. The right renal artery MC goes posterior to the IVC
   b. The left renal vein MC goes anterior to the aorta
   c. Symptomatic, refractory renal fibromuscular dysplasia (FMD) is best treated with PTA and stents
   d. The best conduit for renal artery bypass in a child is the internal iliac artery
   e. Medial type FMD is the MC type and the renal artery is the MC location

Answer c. FMD (eg renal, carotid, iliac, or SMA) is best treated with *PTA <u>only</u>*. Stents are unnecessary.

643. All of the following are true except:
   a. Maintenance of flow to at least one hypogastric artery is indicated for both open and endovascular aorto-bifemoral repairs
   b. Asymptomatic AAA's measuring 4.9 cm should be repaired
   c. Hematemesis 6 months after open AAA repair is worrisome for aorto-enteric fistula (MC aorto-duodenal)
   d. Bloody diarrhea following AAA repair is worrisome for ischemic colitis

Answer b. Asymptomatic AAA's measuring < 5.5 cm should be observed.

644. All of the following are true of chylous ascites following open AAA repair except:
   a. A percutaneous drainage catheter and a high protein / low fat diet effectively treats the majority
   b. NPO and TPN are indicated if refractory to high protein / low fat diet
   c. Surgery should consist of a peritoneovenous shunt
   d. Ligation of the cisterna chyli is indicated if medical therapy fails

Answer c. If surgery is required, ligation of the cisterna chyli should be performed (right side of aorta, just below right renal artery)

645. A 55 yo man presents to the ED with abdominal pain, mild hypotension (90/50), and history of a AAA. What is the most appropriate next step:
   a. Tagged RBC scan
   b. Laparotomy
   c. CT angiogram
   d. U/S in the ED
   e. Formal angiogram

Answer c. The best test for determining AAA rupture (leak) is **CT angiogram** (will show <u>fluid</u> in retroperitoneal space and <u>extra-luminal contrast</u> with rupture). The other diagnostic items listed are not as accurate and take longer to obtain.

276

In the past, hypotension, back-pain, and pulsatile midline mass alone were indications for laparotomy. There is a significant negative laparotomy rate with this (ie there was no rupture) so this approach is falling out of favor. CT angio can generally be performed very quickly in these patients.

646. Initial aortic clamping for a ruptured infra-renal AAA with severe hypotension (70/50), should be:
    a.   Through a left thoracotomy (aorta above the diaphragm)
    b.   At the diaphragmatic hiatus (intra-abdominal aorta, supra-renal)
    c.   At the base of the transverse mesocolon (infra-renal)
    d.   At the iliac arteries

    Answer b. The easiest access for aortic cross-clamping in this patient would be supra-renal at the **diaphragmatic hiatus**. Make an opening in the gastro-hepatic ligament (lesser omentum) and clamp the aorta. Resuscitate the patient while you expose the aneurysm.

    Dissect out the aorta at the base of the transverse mesocolon (just below the left renal vein) and then move your proximal clamp to an infra-renal position (allows perfusion of visceral vessels).

    Permissive hypotension is indicated in this scenario until an aortic cross-clamp is placed.

647. The MC organism in a mycotic aneurysm is:
    a.   Candida
    b.   Staph aureus
    c.   Aspergillosis
    d.   Salmonella
    e.   Histoplasmosis

    Answer b. Mycotic aneurysms are <u>not</u> due to fungi; MC organism - staph aureus

648. Which of the following is the best indication for AAA repair
    a.   5.0 cm AAA in a 50 yo healthy man
    b.   5.0 cm AAA in a 50 yo healthy woman
    c.   5.0 cm AAA in a 85 yo man with renal insufficiency and cirrhosis
    d.   5.0 cm AAA in a 50 yo man with CHF and COPD

    Answer b. The rupture risk is higher in women and the threshold for elective repair is lower (5.0 cm). For high risk patients (multiple co-morbidities) delay until 5.5 cm is indicated. For average male patients, repair at 5.5 cm is indicated.

649. A 65 yo man has a 6.5 cm AAA involving the left renal artery that is not suitable for endovascular repair. On CT scan, the aneurysm wall is significantly thickened. Fibrotic adhesions involve the 3rd portion of the duodenum, the left renal vein, and the IVC. There is mild bilateral hydronephrosis from ureter compression by fibrosis. What is the best approach in this patient:
    a.   Dissecting the duodenum off the aorta and freeing up the ureters
    b.   Leaving the duodenum alone and freeing up the ureters
    c.   Dissecting the duodenum off the aorta and leaving the ureters alone
    d.   Leaving the duodenum and ureters alone

    Answer d. The inflammatory process **resolves** after repair of **inflammatory aneurysms**, so surgery generally revolves around the repair itself and _avoiding injury_ to involved structures (eg duodenum, ureters, IVC, left renal vein).

    A **left retroperitoneal approach** and **supra-renal aortic cross-clamping** will likely help avoid injury, especially to the left renal vein and duodenum which are involved in the fibrotic process.

Note that the inflammatory process is *not* infectious *(ie not a mycotic aneurysm)*.

650. POD 1 from open AAA repair, your patient develops watery diarrhea, distension, and mild LLQ tenderness. CT scan shows thickened edematous mucosal folds in the left colon. The most appropriate next step is:
    a. Palliative care
    b. Repeat laparotomy
    c. IV fluids and antibiotics
    d. Catheter directed papaverine infusion
    e. Soap-suds enema

    Answer c. IVFs and antibiotics. Based on Sx's and the thickened edematous mucosal folds (ie **thumbprinting**) this patient has ischemic colitis, likely from sacrificing the **inferior mesenteric artery** (IMA) during AAA repair. Initial Tx with NPO, IVFs, and broad spectrum antibiotics are appropriate.

    If the patient had **diffuse peritoneal signs**, **unrelenting metabolic acidosis**, **severe sepsis**, **perforation**, or **black colon** (necrotic bowel; seen on flexible sigmoidoscopy), then emergency exploration and colectomy would be indicated (with colostomy and Hartman's pouch).

    During aortobifemoral graft placement, not assuring good flow to at least 1 **internal iliac (hypogastric) artery** can result in **pelvic ischemia problems** (should see good retrograde back-bleeding after opening the internal iliacs if there are good collaterals). The pelvic ischemia problems are usually chronic issues and include vasculogenic impotence, buttock claudication, spinal cord problems, over active bladder and other urinary symptoms, and rectal ischemia (generally not a full thickness injury [Sx's - strictures, pain]).

651. All of the following are indications for re-implantation of the inferior mesenteric artery (IMA) at the time of AAA repair except:
    a. Previous colon surgery
    b. Occluded IMA orifice
    c. Poor back-bleeding (stump pressure < 40 mHg)
    d. SMA stenosis
    e. Dusky looking left colon

    Answer b. Occluded IMA orifice means the IMA does not contribute blood flow to the left colon so reimplantation is unnecessary.

652. You perform an open aortobifemoral bypass for aorto-iliac occlusive disease and get called to the ICU because his right foot is cold. You cannot feel a right femoral or distal pulse. You do feel a left femoral pulse. The most appropriate next step is:
    a. Angiography
    b. Fasciotomy
    c. IV fluids
    d. Re-exploration with laparotomy
    e. Re-exploration with right groin incision

    Answer e. Re-exploration with right groin incision. This patient has vascular insufficiency to the right leg. Because the left femoral pulse is intact, the problem is most likely at the distal anastomosis to the right femoral artery. Heparin should be given (5000 U IV) and the patient should be returned to the OR for right groin exploration.

653. A 55 yo patient presents with hematemesis 6 months after aortic aneurysm repair. EGD is normal. The most appropriate next step is:
    a. Formal angiogram
    b. Tagged RBC scan
    c. CT scan
    d. Tagged WBC scan

e.   MRI

Answer d. This is suspicious for **aorto-enteric** fistula and abdominal CT scan is indicated *(best diagnostic test for aorto-enteric fistula)*. Repair involves extra-anatomic bypass (axillobifemoral bypass), resecting the entire aortic graft, and closure of the hole in the duodenum.

654. Two years after an aortobifemoral graft, your patient presents with an acutely painful right groin. U/S which shows a pseudoaneurysm and a large fluid collection. What is the most likely cause of this patients problem:
        a.   Trauma
        b.   Infection
        c.   Poor surgical technique
        d.   Graft thrombosis

Answer b. Late pseudoaneurysm after vascular bypass graft is most consistent with **graft infection.** The MC organism overall in graft infections is staph epidermidis.

655. Which of the following is the MC Type of endoleak after EVAR:
        a.   I
        b.   II
        c.   III
        d.   IV
        e.   V

Answer b. Type II endoleak is the MC type. It is due to collateral branches filling the aneurysm sac.

656. Which of the following is least favorable for EVAR repair for a AAA:
        a.   Proximal neck 2.9 cm in diameter
        b.   Distal landing zone aorta of 2.0 cm in diameter
        c.   Proximal angulation of 90 degrees
        d.   Bilateral common femoral arteries measuring 11 mm

Answer c. The **angle** between the normal aorta above and aneurysm below must be **< 60 degrees** (termed: **angulation < 60 degrees**) to allow the proximal landing zone to seal properly (would end up with a Type I leak).

657. Which of the following is the most appropriate surveillance:
        a.   U/S for a 3.5 cm AAA every 6 months
        b.   U/S for a 5.6 cm AAA every 6 months
        c.   U/S for a 5.0 cm AAA every 6 months
        d.   U/S for a 5.0 cm AAA every 2 years

Answer c. This aortic aneurysm is approaching repair indications and U/S frequency should be increased to every 3-6 months. Yearly U/S is indicated for aortic aneurysms not near 5.0 cm. Aneurysms > 5.5 cm should be repaired.

658. All of the following are true of pseudoaneurysms except:
        a.   Initial Tx for a femoral artery pseudoaneurysm following arterial angiography is U/S guided thrombin injection
        b.   Tx for a femoral artery pseudoaneurysm following aortobifemoral graft placement is open repair
        c.   Tx for a femoral artery pseudoaneurysm in an IV drug abuser is ligation *without* bypass
        d.   There are no collateral vessels around the hip or knee

Answer d. Circumflex femoral arteries to gluteal arteries exist around the hip and **geniculate collaterals** exist around the knee.

IVDA patients with infected femoral artery pseudoaneurysms can undergo simple ligation (even if it's the common femoral artery – amputation rate is 0% in several large series). Collateral vessels supply the leg.

Initial Tx for a femoral artery pseudoaneurysm following arterial angiography is U/S guided thrombin injection.

Pseudoaneurysm following any surgical bypass requires emergent repair *(high risk of* rupture*).*

659. Six weeks after aortobifemoral graft placement for a complicated AAA, your patient returns to clinic with mild pain in his left groin. His femoral artery tissue was poor on that side and you are worried about a pseudoaneurysm. The study of choice for this is:
   a. MRI
   b. Abdominal CT
   c. Duplex ultrasound (U/S)
   d. Angiogram

   Answer c. Color flow duplex U/S is the most cost effective option to study abdominal aortic and peripheral bypass grafts (estimates blood flow and delineates anatomy).

660. All of the following are true of popliteal artery aneurysms except:
   a. The MC complication is rupture
   b. Thrombosis can occur
   c. They are often bilateral
   d. Emboli can occur

   Answer a. Aneurysms below the inguinal ligament *rarely* rupture. Popliteal artery aneurysms are more likely to have thrombosis (MC) or form emboli.

661. All of the following are true of popliteal artery aneurysms except:
   a. Size > 2 cm is an indication for repair
   b. Presence of intramural thrombus is an indication for repair
   c. Evidence of previous embolization is an indication for repair
   d. Formal angiogram is the diagnostic method of choice

   Answer d. Duplex U/S is the diagnostic method of choice. Formal angiogram may miss these due to intra-mural hematoma although it is used for pre-operative planning (ie figuring out where your bypass is going to go)

662. The MC complication of popliteal artery aneurysms is:
   a. Distal embolization
   b. Compression of adjacent structures
   c. Thrombosis
   d. Rupture

   Answer c. Thrombosis is the MC complication

663. A 50 yo old man with previous right popliteal aneurysm presents with a cool left foot. He has motor and sensation still in the extremity and you feel a left femoral pulse The most appropriate next step is:
   a. Heparin *only*
   b. Catheter directed thrombolysis
   c. Open thrombectomy
   d. Argatroban

   Answer b. Thrombolysis. tPA is indicated (although you would usually give heparin in the ED to help stop propagation of thrombus; heparin is also used in conjunction with tPA). Catheter directed thrombolysis works well in patients with popliteal artery thrombosis as it opens up the popliteal aneurysm thrombosis and also clears distal clot in the trifurcation vessels. If possible, this is the preferred initial Tx for popliteal artery aneurysm thrombosis.

After clearing the thrombus (may take **2-3 days**), definitive surgery should be performed that admission.

Open thrombectomy may be indicated for an acutely **threatened limb** due to popliteal artery aneurysm thrombosis, however, this situation is <u>complicated</u>. It's difficult to clear thrombus from the trifurcation vessels with open thrombectomy. *Combined* percutaneous mechanical thrombectomy (eg AngioJet device) followed by tPA may have a role in these patients.

664. Definitive surgery for the above patient should be:
   a. Endovascular stent placement
   b. Open bypass with saphenous vein graft and interval ligation
   c. Aneurysmorrhaphy with interposition graft
   d. Open bypass with PTFE and interval ligation

   Answer b. Open bypass with saphenous vein graft and interval ligation of the popliteal artery proximal and distal to the aneuryms is the standard operation, although many are trying to treat these lesions with endovascular stents.

   Patients with **compressive Sx's** (*rare*; venous congestion edema, paresthesias, numbness) should undergo **aneurysmorrhaphy with interposition graft** (open aneurysm, place bypass graft in aneurysm sac), as opposed to just exclusion of the aneurysm with bypass. **Geniculate collaterals** can continue to fill the aneurysm sac if it is just ligated, causing recurrent Sx's.

665. A 24 yo non-smoking man presents with left calf pain when playing golf. He can walk 50 yards or so before the pain starts. The pain is relieved with rest. On exam the pulse weakens significantly with plantar-flexion. This most likely represents:
   a. Popliteal entrapment syndrome
   b. Popliteal artery aneurysm
   c. Adventitial cystic disease
   d. Atherosclerosis
   e. Buerger's Disease

   Answer a. Popliteal entrapment syndrome. This can often be **bilateral** and is usually caused by deviation of the popliteal artery around the medial head of the gastrocnemius muscle (Tx: resection of the medial head of the gastrocnemius muscle).

666. A 40 yo non-smoking man presents with left calf pain when playing golf. He can walk 50 yards or so before the pain starts. The pain is relieved with rest. His ABI is 0.6 on the left and normal on the right. CT angio demonstrates a "scimitar sign" and mass in his popliteal fossa. This most likely represents:
   a. Popliteal entrapment syndrome
   b. Popliteal artery aneurysm
   c. Cystic adventitial disease
   d. Atherosclerosis
   e. Buerger's Disease

   Answer c. Cystic adventitial disease (Tx: resection of cyst, possible bypass)

667. The MCC of occlusion at 6 months for a reversed saphenous vein graft used in a lower extremity bypass is:
   a. Hypercoagulable state
   b. Technical error
   c. Intimal hyperplasia
   d. Vein atherosclerosis

Answer c. MCC of failure of a reversed saphenous vein graft for lower extremity bypass in the **intermediate** period (30 days to 2 years) - **intimal hyperplasia**

Early period (< 30 days) - **technical problem**
Late period (> 2 years) - **atherosclerosis in the vein graft**

668. A 60 man has a left sided non-healing 2nd toe ulcer. Angiogram shows a normal superficial artery and a long segment occlusion of the popliteal artery (at the level of the knee) and proximal trifurcation vessels with reconstitution of the anterior tibial artery and run-off to the dorsalis pedis. The patient has had bilateral greater saphenous vein stripping. The most appropriate next step is:
   a. Popliteal-anterior tibial bypass using PTFE
   b. Popliteal-anterior tibial bypass using lesser saphenous vein
   c. 2nd toe amputation only
   d. Syme amputation
   e. Below knee amputation

Answer b. Greater saphenous vein is the best conduit for lower extremity bypass. If that is not available, for bypasses below the knee, **lesser saphenous vein** and **cephalic vein** can be used.

Bypasses to **distal vessels** are usually used _only_ for **limb** (rest pain) or **tissue salvage** (eg non-healing ulcer).

PTFE should _not_ be used for bypasses below the knee.

Because the occlusion is a long segment, PTA-stent is not likely an option here.

669. A 22 yo woman is evaluated in the ED for vague Sx's (N/V) and is found to have an asymptomatic 2.5 cm splenic artery aneurysm. The most appropriate next step is:
   a. Coumadin
   b. Careful follow-up
   c. Exclusion with covered stent placement or open procedure
   d. Splenectomy

Answer c. All **visceral artery aneurysms** (**> 2 cm**, > 1.5 cm for renal artery aneurysms) need repair _except_ for splenic artery aneurysms. The rupture rate for visceral artery aneurysms is 50% for those other than splenic. **Women in child bearing age** should have splenic artery aneurysms repaired due to a specific risk of **rupture with pregnancy**.

The majority of visceral artery aneurysms are repaired using endovascular **covered stents** _(not_ open surgery) and **embolization** (coils / glue).

Laparoscopic excision or exclusion (without splenectomy) is being used more frequently for **hilar splenic artery aneurysms** that are not amenable to endovascular treatment (get proximal control of the splenic artery as a first step).

If both endovascular and laparoscopic treatments are not possible due to a complicated **hilar splenic artery aneurysm**, splenectomy is indicated.

Splenic artery aneurysm is the MC visceral artery aneurysm.

670. You perform a lower arm brachial artery to cephalic vein PTFE loop fistula. In the PACU, the patient has a cold hand with pallor, cyanosis, and mottling. The most immediate next step is:
   a. Return to the OR and band the graft
   b. Formal angiogram
   c. Graft resection
   d. Fistulogram with shunt run-off

Answer a. This patient has severe ischemia and a threatened hand. The most expeditious procedure at this stage is to return to the OR and band the graft, which will improve blood flow to the hand. If that fails, ligate the graft.

671. You take the above patient to the OR and band the graft with vast improvement in the condition of his hand. The most appropriate next step is
    a. Graft resection
    b. Formal arterial angiogram
    c. Graft ligation
    d. Fistulogram with shunt run-off

    Answer b. This patient has an inflow problem which is best assessed with formal arterial angiogram. MC these patients will have a **subclavian artery stenosis** which is treated with **PTA and stent**.

672. You perform a lower arm brachial artery to cephalic vein PTFE loop fistula. There is a palpable thrill and doppler signal at the end of the case. On POD 1, you inspect the graft and there is a poor thrill and poor doppler signal. The most appropriate next step in this patients management is:
    a. Heparin
    b. Fistulogram
    c. Graft ligation
    d. Graft excision

    Answer b. Take the patient back to the OR, de-clot the graft, and perform a **fistulogram** to figure out the issue.

673. You perform a lower arm brachial artery to cephalic vein PTFE loop fistula. Later that day your patient starts to develop hand and arm swelling. Initially you try conservative Tx (eg elevating the arm). The hand continues to swell and now has ulcerations. The most appropriate next step is:
    a. Heparin
    b. Compressive wraps
    c. tPA
    d. Fistulogram and shoot run-off

    Answer d. Arm swelling after AV fistula (or AV graft) placement is due to **venous HTN**. The initial Tx is arm elevation and as collaterals develop, the swelling goes down. If major arm swelling persists, it suggests major outflow obstruction (eg axillary, subclavian, or innominate vein stenosis). Get a fistulogram and look at the shunt run-off and find the obstruction.

674. Fistulogram in the above patient demonstrates an axillary vein stenosis. The most appropriate next step is:
    a. Stent
    b. Graft banding
    c. Graft resection
    d. PTA
    e. Bypass

    Answer d. PTA (percutaneous transluminal angioplasty) of the venous stenosis (outflow obstruction). Venous stenting should generally be _avoided_ outside the thoracic inlet (eg axillary and subclavian veins) and below the common femoral vein (eg popliteal vein) due to poor outcomes.

675. All of the following suggest venous outflow obstruction for an AV fistula except:
    a. Increase in returning line pressure
    b. Acute hand ischemia early following AV fistula placement
    c. High outflow pressure > 200
    d. Increase in re-circulation

Answer b. Acute hand ischemia following AV fistula placement suggests **inflow** obstruction. Arterial angiogram is the best test for Dx.

676. A patient is about to start long term dialysis. The preferred initial access for long term dialysis should be:
   a. Brachiocephalic fistula
   b. Cimino fistula
   c. Tunneled subclavian vein catheter
   d. Forearm AV loop graft

   Answer b. A Cimino should always be tried first although this is not always possible due to issues such as forearm cephalic vein thrombosis and sclerosis.

677. A Cimino fistula is a:
   a. Ulnocephalic fistula
   b. Brachiocephalic fistula
   c. Brachiocephalic AV graft
   d. Radiocephalic fistula

   Answer d. Radiocephalic fistula

678. The MC injured nerve with the above fistula is:
   a. Median
   b. Ulnar
   c. Musculocutaneous
   d. Superficial radial nerve

   Answer d. superficial radial nerve.

679. A 21 yo man is shot in the leg. Five years later he presents to your clinic with right groin discomfort and a "vibration feeling" in his groin. All of the following are true of this patient's most likely condition except:
   a. Heart rate will decrease when the fistula is compressed.
   b. Mild left ventricle hypertrophy
   c. A thrill over the groin is likely present
   d. This is best diagnosed with ultrasound
   e. He will likely need a femoral to popliteal bypass

   Answer e. Open repair is indicated for **acquired AV fistulas** (primary closure of the vein with **lateral venous suture** and a **patch** for the artery; interpose some sartorius muscle between vein and artery so the fistula does not recur).

680. A 56 yo obese man with significant smoking history has multiple large ulcerations on the antero-medial aspect of his left lower leg just above the medial malleolus. The surrounding skin has a brawny appearance. The most effective initial therapy for healing these ulcers is:
   a. Compressive dressings
   b. Duoderm (hydrocolloid)
   c. Wound VAC
   d. Vein stripping

   Answer a. The most effective Tx for venous insufficiency with severe venous ulcers is compressive dressings (eg Unna boot). **Brawny edema** occurs from high capillary venous pressure and leakage of RBCs that are eventually get destroyed with hemosiderin deposition (**brown or brawny appearance**).

681. All of the following are contraindications to vein stripping except:
   a. DVT
   b. Sapheno-femoral and sapheno-popliteal valve incompetence
   c. Venous outflow obstruction
   d. Varicosities with pregnancy

Answer b. Sapheno-femoral and sapheno-popliteal valve incompetence are the indications for vein stripping.

682. Which organ does not contain lymphatics:
   a. Lung
   b. Liver
   c. Spleen
   d. Muscle

   Answer d. Muscle does not contain lymphatics.

683. All of the following are true of suppurative thrombophlebitis except:
   a. Removal of any intravenous catheter is the 1st step in Tx of thrombophlebitis
   b. Continued bacteremia or purulence at the site indicates need for resection of the entire vein.
   c. E. Coli is the MCC of bacterial thrombophlebitis
   d. Antibiotics are indicated

   Answer c. Staph aureus is the MC organism in suppurative thrombophlebitis.

684. Following a prolonged ischemic period (8 hours), you successfully perform a femoral to posterior tibial artery bypass for an acutely threatened leg. Several hours post-op, your patient develops an acutely swollen painful right leg that feels tight to exam. He has pain with passive motion of the leg. The most appropriate next step is:
   a. Fasciotomy
   b. Arterial bypass
   c. Lasix
   d. Heparin

   Answer a. Reperfusion injury resulting in **compartment syndrome** can occur after restoration of blood flow if occlusion time is > 4-6 hours. Tx is **fasciotomy** of the muscle compartments (2 incision, 4 compartment release if in lower leg).

685. The MC injured nerve with lower extremity (calf) fasciotomy is:
   a. Superficial peroneal
   b. Common peroneal
   c. Tibial
   d. Peroneal

   Answer a. The **superficial peroneal nerve** is very superficial at the area between the anterior and lateral compartments near the proximal fibula (fibula head). When performing the 2 incision technique for 4 compartment fasciotomy, the lateral incision comes very close to the superficial peroneal nerve.

686. Which lower leg compartment is most sensitive to compartment syndrome:
   a. Lateral
   b. Anterior
   c. Deep posterior
   d. Superficial posterior

   Answer b. Anterior compartment

687. All of the following are true except:
   a. The MC source for a peripheral or visceral embolus is the heart
   b. The MC obstruction site for a cardiac embolus is the common femoral artery
   c. Strokes MC occur from decreased flow across a carotid stenosis
   d. Cardiac emboli are most commonly the result of atrial fibrillation

Answer c. Strokes MC occur due to embolism of atherosclerotic disease at the carotid bifurcation.

688. A 50 yo woman presents with an acutely cold and painful right foot. Posterior tibial and dorsalis pedis pulses are gone on the right and normal on the left. You cannot feel a right femoral pulse. She has lost sensation and motor function in her right foot. Which of the following is the most appropriate next step
    a.   Catheter directed tPA
    b.   Heparin only
    c.   Femoral artery cut-down and embolectomy
    d.   Careful observation

    Answer c. This patient has a threatened lower extremity (loss of motor function and sensation) and should be taken to the OR for emergent open embolectomy (groin cutdown, transfemoral). This scenario is most consistent with **embolus**.

    If motor function / sensation were still intact and the patient still had a femoral pulse, tPA would be the preferred option as the thrombus / embolus is more likely distal involving the trifurcation vessels (which is better treated with thrombolytics).

    Loss of <u>motor</u> function and/or <u>sensation</u> are *strong indicators of **severe ischemia***

689. A 50 yo woman with a history of atrial fibrillation presents with acute bilateral lower extremity pain. Both lower extremities are cold. You cannot feel a right or left femoral pulse. The most appropriate next step is:
    a.   Aorto-bifemoral bypass graft
    b.   tPA
    c.   Axillo-bifemoral bypass
    d.   Bilateral transfemoral embolectomy
    e.   Heparin

    Answer d. Bilateral transfemoral embolectomy. Given the history, this patient most likely had a embolus to her aortic bifurcation. This is best treated with bilateral femoral cutdowns and <u>*retrograde*</u> embolectomies (use the balloon catheters to break up the clot).

690. A 50 yo man presents with severe buttock claudication after walking 50 feet and impotence despite maximal medical Tx. You cannot feel any femoral pulses. ABI is 0.3 bilaterally. CT angio shows a completely occluded aortic bifurcation with reconstitution of bilateral common femoral arteries. Optimal therapy in this patient is:
    a.   Axillobifemoral bypass with femoral to femoral artery crossover
    b.   Aortobifemoral bypass
    c.   EVAR of the aortic bifurcation
    d.   ASA only
    e.   Stent of bilateral iliac arteries

    Answer b. Leriche syndrome is characterized by buttock claudication, impotence, and loss of femoral pulses. **Aortobifemoral bypass** is the best option. Answer a. could work but would not result in the best long-term outcome (although it may be indicated in patients with a hostile abdomen or prohibitive operative risk – however, none of these were presented in the question). EVAR and bilateral iliac stenting will not work for severe chronic occlusions such as this.

691. A 55 woman presents to a community ED at 3 am with acute abdominal pain. The patient appears to have excruciating pain, however, she is minimally tender and does not demonstrate any rebound or guarding. Past medical history is significant for atrial fibrillation, peripheral arterial disease, and a poorly understood hypercoagulable state. The pain started 2 hours ago. What is the most appropriate next step:
    a.   Angiogram
    b.   CT angiogram
    c.   MRI

d. WBC scan
e. RBC scan

Answer b. CT angiogram. This scenario is worrisome for mesenteric ischemia (from numerous potential causes listed in the past medical history). Formal angiogram would take too long (especially given this is a community hospital) and CT angio would also pick up *other conditions* that might be causing the pain.

692. CT angio in the above patient shows a meniscus sign 3 cm from the origin of the SMA and diffuse edema of the small bowel wall. You give a heparin bolus. In the OR, almost the entire small bowel is mottled as well as the right colon. The duodenum and descending colon appear normal The most appropriate next step is:
    a. Close and obtain a hospice consult
    b. Intra-op direct thrombolytic infusion into the SMA
    c. Bowel resection
    d. SMA embolectomy
    e. Systemic heparin *only*

Answer d. SMA embolectomy (meniscus sign is consistent with an embolus) and assessing the bowel after reperfusion is appropriate here. Obvious non-viable bowel after reperfusion should be resected. *Borderline bowel should be left* in place. A 2nd look operation the next day (24-48 hours) is necessary in determining if the residual bowel is viable or not. Extensive resection of bowel can result in **short-gut syndrome**.

The distribution of ischemia described above is classic for the SMA territory. With SMA embolus, a small segment of jejunum (proximal jejunal branches) and the middle colic artery may be spared as the embolus usually lodges distally.

693. Instead of the above, CT angio shows a 99% stenosis at the SMA origin and diffuse small vessel atherosclerotic disease distally. There is moderate small bowel thickening. The most appropriate next step is
    a. PTA and stent
    b. Heparin *only*
    c. tPA *only*
    d. Open bypass
    e. Palliative care

Answer a. PTA and stent is likely the best option in this patient. Heparin should also be given. Given the small vessels distally, open bypass is not a good option. Also, PTA with stent would restore perfusion quicker than open bypass. Most symptomatic SMA stenotic lesions are treated with PTA and stent. This patient should be followed for signs of infarcted bowel (eg perforation, diffuse peritonitis) after perfusion is restored (may need laparotomy to resect dead bowel).

694. Instead of the above, CT angio shows thickened loops of small bowel with opacification of the superior mesenteric vein and delayed filling of the portal vein. The most appropriate next step is:
    a. Open embolectomy
    b. Heparin *only*
    c. tPA
    d. Open thrombectomy
    e. Catheter-directed papaverine infusion

Answer b. Heparin only is indicated for superior mesenteric vein thrombosis. Thrombectomy does not work. tPA is similarly is associated with *worse* outcomes in mesenteric vein thrombosis. If perforation or diffuse peritonitis occurs, operative exploration would be indicated.

Mesenteric vein thrombosis generally results in patchy or segmental areas of ischemia.

695. A 75 yo woman admitted for dyspnea and pulmonary edema related to a CHF exacerbation develops acute abdominal pain. Exam reveals diffuse tenderness but no peritoneal signs (no rebound, no guarding). CT angio shows diffuse narrowing of the mesenteric blood supply to the small bowel. You start antibiotics. The most appropriate next step is:
    a. Laparotomy
    b. PTA and stent
    c. SMA bypass
    d. Dobutamine and catheter directed intra-arterial papaverine
    e. Heparin only

    Answer d. This patient has **non-occlusive mesenteric ischemia** (NOMI) due to **CHF**. This is results in poor blood flow to the mesentery and spasm. Treatment includes improving **cardiac output** (primary Tx; eg <u>Dobutamine</u>) and reducing spasm (eg <u>papaverine</u>). Antibiotics should also be given.

    Note giving volume (fluid) would <u>not</u> be a good option in this patient (CHF, dyspnea, and pulmonary edema).

696. A 70 yo woman presents with headache, temporal tenderness, and malaise. All of the following are true of this patient's most likely condition except:
    a. It can lead to blindness
    b. It involves giant cells
    c. CEA is indicated
    d. Immediate corticosteroids are indicated
    e. Temporal artery biopsy is indicated

    Answer c. CEA is not indicated for **temporal arteritis**. Temporal artery biopsy is indicated.

697. A 25 yo woman presents with repeated syncope. You cannot feel any pulses in her upper extremities. CT angio shows severe stenosis of her aortic arch and branch vessels. ESR is elevated. All of the following are true of the most likely diagnosis except:
    a. Large blood vessels are involved
    b. Hypertension can occur
    c. It is a granulomatous disease process
    d. PTA works well for this condition
    e. Corticosteroids are indicated

    Answer d. PTA and endarterectomy do <u>not</u> work well for **Takayasu's Arteritis**.

698. Three weeks after left lower extremity bypass with left sided reversed saphenous vein, your patient presents with left sided leg swelling. Duplex U/S is negative for DVT. This most likely represents:
    a. Graft occlusion
    b. Reperfusion injury
    c. HITT
    d. Disrupted lymphatics
    e. Occult DVT

    Answer d. Lymphatic disruption can occur with lower extremity bypass due to groin incisions and taking the greater saphenous vein, leading to lymphedema.

699. All of the following are high risk graft surveillance features on duplex U/S (indicating intervention is needed) when following a lower extremity bypass grafts except:
    a. Peak systolic velocity (PSV) > 300 cm/s
    b. PSV ratio > 3.5 across the stenosis
    c. ABI 0.7
    d. End diastolic velocity > 20 cm/s

e.   > 70% diameter reduction confirmed on angiography

Answer c. ABI 0.7. Although controversial, **graft surveillance** seeks to find critical stenoses in bypass grafts and intervene on them before complete occlusion occurs (complete occlusion is harder to treat effectively and may not re-open). A **higher velocity** means **greater stenosis**.

700. All of the following are true of amputations except:
   a.   Above the knee amputations are more likely to heal compared to below the amputations
   b.   A TCOM of 19 mmHg suggests the stump will heal
   c.   Presence of a proximal pulse suggests the stump will heal
   d.   Healing rate is affected by amputation level

Answer b. A TCOM **< 20 mmHg** suggests the stump will likely <u>not</u> heal. On the other hand, a **TCOM > 40 mmHg** suggests the stump will heal (98%). A TCOM between 20-40 is hard to predict in terms of healing.

701. A 6 month old in the PICU has non-functioning femoral a-line that is removed. Several hours later the child's leg is cool and you cannot feel a femoral pulse. The child can move the leg and sensation seems intact. The most appropriate next step is:
   a.   Femoral artery cutdown and thrombectomy
   b.   Heparin only
   c.   PTA and stent
   d.   Femoral artery cutdown and vein patch angioplasty

Answer b. Heparin. Careful here, children this size have very small vessels and the majority of thrombotic / embolic events can be treated with just heparin. Cutting down on the vessel and opening it often does more harm than good.

702. A 25 yo woman complains of finger pain with cold temperatures. Her fingers turn white, then blue, and then red. She has normal radial, ulnar, and brachial artery pulses. Sx's persist despite gloves and avoiding the cold. The most appropriate next step is:
   a.   Diltiazem
   b.   Metoprolol
   c.   Lisinorpril
   d.   Succinylcholine

Answer a. Diltiazem is the best Tx for refractory **Raynaud's disease**.

703. All of the following are true of thromboangitis obliterans (Buerger's) except:
   a.   It is MC in young men
   b.   It is characterized by thrombotic occlusions of small and medium sized vessels, resulting in severe rest pain and ulceration / gangrene of digits
   c.   It is curable with nicotine cessation
   d.   It involves major occlusions proximal to the brachial and popliteal arteries

Answer d. The major vessels proximal to the brachial and popliteal arteries are *normal* in **Buerger's disease**. Small to medium sized arteries are affected.

ATHEROSCLEROSIS STAGES
- **Normal arterial wall** - intima, media, and adventitia
- **LDL cholesterol** is **oxidized** in blood and **damages** arterial wall
- **Macrophages** repair damage, causing an **inflammatory reaction**
- Macrophages cannot process cholesterol, so **cholesterol builds up** in wall, attracting more macrophages (macrophages become **foam cells** with absorption of LDL)
- Initially starts as a **fatty streak** *(earliest lesion)* and then cholesterol builds up
- **Endothelial injury** is the *central mechanism* in the development of atherosclerosis
- **Smooth muscle proliferation** in media occurs, further narrowing the arterial wall (causes **HTN**)

- **Thrombus** can form on the damaged arterial wall, which if already narrowed, will completely **occlude the vessel** *(etiology of myocardial infarction)*
- RFs: **smoking** (#1), HTN, ↑ LDL or VLDL, DM, age, males, family history
- **Prevention** and **Tx of atherosclerosis:**
  - **Statin drugs** (eg simvastatin, *best preventive Tx for atherosclerosis*)
  - Dietary change - less fat and cholesterol; ↑ omega 3 fatty acids
  - D/C smoking, control HTN, DM control, ASA
- **Homocysteinemia** can ↑ risk of atherosclerosis. Tx: **folate, B-6, B-12**

CONDUITS FOR BYPASS
- Internal mammary artery
- Radial artery
- Internal iliac artery (in <u>children</u>; eg renal artery bypass)
- Greater saphenous *(best vein graft)*, lesser saphenous, or cephalic vein

CEREBROVASCULAR DISEASE
- **Carotid Anatomy**
  - Normal internal carotid artery has **continuous forward flow**
  - Normal external carotid artery has normal **tri-phasic flow** (rapid systolic *antegrade* flow, short *retrograde* reversal of flow in early diastole, and slow *antegrade* flow in late diastole)
  - **1st branch of external carotid artery** (ECA) - superior thyroid artery
  - **1st branch of the internal carotid artery** (ICA) - ophthalmic artery
  - Communication between internal and external carotid arteries is through **ophthalmic artery** (off ICA) and **internal maxillary artery** (off ECA)
  - **Vertebral arteries** - normally come off the subclavian arteries
  - MC <u>diseased intracranial artery</u> - **middle cerebral artery**
  - MC site of <u>stenosis</u> - **carotid bifurcation** (carotid bulb)
  - **Stroke** (cerebral ischemic events) is usually from arterial **embolization** (not thrombosis) from the **carotid bifurcation** (MC) or **internal carotid artery** (ICA)
    - Can also occur from a **low-flow state** through a severe carotid stenosis
    - The **heart** is the 2nd MC source of cerebral emboli
    - MCC of <u>hemorrhagic</u> stroke - **HTN**
  - Most important RF for cerebrovascular disease - **HTN**
  - MC source of **emboli** to the *head* (ie stroke, TIAs) - **carotid bifurcation** (from **atherosclerosis**)
  - MC source of **emboli** to the *extremities* or *viscera* - **heart** (usually due to **atrial fibrillation**)
- **Amaurosis fugax** - temporary occlusion of the **ophthalmic branch** of the ICA (visual changes → shade coming down over eyes; **retinal Sx's**); visual changes are transient
  - See **Hollenhorst plaques** on ophthalmologic exam
  - Sign of **carotid disease** (atherosclerotic emboli are causing the problem)
- **Transient ischemia attacks** (TIAs) → Sx's for < 24 hours
- **Carotid stenosis**
  - **Carotid Duplex U/S** every 6 months
  - **Doppler** measures carotid flow velocities; get **peak systolic velocity** (PSV) for **ICA** and **ICA/CCA ratio**; the *higher velocity the greater the stenosis*

ICA PSV	ICA/CCA PSV ratio	% stenosis
< 125 cm/s	< 2	≤ 50%
125-230 cm/s	2-4	50-79%
> 230 cm/s	> 4	≥ 80%

  - **Angiography** *(best test;* although most operate on just Duplex U/S findings)
- **Carotid endarterectomy** (CEA)
  - CEA indications: **symptomatic** > 50% stenosis, **asymptomatic** > 70% stenosis
  - Timing of CEA after **stroke or TIA**:
    - TIAs or **small, non-disabling** <u>ischemic</u> stroke → CEA within **2 weeks**
    - Moderate to large <u>ischemic</u> stroke → wait **4-6 weeks** (avoids **reperfusion injury** and risk of *intracranial bleeding*)
    - Hemorrhagic stroke → wait **6-8 weeks** (avoids **intracranial bleeding**)

- **Emergent CEA** benefits patients with <u>fluctuating neurologic Sx's</u> or <u>crescendo / evolving TIAs</u>
- **Men** and patients with **hemispheric Sx's** (as opposed to eye/retinal Sx's) derive the greatest benefit from CEA
- Criteria for **shunting during CEA** (some always shunt)
    - **Stump pressure < 50** (back pressure in internal carotid after clamping the common carotid artery)
    - You are operating on patient awake and they have **neuro changes**
    - **EEG changes** (slowing)
    - **Contralateral tight stenosis** or **occlusion**
- Repair the **tightest side** first if the patient has bilateral stenosis
- Repair the **dominant side** first (usually left if right-handed) if the patient has equally tight carotid stenosis bilaterally
- CEA removes **intima** and part of the **media**
- Most important technical concern - getting a **good distal endpoint** (want to avoid an intimal flap)
- **Occluded ICA** (100% occlusion) - *do <u>not</u> repair (CEA is of <u>no</u> benefit)*
- **Facial vein** - can be routinely divided
- The posterior belly of the <u>digastric</u> muscle (cephlad) and <u>omohyoid</u> muscle (caudad) can be divided to improve exposure for CEA
- **Patch closure** of CEA arteriotomy results in:
    - Lowered peri-op stroke and thrombosis risk
    - Decreased long term re-stenosis risk
    - Avoidance of technical issues (eg making arteriotomy too tight, catching the backwall)
- Patients with **dense hemiplegia** and **aphasia** are <u>not</u> likely to benefit from ipsilateral CEA (objective of CEA is to prevent further strokes which wouldn't matter for these patients)
- CEA Cx's:
    - Vagus nerve injury - *MC cranial nerve injury with CEA* → secondary to **vascular clamping** during endarterectomy; Sx's - *hoarseness* (recurrent laryngeal nerve [RLN] comes off vagus); vagus lies between internal jugular and carotid; the <u>RLN</u> and <u>superior laryngeal nerve</u> (both branches of the vagus) can also be directly injured
    - Hypoglossal nerve injury - occurs with high carotid dissection (near digastrics - 2 cm above carotid bifurcation); tongue deviates to the side of injury → *speech and mastication difficulty*
    - Glossopharyngeal nerve injury - rare; occurs with really high carotid dissection → causes *difficulty swallowing*
    - Ansa cervicalis (lower root branches; descendens hypoglossi) - innervate to strap muscles; <u>no</u> deficits with ligation (division helps exposure)
    - Marginal mandibular branch of facial nerve - due to retractor at angle of jaw; get a *droop at the corner of mouth*; often recovers in 3 weeks
    - Neurologic event in PACU after CEA (< 12 hours) → <u>*emergently*</u> back to OR to check for intimal flap or thrombosis (intra-op U/S, angio)
    - Neurologic event >12 hours after CEA → head/neck CT angio (look for thromboembolism)
    - Pseudoaneurysm - pulsatile, bleeding mass after CEA (high risk for **rupture**); Tx - drape and prep before intubation, intubate, then repair (avoid this by taking full thickness bites with sutures)
    - HTN - caused by injury to carotid body; Tx: **nipride** to avoid bleeding
    - Cerebral hyperperfusion syndrome (rare) - HTN (all patients) and headache (from brain edema); can get seizures, neuro deficits, and intra-cerebral hemorrhage; due to impaired cerebral auto-regulation MC occurs within days after CEA (mean **5 days**)
        - RF: **tight stenosis** (if the blood flow to the brain more than doubles after CEA or carotid stent the risk is increased)
        - Tx: **BP control** (IV esmolol best); Keppra or Fosphenytoin (seizures)
    - Myocardial infarction - MCC of mortality following CEA

15% re-stenosis rate after CEA:
> **< 2 years** - MC due to **intimal hyperplasia** (can also be due to incomplete CEA at original procedure)
> **> 2 years** - MC due to **recurrent atherosclerosis**
- **Carotid stenting** with cerebral protection device - indicated for *high-risk patients* (eg previous CEA and **restenosis**, inability to tolerate **general anesthesia**, previous **neck XRT**, previous damage to **contra-lateral vocal cord**, previous ipsilateral **neck surgery**)

■ **Vertebrobasilar artery disease** (vertebrobasilar insufficiency)
- Anatomy: the two **vertebral arteries** arise from the **subclavian arteries** and combine to form a single **basilar artery**; the basilar artery then splits into two **posterior cerebral arteries**
- Usually need basilar artery or bilateral vertebral artery stenosis for Sx's
- Causes - atherosclerosis, spurs, bands
- Sx's: diplopia, vertigo, tinnitus, drop attacks, incoordination
- Tx: **PTA with stent**

■ **Carotid body tumors** (benign): Sx's - painless, pulsatile neck mass anterior to SCM muscle (near carotid bifurcation); from neural crest cells (chemoreceptor cells; is a paraganglioma); can secrete **catecholamines** (Sx's - HTN, tachycardia)
- *Are **extremely vascular** (risk of bleeding with surgery) - <u>avoid</u> biopsy*
- Dx: **CT angio** *(best test)*
- Tx: careful **resection** (stay in <u>periadventitial plane</u> to avoid bleeding)

ABDOMINAL AORTIC ANEURYSMS (AAA)

■ Normal aorta 2-3 cm; 90% of AAA's are infra-renal
■ RFs: males, age, smoking, family history
■ MCC - **atherosclerosis**
■ Sx's: usually found **incidentally**; can present with abdominal / back pain, rupture, distal embolization, or compression of adjacent organs
■ **Rupture**
- MCC of death without an operation
- Sx's: lower back or abdominal pain; can have profound hypotension
- RFs for rupture: HTN, COPD (coughing → expansion), greater size, family history, eccentric shape, females
- Dx: **CT angio** *(best test for suspected leak)* - shows **fluid** in retroperitoneal space and **extra-luminal contrast** with rupture
- MC site of rupture - **left posterolateral wall**, 2-4 cm below renals
- **50% mortality** with rupture if patient reaches hospital alive
■ **Repair** indications:
- **≥ 5.5 cm** for average male patient
- **≥ 5.0 cm** for **women** or those with **high rupture risk** (severe COPD, numerous relatives with rupture, poorly controlled HTN, eccentric shape)
- **Growth > 1.0 cm/yr**
- **Symptomatic**
- **Infected** (mycotic)
- **EVAR** *better* than open surgery for the **elderly**, for **high risk** patients (ie multiple co-morbidities), or those with **"hostile" abdomens**
- For **high risk patients**, delay in repair until **5.5 cm** is warranted (non-symptomatic patients), especially if EVAR not an option
■ Tx: usually use **straight tube graft** (Dacron)
- Ligate bleeding lumbar arteries
- **Inferior mesenteric artery re-implantation** criteria (avoids ischemic colitis):
  > **IMA back pressure < 40 mmHg** (poor back-bleeding)
  > Previous **colonic surgery**
  > **SMA stenosis**
  > If **flow to left colon appears inadequate**
- **Internal iliac artery re-implantation** (ie hypogastric artery):
  > If performing aortobifemoral repair and there is **poor back-bleeding** (absence of retrograde flow which indicates poor collaterals) from bilateral internal iliac arteries (hypogastric arteries) → re-implant (or

bypass) at least **one internal iliac artery** (need to ensure flow to at least one internal iliac artery)

This helps avoid **pelvic ischemia** (usually **chronic** issues - buttock claudication [MC Sx], vasculogenic impotence, spinal cord problems, recto-sigmoid ischemia [generally <u>not</u> a full thickness injury - get strictures, pain], over-active bladder, other urinary symptoms)

- **U/S** is the most cost-effective way of **following AAA's** (**annual U/S**; increase frequency to every 3-6 months as they approach repair indications [eg 0.5 cm below repair indication])
  - **Duplex U/S** (color flow) - most cost effective study for <u>*post-op*</u> **AAA repair** (surveillance; estimates blood flow, defines anatomy) and **peripheral bypass grafts**

- **AAA repair Cx's:**
  - **Mortality** - elective <u>*open*</u> repair: **3-4%**; elective <u>*endovascular*</u> repair **1-2%**
  - MCC post-op death (and MCC <u>early</u> death) - **myocardial infarction**
  - MCC <u>late</u> post-op death - **renal failure**
  - RFs for <u>mortality</u>: **creatinine > 1.8** (#1), CHF, EKG ischemia, pulmonary dysfunction, older age, females
  - **Major vein injury** with proximal cross-clamp - <u>*retro*-aortic left renal vein</u> (left renal vein is usually anterior to the aorta)
  - **Impotence** in 30% secondary to disruption of autonomic nerves and blood flow to the pelvis
  - **Graft infection** rate - 1% (MC - *staph epidermidis*)
  - **Pseudoaneurysm** after graft placement - 1%
  - MC late Cx after aortic graft placement - **atherosclerotic occlusion**
  - **Ischemic colitis** - **diarrhea** (especially **bloody**) after AAA repair is worrisome for **ischemic colitis**; can also have **abdominal pain** (usually **left sided**) and **distension**
    - Inferior mesenteric artery (IMA) often sacrificed (open repair) or covered (EVAR) with AAA repair and can cause **ischemia** (MC site - **left colon**)
    - Dx: **colonoscopy** *(best test)* or **CT scan**
      - Middle and distal rectum are <u>spared</u> from ischemia (middle and inferior rectal arteries are branches off the internal iliac artery)
      - Do <u>*not*</u> use proctoscopy - will <u>*not*</u> see the ischemic area
      - Can occasionally involve parts of the colon other than the left side
    - Initial Tx: NPO, NG tube, IVFs, and broad spectrum antibiotics
    - If the patient has **diffuse peritoneal signs**, **unrelenting metabolic acidosis**, **severe sepsis**, **perforation**, or **black colon** (on flexible sigmoidoscopy - indicates necrotic bowel) → **emergency colectomy** is indicated (with colostomy and Hartman's pouch).
  - **Cold foot** after aorto-bifemoral repair (and no femoral pulse) → Tx: return to OR for **groin re-exploration** (patient has a thrombosed graft branch), balloon thrombectomy, and intra-op angiography to figure out the problem (usually requires revision of the distal anastomosis)
  - **Cold foot** after aorto-bifemoral repair in presence of <u>*normal*</u> proximal pulses is most likely due to **atherosclerotic embolic debris** from aneurysm (no good Tx → embolectomy not effective here)
  - **Chylous ascites** - white drainage; high **triacylglycerides** (> 110 mg/dL) and **lymphocytes** (with WBCs > 500)
    - Can also occur following retroperitoneal lymph node dissection
    - Tx: **drainage catheter** (or repeat paracentesis), conservative Tx for 1-2 weeks (same as chylothorax – low fat, high protein diet; NPO, TPN and octreotide if that fails); generally resolves with conservative therapy
    - If that fails, re-op to <u>ligate</u> **cisterna chyli** area (located on **right side** of aorta just <u>*below*</u> the right renal artery)
  - **Late hemorrhage** or **late pseudoaneurysm** (weeks to years) after AAA repair → Dx: **graft infection** (breaks down suture line)

- **Combined AAA** (> 5.5 cm) and **colon CA**
  - Treat the symptomatic issue 1st (eg AAA with back pain, obstructing colon CA)
  - If elective and in the OR, fix what you came to fix and work-up the incidental finding after
  - If both elective and asymptomatic, Tx the colon CA 1st (get the dirty case out of the way before placing a graft) followed by AAA repair in 2-4 weeks
- **EVAR compared to open repair has:**
  - Less peri-op mortality
  - Less ICU LOS
  - Less hospital LOS
  - Earlier return to normal activity
  - More frequent and ongoing hospital reviews
  - More late interventions
  - No improvement in long term mortality (5 years)
- **Criteria for AAA EVAR** (straight tube graft)
  - **Proximal neck** (landing zone) - ≥1.5 cm in length, ≤ 3 cm in diameter
  - **Distal neck** (landing zone) - ≥1.5 cm in length, ≤ 3 cm in diameter
  - The **angle** between the normal aorta above and aneurysm below must be **< 60 degrees** (termed: **angulation < 60 degrees**)
  - Need a **common femoral diameter** (including the distal internal iliac artery) of at least **8 mm** to allow passage of the deployment device (this needs to be larger for larger grafts)
  - _Exclusion criteria_ - ruptured AAA, mycotic aneurysms, unfavorable anatomy
- **Endoleaks:**
  - **Type I endoleak** - leak at **proximal** or **distal graft attachment sites**
    - Tx: re-balloon area; if that fails, you may need to place another graft more proximal or distal to seal the leak
  - **Type II endoleak** _(MC type)_ - retrograde flow from a **collateral branch** into the aneurysm sac (eg lumbar arteries, testicular artery, inferior mesenteric artery)
    - Tx: in general you can watch these for the first 6 months
      - If leak is persistent and the aneurysm sac is getting larger, you need to try and <u>coil embolize</u> the feeding vessel
      - If no change in aneurysm size or smaller, just follow it
  - **Type III endoleak** - leakage between **different parts of stent grafting** (leakage at the **junction** between components)
    - Tx: place another graft across the junction to seal it
  - **Type IV endoleak** - leakage **through stent graft wall**
    - Tx: place another graft inside the original graft
- **Inflammatory aneurysms**
  - Occurs in 10% of patients with AAA; MC in males
  - _Not secondary to infection - is an inflammatory process (is <u>not</u> a mycotic aneurysm)_
  - Rupture risk is the same as non-inflammatory types
  - Sx's: often have **low back** or **abdominal pain**; weight loss
  - Dx: **CT scan** - **thickened aneurysm wall** above calcifications on CT scan
    - Often get **fibrotic adhesions** to 3rd and 4th portions of **duodenum**
      - **Ureters** (causing **hydronephrosis**), **IVC,** and **left renal vein** can also be involved with the fibrosis and adhesions
    - Have an **elevated ESR** (erythrocyte sedimentation rate)
  - Can place pre-operative **ureteral stents** to help avoid injury (don't always work)
  - Tx: _avoid_ trying to free up all of the involved structures (inflammatory process _resolves_ after resection and graft placement)
    - Goal is to repair aneurysm _without_ damaging the involved structures (**left posteriolateral [_retroperitoneal_] approach works well here**)
- **Mycotic aneurysms**
  - _**Staphylococcus #1,** Salmonella #2_
  - Bacteria infect atherosclerotic plaque, causes aneurysm
  - Sx's: abdominal / back pain, fevers, positive blood cultures in 50%
  - Dx: **CT scan** (peri-aortic fluid, gas, soft tissue edema, lymphadenopathy)
  - Tx: **extra-anatomic bypass** (axillary-femoral with femoral to femoral crossover) and resection of aorta to clear infection

- **Aortic graft infections** (tube graft or aortobifemoral graft)
  - Sx's: fever, elevated WBCs
  - **Staph epidermidis #1** (MC <u>overall</u> and MC <u>late</u>), staph aureus #2 (MC <u>early</u> - 1st 2 weeks), E. coli
  - Dx: **CT scan** (oral / IV contrast; see fluid, micro-bubbles, thickening around graft)
  - Blood cultures are negative in many patients
  - Consider **diagnostic CT-guided sample** of fluid if unsure
  - Tx: **extra-anatomic bypass** through non-contaminated field (eg axillary-femoral bypass with femoral to femoral cross-over) and then resect entire infected graft
  - Some are using **aortic homografts** for aortic graft infections (but <u>not</u> used for aorto-enteric fistula – see below)
  - MC in grafts going to the **groin** (eg aortobifemoral grafts)
  - Most sensitive test for Dx of graft infection - **tagged WBC scan** (although not specific; best for <u>late</u> graft infection Dx)
- **Aorto-enteric fistula** (eg aorto-duodenal fistula)
  - Usually occurs **> 6 months** after abdominal aortic surgery
  - Sx's: **hematemesis** (herald bleed), no bleeding interval, blood per rectum, then **exsanguination** *(classic sequence);* EGD for UGI bleeding is often <u>negative</u>
  - MC site - 3rd or 4th portion of **duodenum** (proximal suture line erodes into duodenum leading to **UGI bleed**)
  - Dx: **CT scan** *(best test)* - peri-graft fluid; thickened bowel wall, graft possibly in bowel lumen, inflammatory change *(are generally <u>not</u> found using arteriography)*
  - Tx: **extra-anatomic bypass** through non-contaminated field (eg axillary-femoral bypass with femoral to femoral cross-over), resect graft with aortic stump closure (place omentum over stump), and then close hole in the duodenum
  - Do <u>not</u> use aortic homograft - the same complication will occur again (still have a proximal suture line which can erode into the duodenum)

PERIPHERAL ARTERIAL DISEASE (PAD)
- **Leg compartments**
  - **Anterior** - deep peroneal nerve (dorsiflexion, sensation between 1st and 2nd toes), anterior tibial artery
  - **Lateral** - superficial peroneal nerve (foot eversion, lateral foot sensation)
  - **Deep posterior** - tibial nerve (plantarflexion), posterior tibial artery, peroneal artery
  - **Superficial posterior** - sural nerve
- MCC PAD - **atherosclerosis**
- **Sx's of PAD** - cramping, pain with exercise (ie intermittent claudication), pallor, dependent rubor, hair loss, slow capillary refill, abnormal nail growth
  - **Severe disease →**
    - If leg is **dependent → **rubor (red) + pain relieved
    - If leg is **elevated →** pallor (white) + pain worsens (blood flow can't be sustained against gravity)
- **Claudication → medical Tx 1st**: smoking cessation *(best Tx),* ASA (helps prevent cardiovascular events), exercise until pain occurs to improve collaterals; cholesterol / HTN / DM management
  - 5-year <u>amputation</u> risk: **1-3%**
  - 5-year need for <u>revascularization</u> risk: **15%**
  - 5-year <u>survival</u>: **70%** (MCC death - myocardial infarction)
  - Increased risk of **cardiovascular events** (MI, stroke, sudden death)
    - Need to be on **ASA or Plavix**
- **Collateral circulation** - forms from abnormal pressure gradients
  - Circumflex iliac arteries to subcostal arteries
  - Circumflex femoral arteries to gluteal arteries
  - **Geniculate arteries** around the knee
- **Leriche syndrome** (need all 3):
    - 1) **No femoral pulses**
    - 2) **Buttock or thigh claudication**
    - 3) **Impotence** (from decreased flow to the internal iliacs)
  - Lesion at aortic bifurcation or above
  - Tx: **aortobifemoral bypass graft**

- MC atherosclerotic occlusion in lower extremities - **Hunter's canal** (distal superficial femoral artery exits here; just above posterior knee); **sartorius muscle** covers Hunter's canal
- **Ankle-brachial index** (ABI - normal is 1.0-1.2)
  - **< 0.9** - start to get **claudication** (typically at same distance each time)
  - **< 0.5** - start to get **rest pain** (usually calf and distal arch of foot)
  - **< 0.4** - **ulcers** (usually starts in toes)
  - **< 0.3** - **gangrene** (usually starts in toes)
  - ABIs can be inaccurate (artificially high) with **diabetes** or **ESRD** due to calcification and incompressibility of vessels; often have to go off **Duplex U/S** (see below), **transcutaneous oximetry** (TCOM < 20 mmHg indicates poor perfusion), and/or **toe pressures** (toe-brachial index; digital arteries are spared from calcification)
  - ABIs based on **return of systolic blood pressure** after application of a blood pressure cuff
  - Ankle pressure can be higher than brachial pressure (ABI > 1)
- **Pulse volume recordings** (PVRs) uses _both_:
  - 1) **Blood pressure cuffs** - used to find **pulse volumes** at the thigh, calf, and ankle levels in the limb; appears as a **waveform** (dampened waveform indicates stenosis)
  - 2) **Duplex U/S** - measures **flow velocities** at each level in the limb, _higher velocity_ means more _significant_ **blockage**
  - Both used to find significant **obstructions** (occlusions) and describe what **level**
- **Arteriogram** is indicated if PVRs and/or ABIs suggest significant disease; can also at times perform **PTA** and **stent**; gold standard in vascular imaging
- **Revascularization indications** for PAD - significant **lifestyle limitation** despite maximal medical Tx, **rest pain** (implies threatened limb, ie ABI < 0.5), or **tissue loss** (eg non-healing ulcers, limb salvage)
  - Get **arteriogram**
  - Fix the most **proximal problem 1st**
  - PTFE (Gortex) - _only_ for bypasses **above the knee** _(PTFE has reduced patency below the knee)_
  - **Reversed saphenous vein graft** - needed for bypasses **below knee**
  - **Dacron** (polyester fiber) - good for aorta and large vessels
  - **Aortoiliac occlusive disease** - most get aortobifemoral graft repair (ABF)
    - Need to ensure flow to at least **1 internal iliac artery** (hypogastric artery); want to see **good back-bleeding** from at least 1 of these arteries, otherwise need a bypass to an internal iliac artery when performing aorto-bifemoral repair to prevent **vasculogenic impotence** and **pelvic ischemia**
  - **Isolated iliac lesions** - PTA and stent 1st choice; if that fails consider **femoral-to-femoral** crossover graft (eg chronically occluded common iliac stenosis in a patient with severe COPD)
  - **Femoro-popliteal grafts**
    - 75% 5-year patency
    - Improved patency rate with surgery for claudication as opposed to limb salvage
  - **Femoral-distal grafts** (peroneal, anterior tibial, or posterior tibial artery)
    - 50% 5-year patency; patency not influenced by level of distal anastomosis
    - Distal lesions more limb threatening because of lack of collaterals
    - Bypasses to **distal vessels** are usually used _only_ for **limb** or **tissue salvage** (eg non-healing ulcer)
    - Bypassed vessel needs to have **run-off below the ankle** (ie target native vessel needs to go past the ankle joint) for this to be successful
  - **Extra-anatomic grafts** (eg axillary to femoral bypass) can be used to avoid hostile conditions in abdomen (eg multiple previous operations in a frail patient)
  - **Femoral-to-femoral crossover graft** - doubles blood flow to donor artery; can get **vascular steal** in _donor_ leg if there is a proximal stenosis (eg iliac stenosis) in the _donor_ leg

- **Swelling** following lower extremity bypass:
  - *Early* (< 24-48 hours) - edema from **reperfusion injury** and **compartment syndrome** (Tx: **fasciotomies** if compartment syndrome)
  - *Intermediate* (3-7 days) - **DVT** (Dx: U/S, Tx: **heparin**)
  - *Late* (> 7 days) - **lymphedema** (Tx: **compression stockings**; *get U/S to rule-out DVT as it can present with Sx's late*)
- Cx's of <u>reperfusion of ischemic tissue</u> - **reperfusion injury** (can lead to **compartment syndrome**), **lactic acidosis, hyperkalemia, myoglobinuria**

- **MCC of <u>failure</u> of reversed saphenous vein grafts →**
  - **Early** (< 30 days) - **technical problem**
  - **Intermediate** (30 days to 2 years) - **intimal hyperplasia**
  - **Late** (> 2 years) - **vein atherosclerosis**
- Best predictor of long term patency - **vein quality**
- Best medical Tx for vein graft <u>patency</u> and <u>decreasing cardiovascular events</u> - **ASA**
- Best technique for <u>graft surveillance</u> (aortic or peripheral bypass graft) - **duplex U/S**
  - RFs for <u>graft occlusion</u> on surveillance (*indications for <u>intervention</u>*):
    Peak systolic velocity (PSV) > 300 cm/s
    PSV ratio > 3.5 across the stenosis
    End diastolic velocity > 20 cm/s
    > 70% diameter reduction confirmed on angiography
- **Late hemorrhage** or **pseudoaneurysm** after aortic or lower extremity bypass graft (weeks to years) - most likely **graft infection** eroding into the suture line (Tx: **resect graft**; bypass through non-contaminated plane)
- MCC graft infection - ***staph epidermidis*** (<u>overall</u> and <u>late</u>)
- MCC <u>early</u> graft infection (1st 2 weeks) - ***staph aureus***
- Most sensitive test for graft infection - **tagged WBC scan**
- **Percutaneous transluminal angioplasty** (PTA)
  - Excellent for common iliac artery stenosis (also place stent)
  - Best for short stenoses
  - Intima usually ruptured and media stretched, pushes the plaque out
  - Requires passage of wire first
  - **PTA + covered stents** increasingly used for lower extremity stenoses
- **Isolated Iliac stenosis Tx - PTA** and **stent** (Tx of choice, 80% 5-year patency)
- **Chronic common iliac artery occlusion** (ie can't stent) in a patient with severe co-morbidities (eg **severe COPD**) - Tx: **femoral to femoral bypass** (fem-fem cross-over)

COMPARTMENT SYNDROME
- Is caused by a **reperfusion injury** to the extremity (occurs with cessation of blood flow and reperfusion > 4-6 hours later)
- Leads to **swelling of muscle compartments** → raises compartment pressures and can lead to **ischemia**
- Is mediated by **neutrophils** (PMNs)
- Sx's: **pain with passive motion** (*1st Sx*), extremity feels **tight** and **swollen** (loss of pulse is a <u>late</u> finding)
- Causes - prolonged OR time for lower extremity bypass; peripheral emboli or thrombosis after restoration of blood flow; trauma (see Trauma chapter)
- For lower extremity, is most likely to occur in **anterior leg compartment** (foot-drop)
- Dx: often based on clinical suspicion; compartment pressure **> 20-25 mmHg** abnormal
- Tx: **fasciotomies** (medial and lateral incisions if lower extremity to get all 4 compartments); leave open 5-10 days; (skin graft after that)
- Can injure **superficial peroneal nerve** with **lateral incision** of lower extremity fasciotomy (MC injured nerve with lower extremity fasciotomy); injury causes decreased foot eversion
- Early post femoral-tibial arterial bypass pain and swelling → Dx: **reperfusion injury**

DIABETIC FOOT ULCERS
- Diabetics can't feel feet (neuropathy), get **plantar ulcers** at pressure areas
- Usually at **toes, metatarsal heads** (MC - 2nd MTP joint), and **heel**

- **Dry gangrene** (non-infectious)
  - See if patient has correctable **vascular lesion**
  - Tx: non-weight bearing, possible antibiotics if cellulitis
  - Can allow to autoamputate if small or just toes
  - Large lesions should be amputated
- **Wet gangrene** (infectious; surrounding erythema [cellulitis], purulence)
  - **Wound Bx** - *best test for organisms*
  - **MRI** - *most accurate test for osteomyelitis*; use bone scan if patient has hardware (eg pacemaker)
  - *Bone Bx is not recommended as this predisposes patients to future osteomyelitis at the Bx site (20% risk)*
  - Tx: early debridement of infected material, keep moist, leg elevation, non-weight bearing, antibiotics (6 weeks if osteomyelitis; may also need bone debridement)
  - *Is a **surgical emergency** if:* 1) **extensive infection** present (eg swollen red toe with pus coming out and red streaks up leg → Tx: ray amputation) *or:* 2) **systemic Cx's** occur (eg septic shock) → *need **emergency amputation** at appropriate level (can be life-saving)*
- **Malperforans ulcer**
  - Older term for plantar ulcers
  - Often associated with **osteomyelitis**
  - Tx: as above but also need **cartilage debridement** of metatarsal head if cartilage is exposed or osteomyelitis is present

AMPUTATIONS

- For extensive gangrene, large non-healing ulcers, or unrelenting rest pain not amenable to surgery
- 50% mortality within 3 years for leg amputation
- **BKA** - 80% heal, 70% walk again, 5-10% peri-op mortality
- **AKA** - 90% heal, 30% walk again, 10-15% peri-op mortality
- Emergency amputation for **extensive infection** or **systemic Cx's** (consider guillotine amputation with staged stump closure)
- Predictors of **healing** following lower extremity amputation:
  - Transcutaneous oxygen measurement (TCOM) **> 40 mmHg** at level of amputation (98% heal)
  - Presence of a **proximal pulse** (eg popliteal pulse, femoral pulse)
- TCOM **< 20 mmHg** - *poor healing rate (most fail)*

ACUTE ARTERIAL EMBOLI

- Often have history of **arrhythmia**; more common than arterial thrombosis
- Patients with emboli usually do not have collaterals, Sx's of chronic limb ischemia, or history of claudication
- Contralateral extremity usually has **normal pulses** (no chronic ischemia)
- Sx's of **extremity ischemia**: pain (MC), paresthesias, paralysis, pallor (white), poikilothermia (cold), pulseless
- Ischemia evolution: **pallor** (white) → **cyanosis** (blue) → **marbling**
- MC source - **heart** (atrial fibrillation (MC); recent MI with left ventricular thrombus, endocarditis, atrial myxoma); #2 aortic atheromatous material (eg recent cardiac catheterization knocks atheromatous material off aorta)
- MC obstruction site for heart embolus - **common femoral artery** (lower extremity gets 70% of heart emboli)
- MC upper extremity site for heart embolus - **brachial artery**
- 10% of heart emboli go to cerebral circulation
- Tx: *open embolectomy* in OR usual; get pulses back, then get intra-op angiogram
  - Consider fasciotomy if ischemia > 4-6 hours
  - Emboli to **aortoiliac bifurcation** (loss of *both* femoral pulses) best treated with bilateral femoral artery cut-downs and bilateral transfemoral *retrograde* embolectomies
  - Acute lower extremity arterial emboli with intact femoral pulse and intact motor / sensation - Tx: **thrombolytics**, heparin

Clinical Distinctions Between
Acute Arterial Embolism and Acute Arterial Thrombosis

Embolism	Thrombosis
Often arrhythmia	Usually no arrhythmia
No prior claudication or rest pain	History of claudication or rest pain
Normal contralateral pulses	Contralateral pulses absent
No physical findings of chronic limb ischemia	Physical findings of chronic limb ischemia (no hair, shiny surface)

ACUTE ARTERIAL THROMBOSIS
- These patients usually do not have arrhythmias; vast majority involves lower extremity
- Most often caused by underlying **chronic PAD** (eg history of claudication, poor pulses in the contralateral leg)
- Often have collaterals and are less likely to have a threatened extremity
- **Threatened limb** (ie loss of sensation or motor function)
  - Tx: go to OR for **open thrombectomy** (safest answer)
- **Limb not threatened** (ie intact motor function and sensation)
  - Tx: go to angiography for **catheter-directed thrombolytics** and/or percutaneous mechanical thrombectomy (eg AngioJet)
  - Mild Sx's (good collateral perfusion) - can consider heparin only
- Thrombosis of **lower extremity graft** (PTFE or vein) → thrombolytics and anticoagulation; if limb threatened → OR for thrombectomy
- Thrombolytics are usually given proximal to or directly into the clot
- Should have a **femoral pulse** before starting thrombolytics for thrombosis - otherwise need open thrombectomy
- **Infants** with loss of femoral pulse and cold foot after a-line or catheterization – technically very hard to operate on femoral artery in an infant and generally thrombosis does not result in limb threatening ischemia; best Tx - **heparin** (non-surgical)

LYTIC THERAPY VS OPEN EMBOLECTOMY / THROMBECTOMY
- Issue most commonly occurs for **lower extremity** ischemia
- **Intact motor function** and **sensation**
  - Most likely has a **distal** clot (eg trifurcation vessels)
  - *Best Tx* - catheter directed **intra-arterial thrombolysis** (tPA + Heparin); infuse through catheter inside clot, run 8-12 hrs, repeat angio (can run for 24-48 hours)
  - Thrombolytics are better here because its **difficult to perform embolectomy for the trifurcation vessels** and more effective to lyse clot with tPA
  - Some are using **percutaneous mechanical thrombectomy** (eg AngioJet) in addition to thrombolytics
  - If **worsening exam** while infusing → OR for embolectomy
  - *Contraindications* – common femoral artery or more proximal clot (ie should be able to feel a femoral pulse before starting tPA)
- **Loss of motor function** or **sensation**
  - Most likely has a more **proximal** clot → *leg is threatened*
  - *Best Tx* - OR for **cut-down** and **open balloon catheter embolectomy**
    Consider fasciotomy if ischemia > 4-6 hrs
  - Also indicated for known common femoral or more proximal clot
  - Thrombolysis would take too long and is less likely to work
  - *Loss of femoral pulse → need open embolectomy*

ATHEROMA EMBOLISM
- Cholesterol clefts that can lodge in small arteries
- MC site of embolization - **renal arteries**
- MC source - **aortoiliac disease**
- **Blue toe syndrome** - flaking of atherosclerotic emboli off aorta or branches
- Patients typically have good distal pulses
- Dx: **CT scan** (chest / abdomen / pelvis; look for source) and **ECHO** (clot or myxoma in heart)
- Tx: may need aneurysm repair or arterial exclusion with bypass

RENAL ARTERY STENOSIS
- Usually caused by **atherosclerosis**
- Can cause HTN and chronic kidney disease
- *No benefit to renal artery stenting compared to comprehensive medical Tx for atherosclerotic renal artery stenosis*
- Fibromuscular dysplasia likely still benefits from PTA

UPPER EXTREMITY
- **Occlusive disease** - proximal lesions usually *asymptomatic* due to **collaterals**
- MC site of upper extremity stenosis - **subclavian artery** (usually asymptomatic)
- **Subclavian steal syndrome**
  - Tight proximal subclavian artery stenosis can result in **reversal of flow** through the **ipsilateral vertebral artery** into the distal subclavian artery
  - Sx's: syncope, vertigo, falls, ocular issues (all vertebrobasilar); arm pain *(rare)*
  - MC Sx's - vertebrobasilar
  - Dx: angiogram
  - Tx: **PTA and covered stent** of subclavian artery stenosis *(best Tx)*; common carotid to subclavian bypass if that fails
  - Subclavian steal can also occur in patients with **previous CABG** with left internal mammary artery to left anterior descending anastomosis (the internal mammary arteries come off the subclavian arteries). Blood is taken away from the heart, causing **angina**. Tx: **subclavian stent**
  - Vascular steal can also occur in patients with **femoral to femoral cross-over grafts** who have **proximal stenosis** in the *donor* artery (eg proximal iliac stenosis in the donor leg); Tx: **PTA and stent**
- **Motor function** can remain in **digits** after prolonged **hand ischemia** because motor groups are in the proximal forearm

MESENTERIC ISCHEMIA
- Overall mortality **60%**; usually involves **superior mesenteric artery** (SMA)
- **CT scan findings** suggestive of intestinal ischemia - vascular occlusion (eg SMA occlusion), small bowel wall thickening, intramural gas (pneumatosis intestinalis), portal venous gas

- Causes of **visceral ischemia**:
  - **Embolic** occlusion (MC) - 50% (MC source - heart)
  - **Thrombotic** occlusion - 25%
  - **Non-occlusive** - 20%
  - **Venous** thrombosis - 5%

- **SMA embolism**
  - MC lodges near **origin of SMA** - heart #1 source (**atrial fibrillation**)
  - Sx's: sudden **abdominal pain out of proportion to exam** *(hallmark)*; hematochezia and peritoneal signs are late findings
  - May have a history of atrial fibrillation, endocarditis, recent MI, or recent angiography
  - Dx: **CT angio** *(usually quicker and rules out other conditions)*; will see a 'meniscus sign' 2-4 cm from SMA origin; formal angiogram *(most definitive test but takes too long)*
  - Tx: *open embolectomy* (standard); resect infarcted (black) bowel
  - **SMA exposure** - divide ligament of Treitz, SMA is to the right of this near the base of the transverse colon mesentery
  - At operation *various degrees of ischemia* are encountered (eg pallor, cyanosis, mottling)
    - Best 1<u>st</u> step is to **restore arterial perfusion** and then **re-assess bowel** before resection
    - Resect obvious necrotic areas (black)
    - *Leave bowel of questionable viability (borderline bowel) with a **second-look operation** after 24-48 hours to re-assess bowel (best)*

- **SMA thrombosis**
  - Often history of chronic problems (Sx's: pain with eating, **food fear**, weight loss)
  - MCC - **atherosclerosis** (often have chronic Sx's of PAD)
  - Sx's: similar to embolism; may have developed collaterals *(less severe Sx's)*
  - Dx: **CT angio** *(quicker, rules out other conditions);* formal angiogram *(most definitive test)*
    - MC have occlusion at **origin** of SMA (**flush occlusion**); atherosclerotic disease in the celiac and inferior mesenteric artery is often present
  - Tx: **thrombectomy** (open <u>or</u> catheter-directed thrombolytics / mechanical thrombectomy); likely need **PTA + covered stent** or **open bypass** after the vessel is opened for any residual stenosis; resection of infarcted bowel if needed
- **Mesenteric vein thrombosis**
  - Usually **short segments** of intestine involved although entire superior mesenteric vein can be thrombosed
  - Sx's: bloody diarrhea, abdominal pain; usually presents subacutely (eg several days of pain)
  - RFs: hypercoagulable state (eg polycythemia vera, protein S deficiency), portal HTN
  - Dx: **CT angio** or angiogram with <u>venous phase</u> contrast (thickened bowel, lack of contrast opacification in superior mesenteric vein, delayed filling of portal vein)
  - Tx: **heparin only** *(no thrombolytics)*; resection of infarcted bowel if present
- **Non-occlusive mesenteric ischemia** (NOMI)
  - Any form of **shock, hypovolemia,** or **pressors** → final common pathway is **low cardiac output** to visceral vessels; also caused by **hypoxia**
  - RFs: prolonged hypotension, CHF, prolonged cardiopulmonary bypass, patients on pressors, medical ICU patients, COPD
  - Sx's: abdominal pain (LLQ) and diarrhea (can be non-bloody)
  - Dx: CT angio or angiogram (shows constricted vessels)
  - Watershed areas: **left colon** most vulnerable (<u>Griffith's</u> point - splenic flexure; <u>Sudak's</u> point - upper rectum)
  - Tx: *volume resuscitation* and *antibiotics (<u>best</u> initial Tx)* - *optimize C.O.*
    - Laparotomy if diffuse peritoneal signs are present (eg rebound tenderness, involuntary guarding)
    - Consider **catheter-directed papaverine** (increases visceral blood flow, give heparin while catheter is in, good temporizing measure)
    - If due to **CHF** - start **Dobutamine** *(best Tx for CHF, <u>not</u> more volume)*

VISCERAL AND PERIPHERAL ANEURYSMS
- **Rupture** - MC Cx of aneurysms <u>above</u> inguinal ligament
- **Emboli** (MC) and **thrombosis** - MC Cx's of aneurysms <u>below</u> inguinal ligament
- **Visceral artery aneurysms** (splanchnic artery aneurysms)
  - RFs: medial fibrodysplasia, portal HTN, pregnancy, arterial disruption secondary to inflammatory disease (eg pancreatitis)
  - Repair <u>all</u> **splanchnic artery aneurysms** (**> 2 cm** need repair; eg hepatic artery, left gastric artery, SMA) when diagnosed (these have a **50%** rupture risk) <u>except</u> **splenic** (< 2% rupture risk, see below)
  - Tx: **covered stent** and **coil embolization** *(preferred);* if that fails need exclusion with bypass or possibly just exclusion if it is a well collateralized vessel (eg left gastric artery)
- **Splenic artery aneurysms** - *MC visceral artery aneurysm*
  - MC in **women**
  - Overall 1-2% risk of rupture *(much lower than other visceral aneurysms)*
  - Indications for repair:
    - **Symptomatic**
    - Patient is **pregnant**
    - Occurs in **women of childbearing age**
    - Size **> 3-4 cm** (high rupture risk)
  - High rate of *pregnancy-related rupture (up to 70%; MC in 3rd trimester)*
  - Tx: endovascular repair with **covered stent** and **coil embolization** *(best Tx)*
    - Can also perform simple laparoscopic **exclusion** (proximal and distal ligation) if in the proximal or middle 1/3 of the splenic artery

> *Do not need splenectomy with these techniques (lots of collaterals around the spleen)*

- **Hilar** splenic artery aneurysms
  - Can be hard to Tx with endovascular techniques
    - Tx: **laparoscopic exclusion** (*without* splenectomy; spleen has good collaterals); get proximal control of the splenic artery 1st
    - If both endovascular and laparoscopic Tx are not possible, splenectomy is indicated.
- **Renal** artery aneurysm (> 1.5 cm need repair) - Tx: **covered stent**
- **Common iliac** (> 3.0 cm need repair) or **common femoral** (> 2.5 cm need repair) artery aneurysms
  - Usually associated with **AAA's**
  - Tx: **covered stent** if isolated
- **Popliteal artery aneurysm**
  - *MC peripheral aneurysm*
  - MCC - **atherosclerosis**
  - Males 50-60's; smokers
  - Leg exam reveals prominent popliteal pulses
  - 50% are **bilateral**
  - 50% have **another aneurysm** elsewhere (MC - AAA)
  - Sx's: most likely to get **thrombosis** (MC) with **limb ischemia** or **emboli**
    - *Rarely rupture*
    - Can also get leg pain from **compression** of adjacent structures (rare)
    - Can present with an **acutely cold lower extremity** from thrombosis
  - Dx: **Duplex U/S** (formal angiogram may miss these due to intramural thrombus although is useful for operative planning)
  - **Indications for surgery**:
    - **> 2 cm**
    - **Symptomatic**
    - **Mycotic**
    - Evidence of previous **distal embolization**
    - Presence of **intramural thrombus**
  - Tx: **exclusion and bypass** for *all* popliteal artery aneurysms (use saphenous vein; arterial ligation proximal and distal to aneurysm)
    - 25% have complication that requires amputation if not treated
    - *Covered stent not recommended for these*
    - Patients with **compressive Sx's** (*uncommon*; eg paresthesias, venous congestion) → perform **aneurysmorrhaphy with interposition graft** (geniculate collaterals can continue to fill aneurysm sac and causes Sx's if just exclusion and bypass is performed)
    - **Acute thrombosis** - catheter-directed **thrombolytics** usual (usually involves trifurcation vessels so open thrombectomy generally not effective); definitive surgery that admission

POPLITEAL ENTRAPMENT SYNDROME
- Sx's: mild **intermittent claudication** in a young patient; often **bilateral**
- Men in 20-30's; *loss of pulses with plantar flexion*
- Dx: **CT angio**
- MCC - medial deviation of popliteal artery around medial head of **gastrocnemius muscle**; others - fibrous bands, enlarged popliteus muscle
- Tx: **resection of medial head of gastrocnemius muscle**; may need arterial reconstruction with saphenous vein graft

CYSTIC ADVENTITIAL DISEASE
- Sx's: **intermittent claudication**; changes in Sx's with *knee flexion-extension*
- Men in 30-50's
- MC area - **popliteal fossa**; occurs in peripheral vessels in proximity of a **joint**
- Dx: **CT angio** ('scimitar sign' - compression of artery by cyst)
- Has **synovial fluid** (mucin); originates from artery **adventitia**
- Tx: **resection of cyst**; vein graft if the vessel is occluded or badly damaged

PSEUDOANEURYSM

- Collection of blood in continuity with the arterial system but <u>not</u> enclosed by all 3 layers of the arterial wall
- MC location - **femoral artery**
- Sx's: groin or leg **pain, swelling,** and/or **bleeding**; erythema if due to infection
- Dx: **Duplex U/S** *(best test)*
- 2 main causes:
    1) **Percutaneous interventions**
    2) **Disruption of a suture line** between graft and artery
- Tx:
    1) If from **percutaneous intervention** → Tx *U/S guided thrombin injection (best Tx)*; need *urgent open repair* if acutely expanding, nerve compression, compromising skin, or failure of conservative Tx (RFs for needing open repair: > 2 cm or on anticoagulation)
    2) If from **disrupted suture line with** <u>recent</u> **bypass** (eg technical error, not getting full thickness bites) → Tx: *emergent operative repair* (can have massive blood loss if this bursts)
    3) <u>Late</u> **pseudoaneurysm** (weeks to years) after bypass graft is MC related to **infection** and suture line breakdown (can have <u>bleeding</u>) → Tx: *complete resection of graft* and bypass through a non-contaminated field
    4) Femoral artery pseudoaneurysm in **IV drug abuser** → Tx: *ligation <u>without</u> reconstruction* (is generally tolerated without need for amputation, even with ligating the **common femoral artery**; collaterals around the hip supply the leg)

BUERGERS DISEASE (thromboangiitis obliterans)

- Young men, **smokers**; can also occur with smokeless **tobacco**
- Sx's: severe **rest pain** with bilateral **ulceration** and **gangrene of digits** (especially fingers)
- Criteria *(need all 5)*:
    - **Age < 45 years**
    - Current (or recent) history of **tobacco** use
    - Distal extremity **ischemia** (claudication, rest pain, ulcers, gangrene)
    - Consistent **angiogram findings** (see below)
    - ***Exclusion*** of autoimmune disease, hypercoagulable state, diabetes mellitus, and proximal source for emboli (Dx: echocardiography, CT angio)
- Dx: **angiogram**
    1) **Corkscrew collaterals** with severe <u>distal</u> disease *and:*
    2) **Normal arterial tree proximal** to popliteal / brachial arteries (ie is a <u>small vessel</u> disease)
- Tx: stop tobacco or will require continued amputations

FIBROMUSCULAR DYSPLASIA (FMD)

- Young white women usual; 50% have **bilateral** lesions; risk of **cerebral aneurysms**
- Sx's: **HTN** (renal artery **stenosis**); **headaches / stroke** (carotid); **claudication** (iliac)
- MC variant - **medial** type fibrodysplasia (85%)
- MC involved vessels - **renal arteries** (MC - right); then **carotid**, iliac, and SMA
- Causes **stenosis**, usually more <u>distal</u> then atherosclerosis
- Dx: **angiogram** *(best test for Dx)* - 'string of beads' appearance (alternating areas of stenosis and dilation)
- Tx: **PTA** <u>only</u> (percutaneous transluminal angioplasty, *best Tx*), open bypass if it fails
    - <u>No</u> endarterectomy
    - Stents <u>not</u> needed

TEMPORAL ARTERITIS

- A **giant cell arteritis** (medium-large vessels; aortic arch + branches including carotids)
- Older white women usual (70's); RF - polymyalgia rheumatica
- Sx's: **headache**, temple tenderness, fever, malaise, visual changes, jaw pain
- ***Blindness*** can occur
- Dx: **temporal artery biopsy** *(best test*; get 2 cm) - shows giant cells
- Tx: *immediate* **corticosteroids** *(can save vision)*

TAKAYASU'S ARTERITIS
- **Granulomatous vasculitis** with _massive_ intimal fibrosis and vascular **narrowing**
- MC involves **aortic arch** and it's **branches** (also pulmonary artery and coronaries)
- Usually in young Asian women (20-30's)
- Sx's: can have antecedent **inflammatory** phase (fever, malaise, elevated ESR) followed by **pulseless phase** (_pulseless_ upper extremities, neuro Sx's [light headedness, seizures, syncope], claudication, angina, abdominal pain)
- Can have **HTN** if the renal arteries are involved
- Dx: **CT angio** (tends to affect **midportions** of vessel); _elevated_ **ESR**
- Tx: **corticosteroids** (immunosuppression if that fails [methotrexate or mycophenolate])
    - Surgery (arterial bypass) _only_ for advanced disease that has failed medical Tx (preferably when inflammation subsides and used for residual fibrosis)
    - _No_ role for endarterectomy or PTA (ineffective)

RAYNAUD'S DISEASE
- Young women; pulses are **normal** (is a small vessel vasospasm disease)
- Progression: pallor (white) → cyanosis (blue) → rubor (red)
- Rubor is **reactive hyperemia**
- Can be precipitated by cold, anxiety, tobacco
- Tx: avoidance of cold; **diltiazem**

ACQUIRED AV FISTULA
- Usually the result of **trauma** (eg GSW)
- Sx's: **arterial insufficiency** (MC; eg claudication)
    - **CHF** (high output cardiac failure due to shunt)
        - Sx's - pulmonary edema, fatigue, tachycardia, left ventricular hypertrophy
        - High heart rate _decreases_ with shunt compression (Branham's sign)
    - **Aneurysm** (dilation of proximal artery)
    - **Limb-length discrepancy**
    - **Low diastolic blood pressure** and **venous hypertension**
- Dx: **Duplex U/S** (best test); may feel **thrill** or hear **bruit** over the area
- Tx: **open repair** → **lateral venous suture**; patch arterial side (may need bypass graft), interpose muscle (eg sartorius muscle if in leg) or tissue between artery and vein so that it does not recur

DIALYSIS ACCESS FISTULAS AND AV GRAFTS
- _Always try and start with a Cimino fistula for dialysis_
- **Cimino fistula** - radial artery to cephalic vein (vein should be ≥ 2.5 mm)
    - Wait **6 weeks** before using → allows run-off veins to mature
    - The cephalic vein is lateral to the radial artery (supine arm)
    - Cx's: sore thumb (venous hypertension); superficial radial nerve injury (MC)
- **Interposition AV graft** (eg brachio-cephalic forearm loop graft)
    - Wait **6 weeks** before using to allow fibrous scar to form (allows percutaneous access without formation of hematoma and potential graft loss)
- MCC of **AV graft** or **fistula** failure overall - **venous obstruction** secondary to **venous intimal hyperplasia**
    - MCC early failure - **technical problem**
    - MCC late failure - **venous intimal hyperplasia**
- **Early thrombosis** after AV graft placement
    - Dx and Tx - de-clot and get fistulogram in OR to figure out the problem; usually a technical issue at venous anastomosis
- **Hand swelling** after AV graft placement
    - Results from **venous HTN**
    - Tx: elevation; generally improves as venous collaterals form
    - If **persistent** or **severe** (eg massive swelling, skin breakdown) it suggests major **venous outflow obstruction** (eg axillary, subclavian, or cephalic vein) →
        - Dx: **fistulogram** with shunt run-off (venogram)
        - Tx: **PTA** of venous stenosis (best Tx)

- Hand **ischemia** after AV graft placement (DASS - dialysis access steal syndrome)
  - Pre-op RF: **digital : brachial index < 0.6** (high risk)
  - **AV grafts** much more at risk than AV fistulas
  - **Mild ischemia** - coolness / numbness / pain with HD - usually reverses (few weeks)
  - **Severe ischemia** usually occurs with upper arm grafts
    - Sx's: pallor, cyanosis, then mottling *immediately* after surgery
    - Associated with **arterial obstruction** (inflow obstruction) proximal to graft (eg subclavian artery stenosis)
    - Tx: acutely can just **band the venous end** of the graft and get an **arterial angiogram** of upper extremity to check for an inflow problem (can ligate the graft if banding does not relieve ischemia)
    - Tx for inflow problem: **PTA and stent** usual (eg subclavian artery stent)
  - **Chronic DASS** (chronic Sx's when getting dialysis) Tx options:
    - *Rule-out inflow problem* - formal arterial angiogram of upper extremity
    - <u>DRIL</u> - distal revascularization (towards hand using a graft) and interval ligation of the artery just distal to the AV graft but proximal to the bypass graft distal anastomosis; fairly aggressive and risky procedure designed to preserve the AV graft
    - <u>RUDI</u> - revision using distal inflow (inflow is placed more distally)
    - <u>PAI</u> - proximal arterial inflow construction (PTA and stent or bypass)
    - <u>Banding</u> venous end of the graft
- **Late venous outflow obstruction** - high returning line (outflow) pressure (> 200) or an increase in re-circulation *(all signs of venous outflow problem and impending graft failure)*
  - Dx: **fistulogram** with shunt run-off to find the obstruction
  - Tx: PTA of venous outflow obstruction (may need to redo venous anastomosis if intimal hyperplasia is the problem)

PRIMARY VENOUS INSUFFICIENCY
- Sx's: edema, ulceration, varicosities, heaviness, bleeding, thrombophlebitis
  - **Brawny edema** - suggests severe disease, occurs from **high capillary venous pressure** and leakage of RBCs that eventually get destroyed with **hemosiderin** deposition (**brown appearance**)
  - **Ulceration** occurs above and posterior to **medial malleoli**
  - Elevation brings relief
- RFs: obesity, low activity or prolonged standing, smoking
- Dx: **Duplex U/S** *(best Dx study)* with patient standing, looking for:
    1) Incompetent **sapheno-femoral valve** - Dx made if relief of muscle pressure proximally (eg thigh) causes retrograde flow in vein
    2) Incompetent **perforator veins**
    3) **DVT** - need to make sure patient does <u>not</u> have a DVT *(DVT is a contraindication to vein stripping and avulsion)*
    4) An incometent **deep system** (ie femoral, popliteal, and trifurcation veins; majority of patients)
  - U/S gives **location, vein size,** and **direction of blood flow**
  - **Normal** venous Duplex U/S - augmentation of antegrade flow (towards the heart) with distal compression (eg calf) or release of proximal compression (eg thigh)
  - <u>Normally</u>, **perforating veins** direct blood from the superficial system to the deep system (the calf muscle pump forces blood into the deep system with walking)
- **Medical Tx 1st** (aimed at **reducing venous hypertension**) - **compression dressings, pentoxifylline**, avoid long standing, weight loss, stop smoking, elevate legs
  - Ulcers < 3 cm usually heal with medical Tx (*Best Tx* - **compressive dressings** [eg **Unna boot**])
- **Surgical Tx** (for failure of medical Tx):
  - < 10% of patients are candidates for surgery (majority have deep venous incompetence)
  - Fundamentals of surgery - **ablation of reflux source** (escape point)
  - Small varicosities **< 1 mm** (eg varicose veins) - Tx: **sclerotherapy**

- Chronic **ulcers**, varicosities **> 4 mm**, or chronic venous insufficiency
    1) If sapheno-femoral valve is <u>competent</u> (ie just have **incompetent perforators**) → *Tx: subfascial endoscopic perforator surgery* (SEPS; ligates perforators, *preferred Tx;* fewer wound Cx's compared to stab avulsion removal of varicosities)
    2) If sapheno-femoral valve is <u>not competent</u> (ie **reflux along entire greater saphenous vein**) → *Tx: greater saphenous vein stripping*
- *Contraindications* to vein stripping and SEPS - **DVT**, venous outflow obstruction, pregnancy (varicosities go away after delivery)

THROMBOPHLEBITIS
- **Superficial thrombophlebitis** - nonbacterial inflammation of superficial vein
    - Sx's: palpable and tender hard **cord**; pain and erythema
    - RFs: peripheral IV, trauma
    - Tx: remove IV; **NSAIDs** and **warm packs**; elevation of extremity
- **Suppurative thrombophlebitis** - same as above *plus* **pus fills vein**
    - Sx's: above + fever, elevated WBCs, fluctuance, red streaking
    - Usually caused by infection following a **peripheral IV**
    - Dx: U/S will show cord; **pus** may be coming out of previous IV site
    - MC organism - **staph aureus**
    - Tx: above + antibiotics initially; resect **entire vein** for continued purulence or sepsis despite antibiotics

LYMPHATICS
- Lymphatics do <u>not</u> contain a basement membrane
- Lymphatics <u>not</u> found in bone, muscle, tendon, cartilage, brain, or cornea
- Deep lymphatics have **valves**
- **Lymphedema**
    - **Primary** (can be congenital or occur later in life): L > R
    - **Secondary**: MC in women after ALND
    - Occurs when lymphatics are obstructed, too few in number, or nonfunctional
    - Sx's: heaviness, fatigue, non-pitting edema, toes look thick and squared off
    - Lymphatic fluid retention leads to **woody edema** secondary to fibrosis in subcutaneous tissue
    - **Cellulitis** and **lymphangitis** secondary to minor trauma are big problems here
    - MC infection - **streptococcus**
    - Dx: lymphoscintigraphy *(best test)* - not all patients need this if Dx obvious
    - MCC of secondary lymphedema - **ALND** in women for breast CA
    - Tx: **graded compression stockings** *(best Tx)*, extremity elevation, antibiotics for infection
- **Lymphangiosarcoma**
    - Raised blue/red coloring; early metastases to lung
    - **Stewart-Treves syndrome** - lymphangiosarcoma associated with breast ALND and chronic lymphedema
- **Lymphocele** following surgery
    - Usually occurs after **groin dissection** (eg after femoral to popliteal bypass)
    - Leakage of **clear fluid**; swelling of groin or a 'knot'; usually 1-3 weeks after surgery
    - Tx: percutaneous drainage (can try a couple of times); lymphocele resection if that fails
    - Can inject **isosulfan blue dye** into foot to identify the lymphatic channels supplying the lymphocele if having trouble locating
- **Lymphedema** following surgery
    - Usually occurs after **lower extremity bypass**
    - **Swollen extremity** *(get duplex U/S to rule-out DVT)*
    - Usually occurs **1-3 weeks** after surgery but can present as long as 1 year out
    - Tx: **compression stockings**

Gastrointestinal Hormones

704. Parietal cells of the stomach secrete:
    a.   Hydrochloric acid (HCL) and intrinsic factor
    b.   Pepsinogen
    c.   Secretin
    d.   Cholecystokinin

Answer a. The parietal cells secrete HCL and intrinsic factor.

705. Chief cells of the stomach secrete:
    a.   HCL and intrinsic factor
    b.   Pepsinogen
    c.   Secretin
    d.   Cholecystokinin

Answer b. Chief cells primarily secrete **pepsinogen**.

706. Intrinsic factor binds:
    a.   Fe
    b.   Cu
    c.   B-12
    d.   B-6

Answer c. Intrinsic factor binds B-12.
Deficiencies in B-12 can occur with:
    1) **Gastric bypass** (intrinsic factor needs acid to bind B-12)
    2) **Terminal ileum resection** (B-12 absorbed there)
    3) **Blind loop syndrome** (bacteria use it up)

707. Omeprazole works by:
    a.   Inhibiting the parietal cell H/K ATPase
    b.   Blocking histamine receptor
    c.   Blocking acetylcholine receptors
    d.   Blocking TSH receptors

Answer a. Omeprazole works by inhibiting the parietal cell H/K ATPase (proton pump). **Ranitidine** works by inhibiting the parietal cell histamine receptor.

708. All of the following are true of gastrin except:
    a.   Is primarily produced in the fundus
    b.   Increases secretion of HCL from parietal cells (via enterochromaffin cells which release histamine)
    c.   Increases secretion of intrinsic factor from parietal cells
    d.   Increases secretion of pepsinogen from chief cells

Answer a. Gastrin is primarily produced by G cells in <u>antrum</u> and <u>duodenum</u>

709. All of the following are true of motilin except:
    a.   The highest concentration of receptors is in the stomach antrum
    b.   Motilin exerts its effect on the migrating motor complex during phase III (peristalsis)
    c.   The primary response is increasing antrum and duodenal motility
    d.   Secretion is stimulated by somatostatin

Answer d. Secretion is motilin is inhibited by somatostatin

GASTRIN
- Produced <u>G cells</u> in *__stomach antrum__ and **duodenum**
- **Secretion stimulated by** - protein, vagal input (acetylcholine), ETOH, antral distention, pH > 3.0
- **Secretion inhibited by** - pH < 3.0, somatostatin, secretin, CCK
- **Target cells - parietal cells and chief cells**
- **Response**:
  - Secretion of **HCL, intrinsic factor** and **pepsinogen** (strongest stimulator for all)
  - ↑s **gastric motility**
- **Proton pump inhibitors** (eg Omeprazole) block H^+/K^+ ATPase of parietal cell (final pathway for H^+ release).
- **Ranitidine** works by inhibiting the parietal cell histamine receptor
- **Parietal cells - release HCl and Intrinsic Factor**
- **Chief cells - release pepsinogen**
- **Intrinsic Factor** - binds B-12 for absorption in the terminal ileum

SOMATOSTATIN
- Produced by <u>D cells</u> in *__stomach antrum__, **small intestine** and **pancreas**
- **Secretion stimulated by** - acid in duodenum
- **Target cells** - *many is "the great inhibitor"*
- **Response**:
  - Inhibits gastrin and HCl release
  - Inhibits release of insulin, glucagon, secretin, CCK, GIP, VIP, motilin
  - ↓s pancreatic and biliary output
  - Slows gastric emptying
  - **Octreotide** (somatostatin analogue) – can ↓ pancreatic, biliary, and small bowel fistula output

CCK (cholecystokinin)
- Produced by <u>I cells</u> of *__duodenum__ (MC site)
- **Secretion stimulated by** - protein and fat in duodenum
- **Response**:
  - **Relaxation of sphincter of Oddi**
  - **Gallbladder contraction**
  - ↑s **pancreatic acinar <u>enzyme</u> secretion** (acinar cells, zymogen granules; *most effective stimulant of pancreatic acinar cells*)
  - ↑ed **intestinal motility**

SECRETIN
- Produced by <u>S cells</u> of *__duodenum__ (MC site)
- **Secretion stimulated by** - acid (pH < 4), fat, bile
- **Secretion inhibited by** - pH > 4.0, gastrin
- **Endocrine** (primarily) and **exocrine** effects
- **Response**:
  - **Inhibits HCl** (primary duty) and **gastrin release**
  - ↑s **pancreatic ductal <u>HCO_3^-</u> secretion**
    - <u>High</u> pancreatic duct output has - ↑ HCO_3^-, ↓ Cl^-
    - <u>Slow</u> pancreatic duct output has - ↓ HCO_3^-, ↑ Cl^-
    - **Carbonic anhydrase** in duct exchanges HCO_3^- for Cl^-

MOTILIN
- Release by <u>M cells</u> primarily from *__duodenum__
- <u>Highest concentration</u> of motilin *__receptors__* - **stomach antrum**, also in duodenum, colon
- **Secretion stimulated by** - duodenal acid, vagus input
  - Released during **fasting** or **inter-digestive phase** (<u>not</u> while eating)
- **Secretion inhibited by** - somatostatin, secretin, pancreatic polypeptide, duodenal fat
- **Primary Response** - increases **motility** of stomach **antrum** and duodenum [initiates **phase III** (<u>peristalsis</u>) of migrating motor complex(MMC)]
- **Erythromycin** acts on this receptor to increase motility

GLUCAGON

- Released by <u>alpha cells</u> of the *pancreas
- **Secretion stimulated by** - ↓ serum glucose, ↑ amino acids (to protect from hypoglycemia with all protein meal), acetylcholine (vagus), catecholamines (beta adrenergic)
- **Secretion inhibited by** - ↑ serum glucose, ↑ insulin, somatostatin
- **Response:**
  - **Relaxes sphincter of Oddi**
  - **Glycogenolysis** and **gluconeogenesis**
  - **Lipolysis** and **ketogenesis**
  - **Proteolysis**
  - **All decreased** → gastric acid secretion, pancreatic secretion, intestinal motility, stomach motility, myenteric motor complexes
- **Alpha** and **beta cells** = G.I. (glucagon and insulin)

INSULIN

- Released by <u>beta cells</u> of the *pancreas
- **Secretion stimulated by** - serum glucose, glucagon, protein ingestion
- **Secretion inhibited by** – somatostatin
- **Response:**
  - **Cellular glucose uptake**
  - **Protein, glycogen** and **fat <u>synthesis</u>** (<u>anabolic</u>)
- **Type I diabetes** - pancreatic beta islet cells destroyed
- **Type II diabetes** - peripheral insulin resistance

OTHER

- **Pancreatic polypeptide**
  - Secreted by islet cells in **pancreas**
  - **Response** - <u>decreases</u> pancreatic endocrine and exocrine function
- **Peptide YY** - released from **terminal ileum** after fatty meal
  - **Response** - <u>decreases</u> gastric emptying, gastric acid secretion, pancreatic function, and gallbladder contraction
- **Bombesin** (gastrin-releasing peptide)
  - Release from post-ganglionic fibers of **vagus nerve**
  - **Response** - <u>increases</u> gastric acid secretion, intestinal motility, and pancreatic enzyme secretion
- **Vasoactive intestinal peptide** (VIP)
  - Produced by cells in **gut** and **pancreas**
  - **Secretion stimulated by** - fat, acetylcholine
  - **Response:** <u>increases</u> intestinal secretion (water, electrolytes) and motility
- **Bowel recovery after surgery**
  - **Small bowel** recovers in <u>24 hours</u>
  - **Stomach** recovers in <u>48 hours</u>
  - **Large bowel** recovers in <u>3-5 days</u>
- **Anorexia** - mediated by hypothalamus (CCK, Bombesin, peptide YY)
- **Deficiencies in B-12** (megaloblastic anemia, pernicious anemia) can occur with:
  1) *Gastric bypass* (intrinsic factor needs acid to bind B-12)
  2) *Terminal ileum resection* (B-12 absorbed there)
  3) *Blind loop syndrome*
- **1st enzyme in protein digestion** - stomach pepsin (from Chief cells)
- **1st enzyme in carbohydrate digestion** - salivary amylase

Esophagus

710. All of the following are true except:
  a. The upper thoracic esophagus is best approached with a right thoracotomy
  b. The MC site of esophageal perforation is the cervical esophagus
  c. The lower esophagus is predominantly smooth muscle
  d. The indentation on EGD at 25 mm from the incisors is likely the diaphragmatic hiatus

  Answer d. The indentation on EGD at 25 mm from the incisors is the aortic arch. The indentation for the diaphragmatic hiatus occurs at 40 cm.

711. All of the following are true except:
  a. The UES pressure at rest and during the early part of the swallow are approximately 60 mmHg and 15 mmHg
  b. LES pressure at rest and during a swallow are approximately 15 mmHg and 0 mmHg
  c. The LES relaxes soon after initiation of a swallow through a vagally mediated process
  d. The lower esophageal sphincter (LES) is normally seen on EGD at about 40 cm from the incisors

  Answer d. The LES is not seen on EGD. It is a physiologic area found with manometry.

712. All of the following are true except:
  a. Diffuse esophageal spasm is characterized by high amplitude repetitive *non-peristaltic* contractions
  b. Nutcracker esophagus is characterized by high amplitude *peristaltic* contractions
  c. Scleroderma of the esophagus is characterized by aperistalsis and high LES pressure
  d. Achalasia is characterized by high LES pressure and absence of peristalsis

  Answer c. Scleroderma of the esophagus is characterized by **aperistalsis** and **low LES pressure** with concomitant massive reflux and severe esophagitis.

713. All of the following are true of achalasia except:
  a. It is caused by proliferation of neuronal ganglion cells
  b. Nitrates and calcium channel blockers have variable success
  c. Balloon dilatation is effective in 80%
  d. These patients are at increased risk for squamous cell CA

  Answer a. It is caused by *destruction* of neuronal ganglion cells

714. The most important step in treatment of a patient with a Zenker's diverticulum is:
  a. Resection of the diverticulum
  b. Division of the superior laryngeal constrictor muscles
  c. Esophagectomy
  d. Division of the cricopharyngeus muscle

  Answer d. The most important step in treatment of a Zenker's diverticulum is performing a **cricopharyngomyotomy**. The anatomic problem with a Zenker's diverticulum is failure of the UES to relax with swallowing (cricopharyngeal dysfunction).

  The diverticulum is usually resected but in some situations when the diverticulum would be too hard to remove, it can be suspended upward such that it drains into the esophagus.

Patients can have cricopharyngeal dysfunction without presenting with a Zenker's diverticulum. Tx is the same (cricopharyngomyotomy).

715. All of the following are true of Zenker's diverticulum except:
   a.   They are a false diverticulum
   b.   The are a pulsion diverticulum
   c.   They are most commonly anterior to the cricopharyngeal junction
   d.   Perforation of these can occur with EGD

   Answer c. They are most commonly posterior to the cricopharyngeal junction.

716. Which of the following is the most sensitive test for GERD:
   a.   24 hour pH study
   b.   Manometry
   c.   Barium Swallow
   d.   EGD
   e.   CT scan

   Answer a. 24 hour pH study (esophageal probe)

717. All of the following are true to Schatzki's Ring except:
   a.   These patients almost universally have hiatal hernias
   b.   These patients usually have GERD
   c.   Dysphagia is the MC symptom
   d.   These lesions should undergo resection

   Answer d. Schatzki's Ring occurs in patients with hiatal hernias. Tx for Sx's includes **ring dilatation** and **PPI**. *Resection of these rings is <u>never</u> indicated.*

718. All of the following are true of laparoscopic fundoplication except:
   a.   The key to hiatal dissection is finding the right crura and the key to the wrap is finding the left crura
   b.   The best test for recurrent reflux or dysphagia following Nissen is barium esophagogram
   c.   The MCC of dysphagia following laparoscopic fundoplication is that the wrap is too tight
   d.   Shortened esophagus requires esophagectomy and gastric replacement

   Answer d. Shortened esophagus requires **Collis gastroplasty** to lengthen the esophageal tube (forms neo-esophagus out of stomach).

719. A 65 yo man undergoes a routine EGD for GERD. After the procedure, he develops severe pain. CXR is negative. The most appropriate next step is:
   a.   Chest CT
   b.   Abdominal CT
   c.   Gastrografin followed by thin barium swallow
   d.   Chest MRI

   Answer c. The Dx study of choice for possible esophageal perforation is **gastrografin** followed by thin **barium swallow**.

720. What is the most likely location for injury in the above patient:
   a.   Cervical esophagus
   b.   Thoracic esophagus
   c.   Abdominal esophagus
   d.   GE junction

   Answer a. The MCC of esophageal perforation is EGD (MC area - **cervical)**

721. Gastrografin swallow in the above patient shows free contrast extravasation from the cervical esophagus. You explore the area through a left cervical incision and find the esophagus is too badly damaged to repair. The most appropriate next step is:
   a.   Esophagectomy
   b.   Place a drain and close the wound
   c.   Esophageal stent
   d.   Palliative care
   e.   Antibiotics only

   Answer b. Non-malignant <u>cervical</u> esophageal perforation should be repaired if possible. If a repair is not possible, just place drains and close the incision with loose skin closure. This area will eventually heal (place J-Tube to feed patient while the area is healing). Note this is only applicable to **cervical** esophageal perforations, *not thoracic esophageal perforations*.

722. A 48 yo male who drinks a case of beer per day devours a large meal, develops nausea, and then vomits. He then develops severe chest pain. All of the following are true of the patient's likely condition except:
   a.   Gastrografin, followed by thin barium swallow is the best study for diagnosis
   b.   The MC location for the problem in the left lower esophagus
   c.   A left thoracotomy is usually the best incision given the MC location
   d.   Simple full thickness esophageal bites are all that is needed for repair

   Answer d. Be careful here. After washing out the vomited material with **Boerhaave's Syndrome**, you need to perform a myotomy to see the extent of the injury in the mucosa. Classically, the mucosal injury will extend farther than the muscle injury. So what you see at first glance is <u>not</u> the full extent of the injury. Layered closure (mucosa layer, then muscle layer) is appropriate. Cover the area with an intercostal muscle flap.

   Depending on the length of time from the perforation event, these patients can present with a septic picture.

   Although swallow studies are the best test for diagnosis, many are diagnosed with CT scan.

723. The above patient's daughter informs you that the vomiting episode occurred over 2 days ago. In the OR, there is significant mediastinitis and severe damage to the esophagus. The most appropriate next step is:
   a.   Place drains and close
   b.   Esophageal stent
   c.   Staple the distal thoracic esophagus and place a cervical esophagostomy
   d.   Omental patch

   Answer c. Staple the distal thoracic esophagus and place a cervical esophagostomy. Unlike the cervical esophagus, just placing drains will <u>not</u> heal the perforated area and also places the patient at great risk for mediastinitis.

   Just performing an esophagectomy at this stage is also an option (as long as the patient is stable) but it was not listed in the answers.

724. Perforation following attempted endoscopic LES dilation is best treated with:
   a.   Primary repair only
   b.   Primary repair with an intercostal muscle flap only
   c.   Esophagectomy
   d.   Primary repair, lower esophageal myotomy on the contralateral side, and intercostal muscle flap

   Answer d. In addition to repair of the perforation, treatment of the achalasia with lower esophageal myotomy is indicated otherwise the area won't heal due to the distal obstuction (ie the non-relaxing LES associated with achalasia).

312

725. An 82 yo frail lady from a skilled nursing facility presents with mild chest pain. She has otherwise been asymptomatic and has never had this pain before. EKG and cardiac work-up are negative however her lower mediastinal silhouette looks wide on CXR and you see a large gastric bubble above the diaphragm. The most sensitive test for a hiatal hernia is:
    a.   CT scan
    b.   Barium swallow
    c.   EGD
    d.   Manometry

Answer b. Barium swallow although many are diagnosed with CT scan.

726. Barium swallow in the above patient shows a large paraesophageal hernia. The most appropriate next step is :
    a.   Observation
    b.   Gastric stent
    c.   Fundoplication
    d.   Partial gastrectomy

Answer a. Observation. Although gastric torsion and necrosis can occur with paraesophageal hernias, the risk is low. Given the frailty of the patient with minimal Sx's, observation is indicated.

727. All of the following are true of Type I hiatal hernia compared to paraesophageal hernias except
    a.   Type I hiatal hernias have a lower esophageal sphincter (and GE junction) that rises above the diaphragm
    b.   Reflux is the MC symptom with paraesophageal hernias
    c.   Paraesophageal hernias have a hernia sac whereas Type I hiatal hernias do not
    d.   Repair of both types (paraesophageal and Type I hiatal hernias) is usually performed using fundoplication
    e.   For Type II paraesophageal hiatal hernias, the lower esophageal sphincter (and GE junction) is in the normal anatomic position

Answer b. The MC symptom for paraesophageal hernias is chest pain.

728. All of the following are true of paraesophageal hiatal hernias except
    a.   Patients can present with anemia
    b.   Barium swallow is the best test for diagnosis
    c.   Are usually caused by traumatic injury
    d.   These can be found with upper endoscopy with retro-flex view
    e.   Organoaxial volvulus is more common than the mesentericoaxial type

Answer c. Paraesophageal hernias are <u>not</u> associated with trauma. They arise due to weakness in the phrenoesophageal membrane (an extension of the transversalis fascia).

729. Treatment of esophageal leiomyoma involves:
    a.   Extra-mucosal enucleation via thoracotomy or VATS
    b.   Segmental resection
    c.   XRT
    d.   Chemotherapy
    e.   Pre-operative endoscopic biopsy

Answer a. Tx of **esophageal leiomyoma** is ***extra-mucosal* enucleation** through a thoracotomy. Notably, you do <u>not</u> want to try and biopsy leiomyomas on EGD - can create mucosal scar tissue and make enucleation difficult and increase the risk of disrupting the mucosa.

730. All of the following are true of esophageal leiomyoma except:
   a. It is the MC benign esophageal tumor
   b. They are MC in the distal 2/3 of the esophagus
   c. They consist of striated muscle
   d. The diagnosis can generally be made with barium swallow

   Answer c. They consist of smooth muscle

731. A 65 yo man with GERD develops mild dysphagia with solid food intake. The most appropriate next step is:
   a. Chest CT scan
   b. EGD
   c. Barium swallow
   d. Manometry
   e. Abdominal CT scan

   Answer c. Barium swallow is the best test for dysphagia.

732. Barium swallow in the above patient shows a slight esophageal stricture. The most appropriate next step is:
   a. Nothing
   b. PPI and periodic dilatation
   c. EGD with biopsy
   d. Endoscopic surveillance
   e. Esophageal stent

   Answer c. EGD with biopsy is needed to rule-out CA

733. EGD with biopsy in the above patient just shows fibrosis consistent with a peptic stricture. The most appropriate next step is:
   a. Extra-luminal resection
   b. Esophagectomy
   c. RF ablation
   d. Esophageal stent
   e. PPI and periodic dilatation

   Answer e. PPI and periodic dilatation

734. Instead of the above, EGD with biopsy shows Barrett's with high grade dysplasia (HGD). The most appropriate next step is
   a. Radiofrequency ablation
   b. Talc sclerotherapy
   c. Close endoscopic surveillance
   d. Alcohol sclerotherapy
   e. Photodynamic therapy

   Answer c. Although in the past HGD was an indication for esophagectomy, it is now recognized that many of these patients do not progress to esophageal CA. The patients can now have either: 1) esophagectomy or 2) close endoscopic surveillance.

   In the future, the local therapies listed above may be options but the current standard of care is esophagectomy or close surveillance.

735. All of the following are true of Barrett's esophagus except:
   a. The hallmark finding is Goblet cells
   b. It generally occurs in the lower esophagus
   c. GERD is a RF
   d. Generally looks like a raised pink lesion
   e. CA risk is not reversed with PPI or fundoplication

Answer a. Barrett's esophagus is characterized by squamous to columnar metaplasia. A subset of Barrett's is intestinal-type metaplasia (which features Goblet cells). Not all patients with Barrett's have this subtype. Intestinal subtype metaplasia .has the highest risk for developing esophageal CA.

736. During routine endoscopic surveillance on an otherwise healthy 50 yo man, a T2 esophageal CA is found. EUS and chest/abdominal CT scans are negative for adenopathy. PET scan is negative. The most appropriate next step is:
    a. Chemo-XRT
    b. Esophageal resection
    c. Esophageal stent
    d. Hospice care
    e. RF ablation

    Answer a. Neoadjuvant **chemo-XRT** is indicated for resectable esophageal tumors T2 or greater.

737. The above patient undergoes chemo-XRT and eventual esophagectomy. POD 6 he develops purulent drainage from his neck incision. In the OR you find drainage emanating from the anastomosis. The most appropriate next step is:
    a. Close the incision primarily with layered closure
    b. Washout the area, place drains, loose wound closure, and WTD dressing changes
    c. Takedown anastomosis, staple the stomach in the neck, and place a cervical esophagostomy
    d. Takedown anastomosis, staple the stomach and return it to the abdomen, place a cervical esophagostomy

    Answer b. Washout, place drains, and loosely close the incision with WTD dressing changes. This area will eventually heal. Note this therapy is appropriate only for significant anastomotic leaks in the _cervical_ esophagus.

    A significant anastomotic leak in the _chest_ (eg fevers, purulent drainage from chest tubes) requires primary repair, redo anastomosis, or complete takedown of the anastomosis (risk of mediastinitis).

738. A 55 yo man presents with dysphagia and weight loss. Esophagogram shows an 'apple core' lesion at the gastro-esophageal junction. Given the likely Dx, all of the following are true except:
    a. The right gastroepiploic artery is the main blood supply to the stomach after trans-hiatal esophagectomy
    b. This patient should have endoscopic U/S (best test for T status)
    c. The most important prognostic factor is depth of lesion
    d. In general, lesions T2 or greater should undergo neoadjuvant chemo-XRT
    e. The MC type of esophageal CA is adenocarcinoma

    Answer c. The most important prognostic factor for esophageal CA devoid of systemic mets is **nodal involvement**.

739. The best test for suspected caustic esophageal injury due to ingestion is:
    a. CXR
    b. Endoscopy
    c. Chest CT
    d. Barium swallow

    Answer b. The best test for suspected **caustic esophageal injury** is upper **endoscopy**. _Do not go past the point of severe injuries as you may cause a perforation - just making the diagnosis and assessing injury here._

ANATOMY AND PHYSIOLOGY

- **Layers**:
    - **Mucosa** (squamous epithelium)
    - **Submucosa**
    - **Muscularis propria**
        - Upper 1/3 esophagus - primarily *striated muscle
        - Lower 2/3 esophagus - primarily *smooth muscle
    - *No* serosa
- **Blood supply**
    - **Cervical** - inferior thyroid artery
    - **Thoracic** - vessels directly off aorta (main supply to esophagus)
    - **Abdominal** - left gastric artery (primary)
- **Innervation**
    - **Right vagus nerve**
        - Travels on **posterior** portion of stomach as it exits chest
        - Becomes **celiac plexus**
        - Has **Criminal nerve of Grassi** → causes persistently high acid levels post-op if left undivided with vagotomy
    - **Left vagus nerve**
        - On **anterior** portion of stomach; goes to **liver** and **biliary tree**
- **Normal manometry**
    - **Pharyngeal contraction with food bolus**   70-120 mmHg
    - **Upper esophageal sphincter** (UES; cricopharyngeus muscle)
        - At **rest**   60 mmHg
        - With **food bolus**   15 mmHg
        - *No pressure drop with food indicates failure of <u>cricopharyngeus</u> to relax*
    - **Lower esophageal sphincter** (LES)
        - At **rest**   15 mmHg
        - With **food bolus**   0 mmHg
        - *Resting LES pressure frequently ≤ 5 with <u>GERD</u>*
    - **Esophageal contraction with food bolus**   30-120 mmHg
        - *Ineffective if < 10 mmHg throughout (ie <u>burned out</u> esophagus)*
- **Normal Distances** (anatomic areas of narrowing, measurements are <u>from incisors</u>, esophagus is **30 cm** total length):
    - **Cricopharyngeus**   15 cm
    - **Aortic arch indentation**   25 cm
    - **Diaphragmatic hiatus**   40 cm
    - *LES is <u>not</u> visible – is a **manometric finding***
- **Upper esophageal sphincter** = <u>cricopharyngeus</u> muscle (circular muscle fibers)
    - Prevents air swallowing; has recurrent laryngeal nerve innervation
    - MC site of **esophageal perforation** - near cricopharyngeus (MCC - EGD)
    - MC site for esophageal **foreign body** - near cricopharyngeus
- **Lower esophageal sphincter** (40 cm from incisors) - relaxation mediated by inhibitory neurons; normally contracted at rest → <u>prevents reflux</u>
    - 1) LES is <u>not</u> an anatomical sphincter *and*;
    - 2) LES is <u>not</u> seen on EGD
    - Is a physiologic zone (3-5 cm) of high pressure found on **manometry**
- **Swallowing stages** (CNS initiates swallow)
    - **Primary peristalsis** - occurs with food bolus and swallow initiation
    - **Secondary peristalsis** - occurs with incomplete emptying and esophageal distention, consists of propagating waves
    - **Tertiary peristalsis** - non-propagating, non-peristalsing, *is <u>dysfunctional</u>*
    - The **UES** and **LES** are *normally* **contracted** between meals to avoid reflux and air swallowing
- **Swallowing mechanism**
    - Soft palate occludes nasopharynx
    - Larynx rises and airway opening is blocked by epiglottis
    - Cricopharyngeus relaxes
    - Pharyngeal contraction moves food into esophagus
    - **LES relaxes soon after initiation of swallow** (vagus induced relaxation; LES pressure goes to 0 mmHg)

- Surgical approach
  - **Cervical esophagus** - **left neck** (left sided course here and avoids non-recurrent laryngeal nerve which is more common on the right side)
  - **Upper ⅔ thoracic** - **right** (avoids the aorta)
  - **Lower ⅓ thoracic** - **left** (left-sided course in this region)
- **Esophageal dysfunction**
  - <u>Primary motility disorders</u> - achalasia, nutcracker, diffuse spasm
  - <u>Secondary motility disorders</u> - GERD (MC), scleroderma
- **Upper endoscopy** (EGD) - *best <u>initial</u> test* for **heartburn** (can visualize esophagitis)
  - Procedure of choice for **foreign body** (Dx and Tx)
- **Barium swallow** (esophagogram) - *best <u>initial</u> test* for **dysphagia** or **odynophagia** (painful swallowing) - better at picking up masses
  - Procedure of choice for **suspected perforation** (gastrografin, then thin barium)
- **Manometry** - *best test to make Dx* of **primary dysmotility disorder** (eg achalasia, diffuse esophageal spasm, nutcracker esophagus) or scleroderma of the esophagus
- **Esophageal foreign bodies**
  - **Adults** MC - food impaction (meat)
  - **Children** MC - coins
  - Dx and Tx: **rigid EGD in OR** (need to intubate 1st)

PLUMMER-VINSON SYNDROME
- Cervical dysphagia, upper esophageal web, and iron-deficient anemia
- Tx: **dilation of web** and **iron**; need to screen for **oral CA**

ZENKERS DIVERTICULUM (pharyngoesophageal diverticulum)
- Caused by **failure of the cricopharyngeus to relax** with swallowing
  - Pharyngeal constrictors push against this, creating high pressure
  - Creates a *pulsion* diverticulum found **posteriorly** (MC) between the **pharyngeal constrictors** and **cricopharyngeus muscle** (Killian's triangle)
- Is a *false* diverticulum (does not contain all layers - <u>no muscle</u>)
- Sx's: **cervical dysphagia**, **regurgitation** of non-digested food, choking from aspiration, halitosis, 'lump in the throat'
- Dx: **barium swallow** (*best test*; shows posterior midline protrusion above UES)
  - Manometry - shows lack of UES relaxation
- *Avoid* **EGD** - risk of perforation
- Tx: *cricopharyngeal myotomy* (key point of surgery); Zenker's itself can either be resected or suspended (removal of diverticula is <u>not</u> necessary)
  - Left cervical incision; leave drains in; gastrografin swallow POD #1

ACHALASIA
- Sx's: **dysphagia** (solids + liquids; nearly all patients), **regurgitation,** and **weight loss**
- Pathology - autoimmune <u>destruction</u> of **neuronal ganglion cells** in myenteric plexus
- **Manometry** *(<u>best test</u> for Dx of achalasia)* shows:
  - 1) **LES fails to relax** with swallowing <u>and</u>;
  - 2) **Loss of peristalsis** (low amplitude and fails to progress)
  - LES pressure is usually high
- **Barium swallow** *(best initial test for dysphagia)* - can get tortuous dilated esophagus and distal tapering (bird-beak appearance); epiphrenic diverticula can occur
- **Upper endoscopy** - *needed in all patients to **rule-out esophageal CA*** at LES *(get Bx)*
- Medical Tx: **balloon dilatation of LES** (80% effective; Cx's - GERD)
  - Nitrates and calcium channel blockers have variable success
  - Botox injection can provide short term relief
- If dilation fails→ Tx: **Heller myotomy** (<u>left</u> thoracotomy [VATS] or laparoscopic, longitudinal myotomy of <u>lower</u> esophagus only; also need partial fundoplication)
- **Post-op Cx's**
  - **GERD** - perform partial wrap to prevent this
  - **Esophageal leak** (pleural effusion, fever)
- Late Cx from achalasia - **esophageal CA** (squamous cell CA; 15 x increased risk)
- *Trypanosoma cruzi* (Chaga's disease) can produce similar Sx's
- **Perforation following balloon dilatation for achalasia** → Tx: left thoracotomy, repair perforation, opposite side longitudinal esophagomyotomy, place drains

DIFFUSE ESOPHAGEAL SPASM
- Sx's: **chest pain** and ***dysphagia**; may have psychiatric history
- **Manometry** *(best test* for Dx of DES) - frequent **high amplitude *_non-peristaltic_* contractions** (unorganized); LES relaxes normally
- Barium swallow - can have corkscrew esophagus
- Pain can be similar to myocardial infarction (check troponins and EKG)
- **Medical Tx** *(best Tx):* **calcium channel blocker** (diltiazem), **Trazodone**, decrease anxiety (psych assessment)
- **Indications for surgery**: reserved for patients with refractory incapacitating episodes of ***dysphagia*** (use surgery as a last resort)
- Surgery: **Heller myotomy** (myotomy of <u>upper</u> *and* <u>lower</u> esophagus - entire thoracic esophagus) - **<u>right</u> thoracotomy** (or VATS); include partial fundoplication
- Surgery usually less effective for esophageal spasm than for achalasia

NUTCRACKER ESOPHAGUS *(MC primary esophageal disorder)*
- Sx's: **chest pain** (MCC of non-cardiac chest pain) and ***odynophagia** (painful swallowing)
- **Manometry** *(best test* for Dx of nutcracker) - very **high amplitude *peristaltic* contractions** (> 180 mmHg); LES relaxes normally
- EKG, CXR, Troponins, and CK-MB → *rule-out <u>myocardial ischemia</u>*
- **Medical Tx** *(best Tx):* **calcium channel blocker** (diltiazem), **Trazodone**, decrease anxiety (psych assessment)
- **Indications for surgery**: reserved for patients with refractory incapacitating episodes of ***chest pain*** (use surgery as a last resort)
- Surgery: **Heller myotomy** (myotomy of <u>upper</u> *and* <u>lower</u> esophagus - entire thoracic esophagus) - **<u>right</u> thoracotomy** (or VATS); include partial fundoplication
- Surgery usually less effective for nutcracker than for achalasia

SCLERODERMA
- Sx's: **heartburn** (from massive reflux) and **dysphagia**
- **Fibrous replacement** of esophageal **smooth muscle** (<u>distal 2/3</u> of esophagus most affected - where most smooth muscle is)
- Complete loss of LES tone
- *Esophagus is the MC organ involved in scleroderma*
- **Manometry** *(best test for Dx)* - shows **low LES pressure** and **aperistalsis**
- **Strictures** can occur (worsens dysphagia) - need Bx to rule-out CA
- Risk of **esophageal adenocarcinoma** in these patients
- Tx: **PPI** (Omeprazole) and **metoclopramide** (Reglan)
- **Indications for operation**: refractory GERD or Cx's (eg ulcers, strictures)
- **Surgery** - esophagectomy usual

GASTROESOPHAGEAL REFLUX DISEASE (GERD)
- Sx's: **heartburn** 30-60 minutes after meals; worse lying down
  - Can also have asthma Sx's (cough), choking, or aspiration
  - Heartburn is from exposure of **esophagus** to **gastric acid**
  - Often associated with a **hiatal hernia** (but <u>not</u> always)
  - RFs - obesity
- Make sure patient does not have another cause for pain (ie unusual Sx's):
  - **Dysphagia / odynophagia** - need to worry about tumors (Dx: barium swallow)
  - **Bloating** (often in diabetics) - suggests aerophagia and delayed gastric emptying (Dx: gastric emptying study)
  - **Epigastric pain** - suggests peptic ulcer, tumor (Dx: EGD)
- MCC of GERD - **incompetent LES** (from **low LES pressure**)
- Most treated empirically with **PPI** without testing (99% effective)
- Failure of PPI despite escalating doses (give it 3-4 weeks) → need **diagnostic studies**
- Dx: 24 hour **pH probe** *(best test for Dx),* **EGD with biopsies** (check histology), **manometry** (resting LES < 6 mmHg suggests GERD; rule-out dysmotility disorders), consider barium swallow (if unusual Sx's, eg dysphagia)
- **Surgical indications**: failure of medical Tx, avoidance of lifetime meds in young patients, refractory Cx's (eg bleeding, esophagitis, stricture)

- Tx: **Nissen fundoplication** → divide short gastric arteries, pull esophagus into abdomen, **approximate crura**, 270- (partial) or 360-degree **gastric fundus** wrap; anchor wrap to the **right crura**
  - Key to **dissection** - finding the **right crura**
  - Key to the **wrap** - finding the **left crura**
  - Mobilize at least **5 cm** of the intra-thoracic esophagus
  - Need at least **2 cm** of <u>free esophagus</u> in the abdomen
  - Wrap over **54 Fr** Bougie to prevent making it too tight
  - Want fundus wrap **2 cm** in length (loose but secure)
  - **Crura approximation** - prevents wrap herniation; repairs weakness of the phrenoesophageal membrane (an extension of the transversalis fascia)
  - Cx's - injury to spleen, diaphragm, or esophagus; pneumothorax
  - **Trouble delivering viscera** from above diaphragm - Tx: **incise hiatus** (left crura at 2 o'clock position), reduce contents, repair later
  - **Collis gastroplasty** - when not enough esophagus exists to pull into abdomen (ie **shortened esophagus**), can staple along stomach cardia and create "new" esophagus (neo-esophagus); wrap ends up going around the neo-esophagus
  - **Partial fundoplication** (eg Toupet, partial Nissen) - posterior 270-degree wrap; used for GERD with concomitant motility disorder (eg achalasia) or poor esophageal contraction
  - MCC of dysphagia following Nissen - **wrap is too tight**
- **Cx's from GERD** - esophagitis, peptic stricture, esophageal shortening, Barrett's esophagus

ESOPHAGITIS
- Usually gets better with PPI; need EGD with Bx if not getting better
- Consider Nissen if refractory to escalating PPI doses

PEPTIC STRICTURE
- MCC of benign esophageal stricture - **GERD**
- Usually right above the EGJ (esophago-gastric junction)
- *Need EGD and Bx to **rule-out malignancy** as a cause of the stricture*
- Medical Tx: **95% effective** (PPI and periodic endoscopic dilatation)
- All peptic strictures have **shortened esophagus** and will need **Collis gastroplasty** if performing a wrap

ESOPHAGEAL SHORTENING
- RFs: peptic stricture, giant hernia, esophagitis, previously failed wraps
- Shortening suggested if EGJ lies **4-5 cm above** diaphragmatic hiatus
- Esophagus should lie (freely) 2 cm below hiatus after dissection for wrap (otherwise need a **Collis gastroplasty**)
- Failure to get sufficient esophageal length can result in **wrap herniation** above the diaphragm (Sx's: both **dysphagia** *and* **reflux**)

SCHATZKI'S RING (lower esophageal ring)
- Almost all patients have an associated sliding **hiatal hernia**
- Ring lies at **squamo-columnar junction** (is a submucosal **fibrosis**) in the distal esophagus
- Sx's: **dysphagia**, food impaction can occur
- Dx: **barium swallow** *(best test)* - shows ring in distal esophagus
  - *Often can <u>not</u> see this with EGD*
- If asymptomatic - *leave alone*
- Tx if symptomatic: **ring dilatation** and **PPI** usually sufficient in majority
  - Surgery if refractory (partial wrap and dilatation of ring)
  - *Do <u>not</u> resect the ring (resection of ring is <u>never</u> indicated)*

BARRETT'S ESOPHAGUS
- **Squamous** <u>metaplasia</u> to **columnar** epithelium (raised, pink lesion)
- Occurs with long-standing exposure to **gastric reflux** (is acquired)
- **Intestinal type** columnar metaplasia is the only type predisposed to esophageal CA
  - Pathology shows **Goblet cells**

- CA risk is increased 50 times compared to general population (adenocarcinoma; relative risk [RR] 50)
- **High grade dysplasia** (HGD) Barrett's esophagus (considered carcinoma in situ)
    - Needs to be confirmed by **2 experienced pathologists**
    - Options:
        1) **Esophagectomy** _or;_
        2) **Endoscopic surveillance** (3 month intervals; 4 quadrant Bx's at 1 cm intervals for entire length of HGD and Bx of any suspicious areas)
    - Some patients with HGD never develop CA (basis for option 2)
    - Cell types other than Barrett's (eg squamous cell CIS) - follow above as well
- **Uncomplicated Barrett's** (eg non-HGD) can be treated like GERD (ie PPI or Nissen) - Tx will decrease esophagitis and further metaplasia
    - Need annual follow-up EGD surveillance for lifetime, even after Nissen
    - _Barrett's CA risk is not reversed with PPI or fundoplication_

HIATAL HERNIA
- **Type I** (99%) - sliding hernia from **dilation of the esophageal hiatus**; associated with GERD; lower esophageal sphincter and GE junction rise <u>above</u> the diaphragm along with the stomach; partially caused by *<u>weakness</u> of the **phrenoesophageal membrane** (an extension of **transversalis fascia**); _do not have a hernia sac_
- **Type II** - paraesophageal hernia; lower esophageal sphincter and GE junction are in the <u>normal</u> anatomic position; has a **hernia sac** _(characteristic feature)_ unlike sliding hernias; stomach herniates through a *<u>defect</u> in the **phrenoesophageal membrane**
- **Type III** - combined I and II
- **Type IV** - entire stomach in chest plus another organ (eg colon, spleen)

PARAESOPHAGEAL HERNIA (Types II - IV)
- Sx's: can be asymptomatic; can have chest pain, retching without vomiting, trouble passing NG tube [Borchardt's triad]), dysphagia, anemia (gastric erosions, chronic blood loss)
- Some risk of incarceration, strangulation, and gastric necrosis
- Can get **gastric volvulus** (torsion) - usually **organoaxial** (GE junction and pylorus are the fixation point); mesentericoaxial type less common
- Paraesophageal hernias have a **hernia sac** _(sliding hiatal hernias do not)_
- Due to a *defect in **phrenoesophageal membrane** (extension of transversalis fascia)
- Dx: **barium swallow** (esophagogram, _best test_)
    - CXR - air-fluid level in chest (stomach)
    - Upper endoscopy - can usually see paraesophageal hernia on retroflex view
- Tx: **Nissen fundoplication** (diaphragm repaired, helps anchor stomach)
    - Repair if significantly symptomatic (risk of incarceration if left alone)
    - _If elderly and frail with minimal Sx's_ → _leave alone_ (observation)

FUNDOPLICATION COMPLICATIONS
- MC intra-op injury - **esophageal perforation** (Tx: repair); can also present post-op as a pleural effusion
- MC Cx overall following fundoplication - **dysphagia**
- **Dysphagia**
    - Dx: **barium swallow** _(best test)_ - figures out problem
    - MC problem - **wrap is too tight** (causes dysphagia early post-op)
        > 95% resolve with **conservative Tx** (edema may be a contributor)
        Tx: **clears** for 1 week, can try to **dilate** after 1 week
        Inability to **swallow liquids** or **foamy salvia** → reoperate
        This Cx is avoided by performing wrap over a 54 Fr Bougie
    - Dysphagia following **redo-fundoplication** - likely from **wrap herniation** above diaphragm (due to **shortened esophagus**)
        Prevent this by performing **Collis gastroplasty**
    - **Late dysphagia**
        Dx: **Barium swallow** _(best test)_ - figures out problem
        Worry about **CA** here

- **Recurrent Reflux**
  - Dx: **barium swallow** *(best test in the situation of recurrent reflux after wrap, normally EGD is the best test for reflux)* - look for wrap disruption and other wrap Cx's
- **Gas bloating** or **delayed gastric emptying**
  - Tx: metoclopramide (Reglan) and simethicone
  - May need **pyloroplasty** if from bilateral **injured vagus nerves**
- **Vagus nerve(s)** - Cx's from injury →
  - Gallstones (cholecystectomy if symptomatic)
  - Delayed gastric emptying (metoclopramide)
  - Gas bloat syndrome in air swallowers (Tx: metoclopramide and simethicone; usually self-limiting)
  - **Both vagus nerves injured** - Tx: pyloroplasty likely needed
- **Esophageal perforation** (can present late as a **pleural effusion**)
  - Dx: **gastrografin swallow** (followed by thin barium) to look for leak
  - Tx: primary repair

LEIOMYOMA
- MC benign esophageal tumor (very low risk of malignant degeneration)
- Consists of **smooth muscle** cells (gray-white swirls)
- Sx's: **dysphagia**
- Usually in **lower 2/3 of esophagus** (where smooth muscle cells are; in muscularis propria [**submucosal**])
- Dx: **barium swallow** *(best test* - characteristic smooth, convex filling defect),
  - Endoscopic U/S - homogenous, hypo-echoic lesion; *overlying mucosa is <u>intact</u>*
  - CT scan (need to rule-out CA)
- *Do <u>not</u> biopsy* → can form scar and make subsequent resection difficult with high risk of disrupting the mucosa
- Tx: if > **5 cm** or **symptomatic** → excision (**extra-mucosal enucleation**) via thoracotomy (or VATS) - do <u>not</u> resect the esophagus; leave the mucosa <u>intact</u>
- **Leiomyosarcoma Tx**: esophagectomy

CAUSTIC ESOPHAGEAL INJURY
- <u>No</u> NG tube. Do <u>not</u> induce vomiting. <u>Nothing</u> to drink
- Intubate patient if having respiratory Sx's (eg stridor, hoarseness)
- <u>Avoid</u> neutralizing agents
- **Alkali** - causes deep liquefaction necrosis, especially if liquid (eg Drano, lye)
  - Worse injury than acid; also more likely to cause CA
- **Acid** - causes coagulation necrosis; mostly causes gastric injury
- **Complications** – esophageal / stomach perforation, necrosis, stricture
- **Chest** and **abdominal CT scan** to look for free air and signs of perforation
- **Endoscopy** to assess degree of injury *(best test)*
  - Do <u>not</u> use with suspected **perforation**
  - Do <u>not</u> go past a site of severe injury (risk of perforation)
- Serial exams and plain films required
- Degree of injury:
  - **Primary burn** (hyperemia)
    - Tx: observation and conservative Tx
    - **Conservative Tx**: IVFs, spitting, antibiotics, PPI, oral intake after 3-4 days; possible serial dilations for strictures (usually cervical)
    - Can also get shortening of esophagus with GERD (Tx: PPI)
  - **Secondary burn** (ulcerations, exudates, and sloughing)
    - Tx: prolonged observation and conservative Tx as above; TPN; keep NPO until able to swallow their own secretions, then clears
    - **Indications for esophagectomy** - sepsis, peritonitis, mediastinitis, free air, mediastinal or stomach wall air, crepitus, contrast extravasation, pneumothorax, large pleural effusion, worsening metabolic acidosis
  - **Tertiary burn** (deep ulcers, charring, and lumen narrowing)
    - Tx: as above, **esophagectomy** usually necessary
    - Alimentary tract not restored until after recovery from injury
- Risk of esophageal **squamous cell CA** later in life

- *All* caustic esophageal **perforations** *require* **esophagectomy** (are not repaired due to extensive damage) - right thoracotomy (allows removal of entire esophagus)

ESOPHAGEAL PERFORATIONS
- MCC overall - **EGD** *(50% of all perforations are iatrogenic)*
- MC site overall - near **cricopharyngeus** (UES; cervical esophagus; is the narrowest point); other sites - indentation of aortic arch, LES
- Sx's: **chest pain** and **dysphagia**
  - Subcutaneous air, respiratory distress, fever → all suggest **free perforation**
- Dx: upright CXR initially (look for free-air or subcutaneous emphysema)
  - **Gastrografin swallow** followed by barium *(best test)* - will make Dx of perforation and location; also the presence of multiple perforations
  - *No EGD for Dx (risk of worsening the injury)*
- **Criteria for non-surgical management** - contained **perforation** by contrast, self-draining, no systemic effects, no distal obstruction (eg no achalasia, stricture, or CA)
  - **Conservative Tx**: IVFs, NPO x 7 days, spit, broad spectrum antibiotics, repeat esophagogram after 7 days, start clears if OK
- **Non-contained perforations** (free perforation):
  - If diagnosed *early* (< 24 hours) and area has minimal contamination → **primary repair** with drains
    - Need **longitudinal myotomy** to see the full extent of injury (mucosal injury usually extends farther than muscle injury)
    - Consider **muscle flaps** (eg intercostal) to cover repair
  - If diagnosed *late* (> 48 hours) *or* area has extensive contamination →
    - **Neck** - *just place* **drains**, this will heal *(no esophagectomy unless for CA)*
    - **Chest** - need 1) **esophagectomy** (place cervical esophagostomy) *or*; 2) **exclusion and diversion** (cervical esophagostomy, staple across distal esophagus, washout mediastinum, place chest tubes); for both **1)** and **2)** need gastric replacement of esophagus late after patient recovers (6-8 weeks)
  - If diagnosed between 24-48 hours - assess contamination and follow either the early or late diagnosis pathways based on findings
- **Esophagectomy** - may be needed for any perforation (contained or non-contained) in a patient with **severe intrinsic disease** (eg burned out esophagus from achalasia, esophageal CA)

BOERHAAVE'S SYNDROME (esophageal perforation after forceful vomiting)
- Sx's: **large meal** and **ETOH**, then **forceful vomiting**, followed by **chest pain**
- Perforation MC in left lateral wall of lower esophagus (90%), 3-5 cm above GE junction; are almost *never* contained perforations
- **Hamman's sign** - mediastinal crunching sound on auscultation (from mediastinal and subcutaneous emphysema)
- *Has* **highest mortality** *of all perforations (40%)* - early Dx and Tx improve survival
  - Survival directly related to time between rupture and surgery (mortality increases 2% / hour)
- Dx: **Gastrografin swallow** *(best test); often diagnosed by CT scan*
  - CXR / AXR - subcutaneous air, PTX, pleural effusion (MC **left**)
- Surgery based on timing of discovery (**left thoracotomy** usual):
  < 24 hours   *repair* unless too damaged
  24-48 hours   assess damage - if OK, repair, if not esophagectomy
  > 48 hours   **esophagectomy** (significant mediastinitis at this point)

ESOPHAGEAL CANCER
- Esophageal tumors are almost always malignant; have **early** invasion of nodes
- Spreads quickly along **submucosal lymphatic channels** (often *advanced stage* when Sx's arise [eg dysphagia])
- Sx's: **dysphagia** (especially solids) and **weight loss**
- RFs: ETOH, tobacco, achalasia, caustic injury, Barrett's, Tylosis (hyperkeratosis and abnormal thickening of skin at the palms and soles)
- Dx: **barium swallow** *(best test for dysphagia)* - apple-core lesion
  - **EGD with EUS** and **Bx** *(best test for T status - depth)*

- **Chest / abdominal CT scan** *(single best test for overall resectability)*
- **Unresectability** - hoarseness (RLN invasion), Horner's syndrome (stellate sympathetic ganglion invasion), brachial plexus invasion, paralyzed diaphragm (phrenic nerve invasion), malignant pleural effusion, invasion of airway / vertebra / other major structure
  - **Nodal disease outside area of resection** (eg supraclavicular or celiac nodes → M1 disease) - *contraindication* to esophagectomy
- Most important prognostic factor - **nodal spread**
  - Spreads quickly along **submucosal lymphatics** (longitudinal)
- MC esophageal CA (U.S.) - **adenocarcinoma** (not squamous)
  - **Adenocarcinoma** - usually in **lower ⅓** of esophagus; **liver** metastases MC; often in background of **Barrett's** (Caucasians, 50-60s)
  - **Squamous cell CA** - usually in **upper ⅔** of esophagus; **lung** metastases MC (African-Americans, 60-70s)
- Pre-op **chemo-XRT** (cisplatin and 5-FU) - indicated for **T2 tumors or greater**; may downstage large tumors and make them resectable
  - T2 = submucosal invasion
- **GE junction tumors** are treated like **esophageal CA**
- **Surgery**:
  1) Patient needs to be able to **tolerate surgery**
  2) Need to have **resectable CA** (eg no distant metastases; no celiac or supraclavicular nodal disease, not invading another structure such as lung)
- **Esophagectomy** - 5% mortality from surgery; curative in 20%
  - Need **6-8 cm margins**
  - **Right gastroepiploic artery** - primary blood supply to stomach after replacing esophagus (have to divide left gastric artery and short gastrics)
  - **Transhiatal approach** - abdominal and neck incisions; bluntly dissect intra-thoracic esophagus; may have decreased mortality from esophageal leaks with the cervical anastomosis
  - **Ivor Lewis** - abdominal incision and right thoracotomy → exposes all of the intra-thoracic esophagus; have an intra-thoracic anastomosis
  - **3-Hole esophagectomy** - abdominal, thoracic, and cervical incisions
  - Need **pyloroplasty** the above procedures
  - **Colonic interposition** - may be choice in young patients when you want to preserve gastric function; 3 anastomoses required; blood supply depends on colon marginal vessels
  - Gastrografin swallow POD #7 to rule-out leak
- Chemotherapy: **5-FU** and **cisplatin**
  - Give <u>pre-op</u> chemo-XRT for tumors **T2 or greater**
  - Give <u>post-op</u> chemo for **≥ T2 or node-positive disease**
- **Malignant fistulas** (broncho-esophageal) - most die within 3 months due to aspiration;
  - Tx - **esophageal covered stent** for palliation

ESOPHAGECTOMY COMPLICATIONS
- **Air Leak** intra-op
  - Performing transhiatal, mobilizing intra-thoracic esophagus, and anesthesiologist states there is an **air leak**
  - Likely tear in **distal trachea** or **left** mainstem
  - Dx: bronchoscopy to find tear
  - Place a long single lumen tube down non-injured bronchus and ventilate (usually need right bronchus mainstem intubation)
  - **Right thoracotomy** to access the distal trachea and proximal left mainstem bronchus
  - Primary repair of the tear
- **Bleeding** intra-op
  - **High** and **dark** (with transhiatal) - <u>right</u> thoracotomy, look for tear in **azygos vein**
  - **Low** and **bright** (with transhiatal) - <u>left</u> thoracotomy, look for **aortic branch** tear
  - **Intra-abdominal** - likely **spleen** if severe
- **Positive** or **close margins** with Ivor Lewis - drape for 3 hole with anastomosis in the neck and resect for additional margin

- **Chylothorax** (see Thoracic chapter)
- **Neck (cervical) anastomosis leak**
  - Sx's: fevers, elevated WBCs, wound infection
  - May have leak on routine gastrografin swallow
  - If **wound infection** or anastomosis looks **completely apart** on gastrografin swallow → go to OR, **open wound**, and assess stomach
    - If stomach looks <u>healthy</u> (not necrotic) → **washout, place drains,** and **loosely close** neck incision; keep NPO *(leak will eventually heal)*
    - If stomach is <u>necrotic</u> (black) - resect necrotic portion and return stomach remnant to abdomen, cervical esophagostomy, late reconstruction with colon (wait 3 months)
  - If **small leak** found on contrast study and **no wound infection** (eg contained leak) → make sure the leak is adequately drained and wait it out *(keep patient NPO)*
- **Thoracic anastomosis leak**
  - If *asymptomatic* and found on routine contrast study → *usually just wait it out (leave drains in, keep patient NPO);* if completely disrupted → reop
  - If associated with *systemic complications* (eg fever, purulent drainage) → reop and washout area (risk of mediastinitis), will need either: 1) primary repair, 2) redo anastomosis, <u>or</u> 3) complete takedown of the anastomosis
- **Cervical wound infection** after esophagectomy
  - Sx's: pus and saliva drainage; surrounding erythema
  - Go to OR and **open wound** (if necrotic stomach, see above); assess for leak
  - Tx: **washout, leave drains, and loosely close**
  - Gastrografin swallow to look for occult leak after washout - if leak is found, Tx as above for small anastomotic leak
- **Anastomotic stenosis** (usually from ischemia) - serial dilation

Stomach

740. All of the following are true except:
   - a. The right gastric artery is a branch off the proper hepatic artery
   - b. The left gastric artery is a branch off the celiac axis.
   - c. A bleeding ulcer from the posterior 1st portion of the duodenum is likely bleeding from the proper hepatic artery
   - d. The short gastrics are branches of the splenic artery

   Answer c. The **gastroduodenal artery** (GDA) is involved in ulcer bleeding in the 1st portion of the posterior duodenum. The **GDA** is a branch of the **common hepatic artery** and comes off just before the right gastric artery.

   The **right gastric artery** is a branch off the proper hepatic artery and comes off just after (distal) the GDA.

741. Which of the following are true:
   - a. Parietal cells are located primarily in the antrum
   - b. G cells are located primarily in the antrum
   - c. Complete vagotomy results in increased liquid emptying and decreased solid emptying
   - d. Diarrhea following vagotomy is due to sustained motor myenteric complexes and is improved with cholestyramine
   - e. Incomplete vagotomy is the MCC of recurrent peptic ulcer after ulcer surgery.

   Answer a. **Parietal cells** are located primarily in the body and fundus.

742. All of the following are true except:
   - a. Dieulafoy's lesion is a submucosal vascular malformation
   - b. Intractable dumping syndrome refractory to a high protein, high fat, low carbohydrate diet is best treated with octreotide
   - c. Menetrier's disease is associated with massive gastric folds, protein loss, diffuse foveolar hyperplasia, achlorhydria, and treatment with Cetuximab
   - d. Large undigestable food particles partially obstructing the pylorus should be treated with gastrostomy
   - e. Gastric lymphoma is primarily treated with chemo-XRT

   Answer d. Phytobezoars can be treated with: Coca-Cola (degrades fiber), papain, cellulase enzymes, meat tenderizer, and EGD. Surgery should be reserved for failure of these therapies

743. The best test for the diagnosis of H. pylori is:
   - a. Histologic examination of endoscopic biopsies of the antrum
   - b. Urease test of biopsies of the fundus
   - c. Urea breath test
   - d. ELISA

   Answer a. The best test for the diagnosis H. pylori is **histologic examination of endoscopic biopsies of the antrum**. If H. pylori is present, Tx with 3 prong therapy should be started (amoxicillin, clarithromycin, proton pump inhibitor).

   H. pylori infection is the most important RF for peptic ulcer disease.

744. The best test for confirming the eradication of H. pylori is:
   - a. Histologic examination of endoscopic biopsies of the antrum
   - b. Urease test of biopsies of the fundus
   - c. Urea breath test
   - d. ELISA

Answer c. A **urea breath test** avoids the necessity of repeat EGD (which is invasive and costs more).

745. A 55 you man undergoes EGD and is found to have a Mallory-Weiss tear. The most appropriate next step is:
    a.   Washout area and place drains
    b.   Angiography and embolization
    c.   EGD treatment
    d.   Open ligation of area
    e.   Graham patch

    Answer c. EGD Tx. A **Mallory-Weiss tear** is a tear in the gastric mucosa after forceful vomiting that can result in **bleeding**. Initial therapy should be EGD with hemoclips. If EGD therapy fails, open ligation of the area is appropriate.

746. A 55 yo man with hematemesis has a bleeding posterior duodenal ulcer on EGD. The most appropriate next step is:
    a.   EGD therapy
    b.   Embolization
    c.   PPI *only*
    d.   GDA ligation
    e.   Graham patch

    Answer a. EGD Tx with hemo-clips. Epinephrine injection and cautery can also be used.

747. The above patient has continued bleeding, requiring 4 units of blood, despite EGD therapy. The most appropriate next step is:
    a.   EGD therapy
    b.   Embolization
    c.   PPI *only*
    d.   GDA ligation
    e.   Graham patch

    Answer d. GDA ligation through a duodenal incision (duodenostomy).

    If the patient had been previously treated with PPI (history of ulcer Tx) and was stable in the OR, **vagotomy** and **pyloroplasty** at the same procedure would also be indicated.

748. A 55 yo man develops severe epigastric pain. CT scan shows free air. You explore him and find a perforated gastric ulcer. The most appropriate next step is:
    a.   Antrectomy including the ulcer and vagotomy
    b.   Whipple
    c.   Ligaton of GDA
    d.   Graham patch
    e.   Stent

    Answer a. Antrectomy including the ulcer and vagotomy. You should _resect_ **gastric ulcers** when you have to operate as there is a high likelihood that this actually represents **gastric CA**.

749. A 55 yo man develops severe epigastric pain. CT scan shows free air. You explore him and find a perforated duodenal ulcer. The most appropriate next step is:
    a.   Antrectomy including the ulcer and vagotomy
    b.   Whipple
    c.   Ligaton of GDA
    d.   Graham patch
    e.   Stent

Answer d. Graham patch. You do not need to resect duodenal ulcers. Patient's with duodenal ulcers essentially have no increased GI CA risk and have actually been shown in several studies to have a _decreased_ risk of GI CA compared to the general population. The mechanism by which duodenal ulcers _decrease_ the risk of GI cancers is not fully understood.

If the patient had been previously treated with PPI (history of ulcer Tx) and was stable in OR, **vagotomy** and **pyloroplasty** at the same procedure is indicated.

750. A 45 yo man has been vomiting copious amounts of fluid for several hours due to gastric outlet blockage from a large gastric or possible duodenal ulcer. You place a naso-gastric tube. All of the following are true for this patient's volume replacement except:
    a.   He likely has a hypochloremic, hypokalemic metabolic alkalosis
    b.   The key is to replace the chloride deficit
    c.   Initial volume replacement should be normal saline
    d.   Maintenance therapy after resuscitation should be lactated ringers

    Answer d. This patient has **gastric outlet obstruction**. This can result in **hypochloremic, hypokalemic metabolic alkalosis**. Adults with severe gastric fluid loss should have their volume replaced initially with **normal saline**. The key is to replace the **chloride deficit**. After volume resuscitation is started, potassium should be given as a separate infusion. Maintenance fluid for ongoing gastric losses is D5 1/2 NS with 20 meq K.

    Tx for obstructing gastric or duodenal ulcer is NG tube suction, PPI, and TPN for up to a week. These usually open up without surgical intervention

    In **children with pyloric stenosis** and severe dehydration, it is important to _hold the potassium_ until adequate urine output is established. Initially, volume resuscitation for severe dehydration is a bolus of **normal saline** (10 cc/kg) and then normal saline 2 x maintenance until the child makes urine. Then change to D5 1/2 NS with 10 meq of K. It may take up to 48 hours to fully resuscitate severely dehydrated children.

751. A 60 yo man undergoes partial gastrectomy and has a Billroth II anastomosis (gastro-jejunostomy). Two months after the procedure he develops severe abdominal pain and non-bilious vomiting. Eventually he has a bilious emesis and the pain is relieved. Which of the following tests is most diagnostic of this patient's symptoms:
    a.   Abdominal CT
    b.   EGD
    c.   Angiography
    d.   HIDA scan

    Answer a. Based on the Sx's, this patient is likely suffering from **afferent loop obstruction**. The best test is an **abdominal CT scan** (shows dilated fluid filled limb that does not fill with contrast). EGD balloon dilatation can be used to relieve the obstruction, with surgery if that fails.

752. A 60 yo man undergoes partial gastrectomy and has a Billroth II anastomosis. Months later he develops mild abdominal pain and steatorrhea. His peripheral blood smear shows megaloblastic anemia. Which of the following tests is most diagnostic of this patient's symptoms:
    a.   HIDA scan
    b.   CT scan
    c.   Angiography
    d.   EGD aspiration
    e.   MRI

    Answer d. EGD aspiration. This patient is suffering from **afferent loop syndrome** (blind loop syndrome) caused by poor motility of the biliary limb and

bacterial overgrowth. Bacteria use up **B-12** which results in **megaloblastic anemia. Steatorrhea** can be aggrevated but the blind loop due to deconjugation of bile acids. EGD with aspiration is used to make the diagnosis.

Tx - **tetracycline** and **metronidazole** (Flagyl) to reduce bacteria; **metoclopramide** (Reglan) or erythromycin to improve afferent limb motility

753. A 60 yo man undergoes partial gastrectomy and has a Billroth II anastomosis. One year later he develops gastric pain and bilious emesis (which does not relieve the pain). EGD reveals bile in the stomach and biopsy shows gastritis. All of the following are true of this condition except:
    a.   The majority of patients with bile reflux do not develop Sx's
    b.   Sx's do not correlate with the amount of bile in the stomach
    c.   Conversion to a Roux-en-Y gastrojejunostomy is a surgical option
    d.   This is more common with a Billroth I compared to Billroth II
    e.   Cholestyramine may help with Sx's

    Answer c. Bile reflux gastritis is more common with a *Billroth II* compared to *Billroth I*. Bile reflux gastritis can present <u>late</u> after gastric surgery.

754. A 60 yo man undergoes partial gastrectomy and has a Billroth II anastomosis. Five days later he develops severe RUQ pain, fever, and hypotension. This is most consistent with:
    a.   Cholecystitis
    b.   Pancreatitis
    c.   Duodenal stump blow-out
    d.   Hepatitis
    e.   Cholangitis

    Answer c. Duodenal stump blow-out - emergent re-exploration, washout, and placement of a lateral duodenostomy tube is indicated for the above patient.

755. The MC nutritional and metabolic disorder following gastrectomy is:
    a.   Calcium deficiency
    b.   Iron deficiency
    c.   B-12 deficiency
    d.   Folate deficiency
    e.   Fat-soluble vitamin deficiency

    Answer b. Iron deficiency

756. All of the following are true of gastric adenocarcinoma except:
    a.   5 cm margins are indicated for resectable tumors
    b.   Resectable cardia tumors are best treated with total gastrectomy
    c.   Stents can be used for proximal, non-resectable lesions causing obstruction
    d.   Gastro-jejunostomy is preferred over total gastrectomy for palliation of non-resectable distal obstructions

    Answer a. 10 cm margins are generally advocated for gastric CA

757. A patient with a history of pancreatitis develops severe bleeding from gastric varices. You do not see any esophageal varices on EGD. U/S shows splenic vein thrombosis. The portal vein is patent. The best Tx for this patient's most likely condition is:
    a.   Splenectomy
    b.   TIPS procedure
    c.   Spleno-renal shunt
    d.   Porto-caval shunt

    Answer a. Gastric varices without esophageal varices are most likely from **splenic vein thrombosis** related to pancreatitis and not cirrhosis. U/S or CT scan are used to demonstrate splenic vein thrombosis. Tx for symptomatic isolated gastric varices related to splenic vein thrombosis is **splenectomy**.

Asymptomatic splenic vein thrombosis should be left alone.

758. All of the following are improved after gastric bypass except:
   a. Diabetes
   b. Hypertension
   c. GERD
   d. Marginal ulcers

   Answer d. Marginal ulcers are a complication of gastric bypass. They occur after any gastro-jejunostomy as the jejunum *lacks* **Brunner's glands** (alkaline mucus) which usually protect the duodenum from acidic gastric secretions.

759. A patient with a BMI of 29 and GERD is best treated with:
   a. Diet modification
   b. Diet modification and medical weight management program
   c. Gastric banding
   d. Gastric bypass
   e. Nothing

   Answer a. Diet modification

760. A patient with a BMI of 34, DM, and GERD is best treated with:
   a. Diet modification
   b. Diet modification and medical weight management program
   c. Gastric banding
   d. Gastric bypass
   e. Nothing

   Answer b. Diet modification and medical weight management program. This patient doesn't quite meet criteria for surgical intervention.

761. A patient with a BMI of 45, HTN, sleep apnea, and significant knee pain would be best treated with:
   a. Diet modification
   b. Diet modification and medical weight management program
   c. Gastric banding
   d. Gastric bypass
   e. Nothing

   Answer d. For patients with this high of a BMI, medical therapy and a weight loss program are very *unlikely* to work, although patients should be started on these programs for education about future dietary habits. The best long term solution for this patient is laparoscopic gastric bypass.

762. The above patient (age 30) undergoes laparoscopic gastric bypass and on POD #5 has significant irritability. Her vital signs are: BP 110/60, HR 130, RR 40. She also complains of vague shoulder discomfort   What is the most appropriate next step:
   a. Abdominal CT
   b. Upper GI series
   c. Re-exploration
   d. Heparin
   e. WBC scan

   Answer c. Re-exploration for leak. *Tachycardia may be the only finding of a leak.* Other Sx's - tachypnea, irritability, left shoulder or flank pain; *late* oliguria and fever *(usually do not have abdominal pain or tenderness).*

763. The above patient eventually recovers. On POD #10, however, she develops sudden severe dyspnea. ABG values are: pO_2 50 and pCO_2 25. The most appropriate next step is:
   - a. Re-exploration
   - b. Chest CT
   - c. Upper GI series
   - d. Heparin
   - e. WBC scan

   Answer d. Start heparin. This patient has likely suffered a PE (dyspnea, hypoxia, hypocarbia). Starting heparin *before* CT angio is indicated if the clinical suspicion is high. Massive PE is the MCC of death following gastric bypass.

764. Following open gastric bypass, how should the incision be closed:
   - a. Non-absorbable fascia closure and skin staples
   - b. Non-absorbable fascia closure, closed suction drain, and skin staples
   - c. Non-absorbable fascia closure, layered vicryls, and skin staples
   - d. Non-absorbable fascia closure, layered vicryls, closed suction drains, and skin staples

   Answer a. Non-absorbable **fascia closure** and **skin** staples. *Drains and sutures in fat should be avoided during laparotomy closure.*

765. A 35 yo woman with previous gastric bypass presents to the ED with crampy abdominal pain. The most important issue to assess for is:
   - a. Appendicitis
   - b. Cholecystitis
   - c. Internal hernia
   - d. Diverticulitis
   - e. Gallstone Ileus

   Answer c. Internal hernia can be devastating. Patients with previous gastric bypass are at high risk for this complication at any point following surgery. Clinical suspicion should remain high.

766. CT scan in the above patient shows a fluid-filled closed loop of small intestine. The most appropriate next step is:
   - a. NPO, bowel rest, NGT and IVFs
   - b. Reglan
   - c. EGD
   - d. Go to the OR

   Answer d. This patient needs immediate abdominal exploration to relieve the **internal hernia**.

767. Which of the following is true of gastric polyps:
   - a. Fundic gland polyps are typically associated with H. pylori infection
   - b. Hyperplastic polyps are typically associated with atrophic gastric mucosa
   - c. Adenomatous gastric polyps have no malignancy risk
   - d. Fundic gland polyps related to PPI have a 10% CA risk
   - e. Fundic gland polyps are the MC gastric polyp

   Answer b. Hyperplastic gastric polyps are usually associated with **atrophic gastric mucosa.**

   Fundic gland gastric polyps are the **MC gastric polyp;** are *rarely* associated with H. pylori; if related to PPI use, *rarely* result in CA.

   Adenomatous gastric polyps have a definite **malignancy risk**.

768. A 50 yo man presents with epigastric pain unrelieved with PPIs. You perform EGD and a mass is found in the stomach mucosa *only*. You biopsy it and it comes back mucosa associated lymphoid tissue. The next appropriate Tx is:
    a. Total gastrectomy
    b. Partial gastrectomy
    c. Chemo-XRT
    d. Tx for H pylori

Answer d. Mucosa associated lymphoproliferative tissue lymphoma (MALT lymphoma) is related to H pylori infection and is considered a *low grade* B cell NHL. Initial Tx is with **3 pronged Tx for H. pylori** (amoxicillin, clarithromycin and PPI) which cures 90% of patients.

769. A 50 yo man presents with epigastric pain unrelieved with PPIs. EGD shows a 6 cm intra-mural hypoechoic mass in the stomach. CT scan does not demonstrate any adenopathy. The biopsy comes back as C-kit positive. What is the most appropriate next step:
    a. H. pylori Tx
    b. Chemo-XRT
    c. WLE with 1 cm margin
    d. Partial gastrectomy
    e. Total gastrectomy

Answer c. Resection with 1 cm margin. This is a **GIST tumor** (gastro-intestinal stromal tumor) based on the C-kit finding.

770. The patient above undergoes resection but intra-op U/S and biopsy shows diffuse liver metastases. The next appropriate Tx is:
    a. Radiation therapy
    b. 5 fluorouracil and cisplatin
    c. Imatinib (Gleevec)
    d. Do nothing

Answer c. Surgical excision with clear margins is the best Tx for **GIST tumors** (75 % benign, 25% malignant). **Imatinib** (Gleevec) a tyrosine kinase inhibitor, has been extremely effective for malignant GIST tumors.

ANATOMY
- **Blood supply**
  - **Celiac trunk** - left gastric, common hepatic, and splenic arteries
  - **Right gastric artery** is a branch off the proper hepatic artery (comes off <u>after</u> the GDA)
  - **Gastroduodenal artery** (GDA) is a branch off common hepatic artery
  - **Right gastroepiploic** is a branch off the GDA
  - **Left gastroepiploic** and **short gastric** are branches of the **splenic artery**
  - **Greater curvature** - right and left gastroepiploic's and short gastrics
  - **Lesser curvature** - right and left gastric arteries
  - **Pylorus** - gastroduodenal artery
- **Mucosa** - simple columnar epithelium
- **Peristalsis** <u>only</u> occurs in the **distal stomach**

GLANDS
- **Cardia glands** - mucus secreting
- **Fundus** and **body glands**
  - **Chief cells** release **pepsinogen** (*1ˢᵗ enzyme in proteolysis*)
    Increase pepsinogen release - acetylcholine (vagus) and gastrin
  - **Parietal cells** release **HCl** and **intrinsic factor**
    Increase HCL release - gastrin, histamine, acetylcholine (vagus)
    Decrease HCl release - **somatostatin**, secretin, CCK
    Intrinsic factor - binds B-12; complex absorbed in **terminal ileum**

> > Pernicious anemia - megaloblastic anemia due to _loss_ of **parietal cells**, _loss_ of **intrinsic factor**, _or_ **atrophic gastritis**
> > **Atrophic gastritis** - chronic loss of gastric glandular cells
> > > Have _low_ HCl (**achlorhydria**; have _elevated_ gastrin), _low_ pepsin, and _low_ intrinsic factor (**pernicious anemia**)

- **Chief cells** and **parietal cells** are located primarily in the fundus and body
■ Antrum and pylorus glands
  - **G cells** release **gastrin** - reason antrectomy helps with ulcer surgery
    Stimulates release - protein, acetylcholine (vagus)
    Inhibits release - H$^+$ in duodenum
  - **D cells** secrete **somatostatin** - primarily _inhibits_ gastrin and acid release
    Inhibits many other GI functions _(the great inhibitor)_
  - **Mucus** and **HCO$_3^-$ secreting glands** - protect stomach
  - **G cells** are located primarily in the **antrum**
■ Duodenum glands
  - **Brunner's glands** - **alkaline mucus** protects duodenum from acid _(jejunum does not have these, can get **marginal ulcers** after roux-en-Y gastro-jejunostomy)_
  - **Somatostatin, CCK,** and **secretin** - all released from duodenum with duodenal **acidification**
■ **Billroth I** - antrectomy with gastro-duodenal anastomosis
■ **Billroth II** - antrectomy with gastro-jejunal anastomosis (has a roux limb)
■ **Rapid gastric emptying** RFs: previous surgery (#1)
■ **Delayed gastric emptying** RFs: diabetes, opiates, hypothyroidism
■ **Trichobezoars** (hair) - hard to pull out; often have psychiatric disorder
  - Tx: EGD generally inadequate; likely need **gastrostomy** and removal
■ **Phytobezoars** (fiber, vegetable matter) - often in _diabetics_ with poor gastric emptying; more common in patients with _previous gastric surgery_
  - Tx: **Coca-cola** (degrades fiber); papain (meat tenderizers) or cellulase enzymes; EGD, diet changes
■ **Dieulafoy's lesion** - large, tortuous, submucosal, arteriole malformation; can **bleed** (Tx: EGD clips)
■ **Menetrier's disease** (hypoproteinemic hypertrophic gastropathy) - massive **gastric folds**, excessive **mucus production** with resultant **protein loss** (hypoproteinemia; and weight loss), and little to **zero acid production** (achlorhydria)
  - Sx's: pain, weight loss, diarrhea
  - Histology - massive foveolar hyperplasia (hyperplasia of surface and glandular mucus cells) and _loss_ of parietal cells
  - RFs - CMV infection in children, H. pylori in adults
  - 24 hour pH study reveals **achlorhydria**
  - Biopsies are indicated to rule-out gastric CA
  - Small increased risk of **gastric CA**
  - Related to _excessive_ transforming growth factor alpha (**TGF-alpha**) production
  - Tx: **high protein diet**, anticholinergic agents, H. pylori eradication, *__Cetuximab__ (blocks epidermal growth factor receptor); gastrectomy may be required in some
■ **Hypergastrinemia** (elevated gastrin level) can be caused by - retained gastric antrum, G cell hyperplasia, pernicious anemia, and renal insufficiency (DDx vs gastrinoma)

MALLORY-WEISS TEAR
■ Secondary to **forceful vomiting**
■ _**Tear** is in **stomach** (not the esophagus)_
  - Usually along the lesser curve, near the GE junction
■ Presents as **hematemesis** following severe retching
■ Bleeding often stops spontaneously
■ Dx/Tx: **EGD** with **hemo-clips**
■ If continued bleeding, may need gastrostomy and over-sewing of the area

GASTRIC VOLVULUS
■ Associated with **paraesophageal hernia**
■ Nausea _without_ vomiting; severe pain; usually **organoaxial volvulus**
■ Tx: reduction and Nissen

ACUTE GASTRIC DISTENSION
- Sx's: severe **abdominal distension** and **pain** → followed by **bradycardia, hypotension, tachypnea,** and **sweating**
- As stomach distends, initiates **vaso-vagal response** (compresses vagus)
- RFs: pancreatitis, recent surgery, psychiatric disorders
- Can be a life threatening complication
- Tx: **NG tube**

VAGOTOMIES
- **Vagotomy** - both **truncal** and **highly selective** will *increase* liquid emptying → vagally mediated receptive relaxation is removed (results in increased gastric pressure that accelerates liquid emptying)
  - **Truncal** vagotomy - divides vagal trunks at level of esophagus; will *decrease* emptying **of solids** (from pyloric constriction)
  - **Highly selective** vagotomy - preserves trunks and divides individual fibers; Criminal nerve of Grassi is divided as well; preserves distal 7 cm "crow's foot" to antrum; have *normal* emptying **of solids**
- Addition of **pyloroplasty** to vagotomy results in *increased* solid emptying
- Other alterations caused by **truncal vagotomy**:
  - **Gastric effects** - decreased acid output by 90%; gastrin will *increase*
  - **Diarrhea** (40%) - *MC problem following truncal vagotomy*
      Caused by **sustained MMCs** (migrating motor complex) forcing **bile acids** into the colon
      Tx: **cholestyramine** and **loperamide**
  - Other non-gastric effects - *decreased* pancreas and biliary function, gallstones

UPPER GASTROINTESTINAL BLEEDING (UGI bleeding)
- RFs: previous UGI bleed, peptic ulcers, NSAID use, smoking, esophageal varices, splenic vein thrombosis, sepsis, burns, trauma, severe vomiting
- If on warfarin, reverse with **prothrombin complex** (or **FFP** *and* IV **Vit K**)
- Dx/Tx: **EGD** (confirm bleeding is from an ulcer); can potentially treat with hemo-clips *(best)*, epinephrine injection, and cautery
  - RFs for **re-bleeding** at the time of initial EGD:
      #1 *spurting blood vessel* (60% chance of re-bleed)
      #2 visible blood vessel (40% chance of re-bleed)
      #3 diffuse oozing (30% chance of re-bleed)
  - Highest RF for **mortality** with non-variceal UGI bleed - *continued or re-bleeding despite EGD*
  - Patients with **liver failure** are likely bleeding from esophageal varices, not an ulcer → Tx: EGD with **variceal banding** or **sclerotherapy**; TIPS if local therapy fails (*vasopressin or octreotide to temporize bleeding until EGD Tx*)
  - UGI bleed but **can't find source with EGD** (eg too much blood, food) → Dx: **angiography**
  - **Slow bleeding** and trouble localizing source → Dx: **tagged RBC scan**

DUODENAL ULCERS
- **MC peptic ulcer** (more common than gastric)
- From increased **acid production**
- RFs: *H. pylori* (#1 risk factor), NSAIDs, tobacco, ETOH, males, uremia, stress (burns, sepsis, and trauma), steroids, chemotherapy
- **H. pylori** - found in 90% of duodenal ulcers
- MC location - **1st portion** of duodenum (bulb); usually **anterior**
  - **Anterior** ulcers <u>perforate</u>
  - **Posterior** ulcers <u>bleed</u> from **gastroduodenal artery**
  - **MC Cx of duodenal ulcers** - <u>bleeding</u> (often minor; life-threatening if GDA)
- Sx's: epigastric pain radiating to back; pain may worsen initially with eating (duodenal acid secretion)
- Dx: **EGD** *(best test)*
- *Best test for H. pylori Dx:* **histologic examination of antral Bx's**
- *Best test for H. pylori eradication* - **urea breath test** (radiolabeled urea given and $^{13}CO_2$ is measured)

- Tx: triple therapy for *Helicobacter pylori* (PPI, amoxicillin, clarithromycin)
- *Surgery for ulcers rarely indicated since PPIs*
- Need to rule out **gastrinoma** if complicated ulcer disease (Zollinger-Ellison syndrome - **gastric acid hypersecretion, peptic ulcers** and **gastrinoma**)
- **Surgical indications:**
  - **Perforation**
  - **Protracted bleeding** despite EGD therapy
  - **Obstruction**
  - **Intractability** despite medical Tx
  - *If the patient has been on a PPI (eg ulcer Tx history) - consider an **acid-reducing procedure** at time of surgery for bleeding or perforation*
- **Surgical options** (acid-reducing surgery)
  - Unlike gastric ulcers, duodenal ulcers have <u>no</u> malignancy potential (most studies show that duodenal ulcers actually <u>decrease</u> stomach CA risk *and* overall GI CA risk) so resection of ulcer is <u>not</u> necessary
  - **Highly selective vagotomy** - <u>lowest</u> rate of Cx's and <u>highest</u> rate of recurrence; no need for antral or pylorus procedure; 10-15% ulcer recurrence (with experienced surgeons; *as high as **30-40% in recent studies***); 0.1% mortality *(very few surgeons perform these - hard procedure to perform effectively)*
  - **Truncal vagotomy** and **pyloroplasty** - 5-10% ulcer recurrence, 1% mortality
  - **Truncal vagotomy** and **antrectomy** - 1-2% ulcer recurrence (<u>lowest</u> rate of recurrence), 2% mortality
  - **Reconstruction** after antrectomy - roux-en-Y gastro-jejunostomy *(best)*; less dumping syndrome and *less* **alkaline reflux gastritis** compared to Billroth I (gastro-duodenal anastomosis) and Billroth II (gastro-jejunal anastomosis)
  - Billroth I and Billroth II are <u>rarely</u> performed anymore
- **Bleeding**
  - MC Cx of duodenal ulcers
  - Major bleeding usually occur in the **1st portion** of the **posterior** duodenum
  - Usually minor but can be life-threatening
  - **Major bleeding**:
    > 6 units of blood in 24 hours <u>or</u>;
    Patient remains hypotensive despite transfusion
  - **Dx + Tx: EGD 1st - hemoclips** *(best)*, cautery, epinephrine injection
    Vasopressin, octreotide, and IV PPI to temporize until EGD
  - **Criteria for surgery <u>following</u> EGD Tx** for bleeding duodenal ulcer (*any* of the following):
    1) **> 4 units of blood** and **still bleeding**
    2) In **shock** despite multiple blood transfusions
    3) **Recurrent bleed** after maximal EGD Tx
    → *all indications for OR*
  - **Surgery** - duodenotomy and **gastroduodenal artery** (GDA) **ligation**
    Avoid hitting common bile duct (posterior) with GDA ligation
    Consider acid-reducing surgery (**vagotomy + pyloroplasty** preferred in this emergent setting) if patient has been on PPI (ulcer Tx history)
- **Obstruction** (gastric outlet obstruction)
  - Tx: *fluid resuscitation 1st* (normal saline); **PPI** and **serial dilation** initial Tx of choice (NPO, TPN) - majority open up with conservative Tx
  - Get **metabolic alkalosis** (hypokalemic, hypochloremic metabolic alkalosis)
  - Need Bx to rule-out CA
  - Surgical options - **antrectomy** and **truncal vagotomy** *(best)*; may include obstructing ulcer in resection if proximal to ampulla of Vater
- **Perforation**
  - 80% will have free air
  - Sx's: sudden sharp epigastric pain; can have generalized peritonitis
  - Pain can radiate to the pericolic gutters (<u>flank</u> pain) with dependent drainage of gastric contents or to the diaphragm (<u>shoulder</u> pain)
  - Tx: **Graham patch** (place **omentum** over perforation)
    Consider acid-reducing surgery if patient has been on PPI (ulcer Tx history)

- Intractability
  - \> 3 months without relief while on escalating doses of PPI
  - Dx based on EGD **mucosal findings**, not Sx's
  - Tx: acid-reducing surgery

GASTRIC ULCERS
- RFs - same as duodenal ulcers *(H. pylori #1)*
- MC location - **lesser curvature** of the stomach body (80%)
- Most have <u>normal</u> acid secretion and <u>decreased</u> mucosal defense
- **Hemorrhage** is associated with *higher* mortality than duodenal ulcers
- There is a significant **gastric CA risk** in patients with gastric ulcers
- Sx's: epigastric pain radiating to the back; relieved with eating but recurs 30 minutes later; melena or guaiac-positive stools
- *Best test for H. pylori* - **histological examination of Bx's from antrum** (70% of gastric ulcers have H. pylori)
- *Best test for H. pylori eradication* - **urea breath test** (radiolabeled urea given and $^{13}CO_2$ is measured)
- Types:
  - Type I - **lesser curve,** between body and antrum; *MC type of gastric ulcer (85%)*
  - Type II - **2 ulcers** (stomach ulcer and duodenal; from *high* acid secretion)
  - Type III - **pre-pyloric** (*high* acid secretion)
  - Type IV - <u>**high**</u> along **cardia,** near **GE junction**
  - Type V - ulcer associated with **NSAIDs**
- Tx: **triple therapy** for Helicobacter pylori (PAC; proton pump inhibitor, amoxicillin, and clarithromycin; 14 days); discontinue smoking, ETOH, and NSAIDs → 99% of ulcers are effectively treated with medical Tx
  - **Refractory** ulcer (switch antibiotics) - PPI, metronidazole, and tetracycline
  - May need to **escalate PPI dose**
  - **Urea breath test** (patient ingests ^{13}C-urea; **urease** in H. Pylori cleaves it and releases $^{13}CO_2$ which is measured in patient's breath [should be *low* if H pylori is eradicated])
- **Surgical indications** - perforation, bleeding not controlled with EGD, obstruction, inability to exclude CA, intractability (> 3 months without relief - based on mucosal findings <u>not</u> Sx's)
- *Ulcer surgery is rare since PPIs*
- Tx: **antrectomy** and **truncal vagotomy** (roux-en-Y gastro-jejunostomy); **include ulcer** in resection (extended antrectomy) - need **separate ulcer excision** if that is not possible *(gastric ulcers are **resected** at time of surgery due to high risk of **gastric CA**)*
  - Omental patch and ligation of bleeding vessels are *poor options* for gastric ulcers due to *high* recurrence of Sx's and risk of **gastric CA** in the ulcer
  - Although Type I and IV ulcers are not generally associated with high acid secretion, an acid reducing procedure (ie vagotomy) is **recommended** to help reduce the risk of recurrent ulcers
- **Cushing's ulcer** - head trauma and gastric ulcer
- **Curling's ulcer** - significant burns and duodenal ulcer

GASTRIC VARICES
- 90% of gastric varices are associated with esophageal varices
- 10% of gastric varices are isolated
- <u>*Isolated*</u> gastric varices →
  - MC from **splenic vein thrombosis** (secondary to **pancreatitis**)
  - Very uncommonly from portal HTN or portal vein thrombosis
  - These can **bleed**
- Dx: **U/S** - make sure splenic vein thrombosis is the problem, not cirrhosis
- Tx: *if symptomatic* → **splenectomy**; *if asymptomatic* → *leave alone*

STRESS GASTRITIS
- Occurs 3-10 days after event; lesions appear in **fundus** *first*
- Tx: **PPI**
- EGD with cautery of specific bleeding points may be effective
- **Chronic gastritis** often associated with *H. pylori*

GASTRIC POLYPS

- **Fundic gland** polyp (*MC type of gastric polyp*; 75%) - associated with **PPIs** or patients who have **FAP**
  - Extremely <u>low</u> malignancy potential for sporadic cases
  - *<u>Not</u> associated with H. pylori*
  - Rarely larger than 1 cm
  - If numerous (> 20) or in a young patient, consider FAP
  - Polyps **> 1 cm** related to **PPI** - remove and consider stopping PPI
  - **> 20 polyps** related to **PPI** - consider stopping PPI
  - Often regress after stopping PPI
  - **FAP** related - 40% dysplasia risk *(<u>all</u> should be removed)*
- **Hyperplastic** polyp
  - Often related to **H. pylori** infection
  - Associated with **inflamed** or **atrophic gastritis**
  - 10% dysplasia risk, 2% CA risk
  - Hyperplastic polyps at **previous gastrectomy sites** and polyps **> 2 cm** have a <u>higher</u> CA risk
  - Tx: **remove polyps > 1 cm** and **H. pylori eradication**
- **Adenomatous** polyp - can be **sporadic** or in association with **FAP**
  - Can be related to **H. pylori** infection
  - Often arise in background of <u>*chronic*</u> **atrophic gastritis**
  - *Definite CA risk (polyps > 2 cm have a 50% CA risk)*
  - 30% have a *synchronous* **stomach adenocarcinoma** in another area
  - Tx: **endoscopic resection** (repeat EGD in 1 year); **eradication of H. pylori**

GASTRIC CANCER

- Sx's: **epigastric pain** (<u>not</u> relieved by eating) and **weight loss**
- MC site - **antrum** (40%)
- Accounts for 50% of CA-related deaths in **Japan**
- Dx: **EGD** *(best test for Dx)*
  - **CT scan** - *overall best test for resectability*
- RFs: **H. pylori** (#1), adenomatous polyps, tobacco, prior gastric surgery, atrophic gastritis, intestinal metaplasia, pernicious anemia, achlorhydria, nitrosamines, blood type A
- **Adenomatous polyps** - high risk for CA; Tx - endoscopic resection, H. pylori Tx
- **Krukenberg tumor** - drop metastases to <u>ovaries</u>
- **Virchow's node** - metastases to <u>supraclavicular</u> nodes
- **Sister Mary Joseph's nodule** - <u>umbilical</u> node metastases
- MC metastatic site - **liver**
- > 90% are **adenocarcinomas**
- Surgical issues
  - Metastases outside resection area - surgery contraindicated unless palliation
  - Splenectomy is generally <u>not</u> performed.
  - **Splenic invasion** - resect stomach + splenectomy en bloc
- **Intestinal-type** gastric CA (MC type; pathology - **glands, Goblet cells**)
  - Surgical Tx: **subtotal gastrectomy** (need **10 cm** margins)
  - **GE junction tumor** (treat like esophageal CA) - Tx: **esophagectomy** with gastric pull-up
  - **Upper 1/3 tumor** (near cardia; proximal) - Tx: *<u>total</u>* **gastrectomy** and esophago-jejunostomy anastomosis (roux limb)
  - **Middle** or **lower 1/3 tumor** (middle or distal) - Tx: *<u>partial</u>* **distal gastrectomy** and gastro-jejunostomy anastomosis
  - 5-YS (all patients) - **25%**
- **Diffuse** gastric CA (**linitis plastica**; poorly differentiated or undifferentiated)
  - Diffuse **connective tissue invasion** throughout stomach; early **lymphatic invasion**; <u>no</u> glands
  - **Less favorable** prognosis than intestinal-type gastric CA
  - Usually beyond resection at time of Dx
  - Surgery:: **total gastrectomy** if resectable due to diffuse nature of linitis plastica
  - 5-YS (all patients) - **10%**
- Chemotherapy (poor response): 5-FU, doxorubicin, mitomycin C

- Metastatic disease outside area of resection → *contraindication* to resection unless performing surgery for palliation
- **Palliation** of gastric CA:
  - **Obstruction** - *proximal* lesions can be **stented**; *distal* lesions can be bypassed with **gastrojejunostomy**
  - Low to moderate **bleeding** or **pain** - Tx: XRT
  - If these fail, consider palliative gastrectomy for obstruction or bleeding

GIST (Gastro-Intestinal Stromal Tumor)
- **MC benign gastric neoplasm** although 25% are malignant
  - If malignant - behave like sarcomas (<u>no</u> nodal metastases)
- Sx's: usually **asymptomatic** but pain, obstruction, and bleeding can occur; weight loss, early satiety; can be <u>large</u> tumors once Sx's arise
- MC location - **stomach** (70%); can also occur in small bowel
- Dx: **CT scan** *(used for determining tumor extent)*
  - **EGD with Bx** (if gastric) - are **C-KIT positive** (immunostaining); tumor may be missed on EGD because it is **submucosal**
  - EUS - **hypoechoic**, smooth edges
- Path: **spindle cells** and connective tissue (mesenchymal tumor, *not epithelial*)
  - **c-Kit** - receptor tyrosine kinase
  - **Malignant** if **> 5 cm** <u>or</u> **> 5 mitoses / 50 HPF** (high powered field)
    <u>Rare</u> nodal spread (< 5%) if malignant
    MC metastasis - **liver**
- Tx: **wedge resection** with 1 cm margins *(no nodal dissection)*
- If malignant - chemotherapy with **Imatinib** (Gleevec; receptor tyrosine kinase inhibitor; side effect - CHF)

MALT (Mucosal-Associated Lymphoid Tissue Lymphoma)
- Is a <u>low</u> grade **B cell NHL** from mucosa lymphoid tissue
- MC location - **stomach** (80%)
  - Usually **confined to stomach** (95% of patients have **stage I-E**)
  - Other sites - other GI tract, lung, Waldeyer's ring (oral tonsils)
- Related to **H. pylori** infection
- *Usually regresses after treatment for H. pylori*
- Sx's: **pain** (similar to ulcer) and **weight loss**
- Dx: **EUS with Bx** (see mass or large folds)
- Tx: **triple-therapy antibiotics for H. pylori** and surveillance (cures 90%)
  - If MALT does not regress → Tx: **XRT** (cures another 90%)
  - <u>Advanced</u> disease (uncommon; nodes other than peri-gastric, Stage III, or Stage IV) → H. pylori Tx + Chemo-XRT (CHOP-R)
- Overall 5-YS - **95%**

GASTRIC LYMPHOMAS
- Have ulcer Sx's; *stomach is the MC location for* **extra-nodal** *lymphoma*
- Usually **non-Hodgkin's lymphoma** (B cell)
- Dx: EGD with Bx (make sure not a GIST tumor)
- Tx: **Chemo-XRT** are the *primary Tx;* surgery for Cx's
- Resection possibly indicated <u>only</u> for stage I disease (tumor confined to mucosa) and then only partial resection is indicated

MORBID OBESITY
- **Central obesity** - worse prognosis
- **Diet** and **medical Tx** for the <u>severely obese</u> has a success rate of only 3% (however patients should still attempt to treat the 3% who lose weight and to prepare them for the lifestyle changes needed after surgery)
- **Best long-term Tx by BMI**:
  - Normal (20-25) - nothing
  - Overweight (26-29) - diet modification
  - Obese (30-34) - diet and medical weight management program
  - Severely obese (35-49) - RYGB
  - Super-obese (≥ 50) - RYGB

Patient Selection for Bariatric Surgery (need all 4)

1) Body mass index >40 kg/m^2 _or_ ;
   Body mass index >35 kg/m^2 with coexisting co-morbidities (eg DM, HTN, GERD)
2) Failure of nonsurgical methods of weight reduction
3) Psychological stability
4) Absence of drug and alcohol abuse

- **Gets better after surgery** - diabetes, cholesterol, sleep apnea, HTN, urinary incontinence, GERD, venous stasis ulcers, pseudotumor cerebri (intracranial hypertension), joint pain, migraines, depression, polycystic ovarian syndrome, non-alcoholic fatty liver disease, quality of life
- Does <u>not</u> get better after surgery - <u>peripheral arterial disease</u> (PAD)
- **Roux-en-Y gastric bypass** (RYGB)
    - Better early weight loss than just banding
    - Mortality rate - 0.5%
    - Need **75-100 cm jejunum** roux limb
    - Perform **cholecystectomy** during operation if stones present
    - Routine **UGI** on post-op day 2
    - **10% failure rate** due to high carbohydrate snacking
    - **Leak** is the most important and frequent major Cx
- **Laparoscopic adjustable gastric banding** (LAGB)
    - Less initial weight loss (years 1-2), after 3-4 years weight loss similar
    - Biggest issue - some patients do not lose _any_ weight with the band
    - _Not a good option for the super-obese_
    - Lower mortality rate compared to RYGB (0.05% vs. 0.5%); fully reversible; can be done as an outpatient
    - MC Cx: **regurgitation** of non-acidic food from upper pouch (**productive burping**); food can also cause obstruction
        Tx: eating less, more slowly and thoroughly
- **Jejunoileal bypass**
    - These operations are no longer done
    - Cx's: **cirrhosis, nephrolithiasis,** and **osteoporosis** (loss of Ca)
    - Need to correct these and perform RYGB if encountered

GASTRIC BYPASS COMPLICATIONS
- **Leak**
    - _**Tachycardia** may be the <u>only indication</u> of leak in these patients_
    - Sx's: tachycardia, tachypnea, irritability, left shoulder or flank pain
        Usually do <u>not</u> have abdominal pain or tenderness
        <u>Late</u> oliguria and fever
    - Peak incidence - **POD 5** (usually occurs in 1st 2 weeks)
    - MC location - **gastro-jejunal anastomosis**
        others - gastric remnant, jejuno-jejunal anastomosis
    - MCC leak <u>overall</u> (and <u>late</u> leak) - **ischemia**
    - MCC <u>early</u> leak - **technical error**
    - If patient has significant clinical findings (**tachycardia, tachypnea**, or **desaturation**) - _skip diagnostic studies and re-operate to look for leak_
    - Dx: UGI, CT scan _(these may <u>not</u> always show the leak)_
    - **Early leak** (not contained) → Tx: **reoperation**
        At reoperation → washout area, try to repair leak, place drains, and place feeding G-tube in the excluded stomach segment
        If not able to repair leak, best option is to just leave drains rather than takedown the anastomosis (will eventually heal; keep NPO)
    - **Late leak** (weeks out from surgery, likely contained) → Tx: **percutaneous drain** and **antibiotics**
        If clinically unstable or uncontained late leak - Tx: reoperation

- **Small bowel obstruction**
  - This is a *surgical emergency* due to the high risk of **internal hernia** (can cause strangulation, infarction, and subsequent **bowel necrosis**); this is a long term potential Cx and should be suspected in anyone with a gastric bypass (can lead to catastrophic loss of small bowel)
  - Sx's: N/V, intermittent crampy abdominal pain
  - **CT scan** shows dilated small bowel with distal decompression; may also see the herniation or a closed loop small bowel obstruction (often in the LUQ)
  - Tx: *re-exploration (surgical emergency)*
  - SBO can also be caused by a variety of kinking / anastomotic issues in addition to internal hernia
- **Dilation of excluded stomach remnant** post-op - hiccoughs, large stomach bubble; has a risk of staple line disruption; Dx: **AXR**; Tx: percutaneous **G-tube** placement in stomach remnant (U/S guidance)
- **Marginal ulcers** - stomach acid in jejunum, which lacks Brunner's glands, causes ulcers (develops in 10%); Tx - **PPI**
- **Stenosis**
  - Sx's - hiccoughs, large stomach bubble, N/V (obstruction Sx's)
  - Tx: **Early** - re-operate (technical problem)
    - **Late** (from ischemia) - usually responds to **balloon dilation**
- **Iron deficiency anemia**
  - *MC metabolic (nutritional) deficiency after gastrectomy*
  - Surgery <u>bypasses</u> duodenum, where most iron is absorbed
  - Also need <u>acidic</u> environment for iron absorption
  - Tx: **oral iron**
- **B$_{12}$ deficiency** - intrinsic factor needs acidic environment to bind B$_{12}$
  - Sx's: pernicious (megaloblastic) anemia, peripheral neuropathy, glossitis
  - Tx: **B-12 shots** every month
- **Calcium deficiency** - bypasses duodenum where most Ca is absorbed
  - Sx's: perioral tingling, hyperreflexia
  - Tx: **Ca** and **Vit D** (helps with absorption)
- **Folate deficiency** (Sx - megaloblastic anemia) - due to poor absorption
- **Wernicke's encephalopathy / polyneuropathy** - can be irreversible; due to **thiamine deficiency** (B1); usually in setting of <u>persistent</u> / <u>frequent</u> **vomiting** (weeks) and a diet with clears and no vitamin supplements
- **Gallstones** - from rapid weight loss; Tx: cholecystectomy if Sx's
- **Pulmonary embolism** - *MCC of **death** after RYGB* (see Hemostasis chapter); prevent with LMWH
- **GI bleeding**:
    <u>Early</u> - usually **gastro-jejunal anastomosis** or excluded gastric remnant
    <u>Late</u> - usually **marginal ulcer**

POSTGASTRECTOMY COMPLICATIONS (most can also occur after **vagotomy** and pyloroplasty)
- **Post-vagotomy diarrhea**
  - *MC Cx following vagotomy*
  - Due to non-conjugated **bile salts** in the colon (osmotic diarrhea)
  - Caused by **sustained postprandial organized MMCs** (myenteric motor complexes)
  - Some have improvement with diet modification (dietary fiber, reducing carbohydrates and milk products, reduce fluids, small meals)
  - Tx: **cholestyramine** and **loperamide**
  - Surgical option (very rarely needed): reversed interposition jejunal graft
- **Recurrent peptic ulcers**
  - MCC - **incomplete vagotomy**; MC due to a missed Criminal Nerve of Grassi off the right vagus nerve posteriorly
- **Dumping syndrome**
  - Can occur after gastrectomy (especially Billroth I – gastroduodenostomy) or after vagotomy and pyloroplasty
  - Occurs from rapid entrance of **carbohydrates** into **small bowel**
  - 95% of cases resolve with medical Tx + dietary changes

- **2 phases**:
  1) Hyperosmotic load causes <u>fluid shift</u> into bowel (**hypotension**, diarrhea, dizziness)
  2) **Hypoglycemia** (diaphoresis, confusion) from reactive insulin increase (this phase *rarely* occurs) 1-3 hours after phase 1
- Dx: **gastric emptying study** (*best test;* radionuclide colloid scintigraphy) - stomach will dump colloid quickly
- Tx: **small**, <u>high</u>-protein; <u>high</u>-fat, and <u>low</u>-carbohydrate meals; *no* liquids with meals and *no lying down* after meals; **octreotide** if that fails *(very effective)*
- **Surgical options** *(very rarely needed)*
  Conversion of Billroth I or II to Roux-en-Y gastrojejunostomy
  Operations to increase gastric reservoir (jejunal pouch) or increase emptying time (reversed jejunal limb)

■ **Bile reflux gastritis** (alkaline reflux gastritis)
- Most patients have evidence of bile in stomach after gastrectomy or pyloroplasty, however, *only* 1-2% develop Sx's (<u>not</u> dependent on amount of bile)
- Sx's: post-prandial **epigastric pain** associated with N/V; **bilious emesis**
  Pain not relieved with vomiting
  Can occur <u>late</u> after surgery (> 1 year)
- Dx: EGD *(best test)* – 1) evidence of **bile reflux** into stomach <u>and</u>; 2) histologic evidence of **gastritis**; HIDA scan shows bile reflux
- Incidence: Billroth II > Billroth I > vagotomy and pyloroplasty
- Tx: **PPI, cholestyramine, metoclopramide** (can be hard to Tx)
- Surgical option: conversion of Billroth I or Billroth II to Roux-en-Y gastrojejunostomy with long afferent limb (60 cm distal to gastrojejunostomy)

■ **Chronic gastric atony** (delayed gastric emptying)
- Sx's: N/V, pain, early satiety
- Dx: **gastric emptying study** *(best test)*
- Tx: **metoclopramide** or erythromycin (prokinetics)
- Surgical option: near-total gastrectomy with Roux-en-Y

■ **Small gastric remnant** (early satiety)
- Actually want this for gastric bypass patients
- Dx: UGI
- Tx: small meals; Surgical option: jejunal pouch construction

■ **Blind loop syndrome** (afferent loop syndrome; biliary limb)
- Caused by **poor motility** and **stasis** in <u>afferent limb</u> after Billroth II or Roux-en-Y
- Can also be caused by a large diverticulum in the small bowel or entero-enterotomy (side to side small bowel bypass)
- Leads to **bacterial overgrowth** (MC - *E. coli*; GNRs) in afferent limb
- Sx's: **pain, steatorrhea** (bacterial deconjugation of bile), **B₁₂ deficiency** (megaloblastic anemia; bacteria use it up), malabsorption
- Dx: **EGD of afferent limb** with **aspirate and culture** for organisms *(best test)*
  D-xylose test (excessive CO_2 in breath confirms Dx)
  Schilling test (failure of intestinal B-12 uptake; urine B-12 level will be *low*)
- Tx: **tetracycline** and **metronidazole** (Flagyl); B-12, low fat diet
  Metoclopramide (Reglan) or erythromycin to improve afferent limb motility
- Surgical option: re-anastomosis with shorter (40 cm) afferent limb

■ **Afferent-loop obstruction** (biliary limb)
- With Billroth II or Roux-en-Y; caused by **mechanical obstruction** of afferent limb (eg kinking, adhesions, stenosis)
- Sx's: **RUQ pain** and **non-bilious vomiting**, pain *relieved* after bilious emesis *(classic)*
- Can cause closed loop obstruction with fever, shock, and perforation
- RFs: long afferent limb with Roux-en-Y
- Dx: **CT scan** *(best test for Dx)* - shows **dilated afferent limb** filled with fluid and does not fill with contrast
  EGD to look for recurrent tumor, fibrosis, food obstruction, tight or twisted anastomosis - best test to figure out what the exact problem is
- Tx: balloon dilation may be possible
- Surgery: re-anastomosis with shorter (40-cm) afferent limb and relieve any obstruction (may require conversion of B-II to Roux en-Y gastro-jejunostomy)

- **Efferent-loop obstruction**
  - Sx's: N/V, abdominal pain
  - Dx: **UGI** *(best test for Dx)*, CT scan
  - Tx: balloon dilation
  - Surgical option: find site of obstruction and relieve it
- **Duodenal stump blow-out** (leak) - found with Billroth II or Roux-en-Y
  - Leak from duodenal stump after gastrectomy
  - Sx's: **RUQ pain, fever, sepsis** (often _sudden_ onset and severe sepsis)
    Can have rapid deterioration
  - Dx: **CT scan** (*best test*; large fluid collection in sub-hepatic space)
  - Tx: re-operate, washout, place **lateral duodenostomy tube**, drains
- **PEG tube Cx's** - insertion into liver or colon
- **Delayed gastric emptying** - Tx: **metoclopramide, erythromycin**

Liver

771. All of the following are true except:
   a. Kupffer cells are liver macrophages
   b. The vast majority of liver damage from hepatitis B is due to cytotoxic T cells
   c. Hepatic stellate (Ito) cells are the major cell type involved in liver fibrosis
   d. Bile is produced mainly by bile canalicular cells
   e. Bile consists of primarily of bile salts (80%)

   Answer d. Bile is produced mainly by **hepatocytes**

772. All of the following are true of liver anatomy except:
   a. The hepato-duodenal ligament is where the common bile duct, portal vein and proper hepatic artery meet
   b. The ligamentum teres carries the obliterated umbilical vein to the undersurface of the liver
   c. The foramen of Winslow enters the lesser sac
   d. The falciform ligament separates the left and right lobes of the liver
   e. The portal vein is posterior to both the bile duct and hepatic artery

   Answer d. The **falciform ligament** separates the medial and lateral aspects of the left lobe.

773. All of the following are true except::
   a. The caudate lobe receives separate right and left portal and arterial blood supplies.
   b. Most primary and secondary tumors are supplied by the portal vein
   c. The MC left hepatic artery variant comes off the left gastric artery and is found in the gastro-hepatic ligament
   d. The MC right hepatic artery variant is comes off the SMA and is found posterior to the portal vein
   e. The middle hepatic vein joins the left hepatic vein before entering the IVC in the majority of patients

   Answer b. Most primary and secondary tumors are supplied by hepatic artery branches.

774. Which of the following would cause the most significant _increase_ is urine urobilin:
   a. Acute hepatitis
   b. Chronic hepatitis
   c. Massive upper GI bleeding
   d. Common bile duct stones
   e. Sepsis

   Answer c. Massive **upper GI bleeding** causes a significant amount of hemoglobin to be reabsorbed in the gut. Hemoglobin is converted to conjugated bilirubin, released in the gut, and eventually broken down to **urobilinogen**. Urobilinogen is reabsorbed, converted to urobilin, and released in urine (turns it yellow). **Hemolytic jaundice** would also cause urine urobilin to increase.

775. Which of the following would cause the most significant _decrease_ is urine urobilin:
   a. Acute hepatitis
   b. Chronic hepatitis
   c. Massive upper GI bleeding
   d. Common bile duct stones
   e. Sepsis

   Answer d. **Common bile duct stones** (or other forms of biliary obstruction) prevent release of conjugated bilirubin into the gut, thus less urobilinogen (and urobilin) would be formed.

776. A diffuse inhomogenous liver, delayed enhancement of the liver periphery, and an enlarged caudate lobe that demonstrates increased contrast enhancement compared to the rest of the liver is most consistent with:
- a. Hepatocellular CA
- b. Adenoma
- c. Focal nodular hyperplasia (FNH)
- d. Budd-Chiari Syndrome
- e. Portal vein thrombosis

Answer d. The description is classic for **Budd-Chiari Syndrome**.

777. All of the following are true of bile acids except:
- a. Primary bile acids include cholic and chenodeoxycholic
- b. Secondary bile acids include deoxycholic and lithocholic
- c. Tertiary bile acids includes urobilinogen
- d. Bile acids are conjugated to taurine or glycine to improve water solubility
- e. The primary bile phospholipid is lecithin

Answer c. Urobilinogen (is not a bile acid) is a breakdown product of conjugated bilirubin in the gut.

778. All of the following are true of spleno-renal shunts except:
- a. They are indicated for Child's A cirrhosis with bleeding as the only problem
- b. These can make ascites worse
- c. These require ligation of the inferior mesenteric vein
- d. These require splenectomy

Answer d. Splenorenal shunts do <u>not</u> require splenectomy.

779. Which of the following is an indication for TIPS:
- a. Persistent coagulopathy (elevated PT and PTT)
- b. Asterixis
- c. Advanced age
- d. Refractory ascites
- e. Caroli's Disease

Answer d. Refractory ascites

780. All of the following are indications for TIPS procedure except:
- a. Worsening encephalopathy
- b. Protracted variceal bleeding
- c. Refractory ascites
- d. Visceral hypoperfusion

Answer a. TIPS (trans-jugular intra-hepatic porto-systemic shunt) does <u>not</u> improve encephalopathy and may worsen it. TIPS allows antegrade flow from the portal vein to the IVC and decompresses the portal system.

781. All of the following are true of cirrhosis with ascites except:
- a. PRN large volume paracentesis is Tx of choice for symptomatic tense ascites despite medical Tx
- b. Ascites from cirrhosis is due to leakage of splanchnic and hepatic <u>lymph</u> into the peritoneum
- c. Pleural effusions with ascites improve with control of the ascites
- d. Umbilical hernias in patients with ascites should be left alone

Answer d. Umbilical hernias with ascites should be repaired (if there is overlying skin necrosis, do this emergently to prevent perforation). If skin necrosis is present at surgery, it should be resected. **Primary closure** should be performed if the skin is <u>infected</u> or <u>perforated</u>. Use **PTFE** (Gortex) **mesh** if not infected or ruptured.

Recurrence rates are higher for primary repair compared to mesh repair of umbilical hernias. Umbilcal hernias in adults are usually **acquired** and occur with conditions that increase **intra-abdominal pressure** (RFs - pregnancy, obesity, ascites). Umbilical hernias in adults are at risk of **incarceration** and **infarction**. Cirrhotic patients with umbilical hernias are *also* at risk for **rupture** through the overlying ischemic skin.

782. A 50 yo man with Child's C cirrhosis (MELD score 21) has refractory ascites despite previous multiple large volume paracentesis procedures and maximal medical Tx. The most appropriate next step is:
    a. Refer for liver TXP
    b. TIPS
    c. Splenorenal shunt
    d. Portacaval shunt

    Answer a. Given the **advanced liver disease** (MELD ≥ 19 or Child's C), this patient is too high risk for TIPS or other shunts *(significant risk of **hepatic failure** due to shunting of blood away from liver)*; **referral for liver TXP is indicated.**

783. A 50 yo man with Child's B Cirrhosis (MELD score 16) has refractory variceal bleeding. He is currently listed for liver TXP. The most appropriate next step is:
    a. Portacaval shunt
    b. Peritoneovenous shunt
    c. TIPS
    d. Liver biopsy
    e. Splenorenal shunt

    Answer c. TIPS is indicated in this patient for **refractory Sx's**. The mortality is much lower for TIPS compared to open shunt placement.

784. A 50 yo man with Child's A cirrhosis is found to have asymptomatic esophageal varices on EGD. The most appropriate next step in this patient is:
    a. Non-selective beta-blocker
    b. Endoscopic variceal band ligation
    c. Observation
    d. Alpha-blocker
    e. TIPS

    Answer a. Non-selective **beta-blocker** (eg Propranolol) is the *first-line therapy* for **prevention of first bleeds** in patients with esophageal varices. If beta-blocker is *not* tolerated and the patient has medium to large sized varices, prophylactic endoscopic variceal band ligation is indicated.

785. A 50 yo man with cirrhosis has refractory ascites. All of the following are true except:
    a. Encephalopathy is a contraindication to TIPS
    b. Spleno-renal shunt would likely be very effective in this patient
    c. Coagulopathy is a contraindication to peritoneovenous shunt
    d. A higher MELD score indicates a higher complication and mortality rate if an open procedure is planned

    Answer b. Splenorenal shunts are only used for Child's A cirrhosis with bleeding Sx's.

786. All of the following are true of liver failure except:
    a. Lactulose serves as a cathartic to remove ammonia forming bacteria and to prevent NH_3 uptake by converting it to NH_4
    b. Neomycin gets rid of ammonia producing bacteria
    c. Increasing total protein intake is important in liver failure
    d. Development of asterixis is a sign that liver failure is progressing and is an early sign of encephalopathy

Answer c. *Decreasing* **protein intake** is important in liver failure to reduce the amount of ammonia in the body, which contributes to encephalopathy.

787. Immediate initial therapy for newly discovered Budd Chiari syndrome is:
    a. Heparin
    b. TIPS
    c. Liver TXP
    d. Mesocaval shunt
    e. Distal splenorenal shunt

    Answer a. Heparin

788. A 25 yo woman develops fever, RUQ pain, jaundice, and ascites 2 weeks after childbirth. This is most likely related to which of the following:
    a. Retained placenta
    b. Hepatocellular carcinoma
    c. Portal vein thrombosis
    d. Budd Chiari Syndrome

    Answer d. (see below)

789. The most appropriate immediate therapy in the above patient is:
    a. Heparin and antibiotics
    b. TIPS
    c. Liver TXP
    d. Mesocaval shunt
    e. Distal splenorenal shunt

    Answer a. Post-partum hepatic vein thrombosis (Post-partum Budd Chiari Syndrome) is rare and related to ovarian vein **thrombophlebitis** (there is an infectious component) that leads to IVC and hepatic vein thrombosis. **SMA arteriogram with venous phase contrast** will identify the lesion. Tx – **antibiotics** and **heparin**

790. A 25 yo man on a remote arctic expedition has had fevers and RLQ pain for the past 7 days. CT scan shows a phlegmon and fat stranding in the RLQ along with air bubbles in the superior mesenteric vein and the portal vein. His LFTs are elevated. This is most consistent with:
    a. Budd chiari syndrome
    b. Mesenteric ischemia
    c. Ischemic colitis
    d. Pylephlebitis
    e. Necrotizing enterocolitis

    Answer d. Pylephlebitis is infection of the **portal system** that usually occurs after diverticulitis or appendicitis. Patients can have fever, elevated LFTs, and air in the portal system. **Liver abscess** can also form. **Portal vein thrombosis** can also occur. Tx - removal of the infectious source, **antibiotics,** and **heparin** (heparin prevents portal vein thrombosis).

791. A 10 yo child with polycythemia vera presents with hematemesis and splenomegaly. EGD shows esophageal varices which are treated with banding. INR, LFTs, and albumin are normal. The patient has had no foreign travel. The most likely Dx is:
    a. Cirrhosis
    b. Budd Chiari
    c. Portal vein thrombosis
    d. Splenic vein thrombosis
    e. Hepatic artery thrombosis

Answer c. Portal vein thrombosis. Given the esophageal varices and normal liver function, this patient has pre-sinusoidal portal HTN and only portal vein thrombosis fits this description. *Portal vein thrombosis is the MCC of UGI bleeding in children aged > 1.*

Splenic vein thrombosis can result in isolated <u>gastric</u> varices (not esophageal) and does <u>not</u> cause portal HTN.

792. The best initial test to diagnose the underlying problem in the above patient is:
    a. MRI
    b. CT scan
    c. Duplex U/S
    d. Angiogram
    e. PET scan

    Answer c. Duplex U/S is the most *cost-effective study* and usually *the initial study* for **portal vein thrombosis**.

793. U/S in the above patient shows chronic extra-hepatic portal vein thrombosis. Recurrent bleeding in the above patient can be treated with all of the following except:
    a. Spleno-renal shunt
    b. Meso-caval shunt
    c. Rex shunt (superior mesenteric vein to intra-hepatic left portal vein bypass)
    d. A standard TIPS procedure

    Answer d. A standard TIPS procedure is intra-hepatic and would <u>not</u> be effective for *extra-hepatic* portal vein thrombosis.

794. A 40 yo woman from Greece presents to the ED with abdominal pain. CT scan shows a calcified cyst in liver that has a double wall. She has positive parasite serology. The most appropriate next step is:
    a. Percutaneous drainage only
    b. Albendazole
    c. Liver resection
    d. Flagyl

    Answer b. You should never perform percutaneous drainage for **echinococcal cysts** as spillage of the cyst can cause a severe anaphylactic reaction. Standard Tx consists of **pre-op albendazole** followed by **resection of cyst.**

    PAIR Tx may be indicated for patients that are *not* operative candidates (<u>P</u>uncture and needle <u>A</u>spiration, <u>I</u>njection of scolicidal agent [30 minutes] and <u>R</u>easpiration).

795. A 45 yo man with recent travel to the middle east develops RUQ pain and a maculopapular rash. CT scan shows an abscess that is best treated with:
    a. Percutaneous drainage and antibiotics
    b. Flagyl
    c. Levofloxacin
    d. Praziquantel

    Answer d. Tx of **schistosomiasis** liver abscess is **praziquantel**.

796. A 45 yo man with ETOH abuse returns from a trip to Mexico and develops fever, chills, and RUQ pain. WBC count is 20. RUQ U/S shows an intra-hepatic fluid collection. Abdominal CT scan shows a large (6 cm) single abscess with a peripheral rim of edema. Given the most likely diagnosis, this condition is best treated with:
    a. Percutaneous drainage and antibiotics
    b. Flagyl
    c. Praziquantel
    d. Liver resection

Answer b. An **amebic abscess** is best treated with **Flagyl**. Amebic colitis is the primary infection (entamoeba histolytica; colitis may be asymptomtic in some patients) that leads to the abscess.

797. Which of the following tests would best confirm the above diagnosis:
   a. Peripheral blood testing for parasites
   b. Serology
   c. MRI
   d. Stool ovum and parasite
   e. AFP

   Answer b. Amebic abscess Dx is based on Sx's, CT scan, and <u>serology</u>.

798. A 45 yo man develops <u>LLQ pain</u>, fever and change in bowel habits from which he recovers with antibiotics. Two weeks later he develops <u>RUQ pain</u>, fever and chills. An abdominal CT scan shows a large abscess which is likely best treated with
   a. Percutaneous drainage and antibiotics
   b. Flagyl
   c. Levofloxacin
   d. Praziquantel

   Answer a. A **pyogenic abscess** is best treated with **percutaneous drainage** and broad spectrum antibiotics These patients usually present with fever and RUQ pain. GNRs are the MC organism in a pyogenic abscess (MC overall - **E. coli**). You should also cover for anaerobes. These patients can also present with multiple abscesses.

   The MC source of liver pyogenic abscess is the **biliary system**.

   Pyogenic liver abscesses can arise weeks after an episode of **diverticulitis**, appendicitis, endocarditis, or other infectious process. Bacteremia seeds the liver, resulting in an abscess.

799. A 30 yo woman on OCPs presents with a minimally symptomatic 4 cm hypervascular lesion on CT scan that is positive (hot) on technetium labeled albumin scan. There is also an enhancing central stellate scar on CT scan. The most appropriate Tx is:
   a. Stop oral contraceptives and repeat CT scan
   b. Resection
   c. Observation only
   d. Cryoablation
   e. Radiofrequency ablation

   Answer c. The above findings are consistent with **focal nodular hyperplasia** (FNH). There is no malignancy or rupture risk so observation only is indicated (<u>no</u> surgery). Sulfur colloid scan or a technetium labeled colloid scan can be used to help differentiate these from adenomas (FNH is hot, adenomas are cold). FNH lesions are thought to be a regenerative process following an intra-uterine vascular injury.

800. A 30 yo woman on OCPs presents with a minimally symptomatic 4.5 cm hypervascular lesion on CT scan that is negative (cold) on sulfur colloid scan. There is no peripheral to central enhancement on CT scan and the lesion appears homogenous. Alpha-feto protein (AFP) level is normal. The most appropriate Tx is:
   a. Stop oral contraceptives and repeat CT scan
   b. Resection
   c. Observation only
   d. Cryoablation
   e. Radiofrequency ablation

Answer b. This lesion is most consistent with **hepatic adenoma**. Because of the size (≥ 4 cm), resection is indicated for rupture and malignancy risk. Formal resection is indicated when resecting hepatic adenomas (eg segmentectomy, lobectomy). If the lesion were smaller, than a trial off OCPs is indicated to see if the lesion gets smaller.

801. All of the following are true of liver hemangioma except:
    a. They are the MC liver tumor
    b. A minimally symptomatic 4 cm hyper-vascular liver lesion that displays obvious peripheral nodular enhancement that progresses centrally suggests hemangioma and no further Tx is necessary
    c. The majority are asymptomatic and resection is rarely indicated
    d. If resection is necessary, hepatic segmentectomy or lobectomy is the preferred operation
    e. High output cardiac failure and thrombocytopenia can occur with large lesions

    Answer d. If resection is necessary, **enucleation** is the preferred operation for liver hemangiomas (+/- pre-op embolization)

802. All of the following are true of polycystic liver disease except
    a. Estrogen and previous pregnancies are RFs for cyst growth
    b. This is often associated with polycystic kidney disease
    c. In rare cases, liver transplantation is indicated
    d. Cyst aspiration and ETOH sclerotherapy has a role
    e. Patients with isolated polycystic liver disease generally have a decreased life expectancy

    Answer e. Patients with isolated **polycystic liver disease** generally have a normal life expectancy.

803. Which of the following is a risk factor for hepatocellular CA
    a. Wilson's disease
    b. Hepatitis A
    c. Hepatitis E
    d. Hepatitis A + E

    Answer a. Wilson's disease

804. A 4 cm hyper-vascular lesion with multiple areas of necrosis associated with an AFP of 500 is most likely represents
    a. Liver adenoma
    b. FNH
    c. Hepatocellular CA
    d. Fibrolamellar CA of the liver

    Answer c. A liver mass that is hyper-vascular with necrosis and a high AFP is most likley **hepatocellular carcinoma (HCC)**. Tx is resection if the tumor is resectable. Fibrolamellar liver CA is <u>not</u> associated with an elevated AFP.

805. A 50 yo man with chronic liver disease has a 4 cm hepatoma in segment 7. You are in the process of assessing resectability and whether or not the patient would survive. Which of the following would still allow this patient to undergo resection
    a. Portal node disease
    b. Peritoneal studding
    c. Child's C cirrhosis
    d. A 2nd lesion in segment 6
    e. Ascites

    Answer d. A 2nd lesion in segment 6. Presence of <u>ascites</u> is a *contraindication*.

806. The most accurate predictor of post-op liver failure in the above patient is:
   a. MELD score
   b. AST
   c. GGT
   d. Lipase
   e. WBC count

   Answer a. MELD score (MELD score ≥ 9 has a 20% risk of mortality)

807. The greatest risk factor for liver failure after resection in the above patient is:
   a. Total bilirubin of 1.5
   b. Portal wedge pressure of 21
   c. Alkaline phosphatase of 300
   d. Creatinine 1.4
   e. Age 65

   Answer b. Portal hypertension with a **portal wedge pressure > 12**

808. POD # 7 after liver resection, the above patient develops abdominal pain. U/S shows a fluid collection around the resected liver bed. The most appropriate next step is:
   a. ERCP
   b. Re-operation
   c. Angio-embolization
   d. Percutaneous drain

   Answer d. Given the timing of the issue, this almost certainly represents a **biloma**. Treatment is a percutaneous drain and this is often definitive.

809. MELD score uses all of the following except:
   a. Creatinine
   b. Bilirubin
   c. INR
   d. Ascites

   Answer d. Ascites. **MELD score** uses **creatinine, INR,** and **bilirubin**

810. In comparing the original Childs score to the Childs-Pugh score, nutritional status was removed and which of the following was added:
   a. INR
   b. Bilirubin
   c. Encephalopathy
   d. Ascites

   Answer a. INR was added as this is a better predictor of hepatic reserve.

811. All of the following are helpful tests for liver function reserve prior to proposed liver resection except:
   a. Indocyanine green clearance test
   b. MELD score
   c. Child-Pugh score
   d. Sulfur colloid scan
   e. INR

   Answer d. Sulfur colloid scan is used to identify FNH (it is not a test of liver function reserve)

812. Which of the following patients is the best candidate for *simultaneous* colon resection and isolated liver metastasis resection:

a. An 80 yo woman with left sided CA and a 7 cm liver metastasis involving segments IVa and II
b. An 80 yo woman with left sided CA and a 3 cm liver metastasis involving segment II only
c. An 40 yo woman with left sided CA and a 3 cm liver metastasis involving segment II only
d. An 40 yo woman with left sided CA and a 7 cm liver metastasis involving segments IVa and II

Answer c. Considerable controversy exits for simultaneous colon CA resection and liver metastasis resection. In general, younger patients not undergoing major hepatectomies have more favorable outcomes with simultaneous resections. The patient for answer C is young and will likely only need a segmentectomy, so she is the best candidate.

Patients not undergoing a simultaneous procedures generally undergo primary resection, chemotherapy, and then re-staging 6-8 weeks later. If the liver metastases are still isolated and resectable, resection should then be performed.

813. All of the following are poor prognostic variables when resecting isolated colorectal CA metastases to the liver except:
 a. 2 years since the primary lesion was resected
 b. Simultaneous colorectal CA and liver metastases
 c. A 6 cm metastasis
 d. CEA of 500
 e. 4 liver tumors

Answer a. A **long disease-free interval** (> 12 months) is considered a good prognostic indicator.

814. All of the following are true of preoperative portal vein embolization except:
 a. The future liver remnant for normal livers should be > 25%
 b. The majority of cases involves right hepatectomy or extended right hepatectomy
 c. If extended right hepatectomy is planned, embolization of segment IV should occur
 d. Compensatory hypertrophy peaks at 6 weeks
 e. Percutaneous embolization is the preferred route

Answer d. Compensatory hypertrophy peaks at **2 weeks**

815. All of the following are true of fibrolamellar liver CA except:
 a. Generally it is associated with elevated AFP
 b. It generally has the best prognosis of all adult liver CA
 c. It is MC in young patients
 d. It is rare
 e. Is associated with neurotensin levels

Answer a. Generally patients with **fibrolamellar liver CA** do not have cirrhosis, viral infection, or an elevated AFP.

ANATOMY AND PHYSIOLOGY
- **Blood supply**
  - **Arterial blood supply**
    - Right, left and middle hepatic arteries (follows hepatic vein system)
      - Most **primary** and **secondary tumors** of liver supplied by <u>hepatic artery</u> (can embolize unresectable tumors)
  - **Hepatic artery variants** (<u>replaced</u> hepatic arteries)
    - **Replaced right hepatic artery** off **superior mesenteric artery** (20%)
      - *MC hepatic artery variant*

Behind **neck of pancreas** (is **posterior** to portal vein)
Posterolateral to CBD
Replaced left hepatic artery off <u>left gastric artery</u>
Found in gastro-hepatic ligament (lesser omentum) medially
- **Portal vein** - from <u>superior mesenteric vein</u> joining <u>splenic vein</u>
No valves in portal vein; normal portal vein pressure is 3 - 5 mmHg
Splits in 2 in liver; provides 2/3 of total hepatic blood flow
<u>Left</u> supplies - II, III, and IV
<u>Right</u> supplies - V, VI, VII, and VIII
Inferior mesenteric vein - enters splenic vein
- **Hepatic veins** - 3 hepatic veins join the IVC
<u>Left</u> - segments II, III, and superior IV
<u>Middle</u> - segments V and inferior IV
<u>Right</u> - segments VI, VII, and VIII
Middle hepatic vein joins <u>left</u> hepatic vein in 80% before IVC
Accessory right hepatic veins - drain medial aspect of right lobe directly into the IVC
Inferior phrenic veins - also drain directly into the IVC
The IVC does <u>not</u> have valves
- **Caudate lobe** - receives separate right and left portal and arterial blood flow; drains directly into IVC via separate hepatic veins
- **Hepato-duodenal ligament** - where common bile duct, portal vein, and proper hepatic artery meet (portal triad)
- **Portal triad** (ie porta hepatis): <u>portal vein</u> *posterior*, <u>common bile duct</u> *lateral*, <u>proper hepatic artery</u> *medial*; portal triad enters liver at segments **IV and V**
- **Pringle maneuver** - porta hepatic clamping; *will not stop hepatic vein bleeding*
- **Falciform ligament**
  - Separates medial and lateral segments of the **left lobe**
  - Attaches liver to anterior abdominal wall
  - Extends to **umbilicus** and carries the umbilical vein remnant
- **Ligamentum teres**
  - Carries the obliterated umbilical vein to undersurface of liver
  - Extends from the falciform ligament
- Line drawn from the middle of the **gallbladder fossa** to IVC (ie portal fissure or **Cantlie's line**) separates right and left liver lobes
- **Foramen of Winslow** - goes into lesser sac; *Anterior* - portal triad; *Posterior* - IVC; *Inferior* - duodenum; *Superior* - liver
- **Glisson's capsule** - the peritoneum that covers the liver
- **Bare area** - posterior-superior surface not covered by Glisson's capsule
- **Gallbladder** - underneath segments **IV and V**
  - These areas may need resection with **gallbladder CA**
- **Kupffer cells** - liver **macrophages**; reticulo-endothelial system
- **Stellate cells** (Ito cells) - major cell type involved in **liver fibrosis**
- **Alkaline phosphatase** - normally located in canalicular membrane
- ***Not made in liver*** → <u>von Willebrand factor</u> and <u>factor VIII</u> (made in endothelium)
- ***Hepatocytes most sensitive to ischemia*** - central lobular (acinar zone III)
- 75% of normal liver (tri-segmentectomy) can be safely resected *without* liver failure – remaining liver will **regenerate** as well

BILIRUBIN
- Breakdown product of **hemoglobin** in **spleen** (Hgb → heme → biliverdin → bilirubin)
- Bilirubin is released into bloodstream, binds albumin, and is transported to the liver
- Conjugated to **glucuronic acid** (enzyme glucuronyl transferase) in **liver** → improves water solubility
- Conjugated bilirubin is then actively secreted into bile and enters gut (see Liver chapter for gut metabolism of conjugated bilirubin)

BILE ACIDS (bile salts)
- **Bile** contains <u>bile acids</u> (80%), <u>phospholipids</u> (15%, MC - lecithin), <u>cholesterol</u> (4%), <u>bilirubin</u>, and <u>proteins</u>
- **Cholesterol** is used to make **bile acids**

- **HMG CoA** → (*HMG CoA reductase*) → **cholesterol** → (*7-alpha-hydroxylase*) → **bile acids**
- **Statin drugs** inhibit HMG CoA reductase
- **HMG CoA reductase** - rate-limiting step for cholesterol synthesis
■ **Bile acids** are conjugated to **taurine** or **glycine** (improves water solubility)
  - **Primary bile acids** (C's) - cholic and chenodeoxycholic
  - **Secondary bile acids** - deoxycholic and lithocholic (dehydoxylated primary bile acids by **bacteria** in gut)
■ **Lecithin** - main biliary phospholipid; solubilizes cholesterol and emulsifies fats in the intestine
■ **Bile salts** serve as mechanism for:
     1) excreting **cholesterol** *and*
     2) **emulsifying lipids** and **fat-soluble vitamins** in the intestine
■ Around **95%** of bile salts are **reabsorbed** through **entero-hepatic recirculation** (see Biliary System chapter)

ACUTE LIVER FAILURE (fulminant hepatic failure)
■ **Acute liver disease + encephalopathy + coagulopathy** (80% mortality)
  - Outcome determined by the course of **encephalopathy**
■ Sx's: N/V, malaise, and jaundice
■ Liver failure leads to inability metabolize **ammonia**, mercaptanes, and false neurotransmitters → get **encephalopathy**
■ **Hepatic encephalopathy Tx**:
  - **Lactulose** - **cathartic** that gets rid of gut bacteria and acidifies colon (prevents ammonia uptake); titrate to 2-3 stools/day
  - **Neomycin** - gets rid of ammonia producing gut bacteria
  - **Limit protein intake** (< 70 g/day) - reduces ammonia
  - **Branched-chain amino acids** - metabolized by skeletal muscle, important energy source in patients with acute liver failure
  - **No** antibiotics unless for a specific infection

CHRONIC LIVER DISEASE (cirrhosis)
■ Chronic hepatocellular destruction and regeneration leads to **fibrosis** and **cirrhosis**
■ MCC - ETOH; others - Hep B, Hep C
■ Sx's: **jaundice** and **ascites**; spider angioma, steatorrhea, palpable liver
  - Development of **asterixis** is sign that liver failure is progressing
■ Best test of liver synthetic function in cirrhosis - **prothrombin time** (PT)
■ **Ascites** - from **hepatic / splanchnic** lymph
  - General medical Tx below controls ascites in 90%
  - Tx: **water restriction** (1-1.5 L/d), **salt restriction** (1-2 g/d), **spironolactone** (counter-acts increased aldosterone seen with impaired hepatic metabolism), and **furosemide**
  - Tx for symptomatic **tense ascites** - PRN **paracentesis**; replace with **25% salt-poor albumin** (IV; 1 g for every 100 cc removed); *best therapy* for large volume tense ascites (*not increasing diuretics*); can remove **4 - 6 L**; make sure these patients are on medical Tx above
  - **TIPS** - indicated for refractory tense ascites (eg frequent trips to ED for paracentesis)
  - **Mechanism** of ascites: *hepatocyte destruction* → *fibrosis and scarring of liver* → *↑ed hepatic pressure* → *portal venous congestion* → *lymphatic overload* → *leakage of splanchnic and hepatic lymph into peritoneum* → *ascites*
  - **Coronary veins** act as collaterals between portal vein and systemic venous system of lower esophagus (azygos veins)
  - **Shunts** can decompress portal system
■ **Encephalopathy**
  - Development of **asterixis** - sign that liver failure is progressing
  - **Rifaximin** (antibiotic) - *decreases* risk of acute hepatic encephalopathy episodes and severity of encephalopathy

- **Hyponatremia** - from volume overload related to renal retention of water and excessive aldosterone and ADH
  - Tx: **salt + fluid restriction**; daily **tolvaptan** (oral vasopressin [ADH] receptor antagonist) _or_ **spironolactone** (should _not_ combine tolvaptan and spironolactone)
  - Correction of hyponatremia with **tolvaptan** results in **improved mental health scores** (_careful monitoring with this drug to prevent Na from being corrected too quickly - can cause central pontine myelinolysis_)
- **Propranolol** prophylaxis against UGI bleed - used for patients with **varices** or previous **UGI bleed**
- **Norfloxacin** (prophylactic antibiotic to prevent SBP) - used if **previous SBP** or with current **UGI bleed** (high risk for SBP)
- **Nutrition** - **branched-chain amino acids** _decrease_ acute hepatic encephalopathy episodes and overall Cx's; also _improve_ nutritional status; cost / palatability are issues
- **Hepatorenal syndrome** - progressive, rapid **renal failure** and **oliguria** despite normal filling pressures in a patient with cirrhosis (_not_ responsive to fluid challenge)
  - _Same_ lab findings as **pre-renal azotemia**
  - Often have a precipitating event (eg GI bleed, over-diuresis, infection)
  - Usually a sign of **end-stage liver disease** that ultimately is only treated with **transplantation** → all other Tx is a temporizing measure
  - Involves dilation of mesenteric vessels and constriction of renal blood vessels
  - Dx:
    - 1st **Volume challenge** (will not work with hepatorenal syndrome, will work with pre-renal azotemia → **main difference** between the two)
    - **Urinalysis** - no protein or RBCs in urine with hepatorenal syndrome
    - Electrolytes from hepatorenal syndrome are the same as pre-renal azotemia (FeNa < 1%, BUN/Cr ratio > 20, Urine Na <20, ect.)
    - **Renal Bx** - shows normal renal tissue
  - Tx: **midodrine** and **octreotide** (_best Tx_, temporizing); **dialysis**
  - Stop diuretics, consider **TIPS**; albumin and vasoconstrictors may be helpful
  - 50% mortality in the short term
  - **Liver TXP** eventually needed

PRE-OP PREPARATION IN CIRRHOSIS (elective case preparation)
- In general, want to avoid elective surgery in these patients
  - Can perform laparoscopic cholecystectomy if symptomatic stones or other indications (_Child's C may be a contraindication_)
  - Umbilical hernia with ascites should be repaired
  - _No_ elective hemorrhoid resection
- _No_ epidural or spinal anesthesia → risk of bleeding
- **Umbilical hernia repair:**
  - Patients with ascites at increased risk for umbilical hernia due to increased intra-abdominal pressure
  - Bowel incarceration and infarction can occur
  - Increased pressure from ascites can lead to ischemia, necrosis, and perforation of **skin** overlying umbilical hernia (can lead to peritonitis and death)
  - **Umbilical hernia with ascites** - do _not_ wait until hernia sac has ruptured to fix; these should be repaired **electively** with prolene mesh (mesh has a lower recurrence rate compared to primary repair [10% vs 1%])
  - If umbilical hernia overlying skin is **perforated, infected,** or **necrotic** → need **emergent repair** (primary closure if infected or perforated; _no_ mesh)
  - **Surgery:**
    - 1st - **removal of ascites** (paracentesis; relieves pressure off umbilical hernia) - replace with IV salt-poor albumin (1 g for every 100 cc removed; use 25% albumin in 50 cc bottle)
    - 2nd - **correct coagulopathy** (_all_ have abnormal PT) - Vit K, FFP, and platelets as needed
    - 3rd - **umbilical hernia repair** - resect necrotic skin area if present, **primary closure** if infected or perforated; **PTFE mesh** (Gortex) if not infected or ruptured
    - 4th - **control ascites** after repair

SPONTANEOUS BACTERIAL PERITONITIS (see Infection chapter)
- Sx's: fever, abdominal pain, PMNs > 250 in fluid, positive cultures
- **E. coli** (#1), pneumococcus, streptococci
- Should be mono-organism; if not, need to worry about visceral perforation (or other *secondary* peritonitis)
- RFs: prior SBP, UGI bleed (variceal hemorrhage), low-protein ascites
- Tx: 3rd generation cephalosporins; patients usually respond within 48 hours

ESOPHAGEAL VARICES
- **Bleed** by rupture; MC in **lower 1/3** esophagus; engorged areas with blue-purple hue; may have cherry red bleeding spots
- Tx for bleeding esophageal varices: **banding** *(best Tx)* and **sclerotherapy** (combined are **95%** effective)
    - **Vasopressin** (splanchnic artery *vaosconstriction*) and **octreotide** (reduces portal pressure by decreasing blood flow) are used to *temporize* until EGD
    - Patients with history of angina receive **nitroglycerine** while on vasopressin
    - Sengstaken-Blakemore esophageal tube - has a balloon used to control variceal bleeding; *risks* - esophageal rupture
- **TIPS** is needed for refractory variceal bleeding (may be needed *emergently*)
- Bleeding varices have a 25% mortality with 1st episode; 50% with re-bleed
- Late Cx's from banding / sclerotherapy - **esophageal strictures**
    - Tx: **dilatation**
- **Propranolol** - may help prevent re-bleeding; *no role acutely*; use in patients with varices or previous UGI bleed
- **Prevention of first bleed** in patient with known esophageal varices:
    - Non-selective **beta-blocker** (eg Propranolol) - *1st line therapy (mainstay)*
    - **Endoscopic variceal band ligation** - indicated for medium to large varices in patients who cannot tolerate beta-blocker

PORTAL HYPERTENSION
- **Pre-hepatic obstruction** - portal vein thrombosis (MCC; accounts for 50% of portal HTN in children); schistosomiasis MCC worldwide
- **Hepatic obstruction** - cirrhosis
- **Post-hepatic obstruction** - Budd-Chiari syndrome (IVC or hepatic vein occlusive disease)
- Normal portal vein pressure: **3 - 5 mmHg**
- **Portal HTN** pressure measurement - uses **hepatic venous wedge pressure**
    - *Assessment of hepatic venous wedge pressure* (HVWP) - go through *internal jugular to a hepatic vein, wedge catheter, and get pressure (wedge pressure > 5 mmHg = portal HTN; > 12 mmHg = clinically **significant** portal HTN)*
- **Coronary veins** act as collaterals between the **portal vein** and the systemic venous system of the lower esophagus (**azygos vein system**)
- Portal HTN leads to esophageal varices, ascites, splenomegaly, and hepatic encephalopathy
- Shunts can decompress portal system
- Portal HTN in **children**
    - Usually caused by *extra-hepatic* **portal vein thrombosis**
    - Portal vein thrombosis is the MCC of **massive hematemesis** in children

BUDD-CHIARI SYNDROME
- Occlusion of **hepatic veins**, often near junction with IVC (may occlude it)
- MC in women
- Sx's: **ascites** (MC), **RUQ pain, hepatosplenomegaly** *(classic triad)*, and **jaundice**
- RFs: **polycythemia vera** (#1), other hypercoagulable states, IVC webs, IVC compression by external tumor, pregnancy
- Dx: **CT scan** with venous phase contrast (shows a diffuse **inhomogenous** mottled liver, **delayed enhancement of the liver periphery**, and an **enlarged caudate** lobe that demonstrates increased contrast enhancement compared to the rest of the liver)
    - **Duplex U/S** - often the initial study (shows no flow in the hepatic veins)
    - Liver Bx *(not needed)* shows sinusoidal dilatation and centrilobular congestion

- Tx: **Heparin** initially, especially if acute thrombosis (prevents clot propagation); long term warfarin
  - **Acute thrombosis** - possible catheter-directed **tPA**
  - **IVC webs** or **outflow obstructive lesion** - angioplasty, possible stent
  - **TIPS** if the patient fails to improve despite above (can make direct retro-hepatic IVC to portal vein shunt if necessary); the shunt needs to go past the area of obstruction
  - *Rarely* a portosystemic shunt is indicated
  - Some patients may require **liver TXP**
- **Post-partum liver failure with ascites** - from **hepatic vein thrombosis** (post-partum Budd Chiari Syndrome) rising from ovarian vein thrombophlebitis (**pelvic thrombophlebitis**)
  - Has **infectious** and **hypercoagulability** components
  - Sx's: RUQ pain, jaundice, ascites
  - **Ovarian vein thrombosis** (often infected - is a **thrombophlebitis**) → leads to IVC thrombus formation → leads to **hepatic vein thrombosis**
    - Related to relative **hypercoagulable state** following pregnancy
    - Patients with hypercoagulable **syndromes** more susceptible
  - Dx: SMA arteriogram with venous phase contrast or CT angio with venous phase contrast
  - Tx: **heparin** and **antibiotics**

PORTAL VEIN THROMBOSIS
- Can cause portal hypertension
- Usually caused by **extra-hepatic** thrombosis of portal vein (eg from a tumor)
- Etiologies - hypercoagulable state, CA, cirrhosis, trauma, pancreatitis, post-splenectomy, can occur after umbilical vein catheterization in children
- Sx's: **ascites** *without* liver failure can occur if not due to cirrhosis; **hematemesis**
  - *MCC of **massive hematemesis in children***
- **Esophageal varices** c   an occur
- Dx: **Duplex U/S** *(most cost-effective study and usually the initial study)*
  - **Angiography** with venous phase contrast *(most sensitive test, nearly 100%)*
  - **CT scan** - shows bowel edema; possible ascites; venous phase contrast will usually show the lesion
  - LFTs and INR are *normal* (does *not* involve the liver)
- Tx: **Heparin** is generally indicated, especially for acute thrombosis, to prevent clot propagation (*avoid* if UGI bleed)
  - Control **UGI bleed** from esophageal varices if present *(no heparin)*
  - Consider **shunt** after first bleeding episode (spleno-renal, meso-caval, or Rex shunt [superior mesenteric vein to intra-hepatic left portal vein bypass])
  - *A standard TIPS procedure does not work for portal vein thrombosis (especially extra-hepatic portal vein thrombosis)*
- **Pylephlebitis** - infection of the **portal system**
  - MC occurs with <u>diverticulitis</u> or <u>appendicitis</u> (may have had a delay in seeking medical care); in children, can occur with <u>omphalitis</u> (infection of umbilical cord stump) or other intra-abdominal infections
  - Sx's: fever, LLQ (diverticulitis) or RLQ (appendicitis) pain; RUQ pain if liver abscess has formed; sepsis
  - Dx: CT scan - **air** in the portal vein and system (may also have thrombotic material); will see **source of infection** (eg <u>appendicitis</u> or <u>diverticulitis</u>); may have **liver abscess**; can also get **portal vein thrombosis**
  - Labs: elevated LFTs and WBCs
  - Tx: **removal of the infectious source** (eg appendectomy or sigmoidectomy), **broad spectrum antibiotics**, and **heparin** (prevents portal vein thrombosis)

TIPS AND SHUNTS
- **TIPS** - transjugular, intrahepatic, portosystemic shunt
  - Decompresses portal system; allows antegrade flow from portal vein to hepatic vein (eventually goes to IVC)
  - PTFE covered stents have better patency than uncovered stents
- *TIPS makes **encephalopathy** <u>worse</u>* (shunted blood bypasses liver metabolism)

- **TIPS indications**:
  - Protracted or refractory **variceal bleeding**
  - Refractory **ascites**
  - **Visceral hypoperfusion**
  - Hepato-renal or hepato-pulmonary syndrome (temporizing)
  - Can be used is selective cases of Budd-Chiari
- TIPS Cx's: encephalopathy, clotting of shunt
- _Contraindications_ to TIPS - encephalopathy; polycystic liver disease and Caroli's disease (intra-hepatic tract can traverse a cyst or the biliary system respectively, causing massive hemorrhage), advanced liver disease (see below), right heart failure (can worsen it), severe pulmonary HTN, HCC involving hepatic veins (dissemination)
- **Advanced liver disease** (MELD ≥ 19 or Child's **C**) - _avoid_ TIPS (significant risk of hepatic failure due to shunting of blood away from liver); refer these patients for **liver TXP**
- _Pre-hepatic portal hypertension is not relieved with TIPS_
- **Distal splenorenal shunt** - low rate of encephalopathy, can leave the spleen
  - _**Need to ligate**_: left adrenal vein, left gonadal vein, inferior mesenteric vein, coronary vein, and pancreatic branches of splenic vein
  - Used only for **Child's A** with just **bleeding** Sx's (rarely used)
  - Can make **ascites _worse_**
  - _Contraindications_ - refractory ascites
  - Do _not_ need splenectomy with splenorenal shunt
- Child's **C** (or MELD ≥19) → _no_ TIPS (refer for liver TXP)
- Child's **A** or **B** with indication for shunt → **TIPS** usual
- Child's **A** that just has **bleeding** → consider **splenorenal shunt** (more durable); otherwise TIPS
- Non-selective shunts (eg porta-caval shunt) - _rarely_ used anymore due to the high rate of encephalopathy
- **Child-Pugh Score** correlates with mortality after open shunt placement (INR replaced nutritional status in the old Child's score)

Child-Pugh Score

	1 point	2 points	3 points
Albumin	> 3.5	3 - 3.5	< 3.0
Bilirubin	< 2.5	2.5 - 4	> 4
Encephalopathy	None	Minimal	Severe
Ascites	None	Treatable with meds	Refractory
INR	< 1.7	1.7 - 2.3	> 2.3

  - Child's **A** (5-6 points)   **2%** mortality with shunt
  - Child's **B** (7-9 points)   **10%** mortality with shunt
  - Child's **C** (10 or greater) **50%** mortality with shunt

- **MELD** score (model for end-stage liver disease) - uses **creatinine, INR, and bilirubin** to grade liver failure; _more accurate_ than Childs-Pugh in **predicting** 1) the **mortality after liver surgery** in patients with cirrhosis, 2) **need for liver TXP** in patients with cirrhosis, _and_; 3) **mortality for patients waiting on the liver TXP list**
  - _Maximum score_ - **40** (all values > 40 are given score of 40)
  - MELD < **15** - _not_ benefited from liver TXP
  - MELD ≥ **15** - benefit from liver TXP
  - MELD ≥ **9** - _no_ liver resection (**20% mortality**)
  - MELD ≥ **15** - _no_ elective general surgery (> **20% mortality**)
  - MELD ≥ **19** - _no_ TIPS (significant risk of **mortality**)
  - _MELD does not take into account hepato–pulmonary syndrome_

- **Indocyanine green clearance test** - used by some centers to test hepatic reserve
- **Peritoneovenous shunt** (LeVeen or Denver shunt) - used for ascites
  - Shunts ascites to venous system
  - *Contraindications* - severe liver failure, previous SBP, previous variceal bleed, coagulopathy
  - Cx's - *disseminated intravascular coagulopathy* (*DIC*)
- **Indications for Liver TXP in End-Stage Liver Disease**
  - Child class **C** or MELD **> 15** - *evaluate for liver TXP*
  - **Indications for TXP:**
    - Recurrent or severe encephalopathy
    - Refractory ascites
    - Recurrent variceal bleeding
    - Hepatorenal _or_ hepatopulmonary syndrome (pulmonary capillary dilation leading to shunting and hypoxia)
    - Hepatocellular CA (no single lesion > 5 cm or ≤ 3 lesions with largest ≤ 3 cm) - should not have gross vascular invasion or metastatic disease
    - Fulminant hepatic failure
  - *Contraindications to TXP*
    - Active substance abuse
    - Sepsis
    - Extra-hepatic malignancy
    - Severe co-morbidity (cardiopulmonary especially)
    - Persistent non-compliance
    - Severe pulmonary HTN (mean > 50, _not_ responsive to prostacyclin)
  - **Liver TXP 1 year survival** - 90% (5-YS - 80%)

LIVER ABSCESSES
- **Pyogenic abscess** *(MC hepatic abscess)*
  - Account for 80% of all abscesses; **15% mortality** due to sepsis
  - Often have **multiple abscesses** (especially if biliary source)
  - Sx's: RUQ pain, fever, chills, weight loss, sepsis
  - MC in **right lobe**
  - MC organism - *E. coli* (*MC class - GNRs*)
  - MCC overall - **contiguous infection** from **biliary tract disease** with ascending infection (related to CBD stones, stricture, CA, biliary stents, manipulation)
  - Can occur following **bacteremia** from other types of **distant infections** (eg diverticulitis, appendicitis, endocarditis)
  - Dx: **CT scan**; high **LFTs** and **WBCs**; positive blood cultures
  - Tx: **CT-guided percutaneous drainage** and broad spectrum **antibiotics** (aerobic and anaerobic); surgical drainage if unstable or continued sepsis
  - *Failure to resolve* → *need to make sure this is not necrotic liver CA*
- **Amebic abscess** (entamoeba histolytica)
  - Sx's: fever, chills, RUQ pain, jaundice, hepatomegaly; 2% mortality
  - Primary infection in colon → **amebic colitis** (reaches **liver** via **portal vein**; this phase may be asymptomatic in some patients)
  - RFs: travel to **Latin America** (Mexico), ETOH; fecal-oral transmission, _males_
  - Positive **antibodies** for *Entamoeba histolytica*
  - Dx: **CT scan** - liver abscess with **peripheral rim of edema**
    - Elevated LFTs and WBCs; MC in **right lobe**, usually a **single abscess**
    - Can usually make Dx based on presentation, CT scan, and serology
  - Tx: *Metronidazole (Flagyl) only* - *most do _not_ require drainage*
    - Aspiration _only_ if patient fails to improve after 72 hrs of medical Tx (looks like anchovy paste)
    - Surgery _only_ if free rupture
- **Echinococcal cyst** (hydatid cyst)
  - Positive **antibodies** to echinococcus
  - Sheep - carriers; dogs - human exposure; often in **Mediterranean** (Greece)
  - ****Do _not_ aspirate percutaneously** → *can leak and cause* **anaphylactic shock**
  - Dx: CT scan shows **ectocyst** (calcified) and **endocyst** (double walled cyst) - can make Dx based on CT scan; MC in **right lobe**

- Pre-op ERCP for jaundice, increased LFTs, or cholangitis to check for communication with the biliary system
- Tx: **pre-op albendazole** (2 weeks) and **surgical removal** (intra-op can inject cyst with alcohol [or other scolicidal agent] to kill organisms, then aspirate out); **need to get all of the cyst wall**
- **PAIR Tx** for patients that are *not* operative candidates (Puncture and needle Aspiration, Injection of scolicidal agent [30 minutes] and Reaspiration)
- *Do not spill cyst contents - can cause **anaphylactic shock***

■ **Schistosomiasis**
- Travel to **Africa**; acquired in **water**; contact through the **skin**
- Sx's: maculopapular **rash**, RUQ pain, can cause **variceal bleeding**
- Dx: **positive serology** (*best test*; ELISA), high **eosinophils**, MC in **right lobe**
- Eventually lodge in **hepatic sinusoids**; can cause **portal HTN**
- 2nd MCC of **esophageal varices** worldwide
- Tx: *praziquantel only*; control of variceal bleeding
- Some types lodge in the **urogenital system** (can cause bladder CA)

BENIGN LIVER TUMORS
■ **Hepatic adenomas**
- Sx's: **RUQ pain** (MC), increased LFTs, mass; *80% are symptomatic*
  50% risk of significant **bleeding** (rupture) - *main reason for resection*
  20% present with hypotension from rupture
- RFs: Women, steroid use, OCPs
- 5% become **malignant**
- MC in **right lobe**
- Dx:
  MRI / CT scan - demonstrates a hypervascular, homogenous tumor
  Sulfur colloid scan - *no Kupffer cells in adenomas, thus **no uptake** (cold)*
  AFP - normal; Tagged RBC scan - normal
  No FNA - bleeding risk
- Tx:
  Minimal Sx's and < 4 cm - stop OCPs and/or steroids; serial CT scans every 4-6 weeks; if *regression* - no further therapy; if *no regression* - resect tumor
  Significantly **symptomatic** or $\geq$ **4 cm** - tumor resection due to bleeding and malignancy risk; embolization if multiple and unresectable
  Not on OCPs or steroids → resection
  Increase in size or worsening Sx's while following → resection
  Surgery - **formal resection** (eg lobectomy, segmentectomy)

■ **Focal nodular hyperplasia (FNH)**
- Has a **central stellate scar** (*diagnostic*, scar enhances with contrast)
- *No malignancy risk; very rare rupture*; usually *asymptomatic*
- Thought to be a regenerative reaction following an intra-uterine vascular injury
- Dx:
  MRI / CT scan - often has characteristic **central stellate scar** (*is diagnostic - scar enhances on CT scan or MRI; not seen with adenoma or hepatoma*); is a hypervascular tumor
  Sulfur colloid scan - has Kupffer cells, will uptake **sulfur colloid** (hot scan; **technetium labeled albumin** can be used as well)
  AFP - normal; Tagged RBC scan - normal
  FNA - not sensitive enough to differentiate FNH vs adenoma
- Tx: ***No surgery*** (*no malignancy or rupture risk*)

■ **Hemangioma**
- *MC hepatic tumor overall*
- Rupture rare; most asymptomatic; women
- ***Avoid*** biopsy → risk of hemorrhage
- Dx:
  MRI / CT scan - shows **peripheral nodular enhancement** that progresses **centrally** (*diagnostic*); is a very hypervascular lesion (very bright on T2 MRI)
  Tagged RBC scan (*best test; can confirm Dx*) - is **positive**

<u>No</u> FNA - significant risk of hemorrhage
- Tx: *__leave alone__* unless significantly symptomatic
- *Surgery - **enucleation** <u>preferred</u> over formal resection if required*
    Pre-op embolization may be considered
    Steroids (possible XRT) for unresectable disease
- Rare Cx's of hemangioma (<u>large</u> lesions, usually seen in <u>children</u>) - consumptive **coagulopathy** and **thrombocytopenia** (Sx's - bleeding issues; Kasabach-Merritt syndrome), **high output CHF** (Sx's - dyspnea)

■ **Solitary cysts**
- Congenital; women, right lobe; walls have a characteristic **blue hue**
- Cx's from these cysts are very rare; vast majority left alone

■ **Polycystic liver disease** (autosomal dominant)
- Often associated with polycystic kidney disease
- Generally, these patients have a **normal life expectancy**
- Only 10% have issues with pain, bleeding, cyst infection, or bile duct obstruction
- RFs for cyst growth - age, female sex, severity of renal cystic disease, prior pregnancies, estrogen therapy (OCPs)
- Tx options (stop OCPs):
    Cyst aspiration - for infection, bile duct obstruction (PAIR ETOH sclerotherapy often used for bile duct obstruction), or pain
    Cyst fenestration - majority done laparoscopically
    Liver resection
    Liver TXP - last resort *(rare)*

METASTATIC LIVER TUMORS (tumors that have metastasized to the liver)
■ Metastases to primary ratio is **20:1** for liver tumors (ie metastases far more common)
■ **Intra-op U/S** - *most sensitive test* for picking up intra-hepatic metastases: **3-5 mm** resolution
- Conventional U/S: 5-10 mm
- CT scan: 5-10 mm
- MRI: 5-10 mm

■ **Colon CA with isolated metastases to liver** - can resect if you leave enough liver for patient to survive
- Liver metastases are supplied by the **hepatic artery** (which would be the route of intra-arterial chemotherapy or embolization for palliation)
- **Resect if completely resectable** and leaves adequate liver function (need **1 cm margin**) - number of tumors, size, and location are not factors if you can get complete resection (even bi-lobar lesions)
- **Wedge vs formal resection** for liver metastases depends on number and location (eg deep metastases to segments 1 and 2 → need left lobectomy and caudate resection)
- *Poor prognostic indicators for metastases to the liver:*
    Disease free interval < 12 months
    > 3 tumors
    CEA > 200 (mcg/L)
    Size > 5 cm
    Positive nodes
    Synchronous primary and liver met
- LFTs are <u>not</u> sensitive indicators for liver metastases
- **Intra-op U/S** - *most sensitive method* for picking up metastases in the liver (detects 3-5 mm lesions)
- **5-YS** after resection for cure of liver metastases - 35% (<u>selected</u> patients)
- **Timing** of resections - the **primary lesion** is usually removed <u>first</u> if staging procedures, followed by chemo, then re-staging in 6-8 weeks. If the liver metastases are still isolated and resectable on re-staging, liver resection is performed.
- **Simultaneous** colon CA resection and isolated liver metastases resection can be considered in **young patients** *(< 70)* <u>not</u> *undergoing major resection* (ie should not be having a lobectomy)

■ **Primary liver tumors** - hypervascular
■ **Metastatic liver tumors** - hypovascular

- **Liver nodule** found at laparotomy for other reasons:
  - **Incidental colorectal CA metastases to liver**
    - If previous CT showed no other nodules, intra-op U/S shows no other nodules, and lesion is amenable to simple wedge → resection
    - **If difficult to take** → just Bx it, finish your procedure, re-stage at 6-8 weeks (chest/abdomen/pelvis CT, LFTs, CEA) and if no other metastases → resection
  - **If not having surgery for colorectal CA** → just wedge or core needle Bx, send for frozen section (may contraindicate resection, eg - pancreatic CA, gastric CA)

HEPATOCELLULAR CARCINOMA (HCC; Hepatoma)
- MC CA worldwide
- RFs: **Hep B** (#1 cause worldwide), Hep C, Hep D + B, ETOH, primary sclerosing cholangitis, Wilson's disease, hemachromatosis, alpha-1 antitrypsin, alfatoxins, hepatic adenomas, anabolic steroids, smoking
- In the U.S., 80% occur in setting of **cirrhosis**
- Sx's: abdominal pain, weight loss, ascites, jaundice
- Dx: **CT scan** (triple phase scanning) or **MRI** - often have mosaic pattern (non-homogenous, necrotic areas, hypervascular)
- Best prognosis - **fibrolamellar** (*best overall*, young patients), clear cell, lymphocytic
- Worst prognosis - **diffuse nodular**
- **Alpha fetoprotein level** (AFP) correlates with tumor size
- *Only 15% can be resected* (multiple exclusion criteria → eg Child's C cirrhosis, porta hepatic lymph node involvement, metastases, not enough liver would be left for survival)
- For tumor removal, need:
  1) **En bloc resection** - can resect multiple tumors in same lobe and some with direct invasion of another organ or peritoneum *and:*
  2) **Retain enough functional liver for survival** (Child's A and a few Child's B cirrhosis patients can undergo resection) - liver failure is a frequent cause of mortality after resection in patients with cirrhosis
- **RFs for mortality** after liver resection: **MELD score** (#1; MELD ≥ 9), portal hypertension (#2; hepatic venous wedge pressure **> 12**), Child's-Pugh score, low platelets, low albumin, high bilirubin
  - MELD ≥ 9 → **20% mortality** after resection
- Hepatectomy **Cx's** - bile leak (Dx: U/S; Tx: percutaneous drain), bleeding, liver failure
- *Contraindications* to liver resection (*any* below):
  - **Nodal disease** (most likely portal nodes)
  - **Metastases** (most likely peritoneal studding)
  - Porto-systemic **encephalopathy,** Child's **C** cirrhosis, **ascites,** or esophageal **varices**
- **Diagnostic laparoscopy** before laparotomy
- Formal resection requires a **1 cm margin**
- Overall 5-YS - 15%; (with resection for cure - 30%)
- Consider **liver transplantation** if tumor is unresectable and the patient has <u>no</u> systemic disease
- Tumor recurrence - most likely in **liver**
- **Palliative Tx** - cryotherapy, radiofrequency ablation, intra-arterial chemo
- 75% of <u>normal</u> liver (tri-segmentectomy) can be safely resected without liver failure - remaining liver will regenerate as well
- **Hepatic sarcoma** - rapidly fatal
- **Fibrolamellar CA** (rare) - best overall prognosis for malignant liver tumors (5-YS – 50%); young patients, generally do <u>not</u> have cirrhosis, viral infection, or elevated AFP; is associated with elevated **neurotensin** levels; can have a central scar (unlike FNH the scar does not enhance with CT scan or MRI)

PRE-OP PORTAL VEIN EMBOLIZATION (prior to hepatic resection)
- 75% of normal liver can be removed (the residual liver regenerates)
- The future liver remnant for **normal livers** should be ≥ **25%**, otherwise morbidity and mortality are greatly increased (generally from **liver failure**)
- The future liver remnant in **compromised livers** (eg cirrhosis) should be ≥ **40%**

- Using a **percutaneous trans-hepatic** route *(best technique)*, coils or particles are introduced into the **portal** branches of the **part of the liver to be resected** to achieve stasis of flow (releases growth factors such as HGF)
- This leads to **compensatory hypertrophy** of the contralateral hemi-liver
- Compensatory hypertrophy **peaks at 2 weeks**; the future liver remnant volume is assessed at 4 weeks.
- The majority of these cases involves a **right hepatectomy** or **extended right hepatectomy** (including segment IV)
- After left hepatectomy or extended left hepatectomy, there is usually sufficient reserve in segments VI and VII such that pre-op portal vein embolization is unnecessary

Biliary System

816. All of the following are true except:
     a. The highest concentration of CCK and secretin secreting cells is in the duodenum
     b. The common hepatic duct becomes the common bile duct after joining the cystic duct
     c. The cystic artery is a branch of the right hepatic artery
     d. The cystic veins drain into the IVC
     e. The common bile duct and hepatic duct blood supply is primarily derived from the right hepatic and gastroduodenal arteries

     Answer d. The **cystic veins** drain into the _right_ branch of the **portal vein**.

817. All of the following are true except:
     a. CCK and vagal neural stimulation _relax_ the normally contracted sphincter of Oddi following meals and cause gallbladder contraction
     b. Active reabsorption of conjugated bile acids occurs in the jejunum
     c. The gallbladder concentrates bile by active absorption of sodium and passive absorption of water
     d. Black gallstones most commonly arise from hemolytic disorders, cirrhosis, ileal resection, or chronic TPN
     e. The gallbladder secretes mucus

     Answer b. _Active_ reabsorption of conjugated bile acids occurs in the **terminal ileum**.

818. Cholesterolosis should be treated with:
     a. Laparoscopic cholecystectomy
     b. Observation
     c. Cholecystectomy and wedge resection of segments IV and V
     d. Chemo-XRT only

     Answer b. Cholesterolosis is the formation of cholesterol deposits on the gallbladder wall and is benign _(no Tx needed)_.

819. Adenomyomatosis and Rokitansky-Aschoff sinuses are MC associated with:
     a. Gallbladder adenocarcinoma
     b. Cholangiocarcinoma
     c. Chronic cholecystitis
     d. A common bile duct stone
     e. Cholesterolosis

     Answer c. Chronic cholecystitis.

820. All of the following are true except:
     a. Discovery of a 2 mm stone on intra-op cholangiography requires common bile duct (CBD) exploration and extraction
     b. ERCP with sphincterotomy and stone extraction is the best Tx for retained CBD stones after cholecystectomy
     c. Diarrhea after cholecystectomy is MC from excess bile salts in the colon
     d. Glucagon _relaxes_ the sphincter of Oddi and can be used intra-op for choledocholithiasis to help flush gallstones out of the CBD
     e. Bile is composed primarily (80%) of bile salts

     Answer a. A CBD stone 2 mm or less will pass on its own. These should be left alone.

821. A 50 yo Asian man presents with chronic RUQ pain, fever, and jaundice. He has the following values: BP 120/80, HR 90, WBC 16, alkaline phosphatase 350, total bilirubin

4. U/S reveals a normal gallbladder and <u>no</u> cholelithiasis. MRCP shows a dilated bile duct system with multiple stones throughout. All of the following are true except:
   a.   These are most likely brown stones
   b.   These are most likely primary biliary stones
   c.   These stones likely occurred from infection and bacterial enzymes
   d.   ERCP with sphincterotomy is the Tx of choice
   e.   Immediate open common bile duct exploration is indicated

   Answer e. ERCP with sphincterotomy is the Tx of choice for **brown** stones (a primary biliary stone due to infection). Pigmented stones contain **calcium bilirubinate**.

822. Several weeks after a motor vehicle accident, a patient presents with jaundice, hematemesis, and RUQ pain. EGD reveals hemobilia. All of the following are true except:
   a.   Angiogram is the best test for diagnosis
   b.   This most commonly arises from an initial arterial pseudoaneurysm
   c.   The MC connection is hepatic artery to bile duct
   d.   Preferred Tx is open ligation

   Answer d. Preferred Tx for a hepatic artery to bile duct fistula is **arterial embolization**. The patients often present with **hemobilia** (blood coming out Ampulla of Vater).

823. A 50 yo male has a 2 cm gallbladder papillary adenoma. The most appropriate next step is:
   a.   Observation
   b.   Cholecystostomy tube
   c.   Cholecystectomy
   d.   Chemo-XRT

   Answer c. In general, **cholecystectomy** is indicated for polyps that are **> 1 cm** and have any of the following: 1) **Sx's**, 2) **age > 50**, 3) presence of **gallstones** *or*; 4) **< 3 polyps** (ie not likely to be cholesterol polyps which are multiple); all have increased **malignancy risk.**

824. A 50 yo woman presents to your office with long standing RUQ pain after eating. The pain occurs about 2 hours after eating and is worse with fatty meals. The pain radiates to her right shoulder. You perform an U/S which shows a normal biliary anatomy and <u>no</u> stones. The most appropriate next step is:
   a.   CCK-CS test
   b.   MR-cholangiopancreaticogram (MRCP)
   c.   Abdominal CT
   d.   Laparoscopic cholecystectomy

   Answer a. Cholecystitis Sx's and lack of gallstones on U/S is suspicious for either **chronic cholecystitis** or **biliary dyskinesia**. Cholecystokinin cholescintigraphy (CCK-CS, uses **HIDA** and **CCK**) is the **most sensitive test** for cholecystitis.

825. All of the following are true of single port (eg robotic) cholecystectomy compared to multi-port laparoscopic cholecystectomy except:
   a.   Return to work is earlier with single port
   b.   Cosmesis is better with single port
   c.   Biliary complications are higher with single port
   d.   There is a learning curve with single port

   Answer c. Biliary complications are <u>not</u> higher with single port.

826. All of the following are true except:

a. The MCC of shock following elective laparoscopic cholecystectomy within the 1st 24 hours is sepsis
b. The best initial test for RUQ pain or jaundice is a RUQ U/S
c. Ceftriaxone can cause sludging and cholestatic jaundice
d. For unstable patients with acalculous cholecystitis, percutaneous cholecystostomy tube is the preferred option
e. The MC type of gallstone is cholesterol stones

Answer a. The MCC of shock following elective laparoscopic cholecystectomy within the 1st 24 hours is **hemorrhage**, MC related to **clips** falling off the **cystic artery**.

827. All of the following increase to risk of conversion from laparoscopic to open cholecystectomy except:
a. Inflammation
b. Elderly patients
c. First time cholecystitis
d. Males
e. Obese patients

Answer c. Repeated attacks of cholecystitis increase the risk of chronic inflammation and difficulty with laparoscopic cholecystectomy.

828. Early cholecystectomy (< 24 hours) compared to delayed cholecystectomy is associated with :
a. Increased mortality
b. Increased morbidity
c. Increased biliary system injury
d. Shorter hospital stay
e. Increased use of biliary drains

Answer d. Shorter hospital stay

829. After a prolonged hospital course following a difficult aortic valve replacement, your patient is now extubated and stable but develops RUQ pain and elevated WBCs. U/S shows a distended gallbladder and no other findings. The appropriate next step is:
a. Laparoscopic cholecystectomy
b. Open cholecystectomy
c. HIDA scan
d. CT scan
e. MRI

Answer c. This is suspicious for **acalculous cholecystitis**. If U/S findings are inconclusive and the patient is stable, HIDA scan is indicated (which will show no filling of the gallbladder in patients with acalculous cholecystitis). Morphine can be given with the test to contract the sphincter of Oddi and help fill the gallbladder (prevents false positive test).

830. All of the following are true of emphysematous cholecystitis except:
a. Delayed cholecystectomy is indicated
b. Clostridium perfringens is a common cause
c. Perforation rate is higher than common cholecystitis
d. Gangrene rate is higher than common cholecystitis
e. It is associated with diabetes

Answer a. *Emergent* *cholecystectomy* is indicated for emphysematous cholecystitis. This is a life-threatening condition.

831. Gallbladder hydrops:
a. Is an inflammatory process
b. Results in a thickened gallbladder wall

c. Results in a shrunken gallbladder
d. Is associated with white bile
e. Has no association with gallstones

Answer d. Gallbladder hydrops is associated with white bile. Long standing obstruction *without* cholecystitis results in overdistension of the gallbladder, bile salt reabsorption, mucus secretion, and formation of a clear mucoid substance (white bile). Tx: **cholecystectomy**

832. A 50 yo patient with cirrhosis (MELD score 13) has had repeated attacks of cholecystitis. The most appropriate therapy in this patient is
    a. Ursodiol
    b. Open surgery
    c. Laparoscopic surgery
    d. Antibiotics only
    e. Percutaneous cholecystostomy tube

Answer c. Although in the past cirrhosis was a contraindication to elective cholecystectomy, it is now recommended for Child's A and Child's B. Child's C cirrhosis elective surgery is *not* recommended (surgical mortality is high in that group). MELD of 13 is approximately Child's B.

833. After ligating and cutting the cystic duct, you notice the remnant cystic duct is exceptionally long (3 cm). The most appropriate next step is:
    a. Leave a drain
    b. Nothing
    c. Re-resect leaving a 1 cm total length
    d. Re-resect leaving a 2 cm total length

Answer b. Cystic duct syndrome was once thought to be due to leaving a long cystic duct. It is now recognized that leaving the duct long does not increase the risk of cystic duct syndrome.

834. The best indication for intra-op cholangiogram is:
    a. To detect occult biliary stones
    b. To identify undiagnosed congenital anomalies
    c. To identify a choledochal cyst
    d. To display correct anatomy and prevent transection of the common bile duct

Answer d. To display correct anatomy and prevent transection of the common bile duct or hepatic duct.

835. During a very difficult laparoscopic cholecystectomy, you perform an intra-op cholangiogram through the cystic duct remnant and notice good distal filling of the CBD, but no filling of the proximal common hepatic duct despite changes in patient position. You convert to open procedure and there are 2 clips on the proximal hepatic duct, a divided hepatic duct, and one clip on the distal common bile duct. The most appropriate next step is:
    a. Whipple
    b. End to end anastomosis with absorbable suture
    c. Hepatico-jejunostomy
    d. Choledocho-jejunostomy

Answer c. The most appropriate step is to perform a **hepatico-jejunostomy**. End to end hepatic duct anastomosis will result in anastomotic **stricture** (due to tension and compromised blood supply) so it is not indicated. Choledocho-jejunostomy would be indicated with CBD transection.

836. Instead of the above injury, the patient has a 2 mm laceration in the common bile duct. The most appropriate next step is:

a. Whipple
b. Primary repair with absorbable suture over a biliary stent
c. Hepatico-jejunostomy
d. Choledocho-jejunostomy

Answer b. Primary repair with absorbable suture over a biliary stent. The stent helps prevent stricture formation and can be removed endoscopically at a later date.

837. The MCC of bile duct injury with laparoscopic cholecystectomy is:
a. Excess caudal traction of the gallbladder fundus
b. Excess cephalad retraction of the gallbladder fundus
c. Misinterpreting intra-op cholangiogram
d. Mistakenly dividing the hepatic duct.

Answer b. *Excess* **cephalad retraction** of the gallbladder fundus.

838. To avoid biliary injury, the best technique for displaying correct anatomy during laparoscopic cholecystectomy is:
a. Cephalad retraction of the gallbladder infundibulum
b. Caudad retraction of the gallbladder infundibulum
c. Medial retraction of the gallbladder infundibulum
d. Lateral retraction of the gallbladder infundibulum

Answer d. Lateral retraction of the gallbladder infundibulum

839. A 55 yo man with previous antrectomy and roux-en-Y gastro-jejunostomy for gastric adenocarcinoma presents to the ED with RUQ pain. U/S shows a dilated CBD (2 cm) and gallstones in the gallbladder. The most appropriate next step is:
a. Ursodiol
b. ERCP
c. PTC tube
d. Choledochotomy
e. Cholecystostomy tube

Answer c. The central issue here is that the CBD is not readily available to ERCP due to the division of the stomach after antrectomy and roux-en-Y gastrojejunostomy. This also applies for patients with previous roux-en-Y gastric bypass. The most expedient way of accessing the CBD in these patients is with a PTC tube. Tools can be used through this tube to remove the stones.

Cholecystectomy should also be performed on this admission.

840. A 30 yo woman presents to your office 7 days after a laparoscopic cholecystectomy and complains of moderate abdominal pain in the RUQ, nausea and vomiting, and very mild jaundice. The most appropriate next step is:
a. RUQ ultrasound
b. Change pain medications
c. ERCP
d. Broad spectrum antibiotics

Answer a. Pain, vomiting, and jaundice after laparoscopic cholecystectomy are unusual. Work-up starts with RUQ U/S (initial study of choice for RUQ pain) and getting LFTs and a CBC.

841. Ultrasound in the above woman reveals an 8 x 8 cm fluid collection in the gall bladder fossa. The bile ducts are normal size. The most appropriate next step is:
a. Broad spectrum antibiotics
b. Re-exploration
c. ERCP
d. Percutaneous drainage

Answer d. Given Sx's and fluid collection, **percutaneous drainage** is indicated.

842. You place a drain in the above patient and it reveals bile fluid. The most appropriate next step in this patient's management is:
   a. ERCP
   b. Exploratory laparotomy
   c. Abdominal CT scan
   d. Broad spectrum antibiotics

   Answer a. Bile fluid is worrisome biliary system injury. Need **ERCP**.

843. ERCP on the above patient shows free extravasation of contrast from the cystic duct remnant. The most appropriate next step is:
   a. Exploratory laparotomy
   b. Broad spectrum antibiotics only
   c. PTC tube
   d. Sphincterotomy and temporary stent

   Answer d. The **clip fell off the cystic duct remnant** and is causing leakage of bile into the abdomen. This problem is effectively treated 95% of the time with **ERCP, sphincterotomy,** and a **temporary stent** (across the leak if possible). Eventually, the cystic duct remnant will scar down.

844. All of the following are true of ERCP complications except:
   a. Retroperitoneal perforations are generally treated conservatively (NPO, antibiotics)
   b. Bile duct perforations are treated with a temporary stent across the perforation
   c. Free perforations of the duodenum are treated with stents
   d. Pancreatitis is the MC Cx following ERCP

   Answer c. Free perforations of the duodenum require open repair. **Contained** retroperitoneal perforations are most often treated conservatively.

845. Which of the following is not criteria for ERCP with gallstone pancreatitis:
   a. Dilated CBD
   b. U/S showing CBD stone
   c. Cholangitis
   d. Elevated bilirubin (> 5) after 24 hours of observation

   Answer a. A dilated CBD is not an indication for ERCP in the setting of **gallstone pancreatitis**. Many patients with gallstone pancreatitis have a dilated CBD and the probability of finding residual stones is low. There is also a 5% complication rate with ERCP (MC - pancreatitis).

   A dilated CBD is criteria for ERCP in patients with **cholecystitis**, as this usually indicates a CBD stone.

846. All of the following are indications for ERCP with gallstone pancreatitis except:
   a. Elevated alkaline phosphatase
   b. Elevated total bilirubin (> 5) after 24 hours of observation
   c. Cholangitis
   d. CBD stone (> 2 mm) present on U/S

   Answer a. Elevated alkaline phosphatase is not an indication for ERCP.

847. A 60 yo woman with no past medical problems presents to the emergency room with jaundice, right upper quadrant pain, and fever. Her blood pressure is 85/45 and her heart rate is 115. You obtain a RUQ U/S which shows a dilated CBD (12 mm) and pneumobilia. The most appropriate next step is:

a. Emergent cholecystectomy
b. Emergent ERCP
c. Emergent PTC placement
d. Fluid resuscitation

Answer d. This patient needs **fluid resuscitation** before any diagnostic studies are performed. IV antibiotics are also indicated after volume resuscitation is started. From the clinical scenario presented, this patient most likely has **cholangitis**. Charcot's triad consists of fever, RUQ pain, and jaundice. Reynolds pentad includes Charcot's triad plus hypotension and mental status changes.

848. The above patient now has a blood pressure of 110/60 and a HR of 100 after aggressive IVFs. The most appropriate next step is:
    a. Emergent cholecystectomy
    b. Emergent ERCP and sphincterotomy
    c. Emergent PTC placement
    d. Hepatico-jejunostomy

Answer b. The most effective Tx for **cholangitis** is decompression of the biliary system. This is most easily done with **ERCP and sphincterotomy**, which not only can decompress the biliary system but can also remove or treat any obstructive lesion (stones most commonly).

849. For gallstone pancreatitis or gallstone induced cholangitis, cholecystectomy should be performed:
    a. Immediately
    b. After the patient recovers and 6-8 weeks after discharge
    c. Three months after the initial diagnosis
    d. After recovery but before discharge

Answer d. After recovery but before discharge. There is a chance of repeated episodes for these conditions so cholecystectomy is indicated.

850. A 75 yo woman from a nursing home presents to the emergency room with crampy abdominal pain. On CT scan, you notice multiple air-fluid levels and distension of her small bowel. Her colon appears decompressed. She also has pneumobilia despite never having surgery before or manipulation of her biliary system. The most appropriate next step is:
    a. Start broad spectrum antibiotics
    b. Exploratory laparotomy
    c. Percutaneous cholecystostomy tube
    d. Endoscopic retrograde cholangiography

Answer b. **Pneumobilia** (in a patient who has never had manipulation of her biliary system) associated with small bowel obstruction is most consistent with **gallstone ileus**. The gallbladder in this patient has eroded into the duodenum (chole-duodenal fistula) and a large gallstone is now causing a small bowel obstruction.

851. The _primary surgery_ for the above patient is:
    a. Whipple
    b. Cholecystectomy
    c. Fistula resection
    d. Longitudinal enterotomy, removing the stone, and running the bowel for other stones.
    e. Ileal resection

Answer d. The primary surgery in this patient is to **relieve the small bowel obstruction**. That involves feeling for the gallstone, opening the ileum proximal to the stone, (longitudinal **enterotomy**, transverse closure), and removing stone.

The secondary procedure, *if the patient can tolerate it*, is cholecystectomy and closure of the hole in the duodenum. **Elderly, infirmed**, and/or severely **septic** patients should just have the stone removed *without* cholecystectomy.

852. The MCC of benign biliary stricture is:
    a.   Cholecystitis
    b.   Previous cholecystectomy
    c.   Gallstones
    d.   Pancreatitis
    e.   Cholangitis

    Answer b. Ischemia following **previous cholecystectomy** is the MCC of benign bile duct stricture. Cautery, clips, and/or aggressive dissection can lead to a devascularized bile duct.

853. A 50 yo woman with a vague history of chronic pancreatitis and liver disease presents with jaundice. The best lab value for determining which disease process is causing her jaundice is:
    a.   AST
    b.   ALT
    c.   GGT
    d.   Alkaline phosphatase
    e.   Bilirubin

    Answer d. Alkaline phosphatase. Chronic pancreatitis can lead to biliary strictures and obstructive jaundice. This would result in an elevated alkaline phosphatase *(the most sensitive indicator of obstructive jaundice)*. Chronic liver disease results in jaundice due to inability to metabolize bilirubin and alkaline phosphatase is generally not elevated with this condition.

854. U/S in the above patient shows dilated proximal bile ducts and a focal mid duct stenosis. The most appropriate next step in this patients work-up is:
    a.   ERCP
    b.   MRCP
    c.   Chemo-XRT
    d.   Exploration

    Answer b. Discovery of a **biliary stenosis** is suggestive of **CA** (either bile duct, gallbladder, or pancreatic), a common bile duct stone, or a benign stricture

    Of the items listed, **MRCP** is the most appropriate next step as this picks up any masses in the gallbladder or pancreas and also provides good reconstruction of the biliary system (anatomy). MRCP is also good at picking up stones. It is not invasive like ERCP (which risks of pancreatitis and perforation) and ERCP may not pick up obvious masses.

855. The above patient is found to have unresectable gallbladder CA growing into the CBD. You feel a biliary stent is appropriate. All of the following are true except:
    a.   Pancreatitis can occur with both metal and silastic stents
    b.   Metal stents have a better long term patency rate compared to silastic
    c.   Complication rates are lower when stents are placed endoscopically compared to percutaneous placement
    d.   Fibrin clot is the primary mechanism of stent obstruction with metal stents
    e.   Silastic stents have a higher stent migration rate compared to metal stents

    Answer d. Tumor in-growth is the primary mechanism of stent obstruction with metal stents

856. The most appropriate surgery for a resectable lower 1/3 bile duct CA would be:

a. Whipple
b. Hepatic lobectomy
c. Local bile duct resection with hepatico-jejunostomy
d. Wide local excision

Answer a. Resectable lower 1/3 bile duct CA should undergo Whipple.

Upper ⅓ (Klatskin tumor, hilar) – Tx: **hepatic lobectomy** if localized to one side
Middle ⅓ - Tx: **resect duct with hepatico-jejunostomy**
Lower ⅓ - Tx: **Whipple**

857. All of the following are risk factors for gallbladder CA except:
a. Gallbladder adenoma
b. Small gallstones compared to large gallstones
c. Porcelain gallbladder
d. Females
e. Obesity

Answer b. Large gallstones have a higher risk of gallbladder CA compared to small stones.

858. A 50 yo woman undergoes routine laparoscopic cholecystectomy and gallbladder adenocarcinoma is found extending into the muscularis propria. Which of the following is true:
a. This patient should undergo partial hepatectomy
b. This patient should undergo wedge resection of segments 4 and 5 (gallbladder fossa) with portal triad lymph node stripping
c. Chemo-XRT only
d. No further therapy

Answer b. (see below)

859. Instead of the above, the gallbladder adenocarcinoma is not involving the muscularis propria. Which of the following is true:
a. This patient should undergo wedge resection of segment 4 and 5 (gallbladder fossa) with portal triad lymph node stripping
b. This patient should undergo partial hepatectomy
c. Chemo-XRT only
d. No further therapy

Answer d. No further therapy

Gallbladder adenocarcinoma confined to the mucosa and lamina propria (stage Ia) can be treated with just **cholecystectomy**.

If it **invades** the **muscularis propria** (stage Ib), you need **wedge resection** of **segments 4 and 5** with 2-3 cm margins and stripping of the portal triad lymph nodes

For tumors that go **beyond** the **muscularis propria** and are resectable (Stage IIa or greater, T3 or T4 tumors), **formal resection** of segments IVb and V is necessary (possible right lobectomy) along with stripping of the portal triad lymph nodes

ANATOMY AND PHYSIOLOGY
■ Gallbladder lies underneath **segments IV** and **V**
■ **Cystic artery** is a branch off **right hepatic artery**, located in triangle of Calot
■ **Right hepatic** (lateral) and retroduodenal branches of the **gastroduodenal artery** (medial) supply the **hepatic** and **common bile duct** [9- and 3-o'clock positions when performing endoscopic retrograde cholangio-pancreatography (ERCP)]; considered longitudinal blood supply

- **Triangle of Calot** (cystohepatic triangle) - cystic duct (lateral), common hepatic duct (medial), liver (superior)
- **Cystic veins** - drain into **right branch** of the **portal vein**, which then goes to the liver
- **Lymphatics** - found on **right side** of common bile duct
- **Innervation**
  - **Parasympathetic** - **left vagus nerve** (anterior trunk); causes **gallbladder contraction** and **relaxation of the sphincter of Oddi**
  - **Sympathetic** - splanchnic and celiac ganglions (T7-T10); _inhibits_ gallbladder contraction
- **Gallbladder**
  - Mucosa is **columnar** epithelium
  - Does _not_ have **submucosa**
  - Common bile duct (CBD) and hepatic duct do _not_ have **peristalsis**
  - Fills by contraction of **sphincter of Oddi** at Ampulla of Vater
  - **Morphine** _contracts_ the sphincter of Oddi
  - **Glucagon** _relaxes_ the sphincter of Oddi
- **Normal sizes**
  - Common Bile Duct (CBD) < 8 mm (< 10 mm after cholecystectomy)
  - Gallbladder wall < 4 mm
  - Pancreatic duct < 4 mm
- _Highest concentration of **CCK** and **secretin releasing cells** - duodenum_
- **Aberrant posterior right hepatic artery** (segments VI and VII)
  - 1% of the population
  - At risk of injury with cholecystectomy (found in Triangle of Calot)
  - Injury can result in **ischemia** to segments VI and VII (Sx's - fevers, pain, ↑ed LFTs, liver abscess)
- **Aberrant posterior right hepatic duct** (from **segments VI and VII**)
  - 1% of the population
  - Enters common bile duct **separately** from right hepatic duct
  - Lies in gallbladder fossa and at **risk of injury** with cholecystectomy
- **Bile excretion**
  - **Increase** bile excretion - CCK, vagal input
  - **Decrease** bile excretion - somatostatin, sympathetic input
- **Gallbladder contraction** - CCK (constant, tonic contraction)
- **Composition and essential functions of bile**:
    1) Fat-soluble vitamin and essential fatty acid absorption
    2) Bilirubin and cholesterol excretion

	Hepatic Bile	Gallbladder Bile
Na (mEq/L)	140-180	225-375
CL (mEq/L)	50-100	1-10
Bile Salts (mEq/L)	1-50	250-350
Cholesterol (mEq/dl)	50-150	300-700

  - **Final bile composition** in gallbladder determined by _active_ reabsorption of **sodium** (Na/K ATPase) with concomitant _passive_ **reabsorption of water** (due to sodium gradient); bile is **concentrated**
  - The gallbladder secretes **mucus**
- **Bile salts** - bile salt pool (6 g)
  - **95%** of excreted bile salts are reabsorbed (**enterohepatic re-circulation**):
    1) **Active resorption** of _conjugated_ bile acids occurs only in **terminal ileum** (45%)
    2) **Passive resorption** of _non-conjugated_ bile acids occurs throughout the **small intestine** (40%) and **colon** (5%)
- **Postprandial emptying** of gallbladder is maximum at **2 hours** (80% emptied)
- Bile is secreted by **hepatocytes** (80%) and **bile canalicular cells** (20%)
- **Conjugated bilirubin** - gives bile its **brownish-yellow** color
- **Urobilinogen** breakdown product of conjugated bilirubin in **gut** (by bacteria); is converted to either **stercobilin** or is _reabsorbed_ and converted to **urobilin**
  - **Urobilin** - released in urine; turns it **yellow**

- **Stercobilin** - gives stool it's **brown** color
- Patients with **obstructive jaundice** have **clay colored stools** from lack of conjugated bilirubin in the gut (also have _very little_ urobilin in the urine); the urine will be **dark brown** (color of cola) from bilirubinemia and **bilirubin** in the urine
- Patients with **GI bleeding** or **RBC hemolysis** (both _increase_ conjugated bilirubin) will have _increased_ **urobilinogen**.

GALLSTONES
- Occur in 10% of the population; vast majority are asymptomatic
- Only 10% of gallstones are radiopaque
- **Non-pigmented** stones
  - **Cholesterol stones** - caused by **stasis, calcium nucleation**, and ↑ **water reabsorption** from gallbladder
  - Also caused by decreased **lecithin** and **bile salts**
  - Found almost exclusively in the gallbladder
  - Most common type of stone found in the United States (75%)
  - Can form after terminal ileum resection from malabsorption of bile salts
- **Pigmented** stones - MC worldwide
  - **Calcium bilirubinate stones** - caused by solubilization of unconjugated bilirubin with precipitation
  - _Dissolution agents (monooctanoin) do not work on pigmented stones_
  - **Black stones**
      - Can be caused by **hemolytic disorders** (eg sickle cell, spherocytosis), **cirrhosis, chronic TPN**
      - Factors for development: ↑ bilirubin load, ↓ hepatic function → get **calcium bilirubinate** stones
      - Almost always form in gallbladder
      - Tx: **cholecystectomy** if symptomatic
  - **Brown stones** (primary CBD stones, formed in ducts, friable; MC in Asians)
      - **Infection** causes deconjugation of bilirubin
          - _E. coli_ most common - produces beta-glucuronidase, which deconjugates bilirubin with formation of **calcium bilirubinate**; also associated with **parasites** (eg _C. sinensis. O. viverrini, A. lumbricoides_)
      - Need to check for ampullary stenosis, duodenal diverticula, abnormal sphincter of Oddi
      - _Most commonly form in **bile ducts** (are primary common bile duct stones)_
      - Can result in biliary strictures and cholangiohepatitis (recurrent pyogenic cholangitis)
      - Tx: almost all patients with primary stones need a biliary drainage procedure - **ERCP with sphincteroplasty** (90% successful)
  - **Cholesterol** stones and **black** stones found in the CBD are considered _**secondary** common bile duct stones_

CHOLECYSTITIS
- **Cystic duct obstruction** caused by a **gallstone**
- Results in gallbladder wall **distention** and **inflammation**
- Sx's: RUQ pain worse 1-2 hours after meal (especially **fatty meals**), N/V, loss of appetite (anorexia)
  - **Referred pain** to the right shoulder and scapula
  - Pain is **persistent** (unlike biliary colic which is transient)
  - **Biliary colic** - transient cystic duct obstruction caused by passage of a gallstone; resolves in 4-6 hours
  - Murphy's sign - patient resists deep inspiration with deep palpation to the RUQ secondary to pain
  - **Suppurative cholecystitis** associated with frank **purulence** in the gallbladder → can be associated with **sepsis** and **shock**
- RFs for stones: age > 40, female, obesity, pregnancy, rapid weight loss, vagotomy, TPN (pigmented stones), terminal ileum resection
- Dx:
  - **U/S** (RUQ) - 95% sensitive for picking up stones (hyper-echoic focus, posterior shadowing, movement of focus with changes in position)

*Best initial evaluation test for **jaundice** or **RUQ pain***
Findings suggestive of **acute cholecystitis** - gallstones, gallbladder wall
thickening (> 4 mm), pericholecystic fluid, sonographic Murphy's
Dilated **common bile duct** (> 8 mm if gallbladder present) suggests CBD
stone and obstruction
Dilated **pancreatic duct** (> 4 mm) suggests stone in Ampulla of Vater
Duct dilation *without* stones → benign or malignant stricture

- **Alkaline phosphatase** and **WBCs** are usually elevated
- Amylase and lipase can be mildly elevated with cholecystitis
- Significant elevations in AST / ALT or amylase / lipase → need to worry about
gallstone <u>pancreatitis</u> and possible <u>cholangitis</u>
- **HIDA scan** (cholescintigraphy) - technetium is taken up by the liver and excreted
into the biliary tract; normally fills the gallbladder
- **CCK-CS test** (cholecystokinin cholescintigraphy; uses **HIDA + CCK**)
    ***Most sensitive test** for cholecystitis*
    Used when gallbladder disease is suspected and U/S is negative (checks
    for **chronic cholecystitis** and **biliary dyskinesia**)
    Technetium (Tc) is given, taken up by liver, and then excreted in biliary
    tract (99mTc-*HIDA* cholescintigraphy, CS)
    Cholecystokinin (CCK) is given to stimulate gallbladder contraction
    Indications for **cholecystectomy** after CCK-CS test:
        1) If **gallbladder not seen** (chronic cholecystitis)
        2) Takes > **60 minutes to empty** (biliary dyskinesia)
        3) **Ejection fraction < 40%** (biliary dyskinesia; 95% get relief after
        cholecystectomy)
- MC organisms in cholecystitis - ***E. coli** (#1)*, Klebsiella, Enterococcus
- Indications for ***emergent*** ERCP (*any* below; likely have **CBD stone**)
  - **Jaundice**
  - **Cholangitis** (eg fever, jaundice, RUQ pain, sepsis)
  - U/S shows a **CBD stone** (> 2 mm stone)
  - **Dilated CBD** *without* gallstone pancreatitis (see below)
  - *Patients should have appropriate **fluid resuscitation** before ERCP*
- Indications for ***pre-op*** ERCP (*any* of following needs to be <u>persistently</u> elevated for >
24 hours to justify pre-op ERCP) - *all are signs a CBD stone might be present:*
  - **Total bilirubin** (> 5)
  - **AST** or **ALT** (> 200) *without* gallstone pancreatitis (see below)
  - *Elevated alkaline phosphatase is <u>not</u> an indication for ERCP*
- **Gallstone pancreatitis** (lipase [best lab test] or **amylase** > 500, see Pancreas chp)
  - Routine ERCP for a <u>dilated CBD</u> with gallstone pancreatitis *is discouraged* since
  the probability of finding residual stones here is low and there is a **5% Cx rate**
  - Similarly, ERCP for elevated <u>AST / ALT</u> with gallstone pancreatitis *is
  discouraged*
  - Emergent or pre-op ERCP should be performed for the other criteria listed above
  - Patients with gallstone pancreatitis should have **cholecystectomy** *after* recovery
  from pancreatitis but on the **same hospital admission** (ie prior to discharge)
- Tx for cholecystitis - **laparoscopic cholecystectomy** (*within* **24 hours** has a lower
rate of Cx's compared to delayed) and **antibiotics**
  - Percutaneous **cholecystostomy tube** (CT or U/S guided) can be placed in
  patients who are very ill and cannot tolerate surgery; cholecystectomy 4-6 weeks
  after recovery usual
  - **Pregnancy** with acute cholecystitis - *NPO and antibiotics only* (cefoxitin; treats
  95%)
  - Best indication for **intra-op cholangiogram** - define <u>anatomy</u> and <u>prevent
  transection</u> of the CBD and hepatic duct
- **Cystic duct stump** - previously thought that the stump should be kept short to prevent
post-cholecystectomy syndrome but recently shown that leaving a long stump does <u>not</u>
increase the risk of stones or stasis post-op
  - The most important technical concern is to identify the cystic duct - gallbladder
  infundibulum junction and ***remove all of the gallbladder***
  - Most cases of post-cholecystectomy syndrome are due to **remnant gallbladder**
  and stone formation

- The cystic duct can be left long if indicated
- **Single port** vs. multiport laparoscopic cholecystectomy
  - Better cosmetic score (especially in women)
  - Less post-op pain
  - Better quality of life overall (improved mobility, earlier return to usual activity, lower anxiety)
  - Longer operative time
  - No difference in bile duct injury or other Cx's
- **RFs for conversion** from laparoscopic to open cholecystectomy - males, elderly, repeated attacks of cholecystitis, previous upper abdominal surgery, inflammation, obesity, multiple co-morbidities (higher ASA class), gallbladder wall thickness > 4 mm
- **Early cholecystectomy** (< 24 hours) vs delayed cholecystectomy for acute cholecystitis is associated with shorter hospital stay and <u>no</u> increase in complication rate, morbidity, or mortality
- **Ceftriaxone** - can cause gallbladder sludging and cholestatic jaundice
- **Diarrhea** after cholecystectomy *(MC Cx following cholecystectomy)* - from excess <u>bile salts</u> in colon (not stored in gallbladder anymore)
- **Air in biliary system** - MC occurs after <u>previous</u> ERCP and sphincterotomy (normal finding)
  - Can also occur with cholangitis or erosion of the gallbladder into the duodenum (ie gallstone ileus)
- **Bacterial infection of bile**
  - **MC route** - usually related to **biliary tract manipulation** (eg ERCP and sphincterotomy)
  - **MC route** (non-intervention related) - dissemination from **portal system**
  - Retrograde infection from bacteria in duodenum is <u>*very rare*</u> unless previous sphincterotomy or ERCP procedure
- MCC of **late stricture** after cholecystectomy - **ischemia**
- **Cirrhosis** - <u>*not*</u> considered a contraindication to cholecystectomy; patients with cirrhosis (Childs A and B) and symptomatic gallstones or other indications for cholecystectomy should undergo **laparoscopic cholecystectomy** (much lower mortality than open procedure, 1% vs. 8%); *Childs C generally <u>not</u> recommended*
- **Pain, vomiting**, or **jaundice** after cholecystectomy - get <u>RUQ U/S</u> *(best initial test)*
- Symptomatic **fluid collection** after cholecystectomy - Dx and Tx: place **percutaneous drain** (if bile → get an **ERCP** to look for leak)
- **Shock** following laparoscopic cholecystectomy
  - **Early** (1st 24 hours) - hemorrhagic shock, clip fell off cystic artery
  - **Late** (after 24 hours) - septic shock from accidental clip on CBD with subsequent cholangitis (usually occurs at median of **7 days**)
- **Porcelain gallbladder** - diffuse calcification of gallbladder wall; high risk for gallbladder CA (15%); Tx - **cholecystectomy**
- **Ursodiol** (UDCA; Actigall) - dissolves gallstones < 2 cm; indicated for either:1) patients with cholecystectomy indications who are too **high risk** for surgery <u>*or*</u>; 2) prevention of stone formation in patients with **rapid weight loss** (eg gastric bypass)
- **Morphine** <u>contracts</u> the sphincter of Oddi (good for HIDA scan)
- **Glucagon** <u>relaxes</u> the sphincter of Oddi (good for trying to get stones to pass intra-op)

PERI-OP CBD STONES
- **ERCP** and **sphincterotomy** - removes CBD stones in > 95%
- < 5% of patients undergoing cholecystectomy will have a retained CBD stone and > 95% of these are cleared with ERCP
- CBD stone ≤ **2 mm** discovered **intra-op** - <u>*leave alone*</u> (will pass on its own)
- **CBD obstruction** found **intra-op** - Tx: <u>*post-op*</u> **ERCP with sphincterotomy**
  - If it's a large stone that you feel cannot be cleared with ERCP, consider laparoscopic CBD exploration (rare)
  - Trouble getting CBD stone to pass into duodenum with CBD exploration - Tx: **glucagon** (relaxes the sphincter of Oddi)
- <u>Retained</u> CBD stone after **cholecystectomy** (jaundice, CBD > 10 mm, CBD stones) - Tx: **ERCP with sphincterotomy**
- <u>Retained</u> CBD stone after **T-tube placement** - Tx: use **choledochoscope** through the T-tube to remove stone

- Retained CBD stone after **roux-en-Y gastro-jejunal anastomosis** (eg gastric bypass or gastric resection)
    - Central issue is that you can <u>not</u> easily access the sphincter of Oddi with ERCP after the roux-en-Y anastomosis
    - Tx: **PTC tube with stone extraction** (*best*; can do this through the PTC tube)
        If gallbladder is still present → many favor <u>laparoscopic</u> cholecystectomy and CBD exploration
- **ERCP Cx's** (5%): pancreatitis (MC, 3%), bleeding (1%), cholangitis (< 1%), perforation
    - **Retroperitoneal perforation** (contained; <u>extra</u>-peritoneal contrast) - conservative Tx (NPO, antibiotics)
    - **Bile duct perforation** - place temporary stent across perforation; will heal
    - **Free perforation of duodenum** (<u>intra</u>-peritoneal extravasation of contrast) - Tx: open repair

ACALCULOUS CHOLECYSTITIS
- Sx's: RUQ pain, N/V; elevated WBCs or fever in an intubated ICU patient
- RFs: major surgery / trauma / burns, long ICU stay, MSOF, prolonged TPN
- Pathology: **bile stasis** (from narcotics, fasting) and increased **viscosity** (from dehydration, ileus) leads to sludging and blockage of cystic duct; **distention** and **ischemia** follow
- Much like mesenteric ischemia, line infections, and UTIs, acalculous cholecystitis can be overlooked in sick, intubated ICU patients (consider this with fever or high WBCs)
- Dx: **U/S** - dilated gallbladder, thickened wall, sludge, pericholecystic fluid, <u>no</u> stones
    - Elevated **WBCs** and **alkaline phosphatase**
- **HIDA scan** is **positive** (*shows <u>no</u> gallbladder filling due to obstructed cystic duct*; use morphine to contract sphincter of Oddi and help fill the biliary system [helps prevent false positive result]; <u>not</u> used in sick ICU patients
- **Perforation** rate, gallbladder **gangrene**, **empyema**, and **mortality** are all higher compared to general cholecystitis
- Tx: **cholecystectomy** and antibiotics
    - **Percutaneous cholecystostomy tube** if the patient is **unstable**

EMPHYSEMATOUS CHOLECYSTITIS
- **Gas** in the gallbladder wall - can see on plain film
- Increased in **diabetics** and elderly **males**; usually secondary to *Clostridium perfringens* (Clostridium welchii, E. coli, and B. fragilis also commonly involved)
- Sx's: severe, rapid-onset abdominal pain, N/V, and sepsis
- **Perforation** rate (20%), gallbladder **gangrene** (75%), and **mortality** (20%) are all <u>higher</u> compared to general cholecystitis
- Tx: **emergent cholecystectomy**; antibiotics (PCN G and clindamycin)

GALLBLADDER MUCOCELE (hydrops gallbladder)
- Long standing obstruction results in overdistension of the gallbladder, bile salt reabsorption, mucus secretion, and formation of a clear mucoid substance (**white bile**)
- *Is <u>not</u> an inflammatory or infectious process (unlike cholecystitis)*
- It can **rupture**
- *There is <u>no</u> malignancy risk (unlike appendix mucocele)*
- Sx's: RUQ pain, N/V
- Dx: **RUQ U/S** *(best test)* - shows a **distended**, <u>thin</u> walled gallbladder (> 5 cm across in anterior-posterior dimension), impacted stones in the infundibulum or neck, and clear fluid content
- Tx: **cholecystectomy**

COMMON BILE DUCT INJURIES
- **Intra-op CBD injury** → open and repair
    - If injury is < 50% CBD circumference - perform **primary repair** over stent
    - If injury is > 50% - need **hepatico-jejunostomy** (MC; or choledocho-jejunostomy)
        Do <u>not</u> try to attach to the duodenum (will not each)
        Do <u>not</u> try primary repair (will get stricture or leak due to tension and compromised blood supply)

- **MCC of CBD injury with laparoscopic cholecystectomy** - _excess cephalad retraction_ of the gallbladder fundus (70% of injuries)
  - You think it's the cystic duct but really it is the CBD brought up from excess traction (considered a **Class III injury**)
  - Minimize risk of injury by visualizing the triangle of Calot (want to see the cystic duct going into the gallbladder)
- **Best way to avoid injury** - **lateral retraction** of the gallbladder infundibulum
- Persistent **RUQ pain, N/V,** or **jaundice** following cholecystectomy → get **U/S** to look for fluid collection
  - _If **fluid collection present**_, may be bile leak → Tx: place **percutaneous drain**; If the fluid is **bilious**, get **ERCP** →
    - If **small** lesion - Tx: **sphincterotomy + biliary stent**; _includes:_ →
      1) **Cystic duct remnant** leak (ie clips fell off)
      2) Small injuries to the hepatic or common bile duct
      3) Leak from a duct of Luschka (< 2 mm)
      Try to place stent **across leak** if possible for all
      Eventually these areas will **scar down** (no surgery is required; biliary stent is temporary)
    - If **large** lesion (eg complete duct transection) - Tx: will require a **hepatico-jejunostomy** (or choledocho-jejunostomy; see below for timing)
  - _If **fluid collection not present**_ and the **hepatic ducts are dilated**, likely have a completely transected CBD with a clip on it (Tx: PTC tube initially, then hepatico-jejunostomy; see below for timing)
  - PTC tube - percutaneous trans-hepatic cholangiography tube
- **Post-op discovery of significant CBD injury** (large lesion, eg complete duct transection)
  - Early Dx (**< 7 days** after cholecystectomy) - re-op for **hepaticojejunostomy**
  - Late Dx (**≥ 7 days** after cholecystectomy) - wait 6-8 weeks after injury before **hepaticojejunostomy** (dense adhesions and friable tissue make surgery too dangerous after 7 days - need to wait)
    - If CBD is obstructed - place PTC tube
    - If fluid collection - place percutaneous drain
- **Sepsis following cholecystectomy** → **fluid resuscitation + antibiotics 1ˢᵗ**
  - May be due to complete transection of the CBD and **cholangitis** → get U/S to look for dilated intra-hepatic ducts or fluid collections (pathway same as above)
- **LFTs** will be elevated with a clip on the CBD causing biliary obstruction
- **Anastomotic leaks** following hepaticojejunostomy → Tx: percutaneous drainage of fluid collection and **ERCP with temporary stent** (leak will heal)

BILE DUCT STRICTURES
- MCC - bile duct **ischemia** following **laparoscopic cholecystectomy** (cautery, clips, and/or aggressive dissection can lead to devascularization, ischemia, and stricture)
- Other causes - chronic pancreatitis, previous cholangitis, gallbladder CA, bile duct CA
- Sx's: **obstructive jaundice** (MC); occasionally present with cholangitis
- Bile duct strictures without a history of pancreatitis or biliary surgery is CA until proven otherwise
- Dx: **MRCP** (_best test for jaundice not caused by stones; magnetic resonance cholangio-pancreatography_) delineates **anatomy** and looks for **mass** → if CA not ruled out with MRCP, need **ERCP** with **brush Bx's**
  - RUQ U/S - 1ˢᵗ test for jaundice (shows dilated proximal ducts, no CBD stones)
- Labs: elevated **alkaline phosphatase** (_most sensitive lab test for obstructive jaundice_) and **total bilirubin**
- Tx: if due to **ischemia** or **chronic pancreatitis** → **choledocho-jejunostomy** (_best long term solution_)
  - If due to CA, follow appropriate work-up
- **Palliation** of malignant biliary obstruction:
  - Expandable mesh **metal stents** have better patency over silastic
  - MCC obstruction in metal stent - tumor in-growth
  - MCC obstruction in silastic stent - sludge deposition
  - Cx's for both metal and silastic stents - pancreatitis, cholecystitis
    - Cx of silastic stents alone - stent migration (slides unlike metal mesh)

- Endoscopic stent placement is the preferred route (better relief of jaundice, lower early mortality); percutaneous placement used as a backup
- 15% of these patients will eventually get a malignant <u>duodenal obstruction</u> - Tx: **duodenal stent**

CHOLANGITIS
- Inflammation (infection) of the biliary system
- MCC - **gallstones**; other causes - strictures, choledochal cysts, duodenal diverticula
- Can also be caused by **indwelling tubes** (eg PTC tube)
- Sx's: **RUQ pain, fever** and **jaundice** (Charcot's triad)
- Reynolds' pentad - Charcot's triad plus <u>mental status changes</u> (eg confusion) and <u>shock</u> (suggests sepsis)
- MC organisms - *E. coli* (#1), *Klebsiella*
- Dx:
  - **U/S** *(usual initial test)* - shows **dilated CBD** (> **8 mm**; > **10 mm** after cholecystectomy) if due to obstruction of the biliary system
  - **Labs** - *elevated* AST/ALT, bilirubin, alkaline phosphatase, and WBCs; positive blood cultures
- Most serious Cx - **renal failure** (related to **sepsis**)
- Tx: *fluid resuscitation + antibiotics initially (stabilize patient <u>before</u> ERCP)*
  - Emergent **ERCP** with **sphincterotomy** and **stone extraction** (decompresses the biliary system - most effective Tx for cholangitis)
      If ERCP fails, place **PTC tube** to decompress the biliary system
      If PTC tube fails, go to OR for intra-op **T-tube** to decompress
  - If cholangitis due to an **infected PTC tube** → **change the PTC tube**
  - If cholangitis due to **stricture** → **ERCP + biliary stent** (PTC tube if that fails)
  - If due to gallstones, need **cholecystectomy** after recovery (*<u>before</u> hospital discharge)*
- Biliary strictures and hepatic abscess are late Cx's of cholangitis

GALLSTONE ILEUS
- **Fistula** between **gallbladder** and 2nd portion of **duodenum**
- **Gallstone** is released causing **small bowel obstruction**
- Sx's: N/V, distension, crampy abdominal pain (**small bowel obstruction**, SBO), and **pneumobilia**; usually seen in **elderly women** (70's)
- Dx: CT scan → **air in biliary tree** (pneumobilia) and **SBO** *(classic findings)*
- MC site of obstruction - **terminal ileum** (usually large gallstone [> 2.5 cm])
- Tx: remove stone through longitudinal enterotomy proximal to obstruction (transverse closure); run bowel for other stones; primary surgery is to remove all of the stones
  - Perform cholecystectomy and fistula resection if patient can tolerate it *(if **old** and **frail** → leave the fistula)*

HEMOBILIA
- Fistula between **bile duct** and **hepatic arterial system** (MC connection)
- Sx's: **hematemesis, jaundice,** and **RUQ pain** *(classic triad)*
- Usually occurs late after **trauma** (mean time - 4 weeks), with **percutaneous liver instrumentation** (MCC, eg PTC tube), or after laparoscopic cholecystectomy and injury to the right hepatic artery
- Dx: **angiogram** *(best test)*; EGD often used as initial study for UGI bleed which will show blood coming out of the Ampulla of Vater
- Tx: **angio-embolization** of culprit vessel; surgical ligation if that is unsuccessful

GALLBLADDER ADENOCARCINOMA
- **MC CA of the biliary tract** although is still rare
- Four times MC than bile duct CA; most have stones
- RFs: **gallstones** *(#1, most important RF, especially <u>large</u> stones)*, porcelain gallbladder, primary sclerosing cholangitis, gallbladder adenomas, obesity, females, choledochal cysts
- Sx's: **jaundice 1st** (bile duct invasion with obstruction) followed by **RUQ pain**

- Dx:
  - **U/S** *(best initial test for RUQ pain or jaundice)* - may show dilated ducts from invasion into the CBD
  - **MRCP** - *best test to get after discovery of a biliary stenosis (obstruction not caused by gallstones)*
- May present as a **mid-bile duct obstruction** not caused by stones (this is gallbladder CA [or bile duct CA] until proven otherwise)
- Pathology
  - 1st spreads to **segments IVb** and **V**
  - 1st nodes involved are the **cystic duct nodes** (right side of portal triad)
  - MC site of metastases - **liver**
  - High incidence of tumor implants in **trocar sites** when discovered after laparoscopic cholecystectomy
  - Laparoscopic approach *contraindicated* for gallbladder CA
  - Overall prognosis <u>poor</u> - only 20% resectable, 80% present as **stage IV** disease
  - Best prognosis - **papillary** sub-type
  - Can be found **incidentally** after cholecystectomy
- Tx:
  - If muscle <u>not</u> involved (confined to <u>mucosa</u> and lamina propria; T1, stage Ia) → **cholecystectomy** is sufficient *(no further therapy after cholecystectomy)*
  - If it **invades muscle** but not beyond (confined to <u>muscularis propria</u>, T2 Stage Ib) - need <u>wedge</u> **resection** of **liver segments IVb** and **V** (ie the gallbladder fossa, 2-3 cm margin)
  - If **beyond muscle** and still resectable (T3 or T4 tumors, Stage IIa or greater) - need <u>formal</u> **resection** of **segments IVb and V** (2-3 cm margin)
    - May need **CBD resection** with **hepatico-jejunostomy** as well
  - Also need **portal triad lymph node stripping** with above resections *(not for T1)*
  - Some recommend **excision of previous laparoscopic port sites** if CA is into the muscle
- 5-YS (all patients) - **5%** (after resection for cure 30%)

BILE DUCT CANCER (cholangiocarcinoma)
- Usually in elderly; males
- RFs: ulcerative colitis, choledochal cysts, primary sclerosing cholangitis, chronic bile duct infection
- Sx's: <u>early</u> - **painless jaundice**; <u>late</u> - **weight loss**; may develop pruritus
- Labs: elevation in **conjugated bilirubin** and **alkaline phosphatase**
- Dx:
  - **U/S** *(best initial test for RUQ pain or jaundice)* - shows dilated ducts
  - **MRCP** *(best test for biliary blockage not caused by stones; defines anatomy, looks for mass)* - is less invasive than ERCP and can pick up a mass
- Invades contiguous structures early (only 15% resectable)
- Discovery of a **focal bile duct stenosis** in patients without a history of biliary surgery or pancreatitis is highly suggestive of CA
- Tx (consider surgery if no distant metastases and tumor is resectable):
  - **Staging laparoscopy** - resectability often determined at time of surgery
  - **Upper ⅓** (Klatskin tumors)
    - **MC type** (75%), worst prognosis, usually unresectable
    - Tx: can try hepatic <u>lobectomy</u> (often extended resection), removal of extrahepatic biliary tree, and hepatico-jejunostomy (right or left hepatic duct) if localized to either the right or left lobe
  - **Middle ⅓** - <u>hepatico-jejunostomy</u>
  - **Lower ⅓** - <u>Whipple</u>
- Palliative stenting for unresectable disease
- 5-YS (all patients) - **5%** (after resection for cure 25%)

OTHER CONDITIONS
- **Adenomyomatosis** - thickened nodules of <u>mucosa</u> associated with: 1) **Rokitansky-Aschoff sinuses** (invaginations or diverticula composed of <u>mucosa</u> going through the gallbladder muscle layer) <u>and</u>; 2) **chronic cholecystitis**
  - <u>Not</u> premalignant; does <u>not</u> cause stones

- Tx: **cholecystectomy** (these patients almost always have chronic cholecystitis)
- **Granular cell myoblastoma** - benign neuroectoderm tumor of gallbladder
  - Can present with Sx's of cholecystitis
  - Tx: cholecystectomy
- **Cholesterolosis** (strawberry gallbladder) - speckled cholesterol deposits on the gallbladder wall; benign *(no Tx necessary)*
- **Gallbladder polyps** (overall 5% are malignant)
  - *In general, cholecystectomy is indicated for polyps that are > **1 cm** and have any of the following: 1) **symptomatic** patient, 2) patients **aged > 50**, 3) associated with **gallstones**, or; 4) **< 3 polyps** (ie not likely to be cholesterol polyps which are multiple); all have increased **malignancy risk***
  - **Cholesterol** polyps (MC type [70%]; are benign) - generally < 10 mm, often *multiple*, pedunculated; usually seen in association with cholesterolosis
  - **Adenomyomatosis** (15%, see above)
  - **Inflammatory** polyps (10%) - generally < 10 mm, from chronic inflammation, benign
  - **Papillary adenoma** (5%) - risk of **malignancy**; Tx: **cholecystectomy**
- **Mirizzi syndrome** - jaundice or other Sx's caused by compression of the common hepatic duct by 1) a stone in the gallbladder infundibulum or; 2) inflammation arising from the gallbladder or cystic duct extending to the contiguous hepatic duct, causing common hepatic duct stricture; Tx: cholecystectomy; may need hepatico-jejunostomy for hepatic duct stricture
- **Indications for asymptomatic cholecystectomy** - patients undergoing liver transplant or gastric bypass procedure (if stones are present)

Pancreas

860. Which of the following pancreatic enzymes is secreted in active form?
   a. Amylase
   b. Trypsin
   c. Chymotrypsin
   d. Pepsin

   Answer a. Amylase is secreted in active form.

861. All of the following are true exocrine functions of the pancreas except:
   a. Secretin primarily causes HCO_3^- release
   b. CCK primarily causes enzyme release and is the most potent pancreatic acinar cell stimulant
   c. Acetylcholine (vagus) increases HCO_3^- and enzyme release
   d. Somatostatin increases pancreatic endocrine and exocrine function

   Answer d. Somatostatin decreases both pancreatic endocrine and exocrine function.

862. All of the following are true of the pancreas except:
   a. Annular pancreas is treated with pancreatic resection
   b. Pancreas divisum associated with pancreatitis is usually first treated with ERCP and sphincterotomy of the minor papilla
   c. The majority of pancreatic adenocarcinomas arise in the head of the pancreas and arise from the main pancreatic duct
   d. MRCP is the best test for CBD stricture complicating chronic pancreatitis (to assess for CA and define anatomy)
   e. ETOH causes acute pancreatitis by impairing enzyme extrusion and causing auto-inactivation

   Answer a. Annular pancreas is treated with duodeno-jejunostomy (MC) or duodeno-duodenostomy, not pancreatic resection.

863. All of the following are true of acute pancreatitis except:
   a. It occurs from impaired extrusion of zymogen granules and activation of degradation enzymes in the pancreas, leading to auto-digestion
   b. ARDS and pancreatic necrosis are from release of phospholipases
   c. MCC of death from pancreatitis is hemorrhage
   d. Coagulopathy and DIC are from release of proteases

   Answer c. The MCC of death in **acute pancreatitis** is **infection** and **sepsis** (MC GNRs).

864. A 55 yo woman presents to the ED with severe abdominal pain. She has no other PMHx. She occasionally drinks. You get routine labs which are significant for an amylase of 3000 and lipase of 3500. AXR is unremarkable. Her WBC count is 17. Her blood pressure is 80/40 and HR is 120. She is afebrile. On exam she is fairly tender in the epigastric area. The most appropriate next step is:
   a. Start IVF's and get an U/S
   b. Start IVF's and get a CT scan
   c. Start IVF's and go to OR
   d. Start IVF's and go to MRI

   Answer a. The initial steps for **acute pancreatitis** are to start giving **IV hydration** (can lose a lot of volume with pancreatitis), keep the patient NPO, and **rule-out gallstones** *(MCC of acute pancreatitis).*

   If there was an obvious CBD stone on U/S, you would go with ERCP, sphincterotomy, and stone extraction *after* resuscitation. **Prophylactic antibiotics** are indicated for severe pancreatitis or if worsening clinically.

865. The above patient worsens clinically so you start antibiotics. Abdominal CT scan shows that 80% of the pancreas does not light up with IV contrast. There is no abscess or air bubbles. The appropriate next step is:
   a. Whipple
   b. Necrotic debridement
   c. Percutaneous drain
   d. Continue current management

   Answer d. Sterile pancreatic necrosis is left alone. Removing sterile necrotic material does not improve outcomes and may worsen prognosis (80% mortality with debridement of sterile necrosis).

866. All of the following have prognostic value for mortality in the above patient except:
   a. Lipase
   b. Age
   c. Glucose
   d. LDH
   e. AST

   Answer a. Lipase is <u>not</u> part of **Ranson's Criteria**, which predicts mortality for acute pancreatitis.

867. A 40 yo man presents 1 week after a MVA with dyspnea. CXR shows a large pleural effusion. Thoracentesis comes back with an amylase of level of 7000. You completely drain the effusion. The most appropriate next step in treatment is:
   a. Pleurodesis
   b. Resection of the fistula
   c. NPO, TPN, and octreotide
   d. Heparin
   e. tPA

   Answer c. Pancreatic pleural effusion (or **pancreatic ascites**) can occur after pancreatitis, trauma, or pancreatic surgery. It is caused by a damaged pancreatic duct or a pancreatic pseudocyst that leaks through the retroperitoneal space resulting in ascites and/or effusion. Initial Tx is the same as a pancreatic fistula (**complete drainage, NPO, TPN, and octreotide**). The majority resolve spontaneously. ERCP with stent is indicated if medical Tx fails.

868. A 50 yo man presents with chronic epigastric pain. CT shows a fibrotic pancreas with areas of edema. EUS-FNA shows a lymphocytic infiltrate. Serum IgG levels are high. The most appropriate next step is:
   a. Chemo
   b. Chemo-XRT
   c. Distal pancreatectomy
   d. Steroids
   e. Whipple

   Answer d. The above is consistent with **autoimmune pancreatitis**; Tx-**steroids**

869. A 50 yo man presents with chronic pain and narcotic use related to chronic pancreatitis. CT scan shows a main pancreatic duct of 9 mm, multiple calcifications, and multiple fibrotic areas. The most appropriate next step is:
   a. ERCP with stent placement
   b. Whipple
   c. Lateral pancreaticojejunostomy
   d. Percutaneous drain

   Answer c. Lateral pancreaticojejunostomy (Puestow procedure). Patients with significantly symptomatic chronic pancreatitis and a dilated main pancreatic duct (> 8 mm) should undergo lateral pancreaticojejunostomy (loop of jejunum is sewn to the main pancreatic duct). ERCP with stent placement is <u>not</u> as effective as an open drainage procedure.

870. A 55 yo man with significant ETOH abuse has an acute episode of pancreatitis. Four weeks later he presents with persistent, refractory emesis and fullness after eating. CT scan shows a <u>new</u> 6 cm simple cystic lesion posterior to his stomach. The next appropriate step for this patient is:
   a. Percutaneous drainage
   b. Pancreatic resection
   c. Conservative treatment including TPN or feeding tube past the ligament of Treitz
   d. Percutaneous cysto-gastrostomy
   e. Open cysto-gastrostomy

   Answer c. Conservative Tx (NPO, TPN) is indicated for patients with a new onset symptomatic **pancreatic pseudocyst**. **Spontaneous resolution** occurs in the majority. You should not operate on pancreatic pseudocysts unless they are mature (> 3 months) <u>*and*</u> are either 1) persistently symptomatic or 2) are growing.

   The 3 month waiting period is required to allow the cyst wall to mature so you can sew to it (**open or laparoscopic cysto-gastrostomy**). The 3 months also allows the cyst to attach to the stomach posterior wall for **endoscopic cysto-gastrostomy.**

   Pseudocysts are <u>*non-epithelialized*</u> sacs and are high in **amylase**.

871. The above patient returns to clinic in 8 weeks. CT scan shows the cyst is the same size. He is tolerating a regular diet and does not have any Sx's. The next appropriate action is:
   a. Percutaneous drainage
   b. Resection
   c. Follow conservatively
   d. Cysto-gastrostomy

   Answer c. Because the cyst is not causing any Sx's and is not growing, the Tx of choice is to follow the lesion. You should not operate on stable (ie no change in size) asymptomatic pseudocysts.

872. Instead of the above, the patient returns to clinic in 8 weeks with continued pain and inability to tolerate a regular diet. Which of the following would <u>not</u> be indicated:
   a. Laparoscopic cystogastrostomy
   b. Endoscopic cystogastrostomy
   c. U/S guided percutaneous drainage catheter
   d. Open cystogastrostomy
   e. Endoscopic transpapillary pseudocyst drainage

   Answer c. Pseudocysts are generally <u>not</u> drained percutaneously due to high **recurrence** (90%) and the potential for seeding an **infection**. *You certainly would <u>not</u> want to leave an indwelling drain in a pseudocyst.*

873. A 50 yo otherwise healthy man presents with epigastric pain. CT scan shows a multi-septated 6 cm cystic lesion in the distal pancreas. The CT scan is otherwise normal. He has no history of pancreatitis, trauma, or pancreatic surgery. The next appropriate step is:
   a. Observation
   b. EUS and FNA
   c. Resection
   d. Chemo-XRT
   e. ERCP

Answer c. Because the cyst is **suspicious for CA** (ie large, multi-septated, not associated with pancreatitis, trauma, or surgery) and because the patient is a **good operative risk**, resection is indicated (there was no indication on CT scan that the mass was unresectable). Based on the mass location, **distal pancreatectomy** +/- splenectomy would be indicated.

874. You are performing a Whipple for a pancreatic head mass. You attempt to pass your finger behind the pancreas from below and get a large amount of blood return when you remove it. You place pressure on the neck of the pancreas and tamponade the bleeding. You have most likely injured the:
   a. Aorta
   b. Inferior vena cava
   c. Celiac artery
   d. Superior mesenteric vein

   Answer d. The **superior mesenteric vein** (SMV) lies directly behind the neck of the pancreas and is the structure MC injured when trying to free this area. Divide the pancreas neck to get to the bleeding.

875. Most significant risk factor for pancreatic adenocarcinoma is:
   a. Tobacco
   b. Alcohol
   c. High fat diet
   d. Nitrosamines

   Answer a. The most significant risk factor for the development of pancreatic cancer is tobacco use.

876. All of the following are risk factors for pancreatic adenocarcinoma except:
   a. BRCA2
   b. Obesity
   c. Caffeine
   d. Hyperglycemia

   Answer c. Caffeine is <u>not</u> a RF (previously thought to be a RF)

877. A 55 yo man in otherwise good health presents with obstructive jaundice. RUQ U/S shows a dilated CBD and no stones. MRCP shows a mass in the head of the pancreas with no adenopathy, vascular invasion, or retroperitoneal extension. PET scan is negative except for the pancreatic mass. The most appropriate next step is:
   a. EUS biopsy
   b. CT guided biopsy
   c. U/S guided biopsy
   d. Surgery

   Answer d. Biopsy is unnecessary in this patient as the tumor appears resectable and the patient would get surgery regardless of the result (a negative biopsy will still result in surgery, a positive biopsy will still result in surgery).

878. Pre-operative biliary stents for pancreatic CA prior to Whipple are associated with:
   a. Decreased peri-op mortality
   b. Decreased peri-op morbidity
   c. Decreased fistula formation
   d. Increased risk of peri-op infections
   e. Shortened hospital stay

   Answer d. Pre-op biliary stents for pancreatic CA prior to Whipple are associated with an increased risk of **peri-op infections** (eg wound infection), increased **pancreatic fistula** formation, and **prolonged hospital stay**. Pre-op biliary stents should be used selectively (eg for severe pain, severe pruritus)

879. A 55 yo woman undergoes Whipple for pancreatic CA. Post-op day 7 she complains of N/V. U/S shows a large fluid collection anterior to the pancreas (9 x 9 cm). The most appropriate next step in management is:
   a. Reglan
   b. Octreotide
   c. Re-operation
   d. Percutaneous drain placement and send the fluid for amylase, lipase, bilirubin, and cytology

   Answer d. The 1st test in a patient with post-op N/V after pancreas surgery is an **U/S**. You should place a percutaneous drain if a fluid collection is present and send the fluid off. This is suspicious for **duct leak**.

880. The fluid above has an amylase of 10,000. The most appropriate next step is::
   a. NPO, octreotide, and follow drainage output
   b. Re-operation with revision of the pancreatic anastomosis
   c. Triple antibiotics
   d. Nothing

   Answer a. Now with a percutaneous drain, you have a controlled **pancreatic fistula**. The vast majority will resolve with conservative Tx.

881. All of the following are true for palliation of metastatic pancreatic adenocarcinoma except:
   a. Biliary stent is the first line Tx for symptomatic obstructive jaundice
   b. Celiac axis block can provide effective pain relief
   c. Whipple is the best option for obstruction
   d. Gastro-jejunostomy is the best option for duodenal obstruction

   Answer c. Whipple should _rarely_ be used as a palliative maneuver. **Biliary stents** are the first line Tx for _palliation_ of symptomatic obstructive jaundice.

882. All of the following are true except:
   a. The MC site of metastases for pancreatic endocrine tumors is the liver
   b. Octreotide scan is effective for locating insulinomas
   c. Functional endocrine tumors generally respond to debulking
   d. Pancreatic endocrine tumors that are most commonly located in the pancreatic head are gastrinoma and somatostatinoma
   e. Octreotide provides effective palliative Tx of all functional pancreatic endocrine tumors except somatostatinoma

   Answer b. Unlike other pancreatic endocrine tumors, octreotide is not effective for locating insulinoma. **Selective arterial calcium stimulation** with **hepatic venous insulin sampling** is the best localizing study for insulinomas not on CT scan (Ca stimulates insulin release from tumor).

883. All of the following are true of insulinomas except:
   a. C peptide should be elevated, otherwise Munchausen Syndrome (self-injection of insulin) should be suspected
   b. Diazoxide can be used for metastatic disease
   c. Blind Whipple may be necessary for a tumor that is not localized
   d. These tumors are evenly distributed throughout the pancreas
   e. This is the MC functional pancreatic endocrine tumor

   Answer c. Blind pancreatic resections should be _avoided_.

884. All of the following are true of gastrinoma except:
   a. Gastrin > 200 pg/ml _and_ BAO > 15 mEq/hr are diagnostic of gastrinoma
   b. Octreotide scan is the best test for localizing the tumor
   c. Vagotomy and antrectomy is indicated for severe symptoms with metastatic disease that has failed maximal medical therapy

d. Approximately 50% have multiple tumors
e. Secretin stimulation results in increased gastrin levels in these patients

Answer c. If medical therapy has failed, **total gastrectomy** is usually the best therapy for severe symptoms *(vagotomy and antrectomy won't work - HCl secreting cells are in the body of stomach, not antrum)*

885. You in the OR for a patient with Zollinger-Ellison syndrome but cannot find a tumor despite Kocher maneuver and opening the lesser sac. The next step is:
   a. Whipple
   b. Distal pancreatectomy
   c. Closure and post-op studies
   d. Proximal duodenotomy

Answer d. 15% of micro-gastrinomas are located in the proximal duodenum

886. A 50 yo woman with a pancreatic mass in the tail of the pancreas develops watery diarrhea and hypokalemia. The most likely diagnosis is:
   a. Glucagonoma
   b. Gastrinoma
   c. Somatostatinoma
   d. VIPoma (VIP – vasoactive intestinal peptide)

Answer d. Watery diarrhea and hypokalemia (without concomitant gastric ulcer disease) is most consistent with **VIPoma**. The diarrhea associated with VIPoma *will not get better* with PPIs whereas the diarrhea found with gastrinoma will get better with PPIs.

The combination of **5-FU** and **alpha interferon** is very effective for metastatic VIPoma.

887. A 50 yo woman with a pancreatic mass develops hyperglycemia, RUQ pain with U/S positive for cholelithiasis, and passage of bulky, oily, foul-smelling stools that seem to float in the toilet.. The most likely diagnosis is:
   a. Glucagonoma
   b. Gastrinoma
   c. Somatostatinoma
   d. VIPoma

Answer c. The above is consistent with **somatostatinoma** (diabetes, gallstones, and steatorrhea).

888. A 50 yo woman with a pancreatic mass develops hyperglycemia and skin lesions. The most likely diagnosis is:
   a. Glucagonoma
   b. Gastrinoma
   c. Somatostatinoma
   d. VIPoma (VIP – vasoactive intestinal peptide)

Answer a. The above is consistent with **glucagonoma** (diabetes and necrolytic migratory erythema).

889. The previous patient is noted to have a 5 cm liver metastasis on pre-op CT scan (confirmed with Bx) that looks resectable and a 1 cm deep liver metastasi that is not resectable. The pancreatic mass in the head of the pancreas looks resectable. The most appropriate Tx is:
   a. Nothing
   b. 5-fluorouracil and XRT
   c. Morphine drip
   d. Resection of the pancreatic mass and the large liver met

Answer d. Debulking surgery is effective palliative treatment for functional endocrine tumors so resecting the large liver mass is indicated if the primary could also be resected.

Non-endocrine tumors (ie adenocarcinoma) of the pancreas with a liver metastasis would be considered *unresectable* and you would <u>not</u> perform a resection.

If the liver mass cannot be resected safely, **radiofrequency** ablation *(coagulation necrosis)* and **cryoablation** (protein / cell membrane *denaturation*) are options.

ANATOMY AND PHYSIOLOGY
- **Head** (including uncinate and neck), **body**, and **tail**
- **Uncinate process** - rests on aorta; is behind SMV and SMA
- **Blood supply**
    - **Head** - <u>superior</u> (off <u>GDA</u>) and <u>inferior</u> (off <u>SMA</u>) **pancreaticoduodenal arteries**; each has <u>anterior</u> and <u>posterior</u> branches
    - **Inferior pancreaticoduodenal artery** is the *1st branch* off the **SMA**
      Middle colic artery is 1st branch going only to bowel
    - **Body** - great, inferior and caudal pancreatic arteries (all splenic artery branches)
    - **Tail** - splenic and dorsal pancreatic arteries
      Venous drainage into the **portal system**
    - **SMA** and **SMV** - **behind** neck of pancreas (*SMV is to right of SMA*)
    - **SMA** and **SMV** - lie **anterior** to the 3rd and 4th portions of duodenum
    - **Portal vein** - forms behind neck of pancreas (SMV and splenic vein)
- **Lymphatics** - celiac and SMA nodes
- **Exocrine** function of pancreas:
    - **Ductal cells** - secrete HCO_3^- (have **carbonic anhydrase**)
      ↑ed flow leads to ↑HCO_3^- and ↓ Cl^-
    - **Acinar cells** - secrete pancreatic **digestive enzymes** and Cl^-
        Enzymes - amylase, lipase, trypsinogen, chymotrypsinogen, carboxypeptidase
        Amylase - only pancreatic enzymes secreted in **active form**
          Hydrolyzes alpha 1-4 linkages of glucose (carbohydrate) chains
        Lipase - converts TAGs to FFAs and mono-acylglycerides
        Enterokinase - *released by duodenum*, converts trypsinogen to trypsin; **trypsin** then activates other pancreatic enzymes including trypsinogen
        Trypsinogen can <u>auto-activate</u> in **acidic environment** (pH < 6)
- **Endocrine** function of pancreas (**islet cells**)
    - **Alpha** cells - **glucagon**
    - **Beta** cells (center of islets) - **insulin**
    - **Delta** cells - **somatostatin**
    - **PP** cells - **pancreatic polypeptide**
    - **Islet cells** with VIP, serotonin, neuropeptide Y, and bombesin also exist
    - Islet cells receive **majority of blood supply** compared to size
    - Blood travels to **islet cells *first***, then travels to acinar cells
    - *Type I Diabetes - failure of the body to produce insulin*
    - *Type II Diabetes - peripheral insulin resistance*
- **Hormonal control** of pancreatic **exocrine function**
    - **Secretin** - ↑s HCO_3^- **release** mostly (**ductal** cells)
    - **CCK** - ↑s **enzyme release** mostly *(most potent **acinar** cell stimulant)*
    - **Acetylcholine** (vagus) - ↑s HCO_3^- and enzyme release
    - **Somatostatin** - ↓s exocrine and endocrine function
    - **CCK** and **secretin** released mostly by cells in **duodenum**
- **Development**
    - **Ventral pancreatic bud** - forms uncinate and inferior portion of pancreas head; contains **duct of Wirsung** (major duct)
    - **Dorsal pancreatic bud** - forms tail, body, and superior aspect of pancreatic head; contains **duct of Santorini** (minor duct)

- **Duct of Wirsung** - major pancreatic duct, merges with CBD before entering duodenum
- **Duct of Santorini** - small accessory pancreatic duct that drains directly into duodenum
- **Ampulla of Vater** - fusion of pancreatic duct and CBD in pancreas, opens into duodenum
- **Sphincter of Oddi** - muscle band at Ampulla entrance to duodenum
    - Controls flow of bile and pancreatic secretions into duodenum
    - Marks transition from **foregut** to **midgut** (where celiac stops supplying gut and SMA takes over, although there are many collaterals here)
    - ERCP with sphincterotomy opens this
    - **CCK** and **IV glucagon** _relax_ the sphincter of Oddi
    - **Morphine** _contracts_ the sphincter of Oddi

ANNULAR PANCREAS
- From **failure of clockwise rotation** of the **ventral pancreatic bud**
- 2nd portion of duodenum is trapped in the pancreas - get **duodenal obstruction**
- Sx's: **feeding intolerance** in infants (N/V; duodenal obstruction)
    - Pancreatitis in adults
- RFs: Down's syndrome
- Dx: **CT scan** - double bubble sign (duodenum and stomach distension)
    - UGI - will show stenosis
- Tx: **duodeno-jejunostomy** (MC; or duodeno-duodenostomy)
    - **Pancreas is _not_ resected**
    - If **pancreatitis** is the problem → ERCP with sphincteroplasty

PANCREAS DIVISUM
- Failed fusion of pancreatic ducts (Wirsung and Santorini)
- Most are **asymptomatic**; some get **pancreatitis** from Duct of Santorini (Accessory Duct) stenosis
- Dx: **ERCP**
    - **Minor papilla** will show long and large duct of **Santorini** (**majority** of the pancreas drains through this duct)
    - **Major papilla** will show short duct of **Wirsung** (inferior portion of the pancreas head drains though this duct)
- Tx: If symptomatic - **ERCP with sphincterotomy** of **minor papilla** (Santorini duct opening), open sphincteroplasty if that fails

HETEROTOPIC PANCREAS
- MC location - **duodenum**
- Usually asymptomatic; surgical resection if symptomatic

ACUTE PANCREATITIS
- MCC - **gallstones** (35%) and **ETOH** (30%)
    - Other etiologies - ERCP, trauma, hyperlipidemia, hypercalcemia, viral infection, medications (eg azathioprine [Imuran], furosemide [Lasix], steroids, cimetidine)
    - **Gallstones** - can obstruct the Ampulla of Vater causing impaired extrusion of zymogen granules and activation of degradation enzymes; leads to pancreatic auto-digestion
    - **ETOH** - causes **impaired pancreatic enzyme extrusion** and **auto-activation** of pancreatic enzymes while still in the pancreas
- Sx's: **abdominal pain** radiating to the back, N/V, and anorexia
    - Can also get **jaundice**, left **pleural effusion**, **ascites**, or **sentinel loop** (dilated small bowel near pancreas as a result of inflammation)
    - **ARDS** - from release of phospholipases
    - **Coagulopathy** and **DIC** - from release of proteases
    - **Pancreatic fat necrosis** - from release of phospholipases
    - **Pseudo-hyponatremia** - can occur with **hyperlipidemia** (hyper-triglyceridemia) from acute pancreatitis (Tx: _nothing_; need to Tx underlying illness)
    - Other Cx's - shock, renal failure
- Mortality rate - **10%**; (hemorrhagic pancreatitis mortality - **40%**)

- MCC death - **sepsis** (MC organism - **E. coli**; MC class - **GNRs**)
- Pancreatitis without obvious cause → need to worry about CA
- **Ranson's** criteria
  - On <u>admission</u>: age > 55, WBC > 16, glucose > 200, AST > 250, LDH > 350
  - After <u>48 hours</u>: Hct *decrease* of 10%, BUN *increase* of 5, Ca < 8, PaO_2 < 60, base deficit - 4 or lower (metabolic acidosis), fluid sequestration > 6 L
  - 8 Ranson criteria met → mortality rate near 100%
- Dx:
  - **Labs** - *elevated* **lipase** *(best lab test),* **amylase**, and **WBCs** (although amylase and lipase are <u>not</u> correlated with severity and are <u>not</u> used in Ranson's)
  - **U/S** - needed to check for gallstones and possible CBD dilatation
  - **CT scan** - use to check for abscess and other Cx's (**necrotic pancreas** will <u>not</u> take up contrast)
  - Mildly increased amylase can be found with sialadenitis (inflammation of salivary gland), cholecystitis, perforated ulcer, bowel obstruction, and intestinal infarction
- Tx: **NPO** and aggressive **fluid resuscitation** (up to 10 L)
  - **ERCP** is needed for **gallstone pancreatitis** with **retained CBD stones** causing duct obstruction → perform sphincterotomy and stone extraction *after* fluid resuscitation
  - Antibiotics for stones, severe pancreatitis, failure to improve, or suspected infection
  - Early **enteral feeding** (< 24-48 hours; naso-jejunal if possible) *reduces* MSOF, infection, need for operative interventions, and mortality compared to TPN
  - Patients with gallstone pancreatitis should undergo **cholecystectomy** when recovered from pancreatitis (on **same hospital admission**)
  - Morphine should be avoided as it can contract the sphincter of Oddi and worsen attack
  - **Surgery** (open debridement) is only indicated for **infected necrosis** or **abscess**; *leave sterile necrosis <u>alone</u>*
  - **Abscess** - Tx: need **open debridement**; percutaneous drainage is not effective for pancreatic abscess *(classic teaching)*
- **Bleeding** - hemorrhagic pancreatitis can track blood through the retroperitoneum (manifests on skin)
  - **Grey Turner sign** - flank ecchymosis
  - **Cullen's sign** - periumbilical ecchymosis
  - **Fox's sign** - inguinal ecchymosis
- **Necrosis** occurs in 15% - *leave sterile necrosis <u>alone</u> (80% mortality with debridement of sterile necrosis)*
  - RF for necrotizing pancreatitis: **obesity**
  - **Infected necrosis** (fever, sepsis, positive blood cultures; may need to sample necrotic pancreatic fluid with CT-guided aspiration to get Dx) → Tx: **surgical debridement**
  - **Gas** in necrotic pancreas = infected necrosis or abscess (need **open debridement**)

PANCREATIC PSEUDOCYSTS
- MCC - **pancreatitis** (both acute and chronic)
  - If <u>not</u> associated with pancreatitis or trauma → need to rule-out CA (eg mucinous cystadenocarcinoma)
- Sx's: **pain** (MC), weight loss, bowel obstruction (compression); can be asymptomatic
- Dx: CT scan *(best test)* - MC occurs in the **head** of the pancreas
  - Appears as a pancreatic fluid collection behind the stomach
  - If thought to be pancreatitis associated, should see signs of acute (edema, fluid) or chronic pancreatitis (shrunken pancreas, calcification, dilated ducts)
- Is a non-epithelialized sac; fluid is high in **amylase**
- Most **resolve spontaneously** (especially if < 5 cm)

- **Pseudocyst criteria** (need all 3):
  - 1) Need history of **pancreatitis, pancreatic surgery,** or **trauma**
  - 2) <u>Not</u> **a complex cyst** (<u>no</u> fronds, papillary projections, or septae; <u>no</u> mass)
  - 3) <u>Not</u> **growing** on serial CT scans

- If above not met, worry about **CA** (eg pancreatic cyst -adenoma or -adenocarcinoma) → Dx: consider **EUS aspiration** of fluid and cytology
- **Serous** fluid - likely serous cystadenoma (benign, can follow)
- **Mucin** in fluid - possible mucinous cyst-adenocarcinoma (need resection)
- **Amylase** in fluid - likely pseudocyst

  ■ Tx:
  - **Asymptomatic** stable pseudocysts - *leave alone*
  - Only need to Tx pseudocysts that are either:
    1) continually **symptomatic after 3 months** *or;*
    2) are **growing** on serial CT scans (worry about CA - need to resect)
  - **Continued Sx's** - *expectant management for 3 months*
    - NPO, TPN or feeding tube past ligament of Treitz, octreotide; some may be able to eat; serial CT scans
    - *Majority resolve on their own*
    - 3 month waiting period also allows the pseudocyst wall to mature and thicken if <u>open</u> cysto-gastrostomy is required (also allows time for the pseudocyst to attach with scar tissue to the posterior wall of stomach which allows <u>endoscopic</u> cysto-gastrostomy)
  - **Interventions** (send fluid, part of cyst wall to rule-out CA)
    - **Open / laparoscopic cysto-gastrostomy** - posterior stomach sewn to cyst wall
    - **Endoscopic cystogastrostomy** - stent placed between stomach and pseudocyst
    - **Endoscopic transpapillary drainage** - stent placed between pseudocyst and main pancreatic duct; generally used if above methods fail (has a higher infection rate)
    - Pseudocysts are generally <u>not</u> drained percutaneously due to high **recurrence** (90%), the potential for seeding an **infection**, and the risk of **fistula**. *You certainly would <u>not</u> want to leave an indwelling percutaneous drain in a pseudocyst.*
- **Cx's of pancreatic pseudocyst** - infection of cyst, portal or splenic vein thrombosis, bowel obstruction
- **Incidental cysts** <u>not</u> associated with pancreatitis, trauma, or surgery should be *resected* (eg worry about **mucinous cystadenocarcinoma**) <u>unless</u> the cyst is purely serous and non-complex (or very small, peripheral, simple cysts)
- **Non-complex, purely serous cystadenomas** have an extremely low malignancy risk (< 1%) and can be <u>followed</u>; are very slow growing
- **Mucinous cysts** have definite malignant potential (ie cystadenocarcinoma) and should be resected
- **Complex cysts** (eg multi-septated, multi-loculated, associated mass / solid components, or frond-like / papillary projections) have definite malignant potential and should be resected
- **IPMNs** (intraductal papillary mucinous neoplasms) - can also present as cystic lesions and may have malignant potential (see pancreatic adenocarcinoma below)
- **Non-pseudocyst cystic lesion management**:
  - **Benign** appearance (eg very small, peripheral, simple cysts) - **surveillance**
  - **Unsure** of findings - **EUS aspiration** (FNA) of fluid and cytology, consider ERCP
  - **Suspicious** findings (eg a mid-duct IPMN, a multi-loculated cyst) - **resection** if good operative risk and lesion is resectable (consider EUS aspiration if poor operative risk to get definitive Dx and guide therapy)

PANCREATIC FISTULAS
- Usually associated with **pancreatic surgery**; can be from **trauma**
- Sx's:
  1) Leakage of fluid from wound after pancreatic surgery (→ place stoma appliance to control drainage; percutaneous drain if fluid collection)
  2) Pancreatic drain with increased drainage after pancreatic surgery
  3) Fluid collection around pancreas from **injured pancreatic duct** (due to surgery, trauma, or pancreatitis → Tx: place percutaneous drain)
- Majority are **asymptomatic**
- Majority **close spontaneously** (especially if low output, ie < 200 cc/d)

- Try to wait these out with **conservative Tx**
- Dx: CT scan; send fluid → can be clear or murky; has high **amylase** (1000s)
- Tx:
    1) **Control drainage** (ostomy or percutaneous drain)
    2) **Antibiotics** for the 1st week
    3) If **high output** (> 400 cc/day) → **NPO + TPN** (distal feedings if J tube)
    4) If **low output** (< 200 cc/day) → let patient eat and avoid Cx's of TPN
    5) **Octreotide** (lowers pancreatic output)
    - If failure to resolve with medical Tx after 6-8 weeks → **ERCP, sphincterotomy,** and **stent** (try to get stent across duct leak if possible)
    - Usually do <u>not</u> have to operate (or re-operate) for pancreatic fistula → *do <u>not</u> rush to re-operate (wait 2-3 months to see if it resolves)*

PANCREATIC ASCITES (also pancreatic pleural effusion)
- Caused by **retroperitoneal leakage** of pancreatic fluid from a pancreatic duct or a pancreatic pseudocyst *(is <u>not</u> a pancreatic-pleural fistula if pleural effusion is present)*
- RFs: **pancreatitis, trauma, pancreatic surgery**
- Can get respiratory issues from pancreatic pleural effusion
- Ascites (or pleural effusion) fluid is high in **amylase** (> 1000)
- *Majority **resolve spontaneously** with conservative Tx*
- Tx: **paracentesis** (or thoracentesis) to drain the fluid followed by conservative Tx (**NPO, TPN,** and **octreotide**)
    - ERCP with stent if above fails

CHRONIC PANCREATITIS
- Corresponds to irreversible **parenchymal fibrosis**
- Exocrine function *decreased*; **endocrine** function (islet cells) usually <u>*preserved*</u>
- MCC - ETOH (80%); 2nd - **autoimmune** disease (Tx: <u>steroids</u>, very effective)
- Sx's: **pain** (MC), **weight loss**, and **steatorrhea** (fat malabsorption)
- Can cause malabsorption of **fat-soluble vitamins**
- Dx: **CT scan** - shrunken pancreas with **calcifications**
    - U/S - pancreatic ducts > 4 mm, cysts, and atrophy
    - ERCP - *most sensitive test* for diagnosing chronic pancreatitis
    - Advanced disease - **chain of lakes** (alternating segments of dilation and stenosis in pancreatic duct)
- Tx: supportive - **pain control** and **nutrition** (low fat diet, **pancrealipase**)
    - TPN for acute episodes
- **Surgical indications** - pain that interferes with quality of life, nutrition abnormalities, addiction to narcotics, failure to rule-out CA, biliary obstruction
- **Surgical options**:
    - **Lateral pancreaticojejunostomy** (Puestow or Frey), for enlarged pancreatic duct > **8 mm** → open along main pancreatic duct and drain into jejunum (dilated duct indicates obstruction within pancreas; most patients improve); more effective then ERCP with balloon / stent
    - **Distal pancreatic resection** - for normal or small ducts and only the distal portion of the gland is affected
    - **Whipple** - for normal or small ducts with isolated pancreatic head disease
    - **Beger-Frey** (duodenal preserving head "core-out") - for normal or small ducts with isolated pancreatic head disease
    - 80% get pain relief with surgery
    - **Diabetes** often a long-term Cx after surgery
    - Bilateral thoracoscopic **splanchnicectomy** or celiac **ganglionectomy** (ETOH ablation) are effective for **pain control** in 80%
- CBD **stricture** found on U/S - causes CBD **dilation**
    - Sx's: **pain** and **jaundice**; can lead to **cirrhosis**
    - Dx: **MRCP** *(best test - finds any masses and delineates anatomy)* and ERCP with brush Bx's (need to rule-out CA if not found on MRCP)
        Make sure the stricture is <u>not</u> pancreatic or biliary system CA
    - Tx: **choledocho-jejunostomy** *(best long-term option; <u>not</u> ERCP with stents)*

- ■ **Splenic vein thrombosis**
  - ● MCC - **chronic pancreatitis**
  - ● Sx's: can get **bleeding** from _isolated_ **gastric varices** that form as collaterals
  - ● Tx: **splenectomy** for _bleeding_ gastric varices; _if asymptomatic_ - **leave alone**
- ■ **Autoimmune pancreatitis**
  - ● Sx's: **pain; obstructive jaundice** due to compression of the intra-pancreatic portion of the CBD is common
  - ● Dx: mononuclear infiltrate (**lymphocytes**); elevated **beta-globulin** and **IgG-4**
  - ● Tx: **steroids** _(very effective)_

PANCREATIC INSUFFICIENCY
- ■ Usually the result of long-standing pancreatitis or occurs after total pancreatectomy (over 90% of the function must be lost)
- ■ Generally refers to exocrine function
- ■ Sx's: **malabsorption** and **steatorrhea**
- ■ Dx: **fecal fat testing**
- ■ Tx: **low-fat diet** and **pancreatic enzymes** (pancrease)

JAUNDICE WORKUP
- ■ **Ultrasound (U/S) 1st**
  - ● **Positive CBD stones, no mass** → ERCP (extraction of stones)
  - ● **No CBD stones, no mass** → MRCP
  - ● **Positive mass** → MRCP

PANCREATIC ADENOCARCINOMA
- ■ Male predominance; usually 6-7th decades of life
- ■ Sx's: **painless jaundice** (tumor in head), then **weight loss** (MC Sx), then **pain**
  - ● Pain as a Sx → still potentially resectable
- ■ RFs: **tobacco #1**, obesity, chronic pancreatitis, diabetes, BRCA2, Peutz-Jegher, Lynch
- ■ _Not_ RFs - ETOH, caffeine
- ■ **CA 19-9** - serum marker for pancreatic CA
- ■ Path
  - ● **Lymphatic spread 1st**
  - ● 70% are in pancreatic **head**; majority arise from **main pancreatic duct**
  - ● 90% are **ductal adenocarcinoma** (_exocrine_ pancreas)
  - ● Others (more favorable prognosis) - **papillary** or **mucinous** cyst-adenocarcinoma
  - ● Most cures with pancreatic head disease
  - ● MC metastatic site - **liver**
- ■ **Unresectable disease** (only 15% resectable):
  - ● Gross invasion or loss of patency of portal vein, SMV, or IVC
  - ● Encasement of the SMA
  - ● Invasion of the retroperitoneum
  - ● Metastases to the peritoneum, omentum, or liver
  - ● Metastases to celiac, SMA, or portal triad nodal system (nodal systems outside area of resection)
- ■ Positive distal peri-pancreatic and peri-duodenal nodes → _still potentially resectable_
- ■ Dx: U/S is the first test if jaundice is the Sx (DDx stones vs other causes)
  - ● Labs: _elevated_ **conjugated bilirubin** and **alkaline phosphatase** _(most sensitive lab test for obstructive jaundice)_
  - ● **MRCP** _(best test for jaundice not caused by stones)_ - good at differentiating dilated ducts secondary to chronic pancreatitis vs. CA
  - ● **Signs of CA** on MRCP - duct with irregular narrowing, displacement, or destruction; double-duct sign for pancreatic head tumors (dilation of both pancreatic duct and CBD); can also detect vessel involvement
  - ● Patients with a **resectable mass** (and no signs of metastatic disease) in the pancreas do **not** need a biopsy because you are taking it out regardless. If the patient appears to have metastatic disease, a Bx is warranted to direct therapy
- ■ **Pre-op biliary stents** - use _only_ if patient is symptomatic (eg severe pain, severe pruritus); pre-op stents are associated with increased **peri-op infections** (eg wound infection), increased **fistula** formation, and prolonged **length of stay**

- Tx:
  - **Resection** if resectable (see above criteria)
  - **Diagnostic laparoscopy** before Whipple - if metastases to peritoneum, omentum, or liver → close and palliate
  - **Whipple** (pancreatico-duodenectomy) removes pancreatic head, duodenum, CBD, and gallbladder, ± antrectomy; then Roux limb of jejunum brought up for →
    - 1) pancreatico-jejunostomy (proximal)
    - 2) choledocho-jejunostomy
    - 3) gastro-jejunostomy (distal)
  - **Distal pancreatectomy** - does _not_ require roux limb (just over-sew pancreas)
    - Often requires concomitant **splenectomy** for en bloc resection
  - **Prognosis** based on vascular and nodal invasion _(ability to get clear margin)_
- 5-YS with resection - **25%**
- Chemo-XRT usual post-op (**gemcitabine** and **5-FU**)
- **High volume centers** (> 12/year) have decreased peri-op mortality
- **Unresectable disease palliation**
  - **Biliary obstruction** - SEMS (self-expanding metal stent) biliary stent
  - **Duodenal obstruction** - SEMS (WallFlex) duodenal stent; if distal duodenum, may need gastro-jejunostomy as it may be hard to reach this area
  - **Pain** - EUS or CT guided **celiac plexus** chemical ablation or bilateral **thoracoscopic splanchnicectomy** (80% get relief); XRT also an option
  - **Steatorrhea** - Tx: pancrealipase
  - _Whipple should rarely be used as a palliative maneuver_
- **Intraductal papillary mucinous neoplasms** (IPMNs)
  - **Main duct type** – majority **malignant**; Tx: formal **resection** (eg distal pancreatectomy or Whipple); 70% harbor CA or high grade dysplasia
  - **Branch duct type** - majority **benign**
    - Indications for **resection** - if symptomatic, > 3 cm, associated with a mass, or has dilatation of the main pancreatic duct
  - Both of the above can present as **cystic lesions**

WHIPPLE COMPLICATIONS
- **Bleeding intra-op behind neck of pancreas** after blunt dissection (most likely injured the SMV) → divide the pancreas to control bleeding
- **Bleeding post-op** after Whipple or other pancreatic surgery - _go to **angio for embolization** (not re-operation)_
  - _**Avoid surgery**_ as the tissue planes are very friable early and pancreatic bleeding is extremely hard to control operatively
- **Delayed gastric emptying** _(MC Cx after Whipple)_ - Tx: metoclopramide (Reglan)
- **Nausea and vomiting** after Whipple - Dx: get **U/S** _(best test)_
  - May represent delayed gastric emptying or anastomotic leak
  - If **fluid collection** is found, place **percutaneous drain** and send off fluid; high amylase (1000s) indicates duct leak - Tx: same as pancreatic fistula (majority resolve conservatively)
- **Pancreatic or bile duct leak** (treated as a pancreatic or bile duct _fistula_ - see pancreatic fistula section)
  - Usually presents as increased drainage from drains placed intra-op (fluid high in amylase or bilirubin) or drainage from wound
  - Tx: **conservative** (NPO, TPN, octreotide, place drains if needed [ensure drainage of fluid collections], stoma appliance if needed)
  - _Do **not** re-operate early on these patients_ - tissue is very friable and will do more harm than good
  - Majority of pancreatic fistulas resolve with conservative Tx
- **Marginal ulceration** (from gastro-jejunostomy; _occurs on **jejunal** side_) - Tx: **PPI**

NON-FUNCTIONAL ENDOCRINE TUMORS
- Represent 30% of pancreatic endocrine neoplasms
- 90% of the nonfunctional tumors are **malignant;** MC metastatic site - **liver**
- More **indolent** and **protracted course** compared with pancreatic adenocarcinoma
- Tx: resect these lesions: metastatic disease precludes resection
- **5-FU** and **streptozocin** may be effective

FUNCTIONAL ENDOCRINE PANCREATIC TUMORS

- Represent 70% of pancreatic endocrine neoplasms
- **Octreotide** for **palliation** - effective for all *except* somatostatinoma
- **Octreotide scan** for **localizing** - good for all *except* insulinoma
- Tumors with predilection for **pancreatic head** - gastrinoma and somatostatinoma
- All tumors can respond to debulking (decreases Sx's)
- MC metastatic site for all - **liver**
- For liver metastases that cannot be resected safely, **radiofrequency** ablation *(coagulation necrosis)* and **cryoablation** *(protein and cell membrane denaturation)* are options (can decrease Sx's)
- **Streptozocin** - toxic to **islet cells** of pancreas
- **Insulinoma**
  - *MC islet cell tumor of pancreas (MC functional pancreatic endocrine neoplasm)*
  - Sx's: Whipple's triad →
    - Fasting **hypoglycemia** (< 50)
    - **Sx's** of hypoglycemia (palpitations, tachycardia, diaphoresis, syncope)
    - **Relief** with glucose
  - 90% are **benign**; are evenly distributed throughout pancreas
  - Dx:
    - Insulin to glucose ratio > **0.4** after fasting
    - Fasting glucose < **50** and fasting insulin > **24**
    - *Should have _elevated_ C peptide and pro-insulin* (if not elevated, suspect Munchausen's Syndrome [self-injection of insulin])
    - *The above are **diagnostic***
  - **CT scan** (or MRI) and **EUS** can be used to localize (finds 80%)
  - Selective **pancreatic arterial calcium stimulation with hepatic venous insulin sampling** - *best test* for localizing a tumor not apparent on CT scan or other studies (Ca^{++} causes release of insulin from tumor in pancreas)
  - Notably, many of these will <u>not</u> light up on octreotide scan
  - Tx:
    - **< 2 cm** - **enucleate** (has pseudo-capsule)
    - **> 2 cm** - **formal resection** (Whipple or distal pancreatectomy)
    - Can have multiple lesions (enucleate each if < 2 cm)
    - Chemo for malignant disease: **5-FU and streptozocin**
    - **Diazoxide** and **octreotide** can help with Sx's (inhibit insulin release)
  - **Trouble finding tumor intra-op** - use **intra-op U/S** to help
    - Still can't find tumor - *avoid blind pancreatic resection* and perform post-op **selective arterial calcium stimulation** with hepatic venous insulin sampling to localize the tumor
- **Gastrinoma** (Zollinger-Ellison syndrome [ZES])
  - 50% **malignant** and 50% **multiple**
  - 75% **sporadic** and 25% **MEN-1**
  - Majority (75%) in **gastrinoma triangle** - common bile duct, neck of pancreas, 3rd portion of duodenum
  - Sx's: <u>refractory</u> or <u>complicated</u> **ulcer disease** (eg multiple ulcers, ulcers extending beyond 1st portion of duodenum, obstruction) and **diarrhea** (diarrhea improved with PPI)
  - Dx *(need both)*:
    1) **Fasting serum gastrin** (> 200; 1000s is usually diagnostic) _and;_
    2) 24-hour **stomach basal acid output** (> 15 mEq/hr)
  - **Secretin stimulation test** - <u>ZES patients</u>: *increase* gastrin (> 200)
    <u>Normal patients</u>: *decrease* gastrin
  - Gastric juice **pH < 2** suggests diagnosis
  - **CT scan** (or MRI) and **EUS** can help localize; look for multiple tumors
  - **Octreotide scan** - *best test for localizing tumor*
  - Tx:
    - **< 2 cm** - **enucleation and regional node dissection**
    - **> 2 cm** - **formal resection** and **regional node dissection**
    - Malignant disease → excise any suspicious nodes
    - *Cannot find tumor intra-op* → perform **proximal duodenostomy** and look inside duodenum for tumor (15% of microgastrinomas there)

Blind pancreatic resections should be <u>avoided</u>
Duodenal tumor - resection with primary closure; may need Whipple if
extensive; be sure to check pancreas for primary
Debulking - can improve Sx's
- Chemo for malignant disease: **5-FU** and **streptozocin**
- Palliation - **octreotide** and **PPI**
- **Metastatic disease with severe Sx's** despite maximal medical Tx → Tx: **total
gastrectomy** (<u>not</u> antrectomy + vagotomy - <u>*won't work*</u> *because HCl secreting
cells are in the fundus and body of the stomach*)

■ **Glucagonoma**
- Sx's: **diabetes** (<u>hyperglycemia</u>) and **dermatitis** (<u>rash</u> - necrolytic migratory
erythema); weight loss
- Dx: fasting glucagon level ($\geq$ 500 -1000 pg/mL)
- Most **malignant**; most in **distal pancreas**
- Tx: resection
- Octreotide
- Zinc, amino acids, or fatty acids may treat skin rash
- Chemo for malignant disease: **5-FU** and **streptozocin**

■ **VIPoma** (Verner-Morrison syndrome)
- Sx's: **watery diarrhea**, **hypokalemia**, and **achlorhydria** (WDHA)
- Hypokalemia from diarrhea
- Dx: fasting VIP levels; should exclude other causes of diarrhea
- Most **malignant**; most in **distal pancreas**, 10% are extra-pancreatic
- Tx: resection
- Octreotide
- Chemo for malignant disease: **5-FU** and **<u>*alpha-interferon*</u>**

■ **Somatostatinoma**
- Very rare
- <u>*Worst*</u> prognosis of all pancreatic endocrine tumors- 85% have metastases at Dx
- Sx's: **diabetes**, **gallstones**, and **steatorrhea** *(classic triad)*
- Dx: fasting somatostatin level
- Most **malignant**; most in **head of pancreas**
- Tx: **resection** and **cholecystectomy**
- Chemo for malignant disease: **5-FU** and **streptozocin**

Spleen

890. All of the following are true of splenic <u>red</u> pulp except:
    a.   Acts as a filter for aged or damaged RBCs
    b.   Contains high concentrations of lymphocytes
    c.   Pitting involves the removal of abnormalities in the RBC membrane
    d.   Culling involves removal of less deformable RBCs

Answer b. The **white pulp** contains high concentrations of lymphocytes.

891. All of the following are true of <u>white</u> pulp except:
    a.   IgG is the most common immunoglobulin in the spleen.
    b.   Serves an immunologic function with high concentrations of lymphocytes and macrophages
    c.   Is the major site of bacterial clearance that lacks pre-existing antibodies
    d.   Is the largest producer of IgM

Answer a. **IgM** is the MC immunoglobulin in the spleen.

892. All of the following are true except:
    a.   Tuftsin acts as an opsonin
    b.   Properdin can activate complement
    c.   Howell-Jolly bodies and target cells increase after splenectomy
    d.   The spleen is commonly involved in platelet disorders
    e.   The splenic artery is a branch off the superior mesenteric artery

Answer e. The **splenic artery** is a branch off the celiac axis.

893. The MCC of spontaneous splenic rupture in the U.S. is:
    a.   Malaria
    b.   Mononucleosis
    c.   Sickle cell anemia
    d.   Hairy cell leukemia

Answer b. Mononucleosis

894. Which of the following is true of hyposplenism:
    a.   The spleen is always normal size
    b.   Howell-Jolly bodies are absent
    c.   These patients are not at risk for PSSS
    d.   Vaccination is recommended
    e.   The MCC is sickle cell anemia

Answer d. Hyposplenism indicates reduced splenic function. Findings are similar to those found after splenectomy. The MCC is sickle cell anemia. It can be associated with an enlarged spleen. These patients are at risk for PSSS so appropriate vaccinations are indicated.

895. A 18 yo girl undergoes splenectomy for ITP. Five days post-op she has a BP of 85/40, temp 101 F, lethargy, abdominal pain, nausea, and vomiting. The patient's blood pressure seems unresponsive to fluid challenge. All of the following are true of this condition except:
    a.   The MCC is withdrawal of exogenous steroids
    b.   ACTH is likely elevated in this patient
    c.   Serum cortisol levels need to be drawn before treatment
    d.   Serum cortisol is likely < 15 in this patient

Answer c. You do not need a serum cortisol before treating **adrenal insufficiency**. Dexamethasone should be given. Note Dexamethasone does not interfere with the ACTH stimulation test for adrenal insufficiency.

896. Certain genetic disorders may require splenectomy to prevent premature destruction of blood elements. The MC congenital disease requiring splenectomy is:
   a. Hereditary spherocytosis
   b. Hereditary elliptocytosis
   c. Protein kinase deficiency
   d. Beta thalassemia minor

   Answer a. The MC congenital abnormality requiring splenectomy is **hereditary spherocytosis**. Splenectomy is curative for this disease.

897. The most appropriate treatment for the above condition:
   a. Immunoglobulin
   b. ASA
   c. Splenectomy
   d. Hydroxyurea
   e. Splenectomy and cholecystectomy

   Answer e. Splenectomy and **cholecystectomy**. Cholecystectomy should be performed at the same surgery.

898. Excluding genetic disorders which involve membrane proteins, the MC congenital abnormality requiring splenectomy is:
   a. Hereditary elliptocytosis
   b. G6PD deficiency
   c. Pyruvate kinase deficiency
   d. Hereditary spherocytosis

   Answer c. The MC non-membrane protein congenital abnormality requiring splenectomy is **pyruvate kinase deficiency**.

899. Continued destruction of blood elements following splenectomy can be related to an accessory spleen. The MC location of an accessory spleen is:
   a. Liver
   b. Kidney
   c. Adrenal gland
   d. Splenic hilum

   Answer d. The MC location of an **accessory spleen** is the splenic hilum. The best test to find an accessory spleen is a **tagged RBC scan**.

900. The MC non-traumatic condition requiring splenectomy:
   a. Immune thrombocytopenic purpura (ITP)
   b. Thrombotic thrombocytopenic purpura (TTP)
   c. Hereditary spherocytosis
   d. Pyruvate kinase deficiency

   Answer a. The MC non-traumatic indication for splenectomy is **ITP.**

901. All of the following are characteristic of ITP except:
   a. With splenectomy, platelets are classically given after ligation of the splenic artery
   b. In children < 10, this often resolves without splenectomy
   c. Enlarged spleen
   d. The primary therapy is steroids

   Answer c. ITP patients have **normal spleens**. ITP is the MC severe platelet problem that involves a normal spleen

902. All of the following are true of lymphoma except:
   a. Non-Hodgkin's lymphoma involving the mediastinum and spleen would be considered stage III disease

b. The MCC of chylous ascites is lymphoma
c. The MC 2nd malignancy following radiation therapy only for lymphoma is breast CA
d. FNA is all that is needed for the diagnosis of lymphoma

Answer d. FNA is not adequate for the Dx of lymphoma as architecture is needed. Core needle Bx or open Bx are indicated.

903. All of the following are common indications for splenectomy except:
a. Splenic abscess (multilocular)
b. Refractory isolated splenic lymphoma
c. Myelofibrosis with myeloid metaplasia causing transfusion dependency
d. Sickle cell anemia

Answer d. The spleen usually infarcts with sickle cell anemia and splenectomy is rarely required.

Splenectomy is used for **multilocilar** splenic abscess due to bleeding risk. **Unilocular** splenic abscess is usually treated with percutaneous drainage.

Splenic abscess is MC due to **hematogenous spread** (MCC - **endocarditis**)

904. A 3 yo undergoes splenectomy for thalassemia major. Six weeks later, the child returns to the ER with a fever of 104 F, chills, rigors, and a systolic blood pressure of 60. The child's WBCs are 20 All of the following are true of the child's most likely condition except:
a. The condition is more common in patients who undergo splenectomy for malignancy or hematologic disease compared to trauma
b. The MC organism involved is N. meningitides
c. Children less then 5 years of age undergoing splenectomy are at higher risk
d. The condition is due to a specific lack of immunity to capsulated organisms

Answer b. The MC organism involved in **Post-Splenectomy Sepsis Syndrome** (PSSS) is **strep pneumoniae.**

Thalassemia major is specifically considered at higher risk
Highest risk for PSSS - **Wiskott-Aldrich syndrome** (immune deficiency resulting in decreased antibody production)

905. Peri-op vaccination for patients undergoing splenectomy should include all of the following except:
a. streptococcus pneumonia
b. haemophilus influenzae
c. neisseria meningitidis
d. escherichia coli

Answer d. E. coli. Vaccinations should be given **2 weeks before** (preferred) *or* **2 weeks after** splenectomy (usually trauma situations)

ANATOMY AND PHYSIOLOGY
- **Vascular supply**
  - **Splenic artery** (off celiac trunk) and **short gastrics** (off splenic artery) are considered end arteries
  - **Splenic vein** is posterior and inferior to splenic artery (behind pancreas); splenic artery is just superior to the pancreas
  - **Operative approach**:
    1) **mobilize spleen** by dividing the **spleno-phrenic, spleno-renal**, and **spleno-colic ligaments** (posterior-lateral)
    2) **divide short gastrics** and **gastro-splenic ligament**
    3) **splenic artery and vein** are then divided, usually separately
  - **Trauma splenectomy** - through midline incision

- **Red pulp** (85%)
  - Acts as a **filter for aged** or **damaged RBCs**
  - **Pitting** - the removal of abnormalities in RBC membrane
    - **Howell-Jolly bodies** - nuclear remnants
    - **Heinz bodies** - hemoglobin
    - **Pappenheimer bodies** - iron (siderocytes)
  - **Culling** - removal of less deformable and old RBCs
- **White pulp** (15%)
  - **Immunologic function**
  - Contains **lymphocytes** and **macrophages**
  - Is the major site of **bacterial clearance that lacks preexisting antibodies**
  - Site of removal for **poorly opsonized bacteria, particles,** and other **cellular debris**
  - Serves as antigen-processing center for **dendritic cells** and **macrophages**; involves **helper T cells** (adaptive immunity)
  - Spleen is the largest producer of **IgM**
  - MC immunoglobulin in spleen - **IgM**
- **Tuftsin** - an **opsonin**; produced in **spleen**
- **Properdin** - an **opsonin**; produced in **spleen**; also activates **complement**
- **Post-splenectomy changes** (most of these changes transient)
  - ↑ed RBCs, WBCs, and platelets
  - Will see **Howell-Jolly, Heinz,** and **Pappenheimer** bodies
  - Will see **spur cells** and **target cells**
  - If platelets > 1-1.5 x 10^6, need ASA
  - Liver picks up some splenic functions
- **Hyposplenism** - reduced splenic function (have the same changes as above)
  - MCC- **sickle cell anemia**, other- celiac sprue, SLE, amyloidosis, ulcerative colitis
  - Can be associated with an enlarged spleen
  - Important to identify these patients as they are at risk for **PSSS** (need appropriate **vaccinations**)
- **Reticuloendothelial system** - monocytes and macrophages
  - Location - spleen, liver (Kupffer cells), lymph nodes, lung (alveolar macrophages)
- **Accessory spleen** - MC found at **splenic hilum**
- **Indication for splenectomy** - idiopathic thrombocytopenic purpura (ITP) far greater than for thrombotic thrombocytopenic purpura (TTP)
- MC non-traumatic condition requiring splenectomy - **ITP**
- MC organ involved in thrombocytopenia - **spleen**
- **Hypersplenism** (with or without splenomegaly) occurs in many disorders (eg portal hypertension, hematologic CA, metabolic disease, congenital hemolytic disease) and results in _decreased_ **RBCs** (anemia), **WBCs** (leukopenia), and **platelets** (thrombocytopenia)
- **Laparoscopic splenectomy** is usually the preferred approach for elective splenectomy

IDIOPATHIC THROMBOCYTOPENIC PURPURA (ITP)
- MC non-traumatic indication for splenectomy
- Many etiologies - drugs, viruses, etc.
- Sx's: petechiae, gingival bleeding, soft tissue ecchymosis (bruising)
- Path
  - **Low platelets** (< 100,000)
  - Caused by **antibodies to platelets** (IgG) - platelets get chewed up by macrophages in spleen leading to bleeding diatheses
  - **Spleen is _normal_ in size and function**
  - Adults can get chronic form
- _In children < **10 years** - ITP usually resolves spontaneously (> 90%)_
  - _Avoid splenectomy in children with ITP_
  - Typically follows **infection** (usually viral; peak **age 5**)
- Diagnosis is one of exclusion
- Tx: **steroids** _(primary Tx)_; immunoglobulin if steroid-resistant
  - **Acute spontaneous bleeding** Tx: **steroids** and **immunoglobulin**; platelets may be required to stop profuse bleeding

- **Splenectomy** indicated for those who <u>fail steroids</u> (eg failed Tx, refractory disease after 3-6 months of therapy, 1st recurrence) → removes IgG production and source of phagocytosis (80% respond after splenectomy)
- Give **platelets** *after* ligating the splenic artery
- **Pre-splenectomy** issues:
  - **Steroids** given at beginning of case (prevent Addisonian Crisis)
  - **Immunoglobulin** 1 week pre-op (prolongs life of platelets)
  - **Immunizations** - S pneumoniae, H. influenza, and N. meningitides (2 weeks before operation best)
- **Post-splenectomy** issues:
  - **Immunizations** if not already given
  - **ASA** for platelets > 1-1.5 x 10^6
  - **Prophylactic Daily Augmentin** for 6 months in children < 10 (helps prevent PSSS)
- **Persistent thrombocytopenia** post-op (recurrent ITP after splenectomy)
  - Dx: look at peripheral blood smear for **asplenic changes** in RBCs (should see Howell-Jolly, Heinz, and Pappenheimer bodies if <u>no</u> spleen is present)
  - If asplenic changes not present, consider **accessory spleen** (MC location is **splenic hilum**; Dx - **RBC scan** *[best test]*)
  - Tx: steroids and immunoglobulin (IV-Ig) if no accessory spleen
  - **Reoperation** if accessory spleen found

THROMBOTIC THROMBOCYTOPENIC PURPURA (TTP)
- Associated with drug reactions, infection, inflammation, autoimmune disease
- **Loss of platelet inhibition** - leads to thrombosis and infarction
  - Is <u>not</u> antibody mediated
- Sx's (*classic pentad):*
  - **Low platelets** (*profound* - high risk for spontaneous bleeding; **petechiae**)
  - **Mental status** changes (eg headaches, seizures)
  - **Kidney failure**
  - **Fever**
  - **Hemolytic anemia** (jaundice; see **schistocytes**)
- Majority (80%) arise from deficiency or inhibition of **enzyme ADAMTS13** (responsible for cleaving large **vWF molecules**); these large vWF molecules go un-cleaved and cause **thrombosis**
- Tx:
  - *Plasmapheresis (primary Tx)* - gets rid of vWF molecules
  - Steroids (immunosuppression; vincristine, cyclophosphamide)
  - 80% respond to medical Tx
  - *Splenectomy <u>rarely</u> indicated*
- Death MC due to **intracerebral hemorrhage** (MC) or acute renal failure

HEMOLYTIC ANEMIAS: MEMBRANE PROTEIN DEFECTS
- **Hereditary Spherocytosis** (autosomal dominant)
  - MC congenital hemolytic anemia requiring splenectomy
  - **Spectrin** deficit (**membrane protein**) deforms RBCs and leads to splenic sequestration (**hypersplenism**)
  - Sx's: anemia, jaundice, **splenomegaly**; pigmented **gallstones**
  - Try to perform splenectomy after age 5 (get through immunizations)
  - Tx: **splenectomy** and **cholecystectomy**
  - Splenectomy curative
- **Hereditary Elliptocytosis**
  - Sx's and mechanism similar to spherocytosis; less common
  - Spectrin and protein 4.1 deficit (membrane proteins)

HEMOLYTIC ANEMIAS: NON-MEMBRANE PROTEIN DEFECTS
- **Pyruvate kinase deficiency**
  - Is the MC congenital hemolytic anemia <u>not</u> involving a membrane protein that requires splenectomy (though not all of these patients need splenectomy)
  - Causes altered glucose metabolism
  - RBC survival enhanced by splenectomy (required in minority of patients)

- **Warm antibody-type acquired immune hemolytic anemia**
  - Is the MC <u>autoimmune</u> hemolytic disease (MC - IgG against RBCs)
  - Splenectomy if refractory to steroids and immunoglobulin
- **Beta thalassemia**
  - MC thalassemia; due to persistent HgbF
  - Major - both chains affected; minor - 1 chain, asymptomatic
  - Sx's: pallor, retarded body growth, head enlargement
  - Most die in teens secondary to hemosiderosis
  - Medical Tx: blood transfusions and iron chelators (deferoxamine, deferiprone)
  - **Splenectomy** (if patient has splenomegaly) may decrease hemolysis
- **G6PD deficiency**
  - Precipitated by infection, certain drugs, fava beans
  - Splenectomy <u>rarely</u> required
- **Sickle cell anemia** - HgbA replaced with HgbS
  - Spleen usually autoinfarcts; splenectomy is <u>rarely</u> required

HODGKIN'S DISEASE
- MC Sx - **painless swollen lymph node in neck**
- Nodal disease has an orderly anatomic spread to adjacent nodes
- Dx: core needle Bx or excisional lymph node Bx (need **architecture**, not just cells);
  - *FNA <u>not</u> adequate for Dx*
  - Bone marrow Bx
  - **PET** or **gallium MRI** of spleen and liver
  - CT scan - does not reliably detect spleen or liver involvement; need 2nd modality (→ **gallium MRI** or **PET**)
- **Staging**
  - I - 1 LN region
  - II - $\geq$ 2 LN regions (non-contiguous) on same side of the diaphragm
  - III - LN regions on <u>**both sides**</u> of the diaphragm (eg abdominal and thoracic)
  - IV - disseminated involvement to 1 or more extra-lymphatic organs (eg liver, bone, lung, ect. *except* spleen)
    - A - asymptomatic
    - B - symptomatic (constitutional Sx's - night sweats, fever, weight loss) → unfavorable prognosis
- Tx: **chemo ± XRT** (ABVD - doxorubicin [Adriamycin], bleomycin, vinblastine, dacarbazine)
- Overall 5-YS: **HL** - 85%, **NHL** - 65%
- Staging laparotomy <u>rarely</u> performed as it does not impact Tx
- Surgery for lymphoma today primarily involves:
  - 1) Getting lymph node tissue for Dx (consider laparoscopic Bx for suspected abdominal lymphoma) <u>and:</u>
  - 2) Tx of chylous effusion
- See **Reed-Sternberg cells**
- **Lymphocyte predominant** - best prognosis
- **Lymphocyte depleted** - worst prognosis
- **MC type** - nodular sclerosing
- **MCC of chylous ascites** - <u>lymphoma</u>
- Patients with lymphoma are at high risk for **2nd malignancies** related to therapy for lymphoma:
  - MC from **prior XRT** and **chemo** - lung CA, leukemia
  - MC from **prior XRT** <u>only</u> - breast CA
  - Also at risk for earlier onset **coronary atherosclerosis** (related to XRT)
- Tx for lymphoma **isolated** to a specific area:
  - **1st or 2nd portions of duodenum** - chemo ± XRT *(<u>No Whipple</u>)*
  - **3rd or 4th portion of duodenum** - wide en bloc resection, then chemo ± XRT
  - **Ileum** or **jejunum** - wide en bloc resection (include nodes), then chemo ± XRT
  - **Colon** lymphoma (MC cecum) - wide en bloc resection (include nodes), then chemo ± XRT
  - **Anal** lymphoma (often in AIDS patients) - chemo ± XRT
  - **Pancreatic** lymphoma - chemo ± XRT

- **Gastric** lymphoma *(MC site for extra-nodal lymphoma)* - surgery only for stage I, otherwise chemo ± XRT
- **Splenic** lymphoma (marginal zone lymphoma; *rare*) - splenectomy, chemo, <u>or</u> watchful waiting
- **Thyroid lymphoma** - chemo ± XRT

NON-HODGKIN'S LYMPHOMA (NHL)
- **Worse prognosis** than Hodgkin's; 90% are **B-cell** lymphomas (40+ types of NHL)
- Sx's reflect involved sites (eg abdominal fullness, bone pain)
- Diffuse nodal and extra-nodal disease usual; non-contiguous spread (generally a **systemic disease** by the time Dx is made)
- Tx - chemo (**CHOP-R**; **C**yclophosphamide, doxorubicin (**H**ydroxy-), vincristine (**O**ncovin), **P**rednisone, **R**ituximab (anti-CD20, kills **B cells**)
- Overall 5-year survival **NHL**- 65%

OVERWHELMING POST-SPLENECTOMY INFECTION (OPSI)
- Post-splenectomy sepsis syndrome (PSSS)
- **Lifetime risk** after splenectomy: 1-2%
- **Increased risk** for OPSI:
  - MC in **children aged ≤ 5** *(the younger the patient, the higher the risk)*
  - MC **within 2 years** after splenectomy (80% of all cases)
  - MC with **non-traumatic causes** for splenectomy (eg malignancy, hemolytic disorders such as thalassemia)
- *Thalassemia major* specifically considered higher risk
- <u>Highest risk</u> for OPSI - **Wiskott-Aldrich syndrome** *(immune deficiency resulting in low antibody production)*
- **Path**
  - Condition is due to a specific lack of immunity to **capsulated organisms** (lack of IgM immunoglobulin)
  - **MC organisms** in OPSI - *streptococcus pneumoniae (#1; pneumococcus), haemophilus influenza, neisseria meningitides, staph aureus*
- **Mortality rate** - **50%** (highest mortality is in **children**)
- **Prevention**
  - Try and delay splenectomy until **after 5 years of age** *(allows antibody formation; child can get fully immunized)*
  - Should be immunized against **pneumococcus, meningococcus,** and **haemophilus influenzae** at least **2 weeks before** elective splenectomy or **2 weeks after** a traumatic splenectomy
  - **Prophylactic Augmentin** for children aged < 10 for 6 months (take every day)
  - Explain to parents they need to bring child to ED for any **fever**
  - **Early broad-spectrum I.V. antibiotics** for suspected infection
  - Antibiotic prophylaxis for **dental procedures** (lifetime)
  - Booster immunization every 3 years for **pneumococcal vaccine**

OTHER CONDITIONS
- **Spontaneous splenic rupture** - mononucleosis (MC U.S patients), malaria (MC worldwide), sepsis, polycythemia vera
- **Splenosis** - splenic implants; usually related to trauma
- **Pancreatitis** - MCC of splenic artery or splenic vein thrombosis
- **MC splenic tumor** (and MC benign splenic tumor) - hemangioma
  - Tx: splenectomy if symptomatic
- **MC malignant splenic tumor** - Non-Hodgkin's lymphoma
- **MCC of malignant splenomegaly** - Non-Hodgkin's lymphoma
- **MC malignant non-blood cell tumor** - angiosarcoma
  - Tx: splenectomy
- **Hairy cell leukemia** - Tx: <u>rarely</u> need splenectomy (Tx: leustatin [cladribine])
- **Felty's Syndrome** - rheumatoid arthritis, splenomegaly, neutropenia; Tx: steroids, rheumatoid arthritis meds; uncommonly need splenectomy
- Almost <u>always</u> need **splenectomy**:
  - **Hereditary spherocytosis**
  - **Hereditary elliptocytosis**

- **Splenic vein thrombosis** with gastric variceal **bleeding**
- **Echinococcal cyst** - Tx: splenectomy after 2 weeks of albendazole
- **Dermoid cyst** (cystic teratoma; has malignancy potential)
- **Splenic abscess** (MC organism - *streptococcus*; followed by staph) - Tx: percutaneous drainage if <u>unilocular</u>; splenectomy if <u>multilocular</u> (significant <u>bleeding risk</u> with percutaneous drainage); splenic abscess in MC related to **hematogenous spread** (MCC – **endocarditis**)

■ <u>*Usually*</u> need splenectomy:
- *<u>Refractory</u>* **Warm antibody type hemolytic anemia**
- *<u>Refractory</u>* **ITP** in adult
- **Isolated splenic lymphoma** (rare; causes splenomegaly)
- **Myelofibrosis with splenic myeloid metaplasia** (spleen acts as bone marrow; get splenomegaly and consumption of blood products)

> Tx: splenectomy if transfusion dependent, is causing pain, or severe thrombocytopenia (all are controversial)

Post-splenectomy changes

- Howell-Jolly bodies (RBC nuclear fragments)
- Heinz bodies (RBC hemoglobin deposits)
- Pappenheimer bodies (RBC iron deposits)
- Target cells (RBCs)
- Spur cells (RBCs, acanthocytes)
- Transient thrombocytosis (high platelets) ASA for platelets $>1\text{-}1.5 \times 10^6$
- Transient leukocytosis (high WBCs)

Small Bowel

906. All of the following are true except:
   a. The 1st branch off the superior mesenteric artery (SMA) is the inferior pancreatico-duodenal artery
   b. The division between the 3rd and 4th portions of duodenum is the SMA
   c. The 2nd and 3rd portions of the duodenum are retroperitoneal
   d. The 3rd portion of the duodenum contains the Ampulla of Vater
   e. The SMA provides blood flow from the 3rd portion of the duodenum to the proximal 2/3 of the transverse colon

   Answer d. The 2nd portion of the duodenum contains the Ampulla of Vater.

907. All of the following are true except:
   a. Brunner's glands secrete alkaline solution
   b. Goblet cells secrete mucus solution
   c. Diarrhea in Carcinoid syndrome is from serotonin
   d. 5-HIAA is the most sensitive test for detecting carcinoid tumors
   e. The primary fuel for small bowel enterocytes is glutamine

   Answer d. Chromogranin A is the most sensitive test for **detection** of carcinoid tumors (almost 100% have it) but it would not give location.

   Brunner's glands are found in the duodenum and secrete **alkaline solution** to serve as a protective barrier to acid coming from the stomach. The jejunum lacks Brunner's glands, which is the reason **marginal ulcers** occur after roux-en-Y gastro-jejunostomy with a long afferent limb.

908. All of the following are true of duodenal diverticula except:
   a. These should be observed unless highly symptomatic
   b. The MC location is the 3rd portion of the duodenum
   c. A chole-duodenal fistula should be ruled out in these patients
   d. The duodenum is the MC small bowel location for diverticula
   e. If biliary obstruction is a significant symptom, hepatico-jejunostomy is indicated

   Answer b. The MC location is the 2nd portion of the duodenum

909. You are considering stricturoplasty in a patient with Crohn's disease. Which of the following is true:
   a. Recurrent surgical Crohn's after stricturoplasty is most likely to occur in previous stricturoplasty sites
   b. A 15 cm stricture is best treated with longitudinal enterotomy and transverse closure
   c. A 5 cm stricture is best treated with side to side anastomosis type stricturoplasty
   d. Longitudinal incision should be made through the anti-mesenteric border

   Answer d. Longitudinal incision should be made through the **anti-mesenteric border**. Strictures < 10 cm are treated with longitudinal enterotomy and transverse closure. Strictures 10 - 25 cm are treated with side to side anastomosis type stricturoplasty. Recurrent surgical Crohn's after stricturoplasty is most likely to occur in *non-stricturoplasty sites*.

910. All of the following are true of Crohn's disease except
   a. The MC site of occurrence is the terminal ileum
   b. Large perianal skin tags are common
   c. Surgery is curative
   d. Perianal fistula are usually treated conservatively
   e. It is more prevalent in smokers

Answer c. Unlike UC, surgery is not curative for Crohn's disease

911. A 35 yo woman with Crohn's disease is started on Infliximab and Flagyl for a peri-anal fistula. All of the following are true of Infliximab therapy except:
    a. The MC serious infection in patients taking Infliximab is tuberculosis
    b. Aggressive surgical resection is indicated for peri-anal fistulas from Crohn's disease
    c. Isoniazid is indicated for patients with a positive PPD
    d. Long term Flagyl is associated with peripheral neuropathy

Answer b. Conservative Tx is indicated for Crohn's peri-anal fistulas.

912. All of the following are true of Crohn's disease except:
    a. Refractory strictures involving the 3rd and 4th portions of the duodenum would likely benefit best from resection with a 2 cm gross margin and duodeno-jejunostomy
    b. Short strictures in the jejunum and ileum can be treated with stricturoplasty to avoid resection and conserve bowel
    c. A Whipple is likely the best treatment for refractory strictures in the 1st and 2nd portion of the duodenum
    d. Creeping mesenteric fat is considered pathognomonic of Crohn's

Answer c. Duodenal Crohn's disease is unusual. Tx for a refractory strictures in the **1st** and **2nd portion** is **gastro-jejunostomy and vagotomy** (no Whipple; also can't really perform stricturoplasty here). Some type of vagotomy is needed to avoid **marginal ulcers** after gastro-jejunostomy.

For refractory strictures in the **3rd and 4th portions** of the duodenum, resection and **duodeno-jejunostomy** is usually indicated. A margin of 2 cm from grossly visible disease is indicated (frozen section is not necessary)

Short strictures in the distal duodenum, jejunum, and ileum can be treated with **stricturoplasty** to avoid resection and conserve bowel.

913. All of the following are true of Crohn's disease except:
    a. The best maintenance Tx for mild Crohn's disease (eg colitis, ileocolitis) is sulfasalazine
    b. The best Tx for acute Crohn's exacerbation is corticosteroids
    c. Aphthous ulcers are the earliest lesion suggestive of Crohn's
    d. The MCC of mortality with small bowel fistula is liver failure
    e. It is MC in patients of high socioeconomic status

Answer d. The MCC of **mortality** with small bowel fistula (in Crohn's or other diseases; also includes other types of fistulas) is **sepsis**. Early drainage of any associated abscess and antibiotics are indicated.

914. A 45 yo woman with Crohn's pancolitis has several areas of dysplasia on surveillance. The most appropriate next step is:
    a. Total procto-colectomy and ileostomy
    b. Continued surveillance
    c. Total procto-colectomy and ileoanal pouch
    d. Segmental colectomy only

Answer a. Total procto-colectomy and ileostomy. Because of the diffuse nature of the Crohn's and the finding of dysplasia, total procto-colectomy is indicated. Pouch formation is contraindicated in Crohn's disease (high risk of complications and pouch failure).

915. A patient undergoes resection of a small bowel carcinoid and an isolated liver metastasis Two years later she develops vague abdominal complaints but you cannot

identify any new lesions on CT scan. The best study to *localize* recurrent carcinoid tumor is:
- a. HIDA scan
- b. MIBG scan
- c. Octreotide scan
- d. MRI

Answer c. Octreotide scan is the most sensitive diagnostic test for <u>localizing</u> a **carcinoid tumor** not apparent on CT scan.

916. All of the following are true of carcinoid tumors except:
- a. The MC site for carcinoid tumor and the site with the highest malignant potential is the ileum
- b. Octreotide is very effective Tx for metastatic carcinoid tumors
- c. Chromogranin A is the most sensitive test for detecting carcinoid tumors (essentially 100% have this)
- d. The 5-YS for carcinoid tumor with metastases is 5%
- e. Acute carcinoid crisis is best treated with octreotide

Answer d. The 5-YS for **carcinoid tumor with metastases** is 35%. Palliation is an important part of Tx for these patients (can survive a long time).

917. All of the following are true of appendicitis except:
- a. The MCC in children is lymphoid tissue
- b. The MCC in adults is fecalith
- c. It is due to a closed loop obstruction
- d. The MC rupture site is the anti-mesenteric border
- e. CT scan has decreased negative laparotomy rate

Answer d. CT scan has <u>not</u> decreased negative laparotomy rate.

918. All of the following are true of appendicitis except:
- a. It is more common in males than in females (3 :1)
- b. Perforation rate is higher in children and the elderly
- c. The appendiceal artery is a branch of the right colic artery
- d. Right lower quadrant pain is due to peritoneal irritation
- e. Nausea, vomiting, visceral pain, and at times diarrhea are due to luminal obstruction and distension of the visceral peritoneum (afferent autonomic nervous system)

Answer c. The appendiceal artery is a branch of the **ileocolic artery**.

919. Laparoscopic compared to open surgery for appendicitis is associated with all of the following except:
- a. Decreased length of stay
- b. Earlier return to work
- c. Lower abscess rate
- d. Lower wound infection rate

Answer c. Abscess rate is about the same for laparoscopic and open procedures.

920. A 9 yo boy presents with abdominal pain, somewhat localized to the RLQ. He is diffusely tender. He has had an upper respiratory tract infection (URI) for a few days. CT scan shows adenopathy near the terminal ileum and cecum. All of the following are true of this patients most likely diagnosis except:
- a. Yersinia, shigella, and campylobacter are frequently involved
- b. This can often occur following an antecedent URI
- c. Emergency appendectomy is indicated
- d. Antibiotics may be indicated
- e. This MC occurs in children

Answer c. This patient has **mesenteric lymphadenitis**, so appendectomy is not indicated. The MC organism involved in mesenteric lymphadenitis is *yersinia enterocolitica.*

921. You perform an appendectomy on a 25 yo man for presumed appendicitis and find a 1 cm tumor at the tip of the appendix. Pathology comes back on the tumor as carcinoid. The most appropriate next step in management is:
    a.   Right hemicolectomy
    b.   Close
    c.   XRT post-op
    d.   Chemotherapy post-op

    Answer b. (see below)

922. You operate on a 25 yo man for presumed appendicitis based on CT scan and find a 2.5 cm tumor at the tip of the appendix. Pathology comes back on the tumor as carcinoid. The most appropriate next step in management is:
    a.   Right hemicolectomy
    b.   Close
    c.   XRT post-op
    d.   Chemotherapy post-op

    Answer a. Appendectomy is adequate treatment for **carcinoid tumors** localized to the appendix as long as they are < 2 cm, not at the base, and there is no evidence of mesenteric lymph node invasion or metastatic disease. If the above criteria not met, perform right hemi-colectomy. Carcinoid tumors have the best 5-YS (85%) of all appendiceal malignancies.

923. All of the following are true of appendiceal tumors except:
    a.   The MC benign tumor is non-malignant carcinoid
    b.   The MC malignant tumor is adenocarcinoma
    c.   The MC presentation for appendiceal adenocarcinoma is bowel obstruction
    d.   The MC malignant subtype is mucinous adenocarcinoma

    Answer c. The MC presentation for appendiceal adenocarcinoma is **acute appendicitis.**

924. All of the following are true of rectal carcinoid except:
    a.   Carcinoid syndrome is common with rectal carcinoids
    b.   For patients with rectal carcinoids > 2 cm, 70% have metastases
    c.   Small (< 2 cm) low rectal carcinoids can undergo local excision
    d.   Muscularis propria invasion requires formal resection
    e.   Alpha interferon is more effective than cyclophosphamide and 5-FU

    Answer a. Carcinoid syndrome is infrequent with **rectal carcinoids.**

    Small (< 2 cm) low rectal carcinoids can undergo local excision. If **large** (> 2 cm) or if invading the **muscularis propria,** low rectal carcinoids require formal resection (eg APR)

925. A patient has a localized adenocarcinoma confined to the junction of the 3rd and 4th portions of the duodenum. Which of the following is most appropriate for this patient:
    a.   Pancreatico-duodenectomy
    b.   Distal pancreatectomy and duodenal resection
    c.   Duodenal resection with duodenal-jejunal anastomosis
    d.   Duodenal resection and splenectomy

    Answer c. The best option for **distal duodenal CA** is to **remove the 3rd and 4th portions of the duodenum** and perform duodenal to jejunal anastomosis (not perform a Whipple). Take the duodenum all the way past the ligament of Treitz.

Adenocarcinoma in the **1st and 2nd portions** of the duodenum usually requires Whipple (high likelihood the Ampulla is involved).

926. All of the following are true of small bowel tumors except:
    a. Adenocarcinoma is the MC malignant small bowel tumor, with a high proportion arising from the duodenum (40%)
    b. The duodenum is the MC location for small bowel adenomas
    c. Ampullary villous adenomas rarely harbor occult CA
    d. Obstructive jaundice with heme positive stools is classic for ampullary villous adenoma (or carcinoma)

    Answer c. Up to 70% of **ampullary villous adenomas** have CA in them.

927. All of the following are true of lymphoma except:
    a. Isolated small bowel lymphoma _outside_ the 1st and 2nd portions of the duodenum is generally resected
    b. Isolated pancreatic lymphoma usually requires Whipple
    c. The MC small bowel site for lymphoma is the ileum
    d. B cell is the MC type of lymphoma (Non-Hodgkin's lymphoma)

    Answer b. Isolated **pancreatic lymphoma** should undergo chemo ± XRT

928. At laparotomy, you find copious amounts of yellowish-gray gelatinous ascites. Which of the follwing is the most likely source:
    a. Ovarian mucinous adenocarcinoma
    b. Appendix mucinous adenocarcinoma
    c. Pancreatic cyst-adenocarcinoma
    d. Choledochocyst

    Answer b. The MCC of **pseudomyxoma perotonei** is **appendix mucinous adenocarcinoma.**

929. The MC source for pseudomyxoma peritonei is the:
    a. Ovary
    b. Stomach
    c. Appendix
    d. Colon

    Answer c. Appendix

930. All of the following are true of a mucocele of the appendix except:
    a. Benign lesions can be left alone
    b. Pseudomyxoma perotonei is the most dreaded complication
    c. These may have malignant or benign etiologies
    d. MCC of death with pseudomyxoma peritonei is small bowel obstruction
    e. Gelatinous ascites with peritoneal implants may be present

    Answer a. Benign mucoceles of the **appendix** should undergo appendectomy. Mucoceles of the appendix can arise from either a retention cyst, mucosal hyperplasia, mucinous adenoma, or mucinous adenocarcinoma. The mucocele fills with mucoid material and can eventually rupture.

    The central issue here is that **endothelial cells** within the mucocele (regardless of benign or malignant etiology) can form implants on peritoneal surfaces. These implants can grow, release mucoid material, form more implants, ect. and eventually cause **bowel obstruction** in a process known as *pseudomyxoma peritonei*. The MCC of death in these patients is **small bowel obstruction**.

    Because of this, all mucoceles should be resected. Most encourage open procedures with discovery of a mucocele. *You want to avoid spillage of the mucocele's contents to prevent __implants__.* If cystadenocarcinoma is found in the appendix, a **right hemi-colectomy** is indicated.

Pseudomyxoma peritonei can on occasion arise from other mucin secreting tumors (eg ovarian mucinous CA) however the **appendix** is the MC source.

931. The most appropriate Tx for pseudomyxoma peritonei is:
    a. IV chemo only
    b. Chemo-XRT
    c. Palliative care only
    d. Peritoneal catheter drainage of mucoid material
    e. Cytoreductive surgery and hyperthermic intra-peritoneal chemotherapy

    Answer e. Cytoreductive surgery and **hyperthermic intra-peritoneal chemotherapy** are appropriate for pseudomyxoma peritonei, especially in young patients. These patients can often go on to live productive lives.

932. All of the following are true except:
    a. The MC malignant tumor of the appendix is adenocarcinoma
    b. Chromogranin A level is the most sensitive test for the diagnosis of carcinoid
    c. The ileum is the MC site for carcinoid tumor
    d. The appendix carcinoid is the site with the highest risk for carcinoid syndrome and metastases
    e. Tricuspid insufficiency is the MC cardiac valve problem in patients with Carcinoid Syndrome

    Answer d. Carcinoid of the **ileum** has the highest risk for carcinoid syndrome and metastases.

933. All of the following are true of appendiceal adenocarcinoma except:
    a. The MC presentation is acute appendicitis
    b. These patients should undergo appendectomy only
    c. Variants can lead to pseudomyxoma peritonei
    d. These tumors have a propensity for early rupture

    Answer b. These patients should undergo **right hemicolectomy**.

934. All of the following are true of intussusception in adults except:
    a. Most commonly there is a malignant lead point
    b. Barium reduction should be performed for ileo-colic intussusception
    c. The MC scenario in adults is the ileum going into the right colon
    d. Cecal adenocarcinoma is the MC lead point in adults

    Answer b. Barium enema and air contrast enema reduction are __not__ indicated for **adult intussusception**. The MC adult scenario is a **cecal adenocarcinoma** forms the lead point and peristalsis takes the tumor and ileum into right colon, forming the intussusception.

935. The most appropriate procedure for most adults with ileo-colic intussusception is:
    a. Barium enema reduction
    b. Manual reduction in the OR
    c. Colonoscopic reduction
    d. Air-contrast reduction
    e. Ileo-colic resection without reduction

    Answer e. Ileocolic resection (+ ileocolic anastomosis) __without__ reduction. Do __not__ reduce in the OR as this increases the risk of tumor spread through veins and lymphatics in the cecum.

936. Concerning short bowel syndrome, all of the following are true except:

a. This is a clinical diagnosis of inability to absorb enough water and nutritional elements to be off TPN
b. The length of bowel in general needs to be at least 75 cm if there is no ileocecal valve in order to live without TPN
c. The length of bowel in general needs to be at least 50 cm if the ileo-cecal valve is present in order to live off TPN
d. High fat diets can help with the syndrome
e. Resection of the jejunum is better tolerated than ileal resection

Answer d. Short gut syndrome is a clinical diagnosis of inability to maintain appropriate hydration and nutrition without the use of TPN. High fat diets will worsen short bowel syndrome. An early low fat, high protein, high carbohydrate diet is indicated to help intestinal adaptation and prevent villous atrophy.

937. You perform laparoscopy on a 25 yo man for presumed appendicitis and find terminal ileitis with edematous mesentery and lymphadenopathy. The cecum is not involved. The ileitis area is non-obstructing. The most appropriate next step in management is:
a. Appendectomy
b. Close
c. Place a drain
d. Ileal resection

Answer a. Patients with **presumed appendicitis** at surgery but instead have terminal ileitis not involving the cecum should undergo **appendectomy** so that confusion of ileitis with appendicitis will not occur in the future. This is the same for ruptured ovarian cyst, endometriosis, thrombosed ovarian vein, Mittelschmerz etc.

Appendectomy is recommended at time of surgery for the above as long as the cecum is not involved in the process (cecal involvement would affect healing after appendectomy).

Regional terminal ileits is usually caused by bacterial or viral infection. In 10% of patients, this actually represents early Crohn's Disease, however, the presence of terminal ileitis does not warrant bowel resection or lymph node biopsy.

938. All of the following are true of small bowel cutaneous fistulas except:
a. The MCC of mortality is sepsis
b. Distal obstruction should be ruled out
c. Cancer recurrence is a possibility
d. They often occur in inflammatory bowel disease
e. Surgery is the primary therapy

Answer e. Conservative Tx is the primary therapy and will help resolve most fistulas.

939. A 65 yo man with previous LAR and chemo-XRT has crampy abdominal pain, nausea, and vomiting. He has the following values: BP 85/50, HR 110, sodium 150. He has not made urine in the past 24 hours. CT scan reveals a small bowel obstruction with a decompressed distal colon. The most appropriate next step is:
a. Emergent surgery and bowel resection
b. Fluid resuscitation
c. Palliative care
d. Colonoscopy

Answer c. Fluid resuscitation is appropriate for this patient at this stage.

940. After fluid resuscitation, you explore the above patient and find a moderate amount of matted small bowel. All of the following are true except
a. Bowel resection could result in short bowel syndrome
b. Biopsies should be taken to check for tumor recurrence

c.   Lysis of adhesions around the matted bowel carries a high risk of bowel injury
d.   Entero-enteric bypass can result in a blind loop and bacteria proliferation
e.   If cancer is found, nothing further should be done

Answer e. If cancer is found, palliation with entero-enteric bypass or possibly even resection should be performed.

941. All of the following are true of appendicitis in pregnancy except:
a.   The highest RF for fetal mortality is appendiceal rupture
b.   RUQ pain is often found in the 3rd trimester
c.   Fetal loss is 5-10%
d.   Premature labor occurs in 10-15%
e.   Laparoscopic approach is strongly recommended if in the 3rd trimester

Answer e. Due to the enlarged uterus, laparoscopy is difficult in the 3rd trimester and an open procedure is often best (mark the site of maximal tenderness before putting the patient to sleep - appendix will be more cephalad than usual).

942. A 25 yo man undergoes open appendectomy for perforated appendicitis and on POD 4 is noted to have stool emanating from his RLQ incision. The most appropriate next step is:
a.   Cecostomy tube
b.   Right hemicolectomy
c.   Stoma device over the inicison
d.   Percutaneous drainage only
e.   Washout, attempt closure of cecum, and place drains

Answer e. This patient has an **appendix stump blow out**. Potential consequences of this include peritonitis, sepsis, abscess, and necrotizing soft tissue infection. Adhesions have not formed yet (too early - only POD 4) so the leak is not likely contained. Washout, attempt closure of cecum, and placement of drains is appropriate.

If this presented on POD 7, treating this as a cecal fistula would be appropriate (60-70% of these will heal on their own with conservative Tx).

943. A 70 yo man presents with a 5 day history of RLQ pain, WBCs 16 with a left shift, and a mild fever. He has mild localized tenderness in his RLQ but no gross peritonitis. CT scan shows a phlegmon near the cecum and you cannot identify an appendix. All of the following are true in this patient's management except:
a.   He should be started on IV antibiotics and bowel rest
b.   If an abscess is identified, it should be drained percutaneously
c.   This patient should undergo emergent surgery
d.   Symptoms can be minimal in this population

Answer c. **Perforated appendicitis** with **delayed presentation** and subsequent phlegmon formation is MC in the elderly who can have reduced Sx's from appendicitis. *Surgery at this time point (well after the time of rupture) has a high Cx rate and should be avoided.*

These patients should be placed on **antibiotics** and **bowel rest**. If an **abscess** is identified, **percutaneous drainage** should be performed.

Interval appendectomy (6-8 weeks after initial presentation) is not recommended by most because: 1) it has a fairly high complication rate and 2) the risk of recurrent appendicitis is low [15%] and can be treated at the time of presentation

ANATOMY AND PHYSIOLOGY

- **SMA** - blood supply from 3rd portion of duodenum to proximal 2/3 transverse colon
- **IMA** - blood supply from the distal 1/3 transverse colon to the upper rectum
- **Duodenum**
  - **Bulb** (1st portion) - 90% of ulcers here; *more distal ulcers think gastrinoma*
  - **Descending** (2nd) - contains Ampulla of Vater
  - **Transverse** (3rd) - under the SMA and SMV
  - **Ascending** (4th) - distal portion held in place by ligament of Treitz
  - **Vascular supply**
    - **Superior pancreaticoduodenal artery** (anterior and posterior branches) - off *gastroduodenal artery*
    - **Inferior pancreaticoduodenal artery** (anterior and posterior branches) - off *SMA (1st branch of the SMA)*
    - Many communications between these artery systems
    - **SMA** eventually becomes **ileocolic artery**
  - **Anatomical features**
    - 2nd and 3rd portions of duodenum are **retroperitoneal**
    - 3rd to 4th portions **transition point** is the acute angle between the aorta (posterior) and SMA (anterior)
- **Jejunum**
  - Apx 100 cm long; long vasa recta off **SMA**; circular muscle folds
  - *Maximum site of all absorption except:*
    - **Iron** (*duodenum*) - have both **heme** and **Fe transporters**
    - **Calcium** (*duodenum*)
    - **Bile acids** (*ileum* - non-conjugated; *terminal ileum* - conjugated)
    - **B$_{12}$** (*terminal ileum*)
    - **Folate** (*terminal ileum*)
  - 95% of all **NaCl** and **water** absorbed in **jejunum** (maximum site)
- **Ileum** - apx 50 cm long; short vasa recta coming off **SMA**; flat appearance
  - Important for **bile acid, B$_{12}$, and folate absorption**
  - Patients at higher risk for *short-bowel syndrome* with ileal resection (including terminal ileum) compared to same length jejunal resection due to loss of bile acid, B$_{12}$, and folate
- **Normal bowel sizes**:
  - Small bowel (3 cm)
  - Transverse colon (6 cm)
  - Cecum (9 cm)
- **Migrating motor complex** (MMC, gut motility)
  - **Phase I** - rest
  - **Phase II** - acceleration and gallbladder contraction
  - **Phase III** - peristalsis
  - **Phase IV** - deceleration
  - *Motilin is the most important hormone in migrating motor complex (**initiates phase III peristalsis**; released during non-eating [inter-digestive] periods)*
- **Intestinal brush border** - microvilli; **intra-membrane enzymes** (eg maltase, sucrase) break down **carbohydrates** and allow absorption
- **Cell types**
  - **Enterocytes** (simple columnar cells) - absorptive cells (primary fuel - **glutamine**)
  - **Goblet cells** - secrete **mucus** (mucin); protective layer
  - **Brunner's glands** (in duodenum) - secrete **alkaline solution**
    - **Protects duodenum** from acid, lubricates, and creates alkaline environment for **activation of enzymes**
    - *Jejunum <u>lacks</u> Brunner's glands – reason **marginal ulcers** occur after gastro-jejunostomy; Tx: PPI*
  - **Peyer's patches** (GALT; gut associated lymphoid tissue; found in gut wall)
  - **IgA** - plasma cells provide IgA to mucosal cells for release into the lumen
  - **Paneth cells** - **host defense** against microbes (release alpha-defensins, lysozymes)
  - **Enteroendocrine cells** - many types; endocrine function on gut
  - **Enterochromaffin cells** (APUD, carcinoid precursor) - release **serotonin** (5-HT); important for gut secretion, peristalsis, nausea

PNEUMOTOSIS INTESTINALIS
- Gas in the bowel wall (is a radiographic or operative finding, not a disease itself)
- Etiologies - COPD, bowel obstruction or incarceration, mesenteric ischemia, NEC, inflammatory bowel states, use of steroids, immunodeficient states (eg chemotherapy [neutropenic typhlitis]), collagen vascular disease
- Readily seen on plain film (usually indicates need for CT scan to check for disease process)
- Can reflect a benign, unrelated issue (eg COPD) or a potentially catastrophic intestinal disease process (eg mesenteric ischemia)
- By itself, is not an indication for surgery

SHORT BOWEL SYNDROME (short gut syndrome)
- Inability to absorb enough water and nutritional elements to be off TPN
- Dx is made on Sx's, not length of bowel
- Usually (75%) results from one massive bowel resection (eg mesenteric ischemia, CA, Crohn's), not multiple resections
  - Children - usually from midgut volvulus, intestinal atresia, or necrotizing enterocolitis
- Sx's: **steatorrhea**, weight loss, nutritional deficiency (lose fat, B-12, electrolytes, water), abdominal pain
  - **Interruption of bile salt resorption** (if terminal ileum gone or just short length) interferes with micelle formation and causes **steatorrhea**
  - **Hyper-secretion of acid** with short bowel → ↓ pH → ↑intestinal motility; interferes with fat absorption → **steatorrhea**
- **Sudan red stain** - checks for fecal fat
- **Schilling test** - checks for B_{12} absorption (radiolabeled B_{12} in urine)
- Normal small bowel length - 600 cm; start to have absorption issues with < 200 cm
- Resection of jejunum better tolerated than ileum (**ileum absorbs bile salts and B-12**)
- Presence of **ileocecal valve** reduces malabsorption as it decreases transit time, allowing for absorption
- Intact **colon** also important (fluid and electrolyte absorption)
- Probably need at least 75 cm to survive off TPN; 50 cm with competent ileocecal valve
- Tx:
  - **Low fat diet**
  - **PPI** (eg Omeprazole; to reduce acid which can cause hypermotility)
  - **Lomotil** (diphenoxylate and atropine) or **loperamide** - slows gut motility
  - **Lactase** (may help if lactose intolerant)
  - **Cholestyramine** (low dose, reduces diarrhea from unabsorbed bile salts)
  - **Octreotide** for refractory cases (reduces GI secretions)
  - **TPN** for acute episodes (chronic TPN leads to cirrhosis)
  - Consider growth hormone and glutamine if still requiring TPN
  - Intestinal adaptation may take 1-2 years
  - Consider **small bowel lengthening** procedure or **small bowel transplant** for refractory cases

CAUSES OF STEATORRHEA
- **Gastric acid**→ ↓ pH→ ↑ intestinal motility, poor fat absorption (eg short gut syndrome)
- **Pancreatic enzyme deficiency** (eg chronic pancreatitis)
- **Bile salt deficiency** (eg terminal ileum resection; biliary obstruction) interferes with micelle formation and fat absorption
- Steatorrhea results in poor nutrition, deficiency of fat soluble vitamins (Vit's A, D, E and K), and deficiency of essential fatty acids (wound healing)

ENTEROCUTANEOUS FISTULA (small or large bowel fistula)
- "FRIENDS" - mnemonic for causes of non-healing fistula: foreign body, radiation, inflammatory bowel disease, epithelialization, neoplasm, distal obstruction, sepsis/Infection
- Categorized by output:

High output:	> 400 cc/d
Medium output:	200-400 cc/d
Low output:	< 200 cc/d

- High-output fistulas are more likely with *proximal bowel* (duodenum or proximal jejunum) and are less likely to close with conservative Tx
- Colonic fistulas are more likely to close than those in the small bowel
- Patients with persistent **fever** → need to check for **abscess** (Dx - fistulogram, CT scan, upper GI with small bowel follow-through)
- Most fistulas are **iatrogenic** and treated conservatively 1st → NPO, TPN, skin protection (stoma appliance), octreotide, PPI, loperamide, and 1 week of antibiotics
- Majority close spontaneously without surgery
- Wait 2-3 months before operating on fistulas (some say 3-6 months)
- Surgery: resect bowel fistula segment, primary anastomosis (80% success)
- **Mortality** (15%) most often related to development of **sepsis** (need early drainage of any associated abscess, antibiotics)

SMALL BOWEL OBSTRUCTION
- **MCC without previous surgery**
  - Small bowel - hernia
  - Large bowel - cancer
- **MCC with previous surgery**
  - Small bowel - adhesions
  - Large bowel - cancer
- Sx's: N/V, crampy intermittent abdominal pain, failure to pass gas or stool, previous surgery or XRT
  - Look for **hernias** and **rectal mass**
  - If still **passing gas** - usually indicates partial bowel obstruction
  - Sx's suspicious of **infarction** or **perforation**: fever, tachycardia, leukocytosis, sepsis, peritoneal signs, continuous as opposed to intermittent pain
- 3rd spacing of fluid into **bowel lumen** occurs - need **aggressive fluid resuscitation**
- Air with bowel obstruction - from **swallowed nitrogen**
- Dx: **CT scan** *(best test)* - air-fluid levels, distended loops of small bowel, distal decompression; if **previous CA** → need CT scan to rule-out recurrence
- Tx: *fluid resuscitation 1st*
  - If strangulation not suspected - NGT, IVFs, bowel rest for 48 hours, correct electrolytes (especially K and Mg); serial exams and X-rays
  - If **strangulated** bowel suspected - go to OR for resection
  - Failure to resolve after 3-5 days → OR for exploration
- **Surgical indications**:
  - Progressing pain
  - Diffuse peritoneal signs (rebound tenderness, involuntary guarding)
  - Failure to resolve after 3-5 days
  - Suspected strangulation, infarction, or perforation
  - Non-reducible hernia (inguinal or ventral)
  - Free air

ENTERO-ENTERIC BYPASS
- May be necessary when resection of bowel for obstruction is unsafe or would result in short gut syndrome (eg previous XRT with matted bowel, previous bowel resections and potential for short-gut, mesenteric fibrosis, diffuse tumor implants, extensive desmoid tumors)
- **Blind loop** is created that can lead to bacterial overgrowth (blind loop syndrome)
  - Can lead to toxic metabolites, steatorrhea, and poor nutrient absorption
  - Sx's: diarrhea, bloating, fever, malaise; positive urea breath test
  - Tx: periodic **metronidazole**; electrolyte, mineral, and vitamin replacement

GALLSTONE ILEUS
- Small bowel obstruction from **gallstone** usually in the **terminal ileum**
- Classically see **air in the biliary tree** and a **small bowel obstruction**
- Caused by a **fistula** between **gallbladder** and 2nd **portion of duodenum**
- Tx: remove stone from terminal ileum
  - Can leave gallbladder and fistula if the patient is old and frail
  - If not old / frail, perform cholecystectomy and close hole in duodenum

MECKEL'S DIVERTICULUM
- Rule of 2's: 2 feet from ileocecal valve; 2% of population; usually presents in 1st 2 years of life with bleeding; is a **true diverticulum**
- Caused by failure of closure of the **omphalomesenteric duct**
- MCC of **painless lower GI bleeds in children**
- **Pancreas tissue** - MC tissue found in Meckel's (can cause **diverticulitis**)
- **Gastric mucosa** - most likely to be symptomatic (MC Sx - **bleeding**)
- **Obstruction** - MC presentation in adults
- **Bleeding** - caused by secretion of gastric juice onto ileum (creates ulcer that bleeds)
  - Segmental resection indicated if bleeding Sx's (is not bleeding from the diverticulum, is bleeding from adjacent ileum)
- **Incidental** → usually not removed unless gastric mucosa suspected (diverticulum feels thick) or has a very narrow neck
- Dx: get a **Meckel's scan** (^{99}Tc) if trouble localizing (mucosa lights up)
- Tx: **diverticulectomy** for uncomplicated diverticulitis
  - Need *segmental* bowel resection for: 1) **bleeding**, 2) **complicated diverticulitis** (eg perforation), 3) **neck > ⅓ the diameter** of normal bowel lumen, *or;* 4) if diverticulitis involves the **base**

DUODENAL DIVERTICULA
- Rule-out **gallbladder disease** (chronic cholecystitis) origin
  - Can be confused with a gallbladder to duodenal fistula (which is how a gallstone ileus occurs; Dx: **CT scan**)
- **Frequency** of diverticula - duodenal > jejunal > ileal
- 70% are in the **2nd portion** of duodenum, often **within 2 cm** of the ampulla (**peri-ampullary**)
- Are a **false diverticulum** (mucosa and submucosa; no muscle); usually on mesenteric border (weakness in bowel wall where blood vessels penetrate)
- *Vast majority (>90%) are asymptomatic*
- Tx:
  - *Observe* unless perforated, bleeding, obstruction (ie diverticulitis), or highly symptomatic (eg pancreatitis or biliary obstruction with jaundice, cholangitis, or choledochlithiasis)
  - Can be difficult cases - underlying concept is figure out something other than a Whipple to Tx symptomatic duodenal diverticula
  - Obstruction with **food** - may be able to remove with EGD
  - **Bleeding** - can be treated with EGD therapy
  - **Perforation** - need resection, consider serosal patch
  - If not **juxta-ampullary** and need operation → Tx: **resection** with primary repair or primary anastomosis
  - **Juxta-ampullary** (ie you don't think you can get primary closure by just resecting it; diverticula is immediately adjacent to or in ampulla):
    - → if **biliary** obstruction - Tx: **hepatico-jejunostomy** (if choledochlithiasis, ERCP can be effective acutely)
    - → if **pancreatic** obstruction - Tx (many options): possible ductoplasty where the duct of Wirsung is opened and sewed to the diverticulum itself; ERCP with stent; some suggest just diversion with gastro-jejunostomy

CROHN'S DISEASE
- Sx's: intermittent **abdominal pain, diarrhea** (not grossly bloody), and **weight loss**
  - Can cause fibrosis, strictures (bowel obstructions), fistulas, and abscesses
  - *MC surgical disease of the small bowel*
- **Transmural** inflammation of GI tract with **skip lesions**
  - Can occur anywhere from **mouth to anus** (usually spares rectum)
  - MC site - **terminal ileum**
  - MC perinanal Sx - large **perianal skin tags** (in 40%; *do not resect*)
  - Crohn's disease usually ***spares* rectum** (unlike UC)
- Can get **toxic megacolon** or **toxic colitis** - fever, tachycardia, ↑ed WBCs, distension
- Extra-intestinal manifestations - growth failure, arthritis, arthralgias, pyoderma gangrenosum, ocular diseases, megaloblastic anemia (folate and B_{12} malabsorption), gallstones, kidney stones

- MC sites for **initial presentation**:
  - **Terminal ileum** (MC) and cecum - 40%
  - Colon only - 35%
  - Small bowel only - 20%
  - Perianal - 5%
  - Isolated upper GI tract - rare
- MC surgical disease of the small bowel
- **Bimodal** age distribution: 20's and 50's
- RFs: Ashkenazi Jews, smokers, northern latitudes, familial inheritance, urban areas, higher socioeconomic status, Accutane (isotretinoin)
- Dx: **enteroclysis** (tube placed through nose to jejunum, barium given, fluoroscopy used to find obstruction); **colonoscopy** with biopsies
- Operative findings - **creeping mesenteric fat** (mesenteric fat wrapping - *considered pathognomonic* of Crohn's; encroachment of mesenteric fat on serosal surface of bowel), thickened mesentery and thickened bowel wall, strictures, skip lesions (segmental disease), rectal-sparing, transmural involvement, cobble-stoning, fistulas; non-caseating granulomas *(hallmark finding)* on path
- *Earliest* lesion suggesting Crohn's - **aphthous ulcers** in colon or small bowel
- Medical Tx: **sulfasalazine** *(best)* and **loperamide** are *best maintenance Tx* for low grade chronic disease (eg colitis, ileocolitis)
  - **Acute Flare Tx** - **corticosteroids** (*best Tx for acute exacerbation*)
    - Add antibiotics (**Cipro + Flagyl**) if fever, high WBCs, or if worried about toxic megacolon or toxic colitis
    - Flagyl *side effects* - **peripheral neuropathy** with chronic use
    - Ciprofloxacin *side effects* - **tendon rupture**
  - **Infliximab** (TNF-α inhibitor) - used for **fistulas** or **steroid-resistant disease** (chronic or flare-ups)
    - Infliximab *side effects*: **TB infection** or reactivation, CHF, multiple sclerosis
  - Low residue diet - avoid fiber in cereal, bread, nuts, vegetables
  - <u>No</u> agents affect the natural course of disease (*avoid* NSAIDs)
  - **TPN** - may induce remission and fistula closure
  - *Avoid* chronic steroids (prednisone) *if possible* - use steroids for acute flares
- **90%** eventually need an **operation**
- 50% recurrence rate requiring another surgery after resection
- *No pouches or ileo-anal anastomosis with Crohn's*
- **Surgical indications** - unlike ulcerative colitis, surgery is <u>not</u> curative; effort should be made to *conserve* bowel in these patient and *avoid* short bowel syndrome
  - **Persistent obstruction** (usually from <u>strictures</u>) - often partial obstruction; conservative Tx initially; persistent obstruction managed by stricturoplasty or segmental resection
  - **Abscess** - Tx: percutaneous drainage
  - Refractory **toxic colitis** or **toxic megacolon** (perforation in 15%) - not very common in Crohn's but can occur
  - **Free perforation** - uncommon
  - **Hemorrhage** - unusual in Crohn's
  - **Closed loop obstruction** (dilated loop of small bowel) - need resection
  - **CA** (Crohn's **pan-colitis** at highest risk)
  - *Any* **dysplasia**
  - Refractory **fistulas**
- **Stricturoplasty** (longitudinal incision through stricture on anti-mesenteric border, close transversely); consider Bx at time of stricture to rule-out malignancy
  - Consider if multiple bowel strictures to save small bowel length
  - For strictures **< 10 cm**, *longitudinal enterotomy with transverse closure* is used (Heineke-Mikulicz type)
  - For strictures **10 - 25 cm**, the segment is folded in half and a *side to side anastomosis* is performed (Finney type)
  - 10% leakage / abscess / fistula rate with stricturoplasty (all of which can usually be treated conservatively)
  - Recurrent surgical Crohn's following stricturoplasty is most likely to occur in <u>non-stricturoplasty sites</u> (90%)
  - *Stricturoplasty is <u>not</u> used for* **colon** *Crohn's disease*

- **Segmental resection**
  - *Do not need clear margins*; just get **2 cm** away from **gross disease**
  - *Exceptions* - refractory **toxic megacolon / colitis, colon perforation,** *or* **pancolitis with dysplasia** will require **total abdominal colectomy** with ileostomy
- **Enterocutaneous fistula** (MC in small bowel)
  - Can usually be treated **conservatively**
  - Dx:
    - **UGI** with SBFT and **barium enema** to rule-out **distal stenosis** (will need resection or stricturoplasty if obstruction present)
    - **CT scan** to rule-out **abscess** (percutaneous drain if present)
  - Tx:
    - **High output** fistulas (> 400 cc/d)- **NPO**, TPN, stoma appliance over fistula
    - **Low output** fistulas (< 200 cc/d) - allow PO; avoids TPN Cx's
    - Continue **maintenance** Crohn's Tx
    - *Add* **Infliximab** and **Flagyl** - both increase fistula closure rate
    - **PPI** (reduces acid which slows down gut), **octreotide** (decreases secretions), and **loperamide** (slows down gut)
    - Conservative Tx for 2-3 months (be patient with these; majority close on their own; some wait 3-6 months)
    - If above fails - resection of involved segment, primary re-anastomosis, and coverage with omentum
- **Peri-anal fistula** (fistulo-in-ano)
  - Tx: **conservative Tx** with draining setons and local wound care best
  - **Infliximab** and **Flagyl** (improve healing)
  - If asymptomatic - *leave alone*
- **Anorectal-vaginal** and **colovesicle fistulas** - *conservative Tx best* with **Infliximab** and **Flagyl** as a first step; may need surgery if persistent
- **Fissures** - *No lateral internal sphincteroplasty with Crohn's* (will *not* heal)
  - See Rectum and Anus chapter for conservative Tx
- **Hemorrhoids** or **perianal skin tags** → ***No resection***
- **Diffuse severe colon disease** - total proctocolectomy and ileostomy the procedure of choice (***No pouches*** *or ilio-anal anastomosis with Crohn's*)
- **Duodenal Crohn's** (get strictures and ulceration; rare)
  - Medical Tx as above, surgery if refractory
  - **1st + 2nd portions** of duodenum
    - Tx: **Gastro-jejunostomy** and **vagotomy** (+ pyloroplasty)
      - Vagotomy to avoid **marginal ulceration**
      - *Stricturoplasty not an option in 1st and 2nd portions of duodenum*
      - *Do not perform Whipple for duodenal Crohn's*
  - **3rd + 4th portions** of duodenum
    - Tx: Resection with **duodeno-jejunostomy** (usual)
      - Could also do a **stricturoplasty** if short stricture
- **Incidental finding** of inflammatory bowel disease at surgery for presumed appendicitis and patient has a normal appendix - Tx: **remove appendix** if cecum not involved (avoids future confounding diagnosis)
- **Cx's from terminal ileum resection** (or severe disease in terminal ileum which has become non-functional for absorption)
  - ↓ed B$_{12}$ and **folate uptake** can result in **megaloblastic anemia**
  - ↓ed **oxalate binding** to calcium secondary to ↑ed intraluminal fat (fat binds Ca) → oxalate then gets absorbed in colon → released in urine → **Ca oxalate kidney stones** (hyperoxaluria)
  - ↓ed **bile salt uptake** causes osmotic **diarrhea** (bile salts) and **steatorrhea** (fat) in colon; Tx - Lomotil and cholestyramine
  - **Bile salt** malabsorption can lead to **gallstones**
- **Crohn's pan-colitis** - same **colon CA risk** as Ulcerative Colitis
  - Surveillance for Crohn's pan-colitis same as for UC

CARCINOID

- Sx's: **abdominal pain** (often mistaken for appendicitis), possible small bowel obstruction
    - Pain from **mass** or **vasoconstriction** and **fibrosis** (desmoplastic reaction)
    - Tricuspid valve insufficiency
- MC <u>benign</u> (although can be malignant) and MC <u>overall</u> **appendix tumor**
    - MC malignant appendix tumor is adenocarcinoma
- **Carcinoid syndrome** (10% of patients) - intermittent **facial flushing** (*kallikrein*) and **diarrhea** (*serotonin*) are hallmark Sx's
    - Caused by bulky **liver metastases** that bypass metabolism (could also be caused by retroperitoneal invasion with systemic venous drainage)
    - **Asthma-like** Sx's (eg bronchospasm) and **hypotension** *(both from bradykinin)*
    - If patient has carcinoid syndrome with a small bowel primary, it indicates **liver metastases** (liver usually clears serotonin, mediators)
    - **Carcinoid crisis** - severe and acute manifestation of the above Sx's, often precipitated by another event (eg anesthesia, surgery, biopsy); Tx - **octreotide**
- Dx: **CT scan**
    - **Chromogranin A** level *(best screening test for Dx*; almost <u>100%</u> have this)
        Highest sensitivity for detecting tumor (but not location)
        Also good to detecting <u>recurrence</u> and <u>response to Tx</u>
        Not as specific as urine 5-HIAA
    - **Octreotide scan** *(best test for localization)*; highest sensitivity to localize tumor
    - **Urine 5-HIAA** (from serotonin breakdown, *not* all carcinoids have this)
        False positive 5-HIAA - fruits
- **Path:**
    - **Kulchitsky cells** (neural crest cells; neuroendocrine) - part of amine precursor uptake decarboxylase system (APUD)
    - **MC sites** (SEER Data) - #1 **ileum**, #2 **rectum**, #3 **appendix** (10% malignant)
    - Site with the *highest* **metastatic** and *highest* **Carcinoid syndrome** rates - **ileum** (35% malignant, 20% Carcinoid Syndrome)
    - Site with the best 5-YS - **appendix** (5-YS: 90%), #2 rectum (5-YS: 75%)
    - Small bowel carcinoid - patients at high risk (20%) for **multiple primaries** and second **unrelated GI malignancies**
- **Debulking** - good for palliation if suffering from carcinoid syndrome
    - If liver metastasis resection performed, also perform **cholecystectomy** for future hepatic arterial embolization of symptomatic metastases
- Chemo - **alpha-interferon**; usually just for unresectable disease
- **Octreotide** - <u>very effective</u> for Tx of carcinoid syndrome Sx's (can be used for **acute Sx's** or **chronically**)
- Appendix carcinoid overall 5-year survival - 90% *(best of all appendix malignancies)*
    - 5-YS for **localized** appendix lesion - 95%
    - 5-YS with **metastases** - 35% *(palliation with octreotide is an important part of Tx for metastatic carcinoid tumors - patients can survive a long time)*
- **Appendix** carcinoid Tx:
    - < 2 cm, base and meso-appendix <u>not</u> involved, <u>no</u> nodes, and <u>no</u> metastases → **appendectomy**
    - ≥ 2 cm, involved base or meso-appendix, positive nodes, or metastases → **right hemicolectomy**
- **Small bowel** carcinoid Tx - segmental resection with lymphadenectomy
- **Colon** and **rectum** carcinoids
    - 15% of all carcinoids; *infrequent* carcinoid syndrome
    - **Metastases** related to tumor size: < 1 cm (rare), 1-2 cm (10%), > 2 cm (70%)
    - 70% of **colon** carcinoids have either local or systemic spread; 25% for **rectum**
    - **Low rectal** carcinoids (ie not able to perform LAR)
        < 2 cm → WLE with negative margins
        > 2 cm <u>or</u> invasion of **muscularis propria** → APR
    - **Colon** and **high rectal** carcinoids
        < 1 cm → endoscopic or trans-anal removal
        ≥ 1 cm <u>or</u> invasion of **muscularis propria** → appropriate segmental resection with lymphadenectomy
    - Rectal carcinoids are more common than colon and have abetter prognosis

- ■ **Duodenal** carcinoids:
  - **Non peri-ampullary** carcinoids
    - Not as aggressive as peri-ampullary and ampullary carcinoids
    - **< 1 cm** - endoscopic removal
    - **1-2 cm** - WLE with negative margins
    - **> 2 cm** - formal resection with lymphadenectomy
  - **Peri-ampullary** carcinoid - _very aggressive_ tumors and **Whipple** is indicated

INTUSSUSCEPTION IN ADULTS
- ■ Often from small bowel or cecal tumors in adults
- ■ Tumor forms lead point, peristalsis then takes tumor and adjacent bowel into distal intestine, forming intussusception (MC intussusception type - **ileo-colic**)
- ■ MC Sx - **obstruction**; MCC - **cecal adenocarcinoma** (ileo-colic intussusception)
- ■ Worrisome in adults as 70% have a **malignant lead point** (eg cecal CA)
- ■ Do _not_ reduce with barium enema in adults → go to OR for resection
- ■ Tx: do _not_ reduce in OR unless confirmed benign cause → just perform **resection** of the area as it is very likely a malignancy (manipulation and reduction can lead to venous metastases); **ileo-colic anastomosis** usual
  - If confirmed benign cause (eg J-tube lead point) or risk of short bowel syndrome (from previous resections) - reduce in the OR (milk it out in a distal to proximal direction) and limit resection

BENIGN SMALL BOWEL TUMORS (rare)
- ■ Benign small bowel tumors are more common than malignant (but still rare)
- ■ **MC benign small bowel tumor** - adenoma (can become CA)
- ■ **Adenomas** - MC in duodenum, usually near ampulla; Sx's - bleeding, obstruction
  - Need resection when identified (often done with endoscopy; for ampullary villous adenomas see below)
  - These are considered _pre-malignant_
- ■ **Ampullary villous adenoma** (are _pre-malignant_)
  - Villous adenoma in the Ampulla of Vater
  - Sx's: obstructive **jaundice** and **heme positive stools** _(classic)_
    - Can cause pancreatitis
  - Dx: get ERCP with Bx's to truly define lesion
    - High **false negative rate** with Bx (ie Bx misses CA harboring in adenoma) - up to **70% have CA** in them on pathology
  - Tx: **endoscopic** or **wide local excision** (will likely end up doing sphincteroplasty or ductoplasty after resection of benign tumor)
    - Send for frozen section to confirm benign (need Whipple if malignant)
    - Do _not_ perform Whipple if benign
- ■ **GIST tumors** (can be malignant) – see stomach chapter
- ■ **Peutz-Jeghers syndrome** (autosomal dominant, STK11 / LKB1 gene mutation)
  - **Hamartomatous polyps** throughout GI tract (small / large bowel, MC in jejunum and ileum
  - Sx's: can cause obstruction (MC 1st presentation - **bowel obstruction**, usually from **intussusception**); bleeding and anemia can occur
  - **Hyper-pigmentation** (melanotic patches, freckles) of **mucus membranes** (oral) and **skin** (hands and feet)
  - Patients have significantly increased risk of **extra-intestinal malignancies** (MC - **breast CA**; others - lung, ovaries, testicles) and a small risk of GI malignancies (related to adenomatous changes in hamartomatous polyp)
  - _No_ significant increased risk of colon CA → _No_ prophylactic colectomy
  - Mean survival - 57 years of age
  - **Screening**
    - EGD and **colonoscopy** every 1-2 yrs; remove polyps if **> 5 cm**, if **hemorrhagic**, or if they look **malignant**
    - Also need screening for uterus, ovary, cervix, breast, testicles

MALIGNANT SMALL BOWEL TUMORS (rare)

- **Adenocarcinoma** (rare) - MC malignant small bowel tumor
  - High proportion in **duodenum** (40%); usually originate at ampulla (**ampullary adenocarcinoma**) from previous ampullary villous adenoma
  - RFs: FAP, Gardner's, polyps, adenomas
  - Sx's: **obstructive jaundice** and **heme positive stools**; bowel obstruction
  - **Small bowel** *(other than duodenum)* - Tx: resection + lymphadenectomy
  - Duodenum:
    - **1st** or **2nd portions** of duodenum → Tx: **Whipple** usual (ampulla usually involved)
    - **3rd** or **4th portions** of duodenum → Tx: resection with **duodeno-jejunal anastomosis** *(not Whipple)*
- **Leiomyosarcoma**
  - Usually in **jejunum** and **ileum**; most extraluminal
  - Can be hard to differentiate compared with leiomyoma (> 5 mitoses/50 HPF, atypia, necrosis)
  - Make sure it is not a **GIST** (check for C-Kit)
  - Tx: resection; _no lymph node dissection_

SMALL BOWEL LYMPHOMA

- MC site - **ileum** (large amount of lymphoid tissue; Peyer's Patches)
- MC type - **B cell** (non-Hodgkin's lymphoma)
- **Post-TXP lymphoma** - increased risk of **bleeding** and **perforation**
- Sx's: pain, weight loss, obstruction, N/V
- RFs: HIV (AIDS), SLE, Crohn's, post-TXP
- Dx: CT scan
- Tx: **wide en bloc resection** (include affected mesentery) with negative margins, mesenteric and para-aortic node sampling outside zone of resection; liver Bx
  - 5-YS - **40%**
  - If in **1st** or **2nd portions** of the duodenum (chemo +/- XRT; _no Whipple_)

STOMAS

- **Parastomal hernias** - highest incidence with **colostomies**; *generally well tolerated and do not need repair unless symptomatic*
- *Candida* - MC stomal infection
- **Diversion colitis** (Hartmann's pouch) - due to lack of short-chain fatty acids
  - Tx: short-chain fatty acid enemas (butyric acid enemas)
- **Ischemia** - MCC of stenosis of stoma
  - Tx: dilation if mild
- **Crohn's disease** - MCC of fistula near stoma site
- **Abscesses** - underneath stoma site, often caused by irrigation device (Tx: drainage)
- **Gallstones** (loss of bile salts) and **uric acid kidney stones** (loss of HCO_3^-) are *increased* in patients with an ileostomy

APPENDICITIS

- Sx's: 1st - **anorexia**; 2nd - **abdominal pain** (periumbilical); 3rd - **vomiting**
- Pain gradually migrates to the **RLQ** as peritonitis sets in (McBurney's point)
  - Periumbilical pain - visceral pain (from distension of appendix; dull ache, N/V)
  - RLQ pain - somatic pain (from peritoneal irritation; localized)
- MC in patients aged **20 - 35**; MC in **males** (3:1)
- Patients can have normal WBC count
- **CT scan** - diameter **> 7 mm** or wall thickness **> 2 mm** (looks like a bull's eye), fat stranding, no contrast in appendiceal lumen
  - Children and females benefit the most from pre-op CT scan (ie these groups have lower negative appendicitis rates at surgery [lower false positive rate] with the use of pre-op CT scan)
  - *CT scan has not changed negative appendicitis surgery rates (10%)*
- MC area to **perforate** - at **midpoint** of anti-mesenteric border
- MCC in children - **lymph node hyperplasia** (can follow a viral illness)
- MCC in adults - **fecalith**

- **Luminal obstruction** followed by (in order): distention of appendix, venous congestion and thrombosis, ischemia, gangrene necrosis, and rupture
  - Is considered a closed loop obstruction
- **Delayed presentation** of perforated appendicitis
  - **Days** (usually 4-5 days) after initial pain episode
  - MC in the **elderly** who can have minimal Sx's
  - CT scan shows **walled-off perforated appendix** (phlegmon)
  - Surgery at this time point (well after the time of rupture) has a high Cx rate and should be _avoided_
  - Tx: **antibiotics** and **bowel rest** *(is a non-operative situation)*
    - 10% failure rate requiring surgery
    - **Percutaneous drainage** if abscess present
    - Follow-up **colonoscopy** to rule-out perforated cecal CA - occasionally, what was thought to be ruptured appendicitis turns out to be a **perforated cecal colon CA**
    - *Interval appendectomy not recommended by most because: 1) it has a fairly high complication rate and 2) the risk of recurrent appendicits is low [15%] and can be treated at the time of presentation*
- **Children** and **elderly** have a higher propensity to **rupture** secondary to delayed diagnosis
  - Children often have **higher fever** and _more_ **vomiting / diarrhea**
  - **Elderly** - Sx's can be minimal (_less_ vomiting / diarrhea); right hemicolectomy if CA suspected
  - *Appendicitis is rare in infants*
- **Perforation** - patient generally more ill; can have evidence of sepsis
- **Fever** or **abdominal pain** after appendectomy - get CT scan, look for abscess (Tx: percutaneous drainage, _not_ re-operation)
- **Drainage of stool** from RLQ incision (appendix stump blow-out; most commonly occurs following **perforated** appendix):
  - **< 7 days** from surgery - re-explore, washout, place drains, consider stapling across cecum if tissue looks good; washout RLQ incision as well (loose closure)
  - **≥ 7 days** from surgery - adhesions prevent safe return to the abdomen at this point; consider it a **cecal fistula** (are generally low output); place stoma appliance and follow (60-70% heal on their own); surgery after 6-8 weeks if it persists; surgery sooner if conservative Tx fails (eg sepsis)
- **Pregnancy** with appendicitis
  - MC problem requiring **surgery** in pregnancy
  - May have **RUQ** pain in 3rd trimester - uterus displaces appendix cephalad with pregnancy; pain may be exacerbated when lying on **right side**
  - Dx: get an U/S 1st (diameter > 7, thickness > 2)
  - Laparoscopic appendectomy if 1st or 2nd trimester; open usual for 3rd
  - If open appendectomy, **mark site of incision over the site of maximal pain** before you put patient to sleep → appendix is displaced **superiorly** by uterus
  - High **appendix rupture** (10-15%), **premature labor** (10-15%), and **fetal loss** (5-10%) rates with appendicitis in pregnancy
  - _Also_ a higher **negative appendicitis rate** (false positive) at surgery compared to non-pregnant women
  - Highest RF for **fetal mortality** - appendiceal rupture

APPENDIX MUCOCELES
- Etiologies - retention cyst, mucosal hyperplasia, mucinous adenoma, mucinous adenocarcinoma
- The **mucocele** fills with mucoid material and can eventually rupture (yellow-gray mucoid material)
- The central issue here is that **endothelial cells** within the mucocele (regardless of benign or malignant etiology) can form implants on peritoneal surfaces. These implants can grow, release mucoid material, form more implants, ect. and eventually cause **bowel obstruction** in a process known as **pseudomyxoma peritonei**
- MCC of death in these patients - **small bowel obstruction**
- Tx: all mucoceles should be resected with **open procedure** (**appendectomy** if benign)
  - Need to _avoid spillage_ of the mucocele's contents to prevent _implants_

- If **mucinous adenocarcinoma** (pathology - Signet ring cells) is found, **right hemicolectomy** is indicated
- The MCC of pseudomyxoma peritonei stems from the **appendix** (*vast majority*); but it can be caused by other **mucin secreting tumors** (eg ovarian mucinous CA - Tx total abdominal hysterectomy and bilateral salpingo-oophorectomy [TAH-BSO])

PSEUDOMYXOMA PERITONEI
- Mucin-secreting cells fill the peritoneal cavity and release **mucin**, which causes **intestinal obstruction** by fibrosis and compression
- Can be **low grade** or **high grade** (Signet Ring cells high grade)
- MCC - **appendix** mucinous denocarcinoma; others (far less common) - ovarian CA
- Dx: **CT scan** - mucoid material filling the abdomen; may have signs of obstruction
- Path - yellow-gray mucoid material
- Tx: 1) **cytoreductive surgery** (removal of <u>primary tumor</u> and secondary <u>implants</u>, removal of <u>peritoneum</u>, removal of <u>omentum</u>; residual tumor deposits should be **< 1 cm**) *and*; 2) **hyperthermic intra-peritoneal chemo** (*heated* mitomycin C; 5-fluorouracil)
- **Appendix mucinous adenocarcinoma** - will need right hemicolectomy
- **Mucinous ovarian CA** - will need TAH-BSO
- These patients can often go on to live very productive lives
- **5-YS**: **80%** for <u>low</u> grade; **60%** for <u>high</u> grade

OTHER APPENDIX
- MC malignant appendix tumor - adenocarcinoma
  - **MC presentation** (40%) - *acute appendicitis*; can also present as SBO or mass
  - **MC subtype** - mucinous adenocarcinoma
- MC benign appendix tumor - non-malignant carcinoid
- Appendix adenocarcinoma - Tx: right hemicolectomy
- Appendix cystadenoma - Tx: <u>open</u> appendectomy
- Appendix cystadenocarcinoma - Tx: right hemicolectomy
- Gastroenteritis - nausea, vomiting, diarrhea
- Regional terminal ileitis - *can **mimic** appendicitis* (RLQ pain)
  - 1) **inflamed mesenteric lymph nodes** (acute mesenteric lymphadenitis) <u>*and;*</u> 2) symmetric inflammation and thickening of **terminal ileum** (ileitis)
  - Use above to differentiate regional ileitis vs. appendicitis (*avoids unnecessary surgery*)
  - Sx's: fever, RLQ pain, N/V, diarrhea, **<u>*no peritoneal signs*</u>**
  - Usually have antecedent **upper respiratory tract infection, pharyngitis**, or exposure to **contaminated food** (other family members may have been sick)
  - Mimics appendicitis although the pain and tenderness is more diffuse without significant guarding or localization
  - MC in **children**
  - 10% is actually early **Crohn's disease**
  - Often caused by Infections – **yersinia (#1)**, campylobacter, salmonella, shigella, strep, mycobacterium
  - Tx: tetracycline or Bactrim (PCN for strep)
  - Finding of regional terminal ileitis does <u>not</u> warrant bowel resection (*course is typically benign*) or lymph node biopsy
  - *If found incidentally at the time of presumed appendicitis, you should perform <u>appendectomy</u> (only if the appendix base at the cecum is <u>not</u> involved) to remove confounding diagnosis in the future*
- At surgery for **presumed appendicitis** but find ruptured ovarian cyst, endometriosis, thrombosed ovarian vein, or regional terminal ileitis <u>not</u> involving cecum → **still perform appendectomy** as long as the appendix base is not involved in the process (*removes confounding diagnosis in the future*)
  - *If the **appendix base** at the cecum is involved in the ileitis or inflammation, <u>avoid</u> appendectomy (risk of perforation and fistula formation)*

- **Typhoid enteritis** (salmonella, foreign travel) - fever, bloody diarrhea, abdominal pain
    - Mesenteric lymphadenopathy and terminal ileitis; enlarged Peyer's patches
    - Tx: antibiotics; if perforation occurs, simple closure of the perforation only (*no segmental resection*)

ILEUS

- Etiologies: **surgery** (MC), electrolyte abnormalities (low **K** and low **Mg**), peritonitis, ischemia, trauma, drugs, pancreatitis
- **Ileus CT scan** - dilatation is uniform throughout the stomach, small bowel, colon, and rectum *without* distal decompression
- **Obstruction CT scan** - there is bowel decompression distal to the obstruction
- Tx: bowel rest, IVFs, NGT, correct electrolytes (K and Mg), ambulation, limit narcotics
- Some use **pro-kinetics** (metoclopramide [Reglan]), **laxatives** (bisacodyl [Dulcolax]), and **opioid antagonists** (Alvimopan) to help prevent prolonged **post-op ileus**

Colon and Rectum

944. All of the following are true except:
    a. The rectal lateral stalks contain the middle rectal arteries
    b. The middle rectal artery is supplied by branches of internal iliac artery
    c. The meandering artery is a direct connection between the proximal SMA and proximal IMA
    d. The middle rectal vein drains into both the inferior mesenteric vein and the internal iliac vein.
    e. The internal anal sphincter is under internal pudendal nerve control (voluntary)

    Answer e. The **internal anal sphincter** is supplied by the pelvic splanchnic nerves, not the pudendal nerve. There is <u>no</u> voluntary control of the internal anal sphincter.

945. All of the following are true except:
    a. Denonvillier's fascia separates the rectum from the prostate and vagina
    b. The main nutrient to colonocytes is short chain fatty acids (eg butyric acid)
    c. The dentate line marks the transition from columnar to squamous epithelium
    d. The pre-sacral fascai separates the rectum from the bladder
    e. Disuse proctitis is treated with short chain fatty acid enemas

    Answer d. The **pre-sacral fascia** (Waldeyer's fascia) separates the rectum from ~~the bladder~~ presacral venous plexus

946. For patients with ulcerative colitis, all of the following improve after colectomy except:
    a. Ocular problems
    b. Arthritis
    c. Anemia
    d. Sclerosing cholangitis

    Answer d. Primary sclerosing cholangitis and ankylosing spondylitis do <u>not</u> get better after colectomy. Interestingly, 70% of all patients with sclerosing cholangitis also have ulcerative colitis (MC associated Dx for sclerosing cholangitis).

947. All of the following are true of ulcerative colitis except:
    a. The MC extra-intestinal manifestation requiring colectomy is failure to thrive
    b. The MC indication for pouch takedown with permanent ileostomy (ie APR) is incontinence
    c. Steroids are the best therapy for acute exacerbations
    d. Low grade dysplasia can be followed
    e. Crypt abscess is consistent with ulcerative colitis

    Answer d. <u>Any</u> **dysplasia** with UC is an indication for **procto-colectomy**.

948. A patient with ulcerative colitis and low grade dysplasia in the upper rectum should undergo:
    a. Low anterior resection
    b. Total procto-colectomy and J pouch formation (ileal-anal anastomosis)
    c. Total procto-colectomy and ileostomy
    d. APR

    Answer b. **Total procto-colectomy** and **J pouch formation** (ileal-anal anastomosis) - the entire colon and rectum need removal; J-pouch preferred

949. A 38 yo woman with ulcerative colitis undergoes J-pouch construction. One month after surgery she presents with bloody diarrhea, urgency, fever, and lower abdominal pain. Which of the following is the most appropriate next step:

a. IVFs and antibiotics
b. Pouch takedown
c. Angiogram
d. Formalin fixation

Answer a. Based on the Sx's, this patient most likely has **pouchitis**. Tx - IVFs and antibiotics (Cipro and Flagyl). Endoscopy with biopsies should be performed to confirm the diagnosis (and rule out undiagnosed Crohn's disease).

950. All of the following are indications for proctocolectomy in patients with ulcerative colitis except:
a. Toxic megacolon worsening after 72 hours of IV steroids and antibiotics
b. Perforation
c. Isolated ulcerative proctitis for 20 years
d. Low grade dysplasia on biopsy

Answer c. Isolated ulcerative proctitis does <u>not</u> have increased CA risk and should not undergo prophylactic colectomy.

951. All of the following are true of colon CA risk and ulcerative colitis except:
a. The greater the extent of inflammation, the higher the colon CA risk
b. The longer the duration of inflammation, the higher the colon CA risk
c. Random biopsies can be effective in surveillance (2-4 random biopsies every 10 cm)
d. Colon CA in these patients is typically preceded by a polyp

Answer d. Colon CA with ulcerative colitis occurs in **flat areas**. This is the reason why random biopsies are recommended.

952. A 60 yo man undergoes open cholecystectomy for cholecystitis and requires increased narcotics to control pain. Five days later, he develops abdominal distension and pain. Plain film shows a distended colon that is 10 cm at the cecum. You start IVF's, place an NG tube, stop narcotics, and keep the patient NPO, however the distension continues. The most appropriate next step in this patient is:
a. Cecostomy
b. Colectomy
c. Neostigmine
d. Nothing
e. Barium enema

Answer c. Neostigmine is effective for **Ogilvie's Syndrome**.

953. The above patient's Sx's continue despite therapy. The most appropriate next step is:
a. Partial colectomy
b. Barium enema
c. Cecostomy
d. Decompressive colonoscopy
e. Total abdominal colectomy

Answer d. Decompressive colonoscopy (If medical Tx fails or if the cecum is > 12 cm - *decompressive colonoscopy is indicated*)

954. A 75 yo woman from a nursing home with long-term constipation requiring laxatives presents with abdominal pain and distension. You get a plain film and the colon is very distended and looks like an 'ace of spades', 'bent inner tube', or inverted U-shape with the medial walls of the loop pointing to the RUQ. She does not have peritoneal signs. You start IV fluid hydration. The most appropriate next step in management is:
a. Flexible sigmoidoscopy
b. Low anterior resection (LAR)
c. Abdominoperineal resection (APR)
d. Do nothing

Answer a. Given the scenario, this patient most likely has a **sigmoid volvulus**. **Flexible sigmoidoscopy** will detorse the sigmoid colon in 80% of these patients.

After detorsion, a **bowel prep** should be given followed by **sigmoidectomy** during the <u>same hospital admission</u>.

955. A 35 yo woman presents with crampy abdominal pain and obstipation. She has had no previous surgery. You get a plain film and the small bowel is distended with air-fluid levels. A loop of bowel that looks like an 'ace of spades' or 'bent inner tube' is pointing to the LUQ. All of the following are true of this patient's most likely condition except
   a.   Right hemicolectomy and primary ileo-transverse anastomosis is indicated
   b.   Detorsion success rate is 20% or less
   c.   One stage surgery without ileosotmy is generally indicated
   d.   Cecostomy is often indicated

   Answer d. Cecostomy is <u>not</u> indicated for cecal volvulus. Right hemicolectomy and primary ileo-transverse anastomosis is indicated *(<u>no</u> ileostomy needed)*

956. In an average male patient, the most distal extent of a T2 rectal cancer which still allows for a low anterior resection with an appropriate margin is:
   a.   8 cm from the anal canal
   b.   6 cm from the anal canal
   c.   4 cm from the anal canal
   d.   2 cm from the anal canal

   Answer d. The most distal rectal tumor extent which would still allow a 2 cm margin is about 2 **cm from the proximal anal canal**. You need a 2 cm rectal cuff above the anal canal which will be resected with the end to end stapler (send the donut in stapler to path as this is part of your margin). In general, it is easier to perform LAR in women compared to men because their pelvic bones are wider.

957. A 60 yo man undergoes LAR for sigmoid adenocarcinoma. The final path report states the tumor invaded the muscularis propria and there was tumor in 2 mesenteric lymph nodes. What is the pathologic TNM classification for this CA?
   a.   T1, N0, M0
   b.   T1, N1, M0
   c.   T2, N0, M0
   d.   T2, N1, M0

   Answer d. Invasion of the **muscularis propria** makes it T2. Involvement of 2 nodes makes it N1 (T2N1M0, stage III).

958. For the above question, following resection what is the appropriate next step:
   a.   5-FU, leucovorin, and oxaliplatin
   b.   5-FU, leucovorin, and oxaliplatin plus XRT
   c.   XRT
   d.   Nothing

   Answer a. Because there was nodal involvement, this patient is stage III and needs chemotherapy (**leucovorin, 5-FU, and oxaliplatin** - FOLFOX). XRT is not indicated for colon CA (unlike some rectal CA's). The FOLFOX regimen has been shown to improve **5-YS** in patients with **stage III** colorectal CA.

959. Six days after a low anterior resection for stage II rectal CA, a CT scan shows an 8 x 8 cm fluid collection near the anastomosis. The next appropriate step is:
   a.   Re-exploration and repair the anastomosis
   b.   Percutaneous drainage and antibiotics
   c.   Abdominoperineal resection

d.   Takedown of the anastomosis with placement of colostomy and Hartman's pouch

e.   Antibiotics only

Answer b. This patient most likely has a leak from his anastomosis and subsequent **abscess** formation. **Percutaneous drainage** is the most appropriate Tx.

960. Instead of the above, CT scan shows a small leak near the anastomosis. The most appropriate next step is:
a.   Re-exploration and repair of the leak at the anastomosis
b.   Percutaneous drainage and antibiotics
c.   Abdominoperineal resection
d.   Takedown of the anastomosis with placement of colostomy and Hartman's pouch
e.   Antibiotics only

Answer e. Antibiotics only

961. A 50 yo woman with mild LLQ pain undergoes a CT scan which shows diverticulitis. She does not have any rebound or guarding.. WBC count is 15 and temperature is 100 F. The most appropriate next step is:
a.   Antibiotics only
b.   Percutaneous drain
c.   Sigmoid resection
d.   Sigmoidoscopy
e.   Barium enema

Answer a. Antibiotics only. These patients need F/U colonoscopy in 6 weeks to rule out colorectal CA. It is not done earlier due to the risk of <u>perforation</u> with acute diverticulitis. This patient could be treated as an outpatient.

You should see diverticula on CT scan otherwise this is likely a perforated CA. A CT scan is recommended for patients with diverticulitis at some point to help rule-out colorectal CA.

962. After 3 days, the above patient's condition worsens. Her WBCs are 30 and she has increased tenderness. CT scan now shows an associated 6 cm abscess. The most appropriate next step is:
a.   Antibiotics only
b.   Percutaneous drain
c.   Sigmoid resection
d.   Sigmoidoscopy
e.   Barium enema

Answer b. Percutaneous drain

963. Instead of the above, CT scan now shows a free perforation with free air and with multiple fluid collections throughout the abdomen. The most appropriate next step is:
a.   Antibiotics only
b.   Percutaneous drain
c.   Sigmoid resection
d.   Sigmoidoscopy
e.   Barium enema

Answer c. Sigmoid resection and **diverting ileostomy**; abdominal washout

964. The distal extent for resection in the above patient should be:
a.   Normal rectum
b.   Lower rectum
c.   Recto-sigmoid junction

d. Lower sigmoid colon

Answer a. Normal rectum

965. After a sigmoid resection with loop ileostomy in the above patient, the stoma appears dark. The most appropriate next step is:
    a. Heparin
    b. tPA
    c. Reoperation and revise
    d. Nitropaste

Answer c. Reoperation and revise. It is very likely that the stoma is being compressed by fascia, has a twist, or has been too devascularized.

966. All of the following are true of colon diverticula except:
    a. Are due to straining
    b. Are pulsion diverticula
    c. MC occur in the sigmoid colon
    d. Can be treated with a high fiber diet and colace
    e. Are true diverticula

Answer e. Lower GI diverticula are **false diverticula**

967. The MCC of colovesicle fistula is:
    a. Inflammatory bowel disease
    b. CA
    c. Diverticulitis
    d. Bladder CA

Answer c. Diverticulitis

968. A 30 yo man with a thickened sigmoid colon with diverticula presents with recurrent urinary tract infections and pneumaturia. The best test for the likely diagnosis is:
    a. CT scan
    b. MRI
    c. Cystoscopy
    d. Colonoscopy

Answer c. Cystoscopy is the best test for **colo-vesicle fistula.** A CT scan is indicated prior to resection but it is not the most sensitive test for Dx.

969. A 50 yo immunocompromised patient has had several recurrent severe episodes of sigmoid diverticulitis. CT scan reveals diffuse colonic diverticuli starting in his cecum and extending to his sigmoid colon. The most appropriate next step is:
    a. Total procto-colectomy and ileostomy
    b. Total procto-colectomy and ileoanal pouch
    c. Sigmoid resection down to normal rectum
    d. Low anterior resection

Answer c. Sigmoid resection down to normal rectum. Only the symptomatic area should be resected. The distal extent of sigmoidectomy for diverticular problems should be normal rectum.

70. All of the following are true of colo-rectal CA with metastases to the liver except:
    a. The most accurate way of identifying liver metastases is intra-op U/S
    b. Metastases to segments I and II likely requires left lobectomy and caudate resection
    c. 5 year survival for resectable liver metastases is about 35%
    d. Four liver metastases is considered unresectable

Answer d Number of metastases does not influence resection as long as all of the lesions are completely resectable and you leave adequate liver reserve.

971. A 55 yo man is undergoing colectomy for adenocarcinoma. When you enter the abdomen, the tumor appears to be invading the 2nd portion of the duodenum near the ampulla. The best management would be:
    a.   Extended right hemicolectomy only and leave the duodenal component
    b.   En bloc extended right hemicolectomy including the portion of the cancer invading the duodenum (even if Whipple is necessary)
    c.   Wedge the duodenum lesion out only
    d.   Close

Answer b. Direct invasion of another structure requires **en bloc resection,** even if you have to perform a Whipple to get en bloc resection.

972. All of the following are true except:
    a.   The MC location for colon cancer is the sigmoid colon
    b.   TRUS is the best method for assessing T and N status of rectal tumors
    c.   CEA is useful for screening for colon CA
    d.   CEA is useful to detect colon CA recurrence and for following response to Tx

Answer c. CEA has <u>not</u> been useful for colon CA screening.

973. A 55 yo man undergoes LAR for a low rectal CA now returns to clinic 6 months later with constipation. You perform anoscopy in the office and notice a mass at the previous suture line. Biopsies show adenocarcinoma. After a metastatic disease work-up, the next appropriate step is:
    a.   Local resection
    b.   Chemotherapy with leucovorin
    c.   5000 rads of XRT
    d.   Abdominoperineal resection (APR)

Answer d. Recurrence at the suture line following LAR demands **APR** unless the patient has metastases that would preclude surgery. You should re-stage patients with recurrence (Abdomen/Pelvic CT, CXR, LFT's, and CEA).

974. In the above patient, 2 days after APR he has severe flank pain. U/S shows significant unilateral hydronephrosis. Given the likely diagnosis, the most appropriate step is:
    a.   Percutaneous nephrostomy tube
    b.   Reop and perform ureterocystostomy
    c.   Trans uretero-ureteral anastomosis
    d.   End to end anastomosis
    e.   Drains only

Answer b. The majority of iatrogenic ureteral injuries involves the **lower third** of the ureter and **bladder re-implantation** in indicated. Given the timing since surgery (**< 7 days**), reoperation is indicated.

975. Instead of the above, on POD #10 he has an elevated serum creatnine and flank pain. U/S reveals a fluid collection. You place a percutaneous drain with the fluid having a creatinine of 15. The most appropriate next step is:
    a.   Percutaneous nephrostomy tube
    b.   Reop and perform ureterocystostomy
    c.   Trans uretero-ureteral anastomosis
    d.   End to end anastomosis
    e.   Leave the percutaneous drain only

Answer e. Leave the **percutaneous drain only** with delayed repair in 6-8 weeks. Want to avoid re-operation $\geq$ **7 days** after surgery due to friable tissue and adhesions (high risk for bowel and tissue injury; also not a good environment to perform ureter to bladder anastomosis). Patients with urine leaks will have an elevated <u>serum</u> creatnine as it is reabsorbed from the peritoneum.

976. A 50 yo man undergoes neo-adjuvant chemo-XRT followed by LAR for rectal CA. Six months later he has severe bleeding from his rectum. He has required several transfusions. All of the following are true except:

    a. Proctoscopy is the initial diagnostic method of choice in this patient
    b. APR is likely needed for radiation proctitis
    c. Dilute formalin fixation of the rectum is for the best Tx radiation proctitis bleeding
    d. Recurrent rectal CA should be considered
    e. This is due to obliterative arteritis

Answer b. You should avoid APR for bleeding from late radiation proctitis. **Formalin fixation** of the rectum usually suffices.

977. All of the following are correct except:

    a. Bevacizumab is a monoclonal antibody to vascular endothelial growth factor
    b. The main 5-FU side effect is ototoxicity
    c. Cetuximab is a monoclonal antibody to epidermal growth factor receptor
    d. Oxaliplatin has less nephrotoxicity compared to cisplatin

Answer b. The main 5-FU side effect is myelosuppression

978. Laparoscopic compared to open resection for colon CA (experienced surgeons) is associated with:

    a. No difference in pathologic margins
    b. Longer hospital stay
    c. Increased operative morbidity
    d. Increased operative mortality

Answer a. No difference in pathologic margins

979. Laparoscopic compared to open resection for colon CA (experienced surgeons) is associated with

    a. Increased blood loss
    b. Longer operative time
    c. Longer hospital stay
    d. Fewer nodes resected

Answer b. Longer operative time

980. An 85 yo man has an extensive rectal villous adenoma with atypia. All of the following are true except:

    a. Trans-anal excision of the tumor is indicated
    b. Abdominal perineal resection (APR) is indicated if the adenoma cannot be completely resected
    c. A T1 CA area with 2-3 mm margins on pathology after resection requires no further Tx
    d. Well differentiated T1 lesions have a better prognosis

Answer b. APR is <u>not</u> indicated for low rectal villous adenomas with atypia (APR is indicated only for CA). Trans-anal excision of the tumor is indicated in this patient.

981. All of the following are true of Familial Adenomatous Polyposis (FAP) Syndrome except:

    a. Patients with FAP have polyps present at birth
    b. Late diagnosis of FAP in a 30 yo requires total colonoscopy, EGD to rule-out adenocarcinoma, and CT scan to look for desmoids tumors

c. Desmoid tumors incorporating significant amounts of mesentery should not be resected
d. In patients who have undergone total proctocolectomy for FAP, the MCC of death is duodenal CA
e. Patients with FAP should undergo screening in their teens

Answer a. Patients with **FAP** have polyps that develop in **puberty**. Patients with FAP should undergo screening in their teens to look for polyps. Total procto-colectomy is indicated at age 20.

Desmoid tumors (eg mesenteric mass) also occur in patients with FAP. If involving significant mesentery, resection is _not_ indicated do to the high incidence of **short bowel syndrome** following resection and **high recurrence rate**. Tx: **Sulindac** and **Tamoxifen** if not easily resectable or for residual disease.

982. A 14 yo boy with the APC gene mutation undergoes sigmoidoscopy and adenomatous polyps are found. Pathology shows no malignancy. The most appropriate next step is:
a. Total proctocolectomy and pouch construction
b. Total proctocolectomy and ileostomy
c. Observation with delayed surgery
d. Remove all of the polyps endoscopically

Answer c. Observation with delayed surgery. Colon CA is very rare in these patients before 20. Most choose to have surgery between a transition in education or between education and work (about 20 yo). This allows maturation of the child (physical, mental, and emotional) before surgery.

983. All of the following are true of hereditary non-polyposis colon cancer syndrome (HNPCC, Lynch Syndrome) and Amsterdam criteria except:
a. Needs to be in 3 primary relatives, over 2 generations, with one person being less than 50 at the time of diagnosis of cancer
b. Colon cancers are right sided predominant and have a better prognosis stage for stage as sporadic colon CA
c. Ovarian, breast, endometrial, and stomach cancer can also occur in these patients
d. These patients have thousands of polyps
e. Involves a defect in mismatch repair genes (hMSH2, hMLH1, hPMS1, hPMS2).

Answer d. These patients do _not_ form thousands of polyps like FAP.

984. Which of the following is recommended screening in patients with HNPCC:
a. Transvaginal U/S and endometrial aspiration biopsy at age 25
b. Transvaginal U/S and endometrial aspiration biopsy at age 35
c. Urine cytology and U/S at age 15
d. Urine cytology and U/S at age 25

Answer b. Transvaginal U/S and endometrial aspiration biopsy at age 35

985. All of the following are true of Familial Juvenile Polyposis except:
a. Prophylactic colectomy is recommended at age 20
b. Hamartomatous polyps form
c. Annual upper and lower endoscopy are recommended
d. It is autosomal dominant
e. There is a small risk of CA

Answer a. _Prophylactic colectomy is not recommended for **Familial Juvenile Polyposis**. If adenomatous changes are found in a hamartomatous polyp, then colectomy is recommended for areas that have polyps (do not necessarily need total proctocolectomy and J-pouch)._

986. All of the following are true of Peutz-Jeghers except:
   a.   These patients are at higher risk of extra-intestinal malignancies
   b.   The MC CA in these patients is breast CA
   c.   These patients form GI tract hamartomatous polyps
   d.   Bowel obstruction is the MC presentation
   e.   Prophylactic colectomy in indicated

   Answer e. Prophylactic colectomy is <u>not</u> indicated for **Peutz-Jeghers**.

987. A 65 yo man undergoes polypectomy from his left colon. During the procedure you see omental fat. The next appropriate step is:
   a.   Left hemicolectomy (one stage)
   b.   Left hemicolectomy and loop ileostomy (two stage)
   c.   Primary repair
   d.   NPO and IV antibiotics

   Answer c. Primary repair is indicated for **free perforation** following colonoscopy (eg seeing omental fat; seeing free air under the diaphragm following polypectomy)

988. All of the following are true of colon polyps except:
   a.   Hyperplastic polyps are the MC colon polyp and are <u>not</u> thought to have increased malignancy risk
   b.   Tubovillous adenomas have the same malignancy risk as villous polyps
   c.   Adenomatous polyps > 2 cm have increased malignancy risk compared to smaller polyps
   d.   Inflammatory polyps (pseudopolyps) are characteristically found in ulcerative colitis

   Answer b. Tubovillous adenomas lower malignancy risk compared to villous polyps and a higher malignancy risk compared to tubular polyps.

989. A 60 yo man presents with moderate lower GI bleeding. His BP is 120/80. NGT returns just bilious fluid. You perform proctoscopy and do not see any hemorrhoids or other sources of bleeding. Which of the following is most appropriate:
   a.   Colonoscopy
   b.   Formal angiogram
   c.   Tagged RBC scan
   d.   Meckel's Scan

   Answer a. Colonoscopy

990. Instead of the above, the patient is having a massive bleed. BP is 90/60 after fluid and blood resuscitation. Which of the following is most appropriate:
   a.   Colonoscopy
   b.   Formal angiogram
   c.   Tagged RBC scan
   d.   Meckel's Scan

   Answer a. The most effective study for a patient with massive lower GI bleeding is still **colonoscopy**.

991. Instead of the above, the patients BP is 70/20 despite fluid and 6 units of pRBCs. Which of the following is most appropriate:
   a.   Continue giving pRBCs only
   b.   Give lactated ringers
   c.   Give platelets only when the platelet count falls below 150
   d.   Give pRBCs, platelets, and FFP in a 1: 1 :1 ratio

   Answer d. Hemostatic resuscitation is appropriate here.

992. The MCC of GI bleeding not apparent on standard upper / lower endoscopy (obscure GI bleeding) is:
   a. Small bowel AVM
   b. Meckel's diverticulum in the ileum
   c. Small bowel Crohn's disease
   d. Aorto-enteric fistula in duodenum

   Answer a. Small bowel AVM (angiodysplasia)

993. A 60 yo woman hospitalized for ARDS and hypoxia is noted to have diarrhea that is guaiac positive along with left sided abdominal pain. She has the following values: BP 100/80, HR 90. The most appropriate next step is:
   a. Tagged RBC scan
   b. Angiogram
   c. CT scan
   d. Colectomy

   Answer c. CT scan. The above scenario is worrisome for **ischemic colitis** related to **hypoxia** (watershed areas are vulnerable). Tx - **IVFs** and **antibiotics**

994. All of the following warrant immediate re-exploration except:
   a. Thick bile colored fluid emanating from a midline wound following small bowel resection on POD 6
   b. Large, copious amount of salmon colored fluid emanating from the midline wound on POD 5 with a bulge under the incision
   c. Stool emanating from RLQ incision following appendectomy on POD 3
   d. Urine emanating from the midline wound on POD 10

   Answer d. Various **leaks** can occur after surgery which can emanate through the **abdominal wound** (eg stool after appendectomy stump blow-out, enterotomy or anastomosis sucus leakage after small bowel resection, urine leak after APR, etc). These are not considered contained. The sequelae after these leaks can be severe (eg peritonitis, sepsis, necrotizing fasciitis, shock, death).

   Management of a leak through an abdominal wound depends on when the leak occurs:
   If < **7 days**, then **reoperation** is generally indicated. Surgery at reoperation depends on the cause but can range from simple washout and placement of drains, to revising an anastomosis or staple line, or resection.

   If ≥ **7 days**, **adhesions** become a problem and reoperation in not advised At this point the leak is now called a **fistula**. Adhesions usually contain these collections at this point. A CT scan is indicated to find any undrained fluid collections. _Exceptions_ to this would be if the patient had sepsis, peritonitis, or fasciitis.

   Leaks controlled with drains (ie not emanating through the abdominal wound) following hepatobiliary or pancreatic surgery generally do not require surgery and should be treated as a fistula. An anastomotic leak following LAR that is not coming through the wound (eg large fluid collection on CT scan) can generally be treated with percutaneous drainage.

   A large amount of pink salmon-colored drainage along with a bulge under the incision is consistent with **fascial dehiscence**. Re-exploration and placement of **retention sutures** is indicated.

995. Erectile dysfunction following LAR is most likely related to injury of:
   a. Pelvic splanchnic plexus
   b. Hypogastric plexus
   c. Pudendal nerve
   d. Genitofemoral nerves

43

Answer a. Pelvic splanchnic plexus (parasympathetic)

996. Retrograde ejaculation following LAR is most likely related to injury of:
    a. Pelvic splanchnic plexus
    b. Hypogastric plexus
    c. Pudendal nerves
    d. Genitofemoral nerves

Answer b. Hypogastric nerves (sympathetic)

997. Ejaculatory failure following LAR is most likely related to injury of:
    a. Pelvic splanchnic plexus
    b. Femoral nerve
    c. Pudendal nerves
    d. Genitofemoral nerves

Answer c. Pudendal nerves (sympathetic)

998. Dysuria and frequency occurring late after LAR is most likely related to injury of:
    a. Pelvic splanchnic plexus
    b. Femoral nerve
    c. Pudendal nerves
    d. Genitofemoral nerves

Answer a. Pelvic splanchnic plexus (parasympathetic; can cause bladder problems)

ANATOMY AND PHYSIOLOGY

- Colon secretes **K⁺** and reabsorbs **Na⁺** (Na/K ATPase) and **water** (1-2 L; mostly right colon and cecum)
- **Layers** - Mucosa (columnar epithelium), Submucosa, Muscularis propria, Serosa
- **Retroperitoneal portions** – ascending, descending, sigmoid colon, and rectum; peritoneum covers anterior portions of upper and middle ⅓ of rectum
- **Vascular supply**
  - **Ascending colon** and **proximal 2/3 of transverse colon** supplied by **superior mesenteric artery** (SMA; eg ileocolic, right colic and middle colic arteries)
  - **1/3 transverse, descending colon, sigmoid colon,** and **upper portion of rectum** supplied by **inferior mesenteric artery** (IMA; left colic, sigmoid branches, superior rectal artery)
  - **Marginal artery** - travels along colon margin, connecting SMA to IMA (provides collateral flow)
  - **Meandering mesenteric artery** (Arc of Riolan) - a short direct connection between the **proximal SMA** and **proximal IMA**; becomes enlarged with either SMA or IMA stenosis *(is a collateral pathway)*
  - *Superior rectal artery* - branch of **IMA**
  - *Middle rectal artery* - branch of **internal iliac** artery (the *lateral stalks* during LAR or APR contain the middle rectal arteries)
  - *Inferior rectal artery* – branch of <u>internal pudendal</u> (off **internal iliac** artery)
  - **Rectal** arteries = **hemorrhoidal** arteries
  - **Internal iliac** arteries = **hypogastric** arteries
- **Watershed areas**
  - **Splenic flexure** (Griffith's point) - SMA and IMA junction
  - **Rectum** (Sudeck's point) - superior rectal and middle rectal artery junction
  - Colon more sensitive to ischemia than small bowel due to **poor collaterals**
- **Venous drainage**
  - Generally follows arterial except inferior mesenteric vein (IMV), which goes to the splenic vein
  - Splenic vein joins SMV to form portal vein behind pancreas neck
  - **Superior rectal veins** drain into **IMV** (and then into the *portal vein*)

- Middle rectal veins drain into both the **IMV** and **internal iliac veins** (dual drainage systems)
- Inferior rectal veins drain into **internal iliac veins** and eventually the *inferior vena cava* (can get isolated lung metastases with low rectal tumors)
  - ■ Nodal drainage
    - **Ascending, transverse, descending,** and **sigmoid** lymphatics follow arterial supply
    - **Superior** and **middle rectum** - drain to IMA nodes
    - **Lower rectum** - primarily to IMA nodes, also to internal iliac nodes
  - ■ **External anal sphincter** - under <u>voluntary</u> *(CNS) control*
    - Is the continuation of the **puborectalis muscle**
    - **Inferior rectal (anal)** branch of *internal pudendal nerve* (sympathetic)
    - The puborectalis is part of the **levator ani muscle group** (striated muscle)
  - ■ **Internal anal sphincter** – <u>no</u> *voluntary control*
    - The continuation of the **muscularis propria** (circular layer, smooth muscle)
    - Innervation by **pelvic splanchnic nerves** (S2-S4, parasympathetic)
    - ***No** pudendal innervation (<u>No</u> voluntary control, normally contracted)*
  - ■ Distances from anal verge (sigmoidoscopy):
    - Anal margin (between anal verge and dentate)   0-2 cm
    - Anal canal (dentate to levator ani muscle-pelvic floor)   2-5 cm
    - Rectum   5-15 cm
    - Recto-sigmoid junction   15-18 cm
  - ■ **Levator ani** - marks transition between anal canal and rectum
  - ■ **Short-chain fatty acids** (eg butyrate) - main nutrient of colonocytes
  - ■ **Denonvilliers' fascia** (*anterior*) - *recto-prostatic fascia* (prostate and seminal vesicles) in men; *recto-vaginal fascia* in women
  - ■ **Recto-vesicle fascia** (*anterior*) - between the rectum and bladder
  - ■ **Waldeyer's fascia** (*posterior*) - *recto-sacral fascia* (**pre-sacral fascia**); separates the rectum from the presacral venous plexus and the pelvic nerves

DISUSE PROCTITIS (diversion proctitis)
- ■ Can occur with Hartman's Pouch
- ■ Sx's: grey mucus drainage from pouch (sloughed dead mucosa), sense of urgency
- ■ Tx: **short-chain fatty acid enemas** (butyrate)

INFECTIOUS POUCHITIS
- ■ Can occur with J-pouch or Kock pouch following total colectomy
- ■ MC long term complication from pouch formation (40%); can be acute or chronic
- ■ Sx's: purulent drainage, diarrhea, hemotochezia; fever, lower abdominal pain, malaise
- ■ Dx: colonoscopy - erythematous, friable pouch (inflammation); confirm Dx and rule-out Crohn's disease
- ■ Tx: **Cipro** and **Flagyl** treat majority; *rarely* need APR (for severe sepsis or if refractory)

COLON CANCER SCREENING
- ■ Screening - at **50** for **normal risk**, at **40** (or 10 years before youngest case) for **intermediate risk** (eg family history of colon CA)
- ■ Screening options - 1) **colonoscopy** every 10 years *or;* 2) **high sensitivity fecal occult blood testing** every 3 years and **flexible sigmoidoscopy** every 5 years *or;* 3) **high sensitivity fecal occult blood testing** annually
  - **Double contrast barium enema** or **CT colonography** every 5 years may be alternatives to above
  - **False-positive guaiac** - beef, vitamin C, iron, cimetidine
  - <u>No</u> colonoscopy with recent MI or splenomegaly; also not with pregnancy if fluoroscopy planned

SIGMOID VOLVULUS
- ■ Sigmoid colon twists itself, causing closed loop obstruction
- ■ Sx's: dull aching pain, distention, and obstipation (failure to pass stool / gas)
- ■ RFs: debilitated, psychiatric patients, elderly, nursing home residents; laxative abuse, high fiber diets (middle east countries)

■ Dx: **CT scan** *(best test)* - bent inner tube, Ace of Spades, or inverted U signs (massively dilated sigmoid colon; edges of the loop inner walls point to the RUQ); bird's beak sign (tapered distal sigmoid colon); signs of large bowel obstruction
■ Tx: **detorse with colonoscopy** (80% reduce, 50% will recur), give bowel prep, and perform sigmoid colectomy during same hospital admission
  - If it doesn't detorse with colonoscopy, go to OR for sigmoid colectomy
■ *Do not attempt detorsion with gangrenous bowel (black on colonoscopy), diffuse peritoneal signs, or perforation → go to OR for sigmoidectomy*

CECAL VOLVULUS
■ Less common than sigmoid volvulus; occurs in 20-30s
■ Sx's similar to small bowel obstruction (SBO)
■ Dx: **CT scan** *(best test)* - closed loop obstruction (dilated cecum in the RLQ) and dilated proximal small bowel; distal colon decompression
■ Can try to detorse with colonoscopy but unlikely to succeed (only 20%)
■ Tx: **right hemicolectomy** with primary anastomosis (no ostomy)
■ If **frail patient and incontinent** → colectomy with ileostomy and mucus fistula or long Hartman's Pouch

ULCERATIVE COLITIS
■ Sx's: **bloody diarrhea, abdominal pain, fever,** and **weight loss**
■ Path:
  - **Mucosal** inflammation (earliest sign - **edema**); involves **colon** and **rectum** only
  - **Spares anus** (unlike Crohn's)
  - Almost universally involves **rectum** (exam - bleeding)
  - Also usually starts in **rectum** and is contiguous *(no skip areas like Crohn's)*
  - **Bleeding** is universal
  - Always need to rule out infectious etiology
  - Backwash ileitis can occur with proximal disease
  - **Crypt abscess** formation
  - **Bimodal** age of onset - 20's and 60's; increased in **Ashkenazi Jews**
■ **Barium enema** - with chronic disease see loss of haustra, narrow caliber, short colon, and loss of redundancy ("lead pipe" colon)
■ Medical Tx: **sulfasalazine** (or 5-ASA) and **loperamide** for maintenance
  - 5-ASA and sulfasalazine can maintain remission in ulcerative colitis
  - Consider azathioprine, cyclosporine, or Infliximab if resistant
  - *Avoid* NSAIDs (can worsen Sx's / cause flares in inflammatory bowel disease)
  - *Avoid* chronic prednisone if possible - use for flares
  - Low residue diet (avoid vegetables, bread, cereal, nuts)
  - **Acute Flare Tx:**
    Steroids *(best Tx for acute exacerbation;* hydrocortisone 100 mg q8)
    Add **Cipro** and **Flagyl** for fevers, elevated WBCs, or if worried about toxic colitis or toxic megacolon
■ **Toxic Colitis** and **Toxic Megacolon**
  - **Toxic Colitis**: > 6 bloody stools/d, fever, tachycardia, hypotension, drop in Hgb, leukocytosis (high WBCs)
  - **Toxic Megacolon**: above plus distension, abdominal pain and tenderness
  - *Initial Tx:* **NG tube, fluids, steroids, bowel rest,** and **antibiotics** (Cipro and Flagyl) - will treat 50% adequately; other 50% require surgery
  - Follow clinical response and abdominal radiographs
  - *Avoid* barium enemas, narcotics, anti-diarrheal agents, and anti-cholinergics
  - *No* colonoscopy with suspected toxic megacolon / toxic colitis - risk of *perforation*

Surgery Indications for Toxic Colitis and Toxic Megacolon

Absolute	Relative
Pneumoperitoneum	Controlled sepsis
Diffuse peritonitis	Worsening megacolon / colitis
Major hemorrhage	Clinical deterioration
Uncontrolled sepsis	Continued blood transfusions
Localized peritonitis + increasing pain and/or colonic distension > 10-12 cm	Failure to improve after 72 h

- Perforation with <u>ulcerative colitis</u> - **transverse colon** more common
- Perforation with <u>Crohn's</u> - **distal ileum** most common
- **Surgical indications**:
  - Significant **hemorrhage**
  - Refractory **toxic megacolon / colitis** (fails to improve after 72 hrs)
  - Persistent **obstruction** or stricture
  - *Any dysplasia* (including low grade)
  - **Cancer**
  - **Failed medical Tx** (continued > 10-12 bloody stools / d)
  - Systemic Cx's (MC is **failure to thrive**)
  - Failure to wean **high dose steroids**
  - **Perforation**
  - Long-standing disease (some controversy here)
- **Emergent / urgent resections** - total proctocolectomy and bring up ileostomy *(<u>no</u> ileo anal anastomosis in urgent setting; perform definitive hook-up later)*
- Surgery is **curative** for UC; unlike Crohn's
- **Elective resections**
  - **Ileoanal anastomosis** - total procto-colectomy with rectal mucosectomy (small segment of rectum remains), J-pouch (from ileum), and ileo-anal (low rectal) anastomosis; <u>not</u> used with Crohn's disease
    - Can protect bladder and sexual function compared to APR
    - Place diverting ileostomy (for 6-8 weeks) while pouch heals
    - Pouch <u>not</u> used if severe rectal disease with incontinence
    - **Leak** (MC major morbidity) - can lead to sepsis (Tx: drainage, antibiotics)
    - **Infectious pouchitis** - Tx: Flagyl
    - Need lifetime surveillance of residual rectal area
    - Many ileoanal anastomoses (15%) eventually need **takedown** (with APR ileostomy) secondary to: 1) **incontinence** (*MC reason for takedown* pouch failure), 2) **CA** or **dysplasia**, or 3) refractory **proctitis / sepsis**
  - **APR with ileostomy** - also an option (total procto-colectomy and anal resection
    - Want ileostomy output < 500-1000 cc/d; use **loperamide** or **Lomotil** to slow output
- **Colon CA risk** (risk based on <u>extent</u> and <u>duration</u> of inflammation)
  - **1% per year** risk of colon CA starting **10 years** after initial Dx of **pan-colitis** (highest risk variant)
  - At **20 years** the case is strong for **prophylactic colectomy** in patients with (any below):
    - **Primary sclerosing cholangitis**
    - **Family history** of colon CA
    - **Young age** at diagnosis
    - **Left sided** colitis
  - CA is more evenly distributed throughout colon compared to general population
  - Colon CA develops in *<u>absence</u>* of polyps
  - Need yearly full colonoscopy starting 8-10 years after diagnosis (random Bx's plus any suspicious areas [> 30 biopsies])
  - **Isolated proctitis** - <u>no</u> increased colon CA risk
  - *Any dysplasia is an indication for total procto-colectomy (30% actually have colon CA)*
- **Extra-intestinal manifestations** of ulcerative colitis
  - MC extra-intestinal manifestation requiring total colectomy - **failure to thrive in children**
  - Do <u>not</u> get better with colectomy → primary sclerosing cholangitis, ankylosing spondylitis
  - Get better with colectomy → most ocular problems, arthritis, and anemia
  - 50% get better → pyoderma gangrenosum
  - **HLA B27** - sacroiliitis, ankylosing spondylitis, ulcerative colitis
  - Can get **thromboembolic disease** (eg DVT, PE, stroke)
  - **Pyoderma gangrenosum** (ulcers, violaceous edges) - Tx: steroids

COLONIC OBSTRUCTION

- **Colon perforation with obstruction** - most likely to occur in **cecum**
- **Closed-loop obstructions** - can be worrisome; can have rapid progression and perforation with minimal distention
  - Competent ileocecal valve can lead to closed-loop obstruction
- **Colonic obstruction** - #1 cancer; #2 **diverticulitis**
- **Pneumatosis intestinalis** - air in the bowel wall, associated with ischemia and dissection of gas into bowel wall (<u>not</u> always an indication for resection)
- **Air in the portal system** - usually indicates significant infection or necrosis of the large or small bowel; often an <u>ominous sign</u> (in adults is usually an indication for resection if due to bowel ischemia)

OGILVIE'S SYNDROME

- Pseudo-obstruction of the **colon**
- RFs: opiate use; bedridden or older patients; recent surgery, infection, or trauma
- Can get a **massively dilated colon** which can **perforate**
  - Small bowel is <u>not</u> dilated (unlike ileus)
  - Rectal exam should reveal an **air-filled rectum**
- Dx: **CT scan** (to rule-out true large bowel mechanical obstruction if not sure)
- Tx: IVFs and replace volume deficit, replace electrolytes (especially **K** and **Mg**); discontinue drugs that slow gut (eg morphine, narcotics); NG tube and bowel rest; **neostigmine** if refractory
  - If **colon > 10-12 cm** (high risk of perforation) <u>or</u> if it fails to resolve with medical Tx (> 24-48 hours) → Tx: **decompression with colonoscopy**
  - If colonoscopy fails to decompress, proceed with **cecostomy** (need colon resection if perforation is found or if bowel is not viable)
- **Neostigmine side-effects** (acetylcholinesterase inhibitor [cholinergic drug]):
  - **Bradycardia** - make sure **atropine** is available
  - Contraindicated in **cardiac disease** (especially bradycardia)
  - Contraindicated in **renal failure**

AMEBIC COLITIS

- *Entamoeba histolytica*; from contaminated food / water with feces that contain cysts
- **Primary infection** - occurs in colon; **secondary infection** - occurs in liver
- RFs: travel to Mexico, ETOH; fecal-oral transmission
- Sx's: similar to UC (dysentery; 3-4 bowel movements/day, cramping, fever)
- Dx: endoscopy → ulceration, **trophozoites** (stool O and P)
- 90% have anti-amebic antibodies
- Tx: **Flagyl**, diiodohydroxyquin

ACTINOMYCES

- Sx's: can present as a mass, abscess, fistula, or induration; suppurative and granulomatous
- MC location – mouth (poor dentition), lung, and **cecum**, (can be confused with CA)
- Pathology shows **yellow-white sulfur granules**
- Tx: **penicillin** or tetracycline, drainage of any abscess

LOWER GI BLEEDING (hematochezia; LGI bleed)

- Stool guaiac can stay positive up to 3 weeks after bleed
- **Hematemesis** - bleeding anywhere from pharynx to ligament of Treitz (UGI bleed)
  - Both melena and hematochezia can occur with UGI bleed
- **Melena** - passage of black tarry stools; need as little as 50 cc of blood
- **Azotemia** (increased BUN) after GI bleed - caused by production of urea from bacterial action on intraluminal blood
- **Hemoglobin absorption** from the GI tract can result in **jaundice** (increased bilirubin)
- **Arteriography** - bleeding must be ≥ 0.5 cc/min
- **Tagged RBC scan** - bleeding must be ≥ 0.1 cc/min
- **Double balloon endoscopy** (push endoscopy) - upper endoscopy using a rigid over-tube to prevent coiling in stomach → gets down to small bowel
- **Video capsule study** being used more frequently for hard to find LGI bleeds (especially small bowel bleeding)

- If **significant bleed**, follow trauma **hemostatic resuscitation** guidelines (PRBCs : FFP : platelets in a 1:1:1 ratio), avoid excessive crystalloids, permissive hypotension (SBP > 70) until bleeding is found and treated
- If on **warfarin** with a significant bleed, reverse with **prothrombin complex** (or **FFP** and IV **Vit K**)
- Dx: **NG tube** (or EGD) to rule out UGI source (make sure you see bile)
  - **Proctoscopy** to rule-out hemorrhoids (perform in **ED**; avoid misdiagnosis of LGI bleed for bleeding hemorrhoids)
  - **Vasopressin** to slow bleeding if hypotensive
  - **Colonoscopy** is usually the _**preferred first step**_ → can be therapeutic and can localize bleeding if surgery is required (ink stain bleed area)
- **Stages** of LGI bleed and **diagnostic studies** (guidelines):
  1) In **persistent shock** (_unstable_ patient, SBP 60's despite blood transfusion):
     - → **Angiography** (find which side of colon) then to OR for **segmental resection** or perform super-select embolization
     - → May need blind total abdominal colectomy if massive bleeding and clinical condition does not allow attempt at localization or if bleeding is not localized on angiography (_life-saving maneuver_; make sure you rule-out **UGI bleed** and **hemorrhoids** 1st)
  2) **Massive LGIB** (SBP < 90 despite blood transfusion) → **colonoscopy** (can Tx with hemo-clips [_best_], cautery, epinephrine injection)
  3) **Moderate LGIB** (BP > 90 → **colonoscopy**
  4) **Mild LGIB** → **colonoscopy**
  5) For 2, 3, and 4 above, if you still can't find it →
     Angiography - bleeding must be > 0.5 cc/min
     Tagged RBC scan - bleeding must be ≥ 0.1 cc/min
     (_most sensitive test;_ but hard to localize exact area)
     Video capsule study
     Meckel scan (technetium-99 pertechnate scintography)
     Push endoscopy (double balloon) - upper endoscopy using a rigid over-tube to prevent coiling in stomach; gets down into small bowel
- **Small bowel bleeding** (uncommon) - **angiodysplasia** (_MCC of obscure GI bleeding; ie not found on upper and lower endoscopy_), tumor, Meckel's, Crohn's
- **Meckel's diverticulum** is the MCC of **painless lower GI bleeding** in **children and teenagers**

DIVERTICULA
- Caused by **straining** (increased intraluminal pressure; often occurs with low fiber diet)
- Herniation of mucosa through the colon wall at sites where arteries enter the muscle
- Circular muscle thickens adjacent to the diverticulum leading to luminal narrowing
- Is a **false diverticula** (_pulsion_ diverticula)
- Most diverticula occur on **left side** (90%) in the **sigmoid colon** (_not in rectum_)
  - **Diverticulitis** is more likely to present on the left side
  - **Bleeding** is more likely with right-sided diverticula (50% of bleeds occur on right)
- Present in 35% of the population
- Tx: recommend high fiber diet

DIVERTICULITIS
- Caused by diverticulum **mucosa perforation** with adjacent fecal contamination
- Denotes infection and inflammation of colonic wall and surrounding tissue
- Sx's: LLQ pain, tenderness, fever, high WBCs
- Dx: **CT scan** (_best test_) - shows bowel wall **thickening** and **fat stranding** (_make sure there are **diverticuli** on CT scan - if no diverticuli most likely represents a perforated CA_); patients in general should have a CT scan at some point to **confirm the Dx**
- Need **follow-up colonoscopy** after episode of diverticulitis to rule-out **colorectal CA**
- **Uncomplicated** diverticulitis → conservative Tx: **levofloxacin** and **Flagyl**; bowel rest for 3-4 days (mild cases treated as an **outpatient**; follow-up CT scan and colonoscopy at some point to rule-out CA); abscess ≤ 4 cm just treated with antibiotics / bowel rest
- **Sx's of complication** - obstipation, fluctuant mass, peritoneal signs, temp ≥ 39 C, WBCs > 20 (all indicate need for hospital _admission_ and a _CT scan_)
  - **Abscess** (_MC Cx_; Tx: **percutaneous drain** if > 4 cm)

- **Free perforation** (diffuse peritonitis) - Tx: LAR and diverting loop ileostomy
- **Obstruction** - conservative Tx and see if it opens up
  - If that fails (try 3-5 days), go to OR for primary resection, place ileostomy
- **Surgery** - for 1) **significant Cx's** (failure of medical Tx, free perforation [eg fecal or purulent peritonitis], or large abscess [> 4 cm] not amenable to percutaneous drainage) *or;* 2) **inability to exclude CA**
  - Need to resect all of the **sigmoid colon** down to the superior rectum (distal margin should be **normal rectum** and *no* diverticuli)
  - Patients with diffuse diverticuli throughout the colon (ascending, transverse, and descending) *only* need the symptomatic area removed (eg diverticulitis or refractory bleeding area); *Do not perform total procto-colectomy*
  - If elective surgery undertaken, wait **6-8 weeks** to allow inflammation to subside
  - *Consider* elective resection for <u>immunocompromised</u> patients (eg diabetes, on steroids), <u>repeated</u> bouts of severe diverticulitis (3 or 4), or patients that required <u>percutaneous drainage</u> (some controversy with these)
- **Right-sided diverticulitis** - 80% discovered at the time of incision for appendectomy
  - Tx: right hemicolectomy and primary anastomosis
- **Colovesicular fistula** (colon to bladder)
  - MC fistula in **men** with diverticulitis
  - Sx's: fecaluria, pneumaturia, UTIs
  - MCC - **diverticulitis** (others - IBD, XRT, colon and bladder CA)
  - Dx: **cystoscopy** (*best test;* <u>not</u> colonoscopy); UA will show enteric contents
  - Tx: if due to diverticulitis → resect involved segment of colon and perform primary anastomosis, close bladder opening (<u>not</u> cystectomy), diverting ileostomy, interpose omentum between bladder and colon
  - If due to CA, en bloc resection is indicated
- **Colo-vaginal fistula** (MC fistula in <u>women</u> with diverticulitis) - similar to above except close the defect in the vagina
- **Inability to exclude CA** → Tx: elective resection
- **Late sigmoid strictures** can form → Tx: balloon dilate; resection if severe

DIVERTICULOSIS BLEEDING
- *MCC of LGI bleeding*
- Usually causes **significant bleeding**
- 75% stops spontaneously; recurs in 25%
- Caused by disrupted **vasa rectum**; creates **arterial bleeding**
- Tx: **endoscopic Tx** (*hemo-clips best*, epinephrine injection, cautery), surgery if that fails
- Patients with **recurrent** diverticular bleeds should have **resection** of area

ANGIODYSPLASIA BLEEDING (AVM's)
- MC on **right side of colon** or in **small bowel**
- Bleeds are usually less severe than diverticular bleeds but are more likely to recur (80%)
- Causes **venous bleeding**
- *Small bowel AVM's are the MCC of **obscure GI bleeding*** (ie not apparent on standard upper and lower endoscopy)
- Soft signs of angiodysplasia on angiogram - **tufts, slow emptying**
- 20% of patients with angiodysplasia have **aortic stenosis** (usually gets better after valve replacement); high incidence in patients with left ventricular assist devices (LVADs)
- Dx: **colonoscopy**
  - If in the **small bowel**, a **video capsule study** or **double balloon endoscopy** are usually indicated to find these
- Tx: **endoscopic Tx** (hemo-clips, cautery, epinephrine), surgery if that fails
  - **Aminocaproic acid** for diffuse disease to control bleeding (short term Tx)
  - **Octreotide** may be effective
  - **Recurrent bleeding** → resection (unless diffuse disease)

ISCHEMIC COLITIS

- Sx's: abdominal pain, hematochezia (LGI bleeding), usually in elderly (70's)
- Etiologies - **low-flow state** (MC; eg recent MI, CHF, sepsis, medical ICU patient, cardiac surgery, severe dehydration, massive diarrhea), **hypoxia** (eg COPD, ARDS), **ligation of inferior mesenteric artery** (IMA) at surgery (eg AAA repair)
- Usually **left sided** (LLQ pain)
- **Splenic flexure** and **upper rectum** are most vulnerable to **low-flow states** and **hypoxia** (watershed areas)
    - **Griffith's Point** (splenic flexure) - middle colic *(off SMA)* and left colic *(off IMA)* junction
    - **Sudeck's Point** - superior rectal *(off IMA)* and middle rectals *(2; off internal iliacs)* junction
    - **Middle and lower rectum are <u>spared</u>** → supplied by middle (off internal iliac) and inferior (off internal pudendal, which is branch of internal iliac) rectal arteries
        Proctoscopy is <u>not</u> sufficient to rule-out ischemic colitis
    - Dx:CT scan- thick edematous mucosa (thumbprint sign); thick colon wall; fat stranding
    - **Endoscopy** *(best test)* → thick, cyanotic, edematous mucosa covered with exudates (do <u>not</u> go past area of injury - risks perforation; just make the Dx and rule out other disease [eg IBD, colon CA])
- Tx: **volume resuscitation and antibiotics** *(best initial Tx)*; bowel rest
    - If **gangrenous colitis** is suspected (diffuse peritonitis, severe sepsis), uncontrolled hemorrhage occurs, or if **perforation** occurs → <u>no</u> colonoscopy and go to OR (sigmoid resection or left hemicolectomy usual)
    - If **necrotic bowel** is found on colonoscopy (**black bowel**) → OR for resection
- **Late strictures** can occur from ischemia - Tx: **dilatation 1st**, resection if refractory

POLYPS

- **Hyperplastic polyps** - MC polyp; <u>no</u> CA risk
- **Inflammatory polyps** (pseudopolyps) - found in ulcerative colitis
- **Tubular adenoma** - MC intestinal neoplastic polyp (75%)
    - Usually pedunculated; **< 5% have CA**
- **Tubovillous** adenoma - **20% contain CA**
- **Villous adenoma** - neoplastic polyp most likely to be symptomatic
    - Usually sessile and larger than tubular adenomas
    - **40% contain CA**
- **Increased CA risk** - > 2 cm, sessile, or villous lesions
- Most colon CA's develop from a polyp
- Polyps have a **left side** predominance
- Most **pedunculated polyps** can be removed endoscopically
- If not able to get all of the polyp (which usually occurs with **sessile polyps**) → need **segmental resection** (stain area with methylene blue so you can find it at the time of resection)
- **High-grade dysplasia** - basement membrane is intact (carcinoma in situ)
- **Intra-mucosal CA** - into muscularis mucosa (carcinoma in situ → still has not gone through basement membrane)
- **Invasive CA** - invades submucosa (T1)
- **Polypectomy** shows **T1 lesion** - polypectomy is adequate if *(need all 3):*
    1) Margins are clear (2 mm)
    2) Is well differentiated
    3) No neuro / vascular / lymphatic invasion
    - *If above not met, need formal colon resection*
- Extensive **low rectal villous adenomas** with atypia - Tx: **transanal excision** (can try mucosectomy) as much of the polyp as possible
    - <u>No</u> APR unless CA is present (if is a T1 tumor, trans-anal excision may still be adequate - see below)
- Pathology shows **T1 lesion** after transanal excision of **rectal villous adenoma** → transanal excision is adequate if *(need all 3):*
    1) Margins are clear (2 mm)
    2) It is well differentiated
    3) It has no neuro / vascular / lymphatic invasion
    - *Need formal resection if above criteria not met*

- Pathology shows **T2 lesion** after transanal excision of **rectal polyp** → Tx: patient needs APR or LAR *(still standard of care)*; pre-op chemo-XRT if T3 or T4
- **Bleeding** after polypectomy - Dx and Tx: **re-scope**
- **Perforation** after polypectomy (Dx: upright CXR, look for free air under the diaphragm) - Tx: **open primary repair**

COLORECTAL CANCER
- 2nd leading cause of CA death
- Sx's: change in bowel habits (**constipation**), small caliber stools, bleeding, iron deficient microcytic anemia, pain
- MC location - **sigmoid colon**
- **Pathology**
  - **CEA** - useful for 1) prognosis (predicts worse prognosis), 2) to detect recurrence, and 3) to follow response to Tx
    Not useful as a screening tool for colon CA
  - Main **gene mutations**: **APC** (tumor suppressor), **p53** (tumor suppressor), **k-ras** (proto-oncogene GTPase or G protein), **DCC** (tumor suppressor)
  - *Better* prognosis - **lymphocytic penetration**
  - *Worse* prognosis - **mucinous** (Signet Ring cell)
  - Associated with **strep gallolyticus** (strep bovis biotype I) and **clostridium septicum** bacteremia - likely represents a marker for colon CA (**colonscopy** is indicated if patients present with these infections)
  - False-positive fecal occult blood test - beef, Vit C, iron, antacids, cimetidine
- **Disease spread**
  - Spreads to **nodes** 1st
  - Most important prognostic indicator - **node status**
  - 5% get drop metastases to **ovaries**
  - MC sites for metastases - **liver** (#1) and lung (#2)
  - Portal vein → **liver metastases**; iliac vein → **lung metastases**
  - **Isolated** liver or lung metastases should be **resected** if resectable and leaves adequate organ tissue behind for function
    - **Liver metastases** - 5-year survival of 35% (selected patients), see below
    - **Lung metastases** - 5-year survival rate of 25% (selected patients)
  - **Rectal CA** - can metastasize to **spine** directly via Batson's plexus (venous)
  - **Colon CA** typically does not go to bone
  - Colorectal CA growing into **adjacent organs** can be resected **en bloc** with a portion of the adjacent organ (eg partial bladder resection)
  - Worse prognosis signs - perforation, ulceration, obstruction
- **Trans-rectal ultrasound** (TRUS) for rectal CA - good at assessing depth of invasion (T status, eg **sphincter** involvement), recurrence, and presence of enlarged nodes (N status)
  - *Best test for T and N status*
  - **T3** and **T4** rectal lesions get neoadjuvant chemo-XRT
- Need **total colonoscopy** to rule-out **synchronous** lesions in patients with colorectal CA
- **Goals of resection**
  - Ultimately resection for all unless stage IV (some stage IV disease may be resected, see below)
  - **En bloc resection** includes: associated **mesocolon**, regional **lymph nodes** (adenectomy), and adequate **margins** (rectal CA ≥ **2 cm**; colon CA ≥ **4-5 cm**; low rectal T1 ≥ **2 mm** - see below)
  - Rectal CA that is **T3, T4,** or has **positive nodes** (stage II or higher) → Tx: *neoadjuvant (pre-op) chemo-XRT 1st* and re-stage
    - **Pre-op chemo-XRT** - produces complete response for some rectal CA's; preserves sphincter in some patients due to tumor shrinkage
  - **T1** or **T2** rectal CA with negative nodes - resection *(no neoadjuvant Tx)*
  - Take **Waldeyer's** and **Denonvilliers fascia** for rectal tumors
  - **Right-sided** colon CA can be treated with primary anastomosis without diverting ileostomy
  - **Rectal pain** with rectal CA → patient needs **APR** (growing into sphincters or pelvic floor)

- Colorectal CA invasion of **adjacent organs** (T4) should be *resected en bloc* (e. partial bladder resection, pancreas, liver, duodenum, any other organ) → this is stage II if nodes are negative and no metastases; should not cut across tumor with resection (even if you have to perform a Whipple)
- **Colon perforation** from obstruction - MC in **cecum** (Law of LaPlace tension = pressure x diameter)
- Suspected **colo-vesicle fistula** → Dx: **cystoscopy** *(best test)*

- **Intra-operative ultrasound** (U/S) - best method of picking up intrahepatic metastases
    - Conventional U/S resolution: 10 mm
    - Abdominal CT: 5-10 mm
    - Abdominal MRI: 5-10 mm (better resolution than CT)
    - *Intra-op U/S: 3-5 mm*

- **Standard resection** techniques:
    - **Right hemi-colectomy** - take ileo-colic and right colic arteries
    - **Transverse colectomy** - take the middle colic artery
    - **Extended right hemicolectomy** - for **hepatic flexure** tumors
        Take ileo-colic, right colic, and middle colic arteries
        Will need to resect most of the transverse colon
    - **Left hemi-colectomy** - take left colic artery
    - **Extended left hemicolectomy** - for **splenic flexure** tumors
        Take left colic and middle colic arteries

- **Low anterior resection** (LAR)
    - Used for **sigmoid** and **rectal** tumors - sigmoid colon and portion of the rectum are resected
    - Take sigmoidal and rectal arteries
    - Leave main inferior mesenteric artery (and left colic) intact to supply left colon
    - Need at least a **2 cm margin** - needs to be at least **2 cm** from levator ani muscles (proximal anal canal) → *if not, perform APR*
    - You need a 2 cm rectal cuff above the anal canal which will be resected with the end to end stapler (send the donut in stapler to path as this is part of your margin)
    - In general, it is easier to perform LAR in women compared to men because thei pelvic bones are wider
    - **Diverting loop ileostomy** recommended for all LARs (controversial; decreases complications of a leak should one occur)
    - Watch for **ureters** (travel over iliac vessels) and **iliac vessels**
    - Watch for **pudendal nerves** (in pelvic sidewall, risk of incontinence and ejaculatory failure) when taking down the **lateral stalks**
    - **Lateral stalks** contain **middle rectal arteries**
    - **Local recurrence** after LAR (at suture line) → Tx: **APR** (re-stage 1st)
    - **Abscess** following LAR → Tx: percutaneous drain

- **Abdominoperineal resection** (APR)
    - Removes rectum and anus with placement of permanent colostomy
    - Can have **impotence** and **bladder dysfunction** after APR
    - *Indicated only for malignant lesions that are not amenable to LAR (not used for benign tumors)*
    - Risk of local recurrence higher with rectal CA than colon CA in general

TNM STAGING FOR COLORECTAL CANCER

Tis: limited to mucosa; not beyond muscularis mucosa
    Carcinoma in situ or *intra-mucosal carcinoma*
T1: invades submucosa
T2: invades muscularis propria
T3: invades subserosa or completely through muscularis propria if no serosa is present
T4: through serosa into free peritoneal cavity (perforates visceral peritoneum) or
    invades adjacent organs / tissues

N0: nodes negative
N1: 1-3 nodes positive
N2: ≥ 4 nodes positive

M1: distant metastases

Stage	TNM Status
Stage 0	Tis, N0, M0
Stage I	T1-2, N0, M0
Stage IIa	T3, N0, M0
Stage IIb	T4, N0, M0
Stage IIIa	T1-2, N1, M0
Stage IIIb	T3-4, N1, M0
Stage IIIc	Any T, N2, M0
Stage IV	Any T, Any N, M1

- **Low rectal T1 lesion** (limited to submucosa) - assess with **TRUS**
  - Can be excised **trans-anally** if:
    - 1) **< 4 cm** in size
    - 2) **< 1/3 circumference**
    - 3) **Negative margins** (need at least **2 mm** margin)
    - 4) **Well differentiated**
    - 5) **No neuro / vascular / lymphatic invasion**
    - *If above not met, need APR or LAR*
- **Low rectal T2** or higher - Tx: APR or LAR
- **Chemo**
  - **Stage III and IV <u>colon</u> CA** (positive nodes or distant metastases) → **post-op chemo**, <u>no</u> XRT for colon CA
  - **Stage II and III <u>rectal</u> CA** → **pre-op chemo-XRT** (neoadjuvant), surgery, then adjuvant chemo
  - **Stage IV rectal CA** → **chemo and XRT +/- surgery** (possibly just colostomy, may want to avoid APR in patients with metastatic disease)
  - Chemo - **5-FU, leucovorin, and oxaliplatin** (FOLFOX, *6 cycles*)
  - Side effects: <u>5-FU</u> - myelosuppression; <u>oxaliplatin</u> - nephrotoxicity, neurotoxicity, ototoxicity (all less than cisplatin)
  - If <u>metastatic</u> disease, *add* **Bevacizumab** (Avastin; monoclonal antibody to vascular endothelial growth factor [VEGF-A]) or **Cetuximab** (Erbitux; monoclonal antibody to epidermal growth factor receptor [EGF receptor])
- **XRT** (5000 rads)
  - Decreases **local recurrence**
  - **XRT damage** (**rectum MC site**) - vasculitis, thrombosis, ulcers, strictures, bleeding
  - **Pre-op chemo-XRT** may help shrink **rectal tumors**, allowing down-staging of the tumor and possibly allowing LAR versus APR
- **5-year survival** for colorectal CA:
  - Stage I - 95%
  - Stage II - 80%
  - Stage III - 65%
  - Stage IV - 10%
- Chemo improves 5-YS for **stage III** colorectal CA (positive nodes, no metastases)
- 20% have a **recurrence** (usually occurs within 1 year)
  - 5% get another primary (metachronous) - *main reason for <u>surveillance colonoscopy</u> after 1 year*
- **Follow-up colonoscopy** at 1 year - mainly to check for a **new primary colon CA** (5% get metachronous lesion)
- **Liver metastases**
  - Liver metastases are supplied by the **hepatic artery** (which would be route of intra-arterial chemotherapy or embolization for palliation)
  - **Resect if completely resectable** and leaves adequate liver function (need **1 cm margin**) - number of tumors, size, and location are not factors if you can get complete resection (even bi-lobar lesions)
  - **Wedge vs formal resection** for liver metastases depends on number and location (eg metastases to *segments 1 and 2* → need left lobectomy and caudate resection; metastases to *segments 5 and 7* → right lobectomy)

- **Poor prognostic indicators** for metastases to the liver:
  - Disease free interval < 12 months
  - \> 3 tumors
  - CEA > 200 (mcg/L)
  - Size > 5 cm
  - Positive nodes
  - Synchronous primary and liver met
- LFTs are not sensitive indicators for liver metastases
- **Intra-op U/S** - *most sensitive method* of picking up metastases to the liver (detects 3-5 mm lesions)
- **5-YS** after resection of isolated liver metastases - 35%

RADIATION PROCTITIS (radiation enterocolitis)
- Risk increased if the patient also receives **chemo**
- **Acute radiation proctitis / enteritis** (1st few weeks; direct damage to **mucosal cells**)
  - Sx's: diarrhea, tenesmus, pain (usually self-limiting process)
  - Tx: conservative Tx (**butyrate enemas** if proctitis) unless perforation (rare)
- **Late radiation proctitis** (months to years; due to **obliterative arteritis** of submucosal vessels)
  - Sx's: **bleeding** (MC), obstruction, fistula, ulcer (get Bx to rule-out CA)
  - Dx: **proctoscopy**
  - **Rectal bleeding** - Tx: dilute **formalin fixation** of rectum *(best Tx)*; argon beam, cautery, epinephrine injection, rectal resection (last resort)
  - **Stricture** with obstruction - Tx: low residue diet, rectal steroids, stricture **dilatation**; local trans-anal excision if refractory (2-3 months); **divert** with ostomy (as a last resort)
  - **Fistulas** Tx - usually conservative Tx
  - *Avoid APR for radiation proctitis*
- **Late radiation colitis or enteritis** (eg XRT for previous ovarian CA; due to **obliterative arteritis**) - Tx: *fluid resuscitation 1st*; surgery if needed (eg refractory bowel obstruction)
  - Results in **fibrosis** and **stricture** formation, leading to **small bowel obstruction**
  - Small bowel resection only when *safe*, otherwise go with entero-enteric bypass (eg for matted bowel)
  - Colon can generally be resected
  - Small bowel fistulas can also form (usually conservative Tx)
  - *Avoid extensive adhesionolysis (risks enterotomy)*
  - *No stricturoplasty*
  - *Corticosteroids are not effective*

FAMILIAL ADENOMATOUS POLYPOSIS (FAP; autosomal dominant; chromosome 5)
- *All have CA by **age 50** (100% lifetime risk); rarely have CA before age 20*
- Mutation in **APC gene** (tumor suppressor) - genetic testing is available and removes necessity of screening family members who do not have the mutation
- *Polyps are not present at birth*
- *Polyps are present in **puberty** (1000's of polyps; carpet the colon)*
- Do not need colonoscopy for surveillance with suspected FAP → just need flexible sigmoidoscopy to check for polyps (in teens)
- Need **total colectomy** prophylactically at **age 20** (colon CA rare before that age)
  - Allows for physical, social, and emotional maturation
  - Many choose a transition in education or from education to employment as a good time for surgery
- Also get **duodenal periampullary polyps** and **adenocarcinoma** → need to check duodenum for polyps and CA with EGD every 1-2 years (remove polyps if found)
- Also get **intra-abdominal desmoid tumors**
- **Newly discovered FAP** (thousands of polyps on sigmoidoscopy) →
  1) Perform **complete colonoscopy** and **metastatic work-up** (CT scan - look for associated **desmoid tumors**, ie Gardner's Syndrome)
  2) Need **EGD** to look for duodenal polyps and CA
  3) Offer genetic counseling to rest of the family

- ■ **Surgery**
  - • Total proctocolectomy, rectal mucosectomy, and ileo-anal pouch
  - • Lifetime **proctoscopy** surveillance of **residual rectal area** and EGD (every 1-2 years) to look for duodenal **polyps / tumors**
  - • **Total proctocolectomy with end ileostomy** also an option
- ■ Following colectomy, the MCC of death with FAP is **peri-ampullary CA of the duodenum** (would need Whipple)
- ■ **Gardner's syndrome** (FAP variant; APC gene)
  - 1) **Colon CA**
  - 2) **Osteomas** (bumps on forehead or other bony protuberances, benign - leave alone)
  - 3) Intra-abdominal **desmoid tumors** - benign but very <u>locally invasive</u>
    - High recurrence rate (70%)
    - Tx: often <u>not</u> amenable to WLE due to local invasion; risk of short bowel syndrome with resection (see Skin and Soft Tissue chapter)
- ■ **Turcot's syndrome** (FAP variant) - **colon CA** and **brain tumors**

LYNCH SYNDROMES (Hereditary Non-polyposis Colon Cancer, autosomal dominant)
- ■ **Fewer polyps than APC** (< 100)
- ■ Defects in **DNA mismatch repair genes** (hMSH2, hMLH1, hPMS1, etc)
- ■ Predilection for **right-sided** and **multiple** colon CA (**80%** lifetime risk)
- ■ **Lynch I** - just colon CA risk
- ■ **Lynch II** - patients <u>also</u> have increased risk of other CA (eg ovarian, endometrial, bladder, stomach)
- ■ **Amsterdam criteria** for Lynch Syndrome - "3, 2, 1" →
  - • At least **3** family members (one of whom is a first-degree relative of the other two [eg parents, siblings, and offspring])
  - • Over **2** generations
  - • **1** relative with cancer before age 50
  - • FAP has been excluded
- ■ 50% get metachronous lesions within 10 years; often have multiple primaries
- ■ Prognosis <u>better</u> stage for stage compared to sporadic colon CA
- ■ Need **total procto-colectomy** with <u>first</u> colon CA operation

Lynch surveillance protocol

CA	Screening Age	Exam	Interval (yrs)
Colorectal CA	20-25	Colonoscopy	1-2
Uterus/Ovaries	**35**-40	Vaginal U/S Aspiration Bx	1-2
Stomach	30-**35**	Upper Endoscopy	1-2
Urinary Tract	30-**35**	Urine cytology and U/S	1

FAMILIAL JUVENILE POLYPOSIS (autosomal dominant)
- ■ Form **hamartomatous polyps**
- ■ Can occur in upper GI tract and in the colon; usually before are 20
- ■ Small risk of adenomatous change and CA formation in the polyp (20%; annual upper and lower endoscopy recommended); *risk of CA <u>not</u> nearly as high as FAP (100%)*
- ■ Should remove these polyps when found
- ■ <u>No</u> prophylactic colon resection for just polyps
- ■ **Adenomatous changes** in the polyps are an indication for colectomy

LAPAROSCOPIC VS. OPEN COLON SURGERY
- ■ Laparoscopy compared to open has (experienced surgeons):
  - • Less blood loss
  - • Longer operative time
  - • Shorter hospital stay (mean 4 days vs 7 days)
  - • No difference in pathologic margins
  - • No difference in number of nodes recovered
  - • No difference in morbidity or mortality

PERIOP MANAGEMENT IN COLORECTAL SURGERY

- **Mechanical bowel prep**
  - <u>No</u> bowel prep if undergoing colon surgery
  - Need bowel prep if undergoing rectal surgery and ileostomy is planned
- <u>No</u> **overnight fasting**
  - Can have clears up to <u>2 hours</u> before surgery and solids up to <u>6 hours</u> before surgery
- Pre-op **carbohydrate drink** <u>2 hours</u> before surgery
- Pre-op **laxatives / prokinetics** (bisacodyl / metoclopramide)
  - Use if colon resection
  - Not used for rectal surgery if ileostomy is planned
- <u>No</u> **NG tube**
- **Epidurals** are encouraged (earlier return of bowel function)
- **Laparoscopic** approach
  - Use if colon case or benign rectal case
  - <u>Not</u> recommended for malignant rectal CA
- <u>No</u> **drains**
- **Immediate mobilization** post-op - out of bed for <u>2 hours</u> on day of surgery
- **Early post-op diet** - oral ad-librium diet (clears, advanced to solids as tolerated by patient)
  - Start clears within <u>24 hours</u> after **colon** or **rectal surgery**
  - Results in earlier return of gut function and decreased length of stay (6 days vs. 9 days)
  - **Alvimopan** (Entereg) - mu-opiod antagonist; decreases LOS by 24 hours
    - *Avoid* in patients on prolonged narcotics pre-op
- **Chewing gum** - promotes earlier return of bowel function

COMPLICATIONS FROM COLORECTAL SURGERY

- **J-pouch bleeding** - Tx: **iced saline** with **epinephrine enemas**
- **Venous plexus** bleeding in pelvis (can be hard to control) - Tx: bone wax or sterile thumbtacks
  - Initially just apply pressure while anesthesia gives resuscitation
- **Anastomotic leaks**
  - Highest rate is for coloanal anastomoses (15%)
  - The lower the anastomosis, the higher the leak rate
  - **Diverting ileostomy** is recommended for all LARs to help complications of a leak (eg sepsis, MSOF, death) should one occur
  - RFs: neoadjuvant chemo-XRT, prednisone, Infliximab
  - *Free leak* (usually presents in <u>first few days</u>; Sx's - fever, tenderness, abdominal pain) - **peritonitis** and possible sepsis can occur as feculent material spreads throughout peritoneum
    - Tx options include **abdominal washout** <u>and</u> either:
    1) Anastomosis takedown and creation of end stoma +/- mucus fistula <u>or</u>,
    2) Primary repair and diverting ileostomy <u>or</u>,
    3) Wide drainage and diverting ileostomy
  - *Contained leak* (usually presents <u>> 7 days</u> after surgery) - CT with oral contrast shows limited contrast leak near anastomosis; often results in an **abscess**
    - Tx:
      - **Percutaneous drain** if significant abscess present (<u>> 4 cm</u>; if just a small contrast leak without significant abscess, a drain is <u>not</u> indicated)
      - Diverting ileostomy (allows area to heal)
      - Antibiotics
    - May result in a fistula or stricture (conservative Tx for up to 6 months)
- **Abscess** - may or may not have associated leak; Tx: **percutaneous drain** if ≥ 4 cm
- **Ureter injury** - can present in the OR or late (Tx depends on when injury is discovered); late can present with yellow-tinged wound drainage, azotemia, or pain from hydronephrosis (ligated ureter)
  - **< 7 days** post-op - reoperate and repair (see Trauma chapter for ureter repair)
  - **≥ 7 days** post-op - place percutaneous drain and wait 6-8 weeks before repair

- > 90% of iatrogenic ureteral injuries occur in the **lower 1/3** of the ureter and re-implantation in the bladder is indicated (ureteroneocystostomy)

- **Bladder dysfunction** (dysuria, frequency)- pelvic splanchnic plexus (parasympathetic)
- **Sexual dysfunction**
  - **Erectile dysfunction** - damage to **pelvic splanchnic plexus** (parasympathetic)
  - **Retrograde ejaculation** - damage to **hypogastric plexus** (sympathetic; T10-L2); MC sexual dysfunction after proctectomy; often resolves
  - **Ejaculatory failure** - damage to **pudendal nerve** (sympathetic; S2-4) in the pelvic sidewall
- **Laparotomy** in the **late post-op period** ($\geq$ 7 days)
  - *This is extremely <u>difficult</u> and <u>dangerous</u> due to dense inflammatory adhesions*
  - Risks include - creation of enterotomies, mesenteric vascular injury, enterocutaneous fistula, and need for massive small bowel resection due to injury
  - If at all possible, surgery should be delayed for at least **6-8 weeks** (eg ureter injury discovered after 7 days)
- **Wound infection** - occurs in 10% undergoing colorectal surgery
  - Sx's: yellow, thick drainage from wound
  - RFs: malnutrition, DM, immunosuppression, age > 60
  - Typically present **POD 5**
  - Tx: open overlying skin, pack wound or place wound vac; allow to heal by secondary intention
- **Perineal wound infection** - RFs include neoadjuvant XRT, prolonged OR time, fecal contamination
  - Tx: open incision to allow drainage, debridement of devitalized tissue, local wound care by packing or wound vac
- **Fascial dehiscence** (Sx's - sudden leak of a large amount of **salmon colored fluid**; bulge under the skin incision [due to intestines])
  - Tx: <u>immediate</u> operative re-exploration, place **retention sutures**
  - Small fascial dehiscence, late after surgery ($\geq$ 7 days) - consider conservative management (eg wet to dry dressing changes)
- **Enterotomy** (inadvertent, iatrogenic) - sucus or green drainage from wound
  - **< 7 days** (this is a <u>leak</u>) → re-operate and repair enterotomy
  - **$\geq$ 7 days** (this is an enterocutaneous <u>fistula</u>) → conservative Tx if fascia is intact and no signs of 1) fasciitis, 2) peritonitis (peritoneal signs), <u>or</u> 3) sepsis (see Small Bowel chapter for management)
- **Dark stoma after APR** - re-operate and revise (indicates vascular compromise; can end up with necrosis or stricture)
- MCC stoma **stenosis** - ischemia, Tx: dilatation
- MCC **fistula** near stoma - Crohn's Disease
- MC stomal **infection** - Candida

Rectum and Anus

999. All of the following are true except:
    a.   Waldeyer's fascia separates the rectum from the sacral venous plexus
    b.   Denonvillier's fascia separates the rectum from the prostate in men and vagina in women
    c.   The rectovesicle fascia separates the rectum from the urethra
    d.   The levator ani marks the transition between rectum and anal canal
    e.   The dentate line marks the transition from columnar to stratified squamous epithelium

Answer c. The recto-vesicle fascia separates the rectum from the bladder

1000. All of the following are true except:
    a.   Anal canal tumors can spread to the inguinal nodes
    b.   Superior and middle rectal areas drain to the IMA nodes
    c.   The lower rectum drains to the IMA and internal iliac nodes
    d.   Above the dentate line (anal canal), tumors only spread to either the IMA or internal iliac nodes
    e.   Below the dentate line (anal margin), tumors drain primarily to the inguinal nodes

Answer d. Anal canal tumors (ie above the dentate line) tend to drain to the **internal iliac** and **inguinal** nodes (eg anal canal squamous cell CA)

1001. All of the following are true except:
    a.   Superior rectal veins drain into IMV
    b.   Middle rectal veins drain into both the IMV and internal iliac veins (dual drainage systems)
    c.   Inferior rectal veins drain into internal iliac veins and eventually inferior vena cava
    d.   The superior rectal artery is a branch of the inferior mesenteric artery (IMA)
    e.   The middle rectal artery is a branch of the IMA

Answer e. The middle rectal artery is a branch of the internal iliac artery

1002. Melanosis coli should be treated with:
    a.   Total abdominal colectomy
    b.   Resection of only the obvious areas
    c.   Palliative care only
    d.   Observation

Answer d. Melanosis coli is a benign condition that involves pigmentation of the colon. It is associated with laxative use and the condition may resolve after it is discontinued.

1003. A 25 yo woman with Crohn's has a peri-anal fistula on routine exam. She has not had any symptoms. The most appropriate next step is:
    a.   XRT
    b.   Endo-rectal advancement flap
    c.   Cutting seton stitch
    d.   Fistulotomy
    e.   Observation

Answer e. Observation. Avoid operating on fistulas in patients with Crohn's as healing is generally poor and complication rates are high. Asymptomatic fistulas in patients with Crohn's can remain dormant for long periods.

1004. Which of the following is the best therapy for a trans-sphincteric fistula that is refractory to a draining seton stitch:

    a. APR
    b. Fistulotomy
    c. Endo-rectal advancement flap
    d. Cutting seton stitch

Answer c. Endo-rectal advancement flap avoids anal incontinence risk.

1005. Which of the following perianal fistula types is least likely to raise concern for a more serious underlying pathology:
    a. A fistula following a peri-rectal abscess in a diabetic patient
    b. Fistula recurrence
    c. Multiple sinus tracts emanating from a fistula
    d. An associated mass

Answer a. A fistula following a peri-rectal abscess in a diabetic patient

Recurrent, multiple, or fistulas with multiple sinus tracts should raise concern for another pathology (eg anal CA, inflammatory bowel disease, STDs)

1006. Which of the following fistula types has the lowest risk of anal incontinence with fistulotomy:
    a. Extra-sphincteric
    b. Posterior inter-sphincteric
    c. Anterior inter-sphincteric
    d. Trans-sphincteric
    e. Supra-sphincteric

Answer a. Extra-sphincteric fistulas are not associated with the sphincter and carry no incontinence risk.

1007. A 55 yo man presents to the ED with anal pain. You try to examine the area in the ED but he is quite tender so you take him to the OR for EUA (exam under anesthesia) and find an abscess. All of the following are true of this condition except:
    a. A supra-levator abscess must be drained transrectally
    b. An inter-sphincteric horseshoe abscess requires a horseshoe-type incision
    c. These are usually caused by an obstructed gland
    d. Antibiotics are indicated for patients with prosthetic hardware
    e. Diabetes is a RF

Answer b. A **horseshoe abscess** does not require a significant incision, just enough to relieve the abscess

1008. A 50 yo man presents with peri-anal pain for 48 hours. On exam you find a small tender bluish-purple mass. The most appropriate therapy is:
    a. Lance open the hemorrhoid
    b. Elliptical incision
    c. NTG cream
    d. Ca cream
    e. Botox

Answer b. Elliptical incision (see below)

1009. Instead of the above the patient has had pain for 96 hours. The most appropriate therapy is:
    a. Lance open the hemorrhoid
    b. Elliptical incision
    c. NTG cream
    d. Ca cream
    e. Botox

Answer a. Lance open the hemorrhoid

Thrombosed external hemorrhoid → Tx:

If **< 72 hours** of Sx's - <u>surgery</u> with elliptical excision

If **> 72 hours** of Sx's - <u>lance</u> open only (pain of surgery worse than hemorrhoid itself at this point; hemorrhoid will become fibrosed)

1010. Eight days after internal hemorrhoid resection your patient is alarmed by a small amount of blood smear on toilet paper. Which of the following is true:

    a.   This is likely a bleeding diverticulum

    b.   This is likely ischemic colitis

    c.   This is likely a peptic ulcer

    d.   The patient would likely benefit from fiber supplements

Answer d. This patient has **sloughing of eschar** from his **hemorrhoidectomy site**. **Fiber supplements** and **improved hydration** help avoid local trauma.

Severe bleeding (rare; eg toilet bowel full of blood, possible hypotension) would require an exam under anesthesia (EUA) with suture ligation of the bleeding area.

1011. A 60 yo woman presents with severe perianal pain and bleeding from large hemorrhoids that she is normally able to manually reduce. On exam, you find a large swollen mass of hemorrhoidal tissue that you are unable to deliver back through the anus. The most appropriate next step is urgent:

    a.   Stab incision

    b.   Elliptical excision

    c.   3 quadrant resection

    d.   EUA and manually reduce in the OR

    e.   Banding

Answer c. Strangulated quaternary hemorrhoids should be resected to prevent necrosis (urgent hemorrhoidectomy with 3 quadrant resection).

The dentate line separates internal from external hemorrhoids.

1012. A 32 yo man undergoes discectomy for a ruptured lumbar disc. He has required heavy narcotic use and POD 5 he is noted to have blood in his stools. Which of the following is true:

    a.   The patient likely has a aorto-enteric fistula

    b.   The patient is likely bleeding from a sigmoidal artery

    c.   The patient likely has a colon cancer

    d.   The patient likely needs stool softeners

Answer d. This patient most likely has an **anal fissure** related to constipation and straining from large hard stools. Surgery (especially back surgery) can cause this problem which is compounded by heavy narcotic use.

1013. A 50 man presents with pain on defecation and some red streaking after bowel movements for the past 3 weeks. Anal exam reproduces the symptoms and you notice some piled up anoderm in the posterior midline along the anal margin. There is a small tear there as well. The initial treatment for this patient is:

    a.   Topical NTG cream

    b.   Topical calcium channel blocker

    c.   Botox

    d.   Lateral internal subcutaneous sphincterotomy

    e.   Topical evening primrose oil

Answer a. The initial Tx of **anal fissure** (piled up anoderm is the **sentinel pile** associated with these) is medical with Sitz baths, stool softeners, increasing fluid intake, and **topical nitrate cream**.

Anal fissures that are not in the midline (ie **lateral fissures**) should raise
suspicions of other pathologies (eg anal CA, inflammatory bowel disease, STDs)

1014. Despite 3 months of therapy, the above patient has continued symptoms. The most
appropriate next step is::
   a.   Topical NTG cream
   b.   Topical calcium channel blocker
   c.   Botox
   d.   Lateral internal subcutaneous sphincterotomy

   Answer b. Topical calcium channel blocker is indicated for refractory cases (>
   3 months)

   Surgical indications for anal fissure (lateral internal sphincterotomy) - failure to
   improve after 2 cycles of calcium channel blocker (patients that have failed
   around 6 months of medical Tx)

1015. For anal fissures that have failed over 6 months of aggressive medical therapy, which
of the following has the highest healing rate:
   a.   Botox injection
   b.   Lateral internal subcutaneous sphincterotomy
   c.   Fibrin glue
   d.   Colace

   Answer b. Lateral internal subcutaneous sphincterotomy (90% healing
   rate), Botox (60% healing rate), poorer results with fibrin glue.

1016. The most serious complication of lateral internal subcutaneous sphincterotomy is:
   a.   Anal incontinence
   b.   Infection
   c.   Persistent pain
   d.   Bleeding

   Answer a. Anal incontinence

1017. All of the following are true of procidentia except:
   a.   Initially treated with laxatives
   b.   Initially treated with high fiber diet and stool softeners
   c.   Is secondary to pudendal neuropathy
   d.   The Altemeier procedure is good for frail patients

   Answer a. Laxatives are *contraindicated* in patients with **rectal prolapse**
   (procidentia). Conservative medical Tx (high fiber diet and stool softeners) is
   indicated for rectal prolapse that reduces spontaneously. Patients that have to
   manually reduce or who cannot reduce the prolapse (incarcerated rectal
   prolapse) require surgery.

1018. An 82 yo multiparous woman from a nursing home has severe dementia, COPD, and
requires oxygen. She presents with fecal incontinence and on exam her rectum slides
below her anus. You are able to reduce it manually. The most appropriate surgical
strategy in this patient would be:
   a.   Perineal rectosigmoidectomy
   b.   Open low anterior resection (LAR) and pexy
   c.   Laparoscopic low anterior resection and rectopexy
   d.   Anterior mesh rectopexy

   Answer a. This patient has **rectal prolapse** (procidentia). For elderly and frail
   patients, the **Altemeier procedure (perineal rectosigmoidectomy)** avoids a
   laparotomy. The redundant rectum and sigmoid are manually prolapsed through
   the anus, are resected with primary anastomosis and then returned to the pelvis.

For young and fit patients, **LAR** (**recto-sigmoid resection** with pexy of the residual colon, laparoscopic or open) offers the best chance of long-term success (< 10% recurrence).

1019. The MCC of solitary rectal ulcer syndrome is:
      a.   Rectal CA
      b.   Internal intussusception
      c.   HPV
      d.   HIV
      e.   Lymphoma

Answer b. Solitary rectal ulcer syndrome is caused by **internal intussusception** (Sx's: straining, rectal pain, bloody mucus discharge, tenesmus, constipation; see an ulcer in the anterior rectum on colonoscopy). Repeated damage to rectal mucosa causes the ulcer. Can be misdiagnosed as CA (get Bx to confirm); Tx- high fiber diet, stool softeners, and defecation training

1020. Several years after APR for low rectal CA, your patient develops a bulge near his end colostomy site. He is otherwise asymptomatic. The next appropriate step is:
      a.   Observation
      b.   Relocate colostomy
      c.   Tighten the fascia around the colostomy site
      d.   Place mesh to fill the fascia defect

Answer a. Asymptomatic **parastomal hernias** should be observed. These are generally well tolerated.

1021. A 32 yo woman suffers from severe fecal incontinence after vaginal delivery. All of the following are true except:
      a.   Initial treatment is with a high fiber diet and bulk
      b.   Vaginal delivery is the MC traumatic cause of fecal incontinence
      c.   The external sphincter is tightened with anterior sphincteroplasty
      d.   Surgery should be considered after 2-3 weeks of medical therapy.

Answer d. Surgery should be considered after **2-3 months** of medical therapy.

Anal incontinence from damage to the external anal sphincter following vaginal delivery (a type of **abdomino-perineal descent**) that is refractory to medical Tx is best treated with **anterior sphincteroplasty** (anterior portion of external anal sphincter is tightened).

1022. Which of the following is the MCC of anorecto-vaginal fistula:
      a.   Inflammatory bowel disease
      b.   XRT
      c.   Adenocarcinoma
      d.   Diverticulitis
      e.   Obstetrical trauma

Answer e. Obstetrical trauma

1023. A 32 yo woman has stool and flatus emanating from her vagina 1 week following vaginal delivery. All of the following are true except:
      a.   These are usually in the lower 1/3 of the vagina
      b.   Endorectal advancement flap is the primary surgical treatment for low recto-vaginal fistulas
      c.   Surgery should be considered after 2-3 weeks for the above patient
      d.   If an abscess is present, it should be drained

Answer c. Surgery should be considered after **2-3 months**. The majority of recto-vaginal fistulas heal spontaneously.

1024. A 50 yo man presents with a 4 cm anal mass above the dentate line and bleeding. Biopsy comes back as cloacogenic cancer (T2). The most appropriate next step is:
   a. Abdominoperineal resection
   b. Laser fulgration
   c. Chemo-XRT (5-FU and mitomycin, plus XRT)
   d. Low anterior resection

Answer c. The most appropriate Tx of **anal canal squamous cell CA** (cloacogenic CA is a variant of squamous cell CA) is the **Nigro protocol**, which consists of **5-FU** and **mitomycin**, plus **XRT**. This cures 80%.

Surgery is not the initial Tx of choice.

1025. Which of the following is true of the inguinal nodes for the above patient:
   a. They are rarely involved in this type tumor
   b. Positive inguinal nodes confer a worse prognosis compared to iliac nodes
   c. Positive iliac nodes confer a worse prognosis compared to inguinal nodes
   d. Bilateral inguinal lymph node dissection is indicated if they are clinically positive

Answer b. Positive inguinal nodes confer a worse prognosis compared to iliac nodes. If they are positive for tumor, they should be included in the XRT field with the Nigro protocol (not inguinal lymph node dissection).

Poor prognostic factors for anal CA - tumor size, depth, grade, and nodal status (inguinal nodes have worse prognosis compared to internal iliac nodes)

ANATOMY
- **Anal canal** - area proximal to dentate
- **Anal margin** - area between the dentate line and anal verge
- **Dentate line** - transition from **columnar** to **stratified squamous epithelium**
- **Anus arterial supply** - inferior rectal artery
- **Anus venous drainage**
  - Above dentate - internal hemorrhoid plexus
  - Below dentate - external hemorrhoid plexus
- **Nodal Drainage**
  - **Superior** and **middle rectum** - IMA nodes
  - **Lower rectum** - IMA nodes (primarily), also to internal iliac nodes (pelvic nodes)
  - **Anal canal** (above dentate) - internal iliac nodes and inguinal nodes
    - *Anal canal CA (eg squamous cell CA) can metastasize to inguinal nodes*
  - **Anal margin** (below dentate) - inguinal nodes
- **Anal verge** is the opening of the anus to the skin surface of the body
- **External anal sphincter** is the continuation of the **puborectalis muscle**
- **Internal anal sphincter** is the continuation of the **muscularis propria**
- **Central tendon** - separates vagina and external sphincter

HEMORRHOIDS
- Caused by straining
- Left lateral, right anterior, and right posterior hemorrhoidal plexuses
- **External hemorrhoids** cause pain when they thrombose
  - Distal to the **dentate line**
  - Covered by sensate squamous epithelium
  - Sx's: pain, swelling, and itching
- **Internal hemorrhoids** cause bleeding or prolapse
  - **Primary** - slides below dentate with strain
  - **Secondary** - prolapse that reduces spontaneously
  - **Tertiary** - prolapse that has to be manually reduced
  - **Quaternary** - not able to reduce
- Tx: bulk **fiber** and **stool softeners** (prevent straining); sitz baths, water hydration, lidocaine jelly

- **Thrombosed external hemorrhoid** → Tx:
  - If **< 72 hours** of Sx's - <u>surgery</u> with elliptical excision
  - If **> 72 hours** of Sx's - <u>lance</u> open only (pain of surgery worse than hemorrhoid itself at this point; hemorrhoid will become fibrosed)
- **Surgical indications:** recurrent bleeding, multiple thromboses, large external component, moderate to severe pain
- **External** hemorrhoids - resect with **elliptical excision**
  - *Do <u>not</u> band <u>external</u> hemorrhoids (painful)*
- **Internal** hemorrhoids
  - **Primary** and **secondary** - banding (in office)
  - **Tertiary** and **quaternary** - 3 quadrant resection (some use <u>stapler</u>)
      - Need to resect down to the **internal anal sphincter** *(do <u>not</u> go through it)*
      - Take mucosa and submucosa along with venous plexus
      - Post-op - sitz baths, stool softener, high-fiber diet, lidocaine jelly
      - *Strangulated* quaternary hemorrhoids need ***urgent surgery*** to avoid necrosis (Sx's: swollen non-reducible hemorrhoidal tissue, pain and bleeding)
- **Cx's**
  - **Urinary retention** (MC Cx following hemorrhoidectomy, 20%)
      - **Pelvic musculature spasm** after local anesthesia wears off
      - Tx: place **urinary catheter**
  - **Eschar can slough off** causing **light bleeding** <u>late</u> post-op (eg blood on toilet paper)
      - MC occurs **5-10 days** after banding or hemorrhoidectomy
      - Tx: **stool softeners, fiber supplements** and **water hydration** to avoid local trauma; avoid ASA *(does <u>not</u> require EUA)*
  - **Significant bleeding** *(rare; eg toilet bowel full of blood)* needs exam under anesthesia and suture ligation of bleeding area
  - **Sepsis** - *very rare after hemorrhoidectomy* (Sx's - severe perianal pain, fevers, urinary retention, immunocompromised patient); Tx: IVFs, broad spectrum antibiotics, and EUA (look for abscess or necrotizing soft tissue infection)

RECTAL PROLAPSE (procidentia)
- Starts 6-7 cm from anal verge
- Secondary to pudendal neuropathy and laxity of the **anal sphincters**
- Sx's: protruding mass, incontinence, constipation, straining, tenesmus, bleeding
- RFs: multiparous females, straining, chronic diarrhea, laxative abuse, redundant sigmoid colons, COPD (coughing), elderly
- Types:
  - **Full-thickness** rectal prolapse - entire rectum protrudes through anus
  - **Mucosal** prolapse - just rectal mucosa (not entire wall)
      - **Solitary rectal ulcer syndrome** - anterior rectum mucosa is forced into the anal canal; repeated damage results in ulcers (can be multiple)
  - **Internal intussusception** - the rectum collapses on itself
- Medical Tx: **high-fiber diet**, **stool softeners**, and **hydration** (prevent straining); defecation training; *avoid* laxatives
- Surgery:
  - Indicated for **full thickness prolapse** <u>only</u> (all layers of bowel wall) **and** have to **manually reduce** or **can't manually reduce**
  - Old frail lady → **Altemeier** procedure (**perineal rectosigmoidectomy**; pull rectum / sigmoid out anus, resect with primary anastomosis)
  - Good condition patient → **low anterior resection** (LAR, laparotomy) and **pexy** of residual colon

CONDYLOMATA ACUMINATA
- Cauliflower mass; papillomavirus (HPV)
- Tx: laser surgery

ANAL FISSURE

- Sx's: **pain** with defecation (straining bowel movements); bright red anal **bleeding**
- Often a history of **constipation**
- Can occur after back or perineal surgery; heavy narcotic use
- Caused by a **split in the anoderm** from large, hard stools
- 90% in **posterior midline**
- Chronic ones usually have a **sentinel pile**
- **Rectal exam** to confirm Dx (will see anoderm split; **pain** reproduced with **exam**)
- *Early medical Tx* (**< 4 weeks** of Sx's):
  - **Sitz baths**
  - **Bulk fiber**
  - **Water hydration**
  - **Colace**
  - **Lidocaine** ointment to the skin tear
  - Anal *topical* **nitroglycerine** cream *(glyceryle trinitrate; 6 week cycles)*
  - *90% of acute fissures heal with medical Tx*
  - *Avoid suppositories (cause irritation, pain)*
- *Late medical Tx* (**> 3 months** of Sx's; indicates difficult or refractory case)
  - Anal *topical* **diltiazem 2%** *(calcium channel blocker) for 6 weeks*
- **Surgical indications** (failure to improve after 2 cycles of calcium channel blocker; have failed around 6 months of medical Tx)
- Surgical Tx:
  - **Lateral subcutaneous internal sphincterotomy**
    - Feel for groove between internal and external anal sphincter
    - Use 11 blade to make a transverse cut through internal sphincter
    - Considered the most effective Tx for anal fissures
    - Do *not* go past the dentate line
    - Do *not* cut the external sphincter
    - Do *not* cut the mucosa
    - Do *not* perform in patient's with Crohn's' disease
    - 90% healing rate
    - *Fecal incontinence is the most serious Cx of surgery (1%)*
  - **Botulinum toxin injection** (Botox) - 60% overall healing rate
- **Lateral** or **recurrent fissures** - worry about inflammatory bowel disease, STDs, and anal CA

ANORECTAL ABSCESS

- Can cause severe peri-rectal pain
- Caused by obstructed **anal glands**
- Exam under anesthesia (EUA) - best for finding and treating a peri-anorectal abscess
- **Perianal, intersphincteric,** and **ischiorectal abscesses** are drained through the skin (all are below the levator ani muscles)
- **Supralevator abscesses** (above levator ani muscles) need to be drained transrectally
- **WTD dressings** and try to heal from the bottom up
- **Intersphincteric** and **ischiorectal abscesses** can form horseshoe abscess
  - A Horseshoe abscess does *not* need an extensive incision, will drain through the opening you make
- Broad spectrum antibiotics indicated for cellulitis, DM, immunosuppression, or prosthetic hardware

RECTOCELE

- Rectum bulges into vagina with bowel movements; RFs - vaginal delivery, straining
- Tx: bulk fiber, hydration, colace (treats *majority*)
- Surgery - reinforce the **rectovaginal septum** (variety of techniques)

CYSTOCELE

- Bladder bulges into vagina; RFs - vaginal delivery, straining bowel movements
- Tx: *mild* Sx's - observation; *significant* Sx's - transvaginal reinforcement of the **pubocervical fascia**

ANAL INCONTINENCE

- **Neurogenic** (gaping hole with laxity of levators, eg spinal cord injury) - no good Tx (possible colostomy)
- **Damage to sphincter mechanism** (a type of **perineal descent**)
  - Trauma to levator ani, puborectalis, and external anal sphincter muscles
  - Anus falls below **levators**
  - MCC - **vaginal childbirth**
  - Medical Tx: bulk fiber, colace, hydration (limit to 1 BM/day; _avoid_ straining)
  - Surgery - **anterior anal sphincteroplasty**
    - Tightens **external anal sphincter muscle**
    - **Pudendal nerves** in lateral walls - _avoid_ dissection there
  - **Stenosis** post-op (MC Cx)
    - Tx: sitz baths, bulk, lidocaine jelly, stool softeners, water hydration
    - **Anal dilatation** under anesthesia over several weeks

ANAL CANCER

- Association with **HPV** and **XRT**
- The **dentate line** is an important landmark for how SCCA is treated
  - Anal canal - above dentate line
  - Anal margin - below dentate line
- **Anal canal** lesions _(above dentate line)_
  - Sx's: pruritus (itching), bleeding, palpable mass
  - **Squamous cell CA** (eg epidermoid CA, mucoepidermoid CA, cloacogenic CA, basaloid CA)
    - RFs: HIV, HPV, immunosuppression
    - Tx: **Nigro protocol** (chemo-XRT, _5-FU and mitomycin_), _not_ **surgery**
    - Chemo-XRT cures 80%
    - Surgery for treatment failures or recurrent cancer
    - Poor prognostic factors - tumor size, depth, grade, and nodal status (inguinal nodes have worse prognosis compared to internal iliac nodes)
  - **Adenocarcinoma**
    - Tx: APR usual; WLE if < 4 cm, < ⅓ circumference, limited to submucosa (T1 tumors - 2 mm margin needed), well differentiated, and no vascular/ neuro / lymphatic invasion
    - Post-op chemo-XRT same as rectal CA
  - **Melanoma**
    - Anal canal is the 3rd MC site for melanoma (skin #1, eyes #2)
    - ⅓ has spread to mesenteric lymph nodes
    - Hematogenous spread to liver and lung is early and accounts for most deaths
    - Symptomatic disease - usually have metastatic disease
    - MC Sx - **rectal bleeding**
    - Most tumors are lightly pigmented or not pigmented at all
    - Tx: APR usual; use standard melanoma depth criteria
- **Anal margin** lesions _(below dentate line)_ - much better prognosis than anal canal lesions; _Tx is similar to_ **skin CA**
  - RFs: HIV, HPV, immunosuppression
  - **Squamous cell CA**
    - Ulcerating, slow growing; men with better prognosis
    - Metastases - go to **inguinal nodes**
    - Lesions **< 5 cm** - Tx: **WLE** (need 0.5 cm margin)
    - Lesions **> 5 cm**, if involving the **anal sphincter**, if **positive nodes**, or if **recurrence** → Tx: **chemo-XRT** (5-FU and cisplatin; _trying to preserve the anal sphincter here and avoid APR_)
    - Need inguinal node dissection if clinically positive
    - _Sphincter preservation in 80%_
    - 5-year survival with positive nodes - 80%
  - **Basal cell CA** - central ulcer, raised edges, rare metastases
    - Tx: WLE usually sufficient, only need 3 mm margins; rare need for APR unless sphincter is involved

AIDS ANORECTAL PROBLEMS
- **Kaposi's sarcoma** - see nodule with ulceration; MC CA with AIDS
- **CMV** - can see shallow ulcers; Tx - ganciclovir
- **HSV** - MC rectal ulcer; Tx - acyclovir
- **B cell lymphoma** - can look like abscess or ulcer; Tx - chemo +/- XRT
- Need Bx's of ulcers and anal lesions to rule-out CA and figure out above

NODAL METASTASES
- **Superior** and **middle rectum** - IMA nodes
- **Lower rectum** - primarily IMA nodes, also to internal iliac nodes
- **Anal canal** - internal iliac nodes; also to inguinal nodes
- **Anal margin** - inguinal nodes

PERIANAL FISTULAS (fistula-in-ano)
- Sx's: usually history of abscess, now with soiling and drainage
- **Inter-sphincteric (70%)** - arise from a **peri-anal abscess**
  - Located between the internal and external anal sphincters
  - Tx: **fistulotomy** (open tract and curettage out fistula, healing by secondary intention); very small risk of anal incontinence
- **Trans-sphincteric (20%)** - arise from an **ischio-rectal abscess**
  - Goes through external anal sphincter
  - *Upper 2/3* of external anal sphincter Tx - **draining seton stitch** (allows drainage and promotes fibrosis of tract); consider **endorectal advancement flap** if refractory *(No fistulotomy - risk of incontinence)*
  - *Lower 1/3* of external anal sphincter Tx - **draining seton stitch** safest, may consider **fistulotomy**; biggest issue here is risk of incontinence
- **Supra-sphincteric (< 5%)** - arise from a **supra-levator abscess**; often have inter-sphincteric component
    Tx: **draining seton stitch** or **endo-rectal advancement flap**
- **Extra-sphincteric (< 5%)** - usually the result of trauma, Crohn's, colon CA, XRT, or diverticulitis; *these bypass* the anal canal
  - Tx: **fistulotomy** *(no risk of anal incontinence)*
- **Draining setons** should be strongly considered for: 1) recurrent or multiple fistulas, 2) anterior fistulas in women, *or* 3) patients with inflammatory bowel disease, previous sphincter injury, or impaired continence
- Recurrent, multiple, or fistulas with multiple sinus tracts should raise concern for another pathology (eg anal CA, inflammatory bowel disease, STDs)
- *Should avoid fistulotomy in patients with Crohn's*
- *Avoid cutting setons in general*
- Tx of **persistent fistulo in ano** - endorectal advancement flap
- Tx for **asymptomatic** fistula-in-ano with Crohn's - *observation*
- The most serious Cx that can occur from fistula surgery is **anal incontinence** as a result of damage to the **external anal sphincter**
- Patients with **inflammatory bowel disease** (ie Crohn's or UC) suffering from **active proctitis** or **inflamed peri-anal disease** should not undergo endo-rectal advancement flap due to poor healing
- **Endo-rectal advancement flap** includes the **mucosa** and the **internal anal sphincter muscle** layer
- **Goodsall's Rule**
  - **Posterior fistulas** (90% of fistulas) connect to anus at posterior midline
  - **Anterior fistulas** connect to anus in a straight line
  - Fistulas that are not posterior and in midline → need to rule-out inflammatory bowel disease and CA

RECTOVAGINAL FISTULAS (ano-vaginal fistula)
- Etiologies: **obstetrical trauma** (MCC), diverticulitis, inflammatory bowel, XRT, CA
- **Simple** - low to mid-vagina (usually from **obstetrical trauma**)
  - Many obstetrical fistulas heal spontaneously (give it 2-3 months)
  - Tx: **endo-rectal advancement flap** (is a trans-anal approach) if it fails to heal (flap of rectal mucosa and internal sphincter is advanced and used to cover the fistula hole)

- **Complex** - high in vagina (usually from **diverticulitis**)
  - Tx: **abdominal** or combined **abdominal / perineal approach** usual; **resection and anastomosis of rectum**, close hole in vagina, interpose omentum, diverting ileostomy

PARASTOMAL HERNIA
- Increased in **colostomies** compared to ileostomies
  - 50% five-year incidence for colostomies
- RFs: fascial opening too large; stoma lateral to rectus sheath, obesity, COPD, Age
- *Do not fix these unless significantly symptomatic - generally well tolerated* (< 10% need repair)
- Absolute repair indications - obstruction; incarceration with strangulation, severe pain
- Relative repair indications - incarceration, severe prolapse
- Tx: **observe** unless causing significant Sx's
  - If surgery needed, ***relocate the ostomy** to the rectus muscle (preferred)*
  - **Prolapse** - keep stoma at same site, fix mesentery (ostomy is in rectus and the fascia is intact but bowel is prolapsing through)

Hernias and Abdominal Wall

1026. A 40 yo woman with previous open gastric bypass has a ventral hernia. Laparoscopic ventral hernia repair compared to open ventral hernia repair is associated with:
   a. Higher recurrence rate
   b. Increased infection rate
   c. Longer operative time
   d. Longer hospital stay
   e. Higher overall complication rate

   Answer c. Longer operative time

1027. You attempt laparoscopic ventral hernia repair in the above patient. While attempting abdomen entry you make an enterotomy. Which of the following is most appropriate:
   a. Repair the enterotomy and repair the hernia
   b. Repair the enterotomy, repair the hernia, and keep the patient on antibiotics for 6 weeks
   c. Repair the enterotomy, close the incision, and try again in 6 weeks
   d. Create an external ostomy

   Answer c. Repair the enterotomy, close the incision, and try again in 6 weeks

1028. You bring the above patient back and due to hostile abdominal conditions you perform an open mesh ventral hernia repair. Three weeks later she presents with mild pain. There is a firm rounded structure deep to the incision. The most appropriate step is:
   a. Wound vac
   b. Observation
   c. Reoperation
   d. Antibiotics
   e. Place a drain

   Answer b. Observation. This most likely represents a **seroma** which usually reabsorb on their own. Percutaneous drainage should be avoided if possible due to the risk of bacterial contamination of the mesh.

1029. All of the following are true of inguinal anatomy except:
   a. The MC organ found in women with sliding hernias is ovary
   b. The MC organ found in men with sliding hernia is cecum
   c. The MC Cx following hernia repair is urinary retention
   d. The shelving edge is formed by the internal abdominal oblique fascia

   Answer d. The **external abdominal oblique fascia** forms the **shelving edge**

1030. All of the following are true of inguinal anatomy except:
   a. The cremasteric muscles arise from the internal abdominal oblique muscle
   b. Direct hernias are medial to the inferior epigastric muscles
   c. The genital branch of the genitofemoral nerve enters the inguinal canal through the external (superficial) ring
   d. The round ligament is found in the inguinal canal of females

   Answer c. The **genital branch of the genitofemoral nerve** enters the inguinal canal through the **internal (deep) ring** before descending into the scrotum where it provides sensation to the scrotum and motor to the cremasteric muscle.

031. All of the following are true of inguinal cord structures except:
   a. The vas deferens is usually medial
   b. The genital branch of the genitofemoral nerve is posterior
   c. The ilioinguinal nerve is anterior
   d. The ilioinguinal nerve enters inguinal canal through the deep (internal ring)
   e. The genital branch of the genitofemoral nerve exits the inguinal canal through the external (superficial) ring

Answer d. The **ilioinguinal nerve** enters the cord after piercing through the internal abdominal oblique muscle near the iliac crest. It does not travel through the internal (deep) ring. It provides sensation to the skin at the base of the penis and upper scrotum (skin over mons pubis and labium majorum in women).

1032. All of the following are true of inguinal hernia repair except:
    a.   The vas deferens runs medial to the cord structures
    b.   Patients with severe COPD can undergo local inguinal hernia repair with injection of the ilioinguinal nerve
    c.   Testicular atrophy following inguinal hernia is most commonly due to thrombosis of the spermatic artery
    d.   The most commonly injured nerve with laparoscopic inguinal hernia repair is the lateral femoral nerve

Answer c. Testicular atrophy following inguinal hernia is most commonly due to **thrombosis of the spermatic veins**. This injury most commonly occurs during dissection of a **large scrotal hernia sac**.

The **femoral branch of the genitofemoral nerve** (ie the lateral femoral nerve) is the MC injured nerve with laparoscopic inguinal hernia repair and can cause post-op pain (neuralgia). Neuralgia should first be treated with lidocaine and steroid injection. Neurectomy should be performed if that fails.

1033. All of the following are true of hernias in adults except:
    a.   Indirect inguinal hernias are the most common type in men
    b.   Direct inguinal hernias are the most common type in women
    c.   Umbilical hernias are more common in women
    d.   Femoral hernias are more common in women
    e.   Obturator hernias are more common in women

Answer b. Direct inguinal hernias are *rare* in women. **Indirect inguinal hernias** are the MC type in both **men** and **women**

1034. A 55 yo man returns to clinic following Lichtenstein (mesh) hernia repair with a persistent right groin burning pain that radiates to the scrotum. You perform a physical exam and obtain a CT scan, both of which show no signs of hernia recurrence or infection. The pain seems to be reproduced with tapping just medial to the anterior superior iliac spine. This most likely represents injury to the:
    a.   Ilioinguinal nerve
    b.   Genitofemoral nerve
    c.   Sciatic nerve
    d.   Lumbosacral plexus nerves

Answer a. The MC injured nerve (or entrapped nerve) with inguinal hernia repair is the **ilioinguinal nerve**.

1035. Initial Tx for the above patient should be:
    a.   Open inguinal re-exploration
    b.   Nerve blocks
    c.   Laparoscopic re-exploration
    d.   Neurectomy

Answer b. Tx is with **ilioinguinal nerve block**, which can be therapeutic and diagnostic. If the pain recurs after nerve blocks (local anesthetics and steroids) and NSAIDs, **neurectomy** is indicated.

1036. A 55 yo man returns to clinic following Lichtenstein (mesh) inguinal hernia repair that involved a large scrotal hernia sac. He reports having a tender and enlarged right testicle. The most appropriate next step is:

a. MRI
b. Re-exploration
c. U/S
d. Antibiotics only
e. PET scan

Answer c. U/S - this patient most likely has **ischemic orchitis** due to disruption and thrombosis of the **testicular veins**. U/S will show no or poor blood flow to the testicle.

1037. All of the following are true of laparoscopic mesh inguinal hernia repair compared to open mesh inguinal hernia repair except
a. Recurrence rate is higher
b. Overall complication rate is higher
c. Return to work is earlier
d. Initial pain is less
e. Major complication rate is lower

Answer e. Major complication rate is higher for laparoscopic mesh inguinal hernia repair (eg injury to bowel, major blood vessel).

1038. At reoperation for a recurrence of an inguinal hernia following laparoscopic repair, the most common location for the recurrent hernia is:
a. Lateral
b. Medial
c. Anterior
d. Posterior

Answer b. Laparoscopic mesh hernia repair has a 5% recurrence. The MCC is **separation of the mesh from the fascia medially**. This is usually due to **making the mesh too small**.

You need at least a 3 cm overlap of the fascia and mesh with adequate fascia fixation (*avoid* making the mesh too small and make sure it's attached medially; need it tension free)

1039. A 65 yo woman presents with a tender mass just <u>below</u> the inguinal ligament. This most likely represents:
a. An inguinal hernia
b. An obturator hernia
c. A ventral hernia
d. A femoral hernia

Answer d. A mass below the inguinal ligament is consistent with a **femoral hernia**.

1040. You explore the above patient through an inguinal approach and find necrotic bowel which you resect. The most appropriate next step is:
a. Use mesh to repair the hernia
b. Place a wound vac in the inguinal incision
c. Cooper's ligament repair
d. Just close with skin overlying the area

Answer c. Cooper's ligament repair (pectineal ligament repair)

These patients can also present with small bowel obstruction and the diagnosis is made at the time of laparotomy (always check for hernias in patient's with small bowel obstruction). In that situation you can perform a pectineal ligament repair from inside the abdomen.

1041. The most important technical priority in the above patient is:

a. Dividing the inguinal ligament
b. Dividing the pectineal ligament
c. Closing the empty space between the femoral vein (lateral) and lacunar ligament (medial)
d. Approximation of the conjoined tendon to the shelving edge

Answer c. Closing the space between the femoral vein and lacunar ligament.

Femoral hernia boundaries:
> **Superior** - inguinal ligament
> **Inferior** - pectineal ligament
> **Medial** - lacunar ligament (attaches to pubis; connect the inguinal and pectineal ligaments)
> **Lateral** - femoral vein

1042. Which of the following would <u>not</u> be a good option for repair of a femoral hernia:
a. Pectineal ligament repair
b. Infra-inguinal approach, mesh repair
c. Pre-peritoneal approach, mesh repair
d. Approximation of the conjoined tendon to the free edge of the inguinal ligament

Answer d. This repair would not obliterate the space between the femoral vein and lacunar ligament.

1043. During repair of a femoral hernia through an inguinal approach, you try to reduce the bowel but are unsuccessful. The most appropriate next step is:
a. Pull on the bowel until it gives
b. Resect the bowel through a femoral exploration
c. Divide the rectus muscle
d. Divide the inguinal ligament

Answer d. If you are unable to reduce the bowel for a **femoral hernia** through an inguinal approach, **divide the inguinal ligament**, reduce the bowel (making sure its viable 1st), and then repair the inguinal ligament.

1044. All of the following are true except:
a. Femoral hernias are MC in females
b. Pediatric umbilical hernias are MC in males
c. Adult umbilical hernias are MC in women
d. Direct inguinal hernias are the MC type in men
e. Indirect inguinal hernias are the MC type in women

Answer d. Indirect inguinal hernias are the MC type in both men and women

1045. In which of the following patients is observation an option:
a. A 42 yo man with a minimally symptomatic inguinal hernia
b. A 32 yo woman with an asymptomatic femoral hernia
c. An 80 with severe COPD with a direct inguinal hernia that contains a large neck and is reducible
d. A premature infant with an inguinal hernia who is ready to be discharged home in the next few days.

Answer c. It should be remembered that inguinal hernias cause death in over 2000 patients in the US each year so they are not benign. Recent studies suggest observation, however the vast majority of these patients cross-over to surgery at some point. Elective repair carries a *far lower complication and mortality rate* compared to emergency repair (which is usually for an acutely incarcerated hernia or a chronically incarcerated hernia that becomes painful; both of these scenarios can result in bowel infarction).

All of the above hernias should be electively repaired with the exception of the elderly gentleman with severe COPD. The hernia has a large neck and is reducible. Given his high operative mortality risk, observation is an option.

1046. All of the following are true of adult umbilical hernias except:
   a.   A 50 yo man with a small reducible umbilical hernia should undergo repair
   b.   Incarceration risk is much higher in adults than in children
   c.   Patients with cirrhosis and ascites should not undergo repair
   d.   Mesh closure has lower recurrence rates
   e.   Pregnancy is a RF

Answer c. Patients with **umbilical hernias** who have **cirrhosis** and **ascites** should undergo repair. Umbilical hernias and ascites can stretch the overlying skin making it ischemic. This leads to perforation, infection, and peritonitis.

Most adult umbilical hernias are acquired (RFs - pregnancy, ascites, obesity, aortic aneurysms) and the vast majority should undergo repair. _Watchful waiting is not recommended for adult umbilical hernias._

1047. A 65 yo woman presents with a tender medial thigh mass. The pain increases with internal rotation of the thigh. This most likely represents:
   a.   A Spigelian Hernia
   b.   An obturator hernia
   c.   A lumbar Hernia
   d.   A Richter's Hernia

Answer b. This scenario is consistent with an **obturator hernia**. The Howship-Romberg sign is pain with internal rotation of the thigh (classic for obturator hernia).

1048. A 25 yo woman undergoing bilateral tubal ligation has an insufflation pressure of 0 mmHg at the start of the case. The most appropriate next step is:
   a.   Convert to open procedure
   b.   Make sure the stopcock is closed
   c.   Reposition the insufflation needle
   d.   Obtain a new laparoscopic set-up
   e.   Change the insufflation tubing only

Answer b. Make sure stopcock is closed (meaning closed to the atmosphere)

1049. Instead of above, the pressure is 20 mmHg. The most appropriate next step is:
   a.   Convert to open procedure
   b.   Reposition the insufflation needle
   c.   Obtain a new laparoscopic set-up
   d.   Change the insufflation tubing only

Answer b. Reposition the insufflation needle. It is most likely still in the abdominal wall.

1050. An 80 yo woman on Plavix for a coronary stent placed years ago presents with acute abdominal pain after a coughing spell. Her BP is 90/50 and HR 100. She has had no previous surgery. You feel a mass-like area in her lower abdominal wall. The most appropriate next step is:
   a.   Open exploration and ligation
   b.   Angioembolization
   c.   Laparotomy
   d.   Platelets
   e.   Heparin drip

Answer d. Platelets. This patient has a **rectus sheath hematoma** related to her age, anticoagulation, and coughing fit. These bleeds can be life-threatening.

The first step in management is reversal of anticoagulation. If that fails, angio-embolization is indicated. Hematomas below the arcuate line (just below the umbilicus) tend to cause more severe bleeding and can also be confused with an intra-abdominal process. CT scan is the best test for diagnosis.

1051. All of the following are true except:
   a. The anterior and posterior rectus sheath are intact above the arcuate line (linea semicircularis)
   b. The arcuate line is a few centimeters below the umbilicus
   c. Spigelian hernias generally occur through or near the linea semicircularis
   d. Above the arcuate line, the internal abdominal oblique fascia contributes to both the anterior and posterior rectus sheath
   e. Below the arcuate line, the internal abdominal oblique fascia contributes only to the anterior rectus sheath

   Answer c. Spigelian hernias generally occur through the **linea semilunaris**. These tend to be small and a palpable bulge is uncommon. CT scan can aid in Dx. Spigelian hernias are at high risk for **incarceration** due to a small hernia neck. Below the arcuate line, the rectus muscle lies on the transversalis fascia _only_.

INGUINAL ANATOMY
- **Round ligament** - located in the **inguinal canal** of women
- **External abdominal oblique fascia**
  - Forms **inguinal ligament** (shelving edge) at inferior portion of inguinal canal
  - Also forms roof of the inguinal canal (anterior portion)
  - You cut through this to get to the inguinal canal
- **Internal abdominal oblique fascia**
  - Muscle portion forms **cremasteric muscles**
  - Fascia combines with transversalis fascia to form the **conjoined tendon,** which serves as the floor of the inguinal canal
- **Transversalis fascia** - along with internal abdominal oblique fascia forms conjoined tendon and the iliopubic tract
- **Conjoined tendon**
  - Composed of the aponeurosis of the internal abdominal oblique fascia and transversus abdominis fascia (transversalis fascia)
  - Forms the inguinal canal floor
  - Beneath this are the femoral vessels
  - Also forms iliopubic tract in some (found posterior to inguinal ligament and anterior to pectineal ligament; curves over femoral vessels; _not always present_)
- **Inguinal ligament** (Poupart's ligament; shelving edge)
  - Arises from the inferior portion of the **external abdominal oblique fascia**
  - Runs from anterior superior iliac spine to the pubis
  - This is anterior to where the femoral vessels exit the pelvis
  - Forms inferior portion of inguinal canal
- **Lacunar ligament**
  - Where inguinal ligament splays and insert into pubis
  - Connects the inguinal and pectineal ligaments (forms an arc)
  - Femoral vessels / nerve go through arc (between inguinal - pectineal ligaments)
- **Pectineal ligament** (Cooper's ligament)
  - Posterior to the femoral vessels (lies right against the bone)
- **Internal ring** - entrance to inguinal canal from peritoneum
- **External ring** - exit from inguinal canal into scrotum
- **Vas deferens** - runs medial to cord structures
- **Spermatic cord** structures:
  - Testicular artery
  - Pampiniform plexus
  - Vas deferens
  - Cremasteric muscle
  - Ilioinguinal nerve (anterior)
  - Genital branch of the genitofemoral nerve (posterior)

INGUINAL HERNIAS

- **Hesselbach's triangle** - rectus muscle, inferior inguinal ligament, and inferior epigastric vessels
  - **Indirect hernias** are superior / lateral to the epigastric vessels
  - **Direct hernias** are inferior / medial to the epigastric vessels
- **Indirect hernias** (MC type)
  - From persistently **patent processus vaginalis**
  - Higher risk of **incarceration** compared to direct
  - MC type in **males** and **females**
- **Direct hernias**
  - Very <u>rare</u> in females
  - From weakness in abdominal wall
  - Higher **recurrence** rate compared to indirect
- **Pantaloon hernia** - direct and indirect components
- **Inguinal hernia RFs** (adults): age, obesity, heavy lifting, COPD (coughing), chronic constipation, straining (BPH), ascites, pregnancy, peritoneal dialysis
- **Incarcerated hernia** - can lead to bowel strangulation; should be repaired emergently if it can't be reduced
- **Sliding hernias** - retroperitoneal organ makes up part of the hernia sac (MC in males)
  - **Females** - **ovaries** (MC) or fallopian tubes
  - **Males** - **cecum** (MC) or sigmoid MC
  - Bladder can also be involved
- **Females with ovary in the canal**
  - Ligate the **round ligament** (lets ovary fall back into pelvis)
  - Return ovary to peritoneum
  - Bx ovary if looks abnormal
- **Hernias in infants and children** (up to age 18)
  - Just perform high ligation (nearly always indirect)
  - Open sac prior to ligation to make sure nothing important is in there
- **Lichtenstein repair** = mesh
  - Mesh goes from the conjoined tendon to the inguinal ligament (reconstructs floor of the inguinal canal)
  - Hernia recurrence is <u>decreased</u> with use of **mesh** (decreases tension) compared to non-mesh repairs
- **Bassini repair** - approximation of the conjoined tendon (superior) to the free edge of the inguinal ligament (shelving edge, inferior)
- **Cooper's ligament repair** (pectineal ligament repair) - approximation of the conjoined tendon (superior) to the pectineal ligament (inferior)
  - Need a <u>relaxing incision</u> in the external abdominal oblique fascia
  - Requires a lateral transition stitch between the conjoined tendon, pectineal ligament, and inguinal ligament (avoid compressing the femoral vein with this stitch which would result in venous thrombosis [ie femoral vein DVT])
  - Can use this for **femoral hernia** repair
- **Observation criteria** – *most inguinal hernias should be <u>repaired</u>*
  - Elderly <u>infirmed</u> patients or patients with <u>high operative risk</u> with **minimally symptomatic <u>direct</u>** hernias that have a **wide neck** and are **easily reducible** may be observed.

INGUINAL HERNIA REPAIR COMPLICATIONS (see Pediatric Surgery chp for children)

- **Urinary retention** - MC Cx following hernia repair
  - Tx: urinary catheter, leg bag if persistent, will get better
- **Recurrence rate** - 1%, lower with mesh
- **Wound infection rate** -1%
- **Cord lipomas** - remove
- **Severe COPD** with incarcerated inguinal hernia →
  - Can repair under **local** with anesthetic injection into **ilioinguinal nerve** (medial to anterior superior iliac spine) and direct groin injection; can also go with spinal anesthesia
- **Trouble reducing** incarcerated inguinal hernia at time of repair → **divide inguinal ligament** at internal ring (*best option*; repair it after)

- You find a **femoral hernia** when exploring inguinal hernia and can't reduce contents → Tx: **divide inguinal ligament** to free up bowel; end up with **Cooper's ligament repair** (pectineal ligament repair)
- You find **pneumointestinalis** (air in the bowel wall) when reducing an inguinal hernia in OR → *Do not resect* unless the bowel is necrotic (black); pneumatosis intestinalis can occur with just strangulation which does not require resection
- **Testicular atrophy** (from ischemic orchitis) - MC from dissection of the distal part of the hernia sac (beyond pubic tubercle) with disruption and thrombosis of the **spermatic cord veins**
  - RFs: open redo hernia repair, large hernia sac, indirect hernias
- **Ischemic orchitis**
  - Sx's: large, indurated, painful testicle; usually within 1st week
  - Can progress to testicular atrophy
  - From thrombosis of **spermatic cord veins** (pampiniform plexus)
  - RFs: excision or dissection of a **large hernia sac**; open redo inguinal hernia repair, indirect hernias
  - Dx: **U/S** (shows no blood flow to testicle)
  - Tx: **NSAIDs**, pain control, re-assurance
  - *Avoidance* - divide the hernia sac and leave the distal portion of the sac intact *without* dissection (eg leave the large portion of the hernia sac in the scrotum); *avoid* dissection of the spermatic cord past the pubic tubercle
- **Pain** after inguinal hernia repair
  - Residual pain occurs in 10% after inguinal hernia repair (majority resolved with conservative measures)
  - Usually from compression of **ilioinguinal nerve**
  - Tx: local anesthetic infiltration of the ilioinguinal nerve (lidocaine + steroids) can be diagnostic and therapeutic (inject near anterior superior iliac spine)
  - If that doesn't work, go in and **resect nerve** (neurectomy)
- **Ilioinguinal nerve** injury
  - MC nerve injury after **open** inguinal hernia repair
  - Enters the cord after piercing through the internal abdominal oblique muscle near the iliac crest. *It does not travel through the internal (deep) ring.*
  - Sx's: pain / numbness on ipsilateral **penis base, upper scrotum** (mons pubis and labia majorum) and upper **inner thigh**; can lose cremasteric reflex (provides some sensory fibers)
  - Nerve usually injured at **external ring** (superficial ring)
  - Nerve is **anterior** to cord structures
  - Tx: **local anesthetic infiltration** (nerve block) of the ilioinguinal nerve (lidocaine + steroids) can be diagnostic and therapeutic *(avoid early reoperation)*
  - If that doesn't work go in and **resect nerve** (neurectomy; near iliac crest)
- **Genitofemoral nerve** injury
  - MC nerve injury with **laparoscopic** inguinal hernia repair (MC - **femoral branch**)
  - The **femoral branch** does not enter ther inguinal canal
  - The **genital branch** enters the inguinal canal through the **internal ring** (deep ring) before descending into the scrotum through the external (superficial) ring
  - **Femoral** branch (*MC injured branch*; lateral femoral nerve) - goes to upper **lateral thigh** (sensory); runs lateral to femoral / iliac vessels
  - **Genital** branch - branches to **cremaster** (motor) and **lower scrotum** (sensory) runs posterior / inferior to cord; responsible for majority of **cremasteric reflex**

LAPAROSCOPIC INGUINAL HERNIA REPAIR
- Best indications - **bilateral** or **recurrent** inguinal hernia (hard to justify for first time hernias)
- Inferiorly, make sure to staple mesh to **inguinal ligament** - avoid area where spermatic cord and epigastric vessels enter inguinal canal (although you need staples medial to this to avoid recurrence)
- 5% recurrence
- MCC of **recurrence** after laparoscopic hernia repair → **medial separation of mesh** from fascia at inguinal ligament (MCC - mesh is **too small**)
- Need at least a 3 cm overlap of fascia and mesh with adequate fascia fixation (*avoid* making mesh too small and make sure its attached medially; need it tension free)

- Laparoscopic inguinal hernia repair compared to open repair has:
  - Reduced immediate post-op pain
  - Earlier return to work
  - Increased **complication rate** overall, especially **life threatening** (anesthetic related and injury to blood vessels / bowel [eg placement of trocars])
  - Increased risk for **recurrence** for first time hernias (10% vs 5% for open repair)
- MC nerve injury - **genitofemoral nerve injury** (MC branch - lateral femoral nerve)

FEMORAL HERNIA
- Sx's: **mass** just _below_ inguinal ligament
- MC in **females**
- Femoral canal boundaries:
  - **Superior** - inguinal ligament
  - **Inferior** - pectineal ligament
  - **Medial** - lacunar ligament (attaches to pubis; connects the inguinal and pectineal ligaments)
  - **Lateral** - femoral vein
- Femoral canal structures - **NAVEL** (lateral to medial) - femoral nerve, femoral artery, femoral vein, empty space, lymphatics / lacunar ligament
- High risk of **incarceration** → may need to **divide inguinal ligament** to reduce bowel
- Hernia passes **posterior** (deep) to the inguinal ligament
- Have characteristic **bulge** on anterior-medial thigh below inguinal ligament
- Tx: **pectineal ligament** repair (Cooper's Ligament repair) or can place mesh if bowel not compromised (key maneuver - **closing the space lateral to lacunar ligament**)
  - Can also use a direct infra-inguinal incision over the bulge
- _No_ mesh if bowel compromised (eg perforation, necrotic bowel, bowel resection)

OTHER HERNIAS
- **Umbilical hernia**
  - Pediatric umbilical hernias (congenital) - MC in **males**
  - Adult umbilical hernias (majority acquired) - MC in **females** (due to pregnancy)
  - RFs (children) - African-Americans
  - RFs (adults) - obesity, ascites, pregnancy, aortic aneurysms
  - Tend to **close spontaneously** in children (especially if < 2.5 cm)
  - Delay repair until **age 5** unless symptomatic (rare)
  - Risk of **incarceration** is in adults, _not_ children
  - Adults with umbilical hernias (even small ones) should undergo **repair** (watchful waiting _not_ recommended)
  - For adults, the risk of **recurrence** is _lower_ with the use of **mesh**
  - see Liver chapter for umbilical hernias in cirrhosis
- **Spigelian hernia**
  - Occur at lateral border of rectus muscle, adjacent to or through the **linea semilunaris**
  - Almost always **inferior** to (below) the arcuate line (linea semicircularis)
  - Occurs between the muscle fibers of the internal abdominal oblique muscle and insertion of the external abdominal oblique aponeurosis into the rectus sheath
  - Sx's: abdominal **pain**, may present with **small bowel obstruction** (high risk of **incarceration**); are often **small** and usually can _not_ feel a bulge (are posterior to the external abdominal oblique muscle)
  - Dx: often diagnosed on **CT scan**
- **Obturator hernia** (anterior pelvis)
  - Herniation through the **obturator canal** (formed from ischium and pubic bones)
  - MC in **females**; elderly, multiparous, recent weight loss
  - Sx's: tender medial thigh mass, small bowel obstruction
  - **Howship-Romberg sign** - inner thigh pain with internal rotation (classic)
  - High risk of incarceration and strangulation
  - Dx: CT scan - bowel gas below superior pubic ramus
  - Dx usually made at time of surgery for small bowel obstruction
  - Tx: operative reduction, may need mesh; check other side for same defect
  - High mortality (10%) related to gangrenous bowel and advanced age of patients
- **Sciatic hernia** (posterior pelvis)

- Herniation through greater sciatic foramen; high rate of strangulation
■ **Incisional hernia** - hernia most likely to recur; MCC - inadequate fascial closure

RECTUS SHEATH
■ **Anterior rectus sheath** - complete
■ **Posterior rectus sheath** - is absent inferior to (below) the semicircularis line (arcuate line)
■ Superior to (above) the arcuate line, the internal abdominal oblique fascia splits to help provide the aponeurosis for both the anterior and posterior rectus sheaths
■ The internal abdominal fascia moves anterior below the arcuate line
■ Below the arcuate line the rectus muscle rests on the transversalis fascia only
■ The arcuate line is located a few centimeters below the umbilicus
■ **Rectus sheath hematomas**
   ● Prevalence has increased with the use of **blood thinners** (eg Plavix, warfarin)
   ● Now occurs in **elderly** on blood thinners with minor process (eg sneezing, coughing)
   ● MC involves **epigastric artery**
   ● Dx: CT scan
   ● If <u>above</u> the arcuate line - will not cross the midline (less bleeding)
   ● If <u>below</u> the arcuate line - can cross the midline (more severe bleeding)
   ● Painful abdominal wall mass; more prominent and painful with flexion of the rectus muscle (Fothergill's sign)
   ● If <u>below</u> the arcuate line, can feel like an intra-abdominal process
   ● Tx: reverse anti-coagulation, pRBCs, **angio-embolization** if expanding, open ligation if that fails

MESENTERIC TUMORS
■ Of the primary tumors, most are cystic
   ● **Malignant tumors** - closer to the **root** of the mesentery
   ● **Benign tumors** - usually more **peripheral**
■ Malignant - **liposarcoma** (#1), leiomyosarcoma
■ Dx: CT scan
■ Tx: resection

RETROPERITONEAL TUMORS
■ 15% in children, others in 5-6th decade
■ Malignant > benign
■ MC malignant retroperitoneal tumors - #1 **lymphoma**, #2 liposarcoma
■ Sx's: vague abdominal and back pain; leg neurologic dysfunction
■ **Retroperitoneal sarcomas** (see Skin and Soft Tissue chapter)
   ● < 25% resectable; local recurrence in 40%
   ● Have pseudocapsule but cannot shell out → would leave residual tumor
   ● Metastases go to lung

OMENTAL TUMORS
■ MC omental solid tumor is **metastatic disease**
■ Omentectomy for metastatic CA has a role for some CA (eg ovarian CA)
■ Omental cysts are usually asymptomatic, can undergo torsion
■ <u>Primary</u> solid omental tumors are rare; 1/3 are malignant
   ● <u>No</u> Bx → can bleed
   ● Tx: resection

OMENTAL TORSION
■ Twisting of omentum around its vascular pedicle
■ Primary omental torsion is very rare
■ Is usually secondary torsion (due to tumor, adhesions, hernia sac, or inflammation)
■ Can *mimic* other disease (eg appendicits, cholecystitis, PID)
■ Tx: untwisting of omentum (may need resection if infarcted)

PERITONEAL MEMBRANE
- Blood is absorbed through fenestrated lymphatic channels in peritoneum
- Most drugs are <u>not</u> removed with peritoneal dialysis
- NH_3 and Ca are removed with peritoneal dialysis
- Movement of fluid into the peritoneal cavity can occur with hypertonic intra-peritoneal saline load (mechanism of peritoneal dialysis); can cause hypotension

CO_2 PNEUMOPERITONEUM (normal pressure 10-15 mmHg)
- Cardiopulmonary dysfunction can occur with intra-abdominal pressure > 20 (try to keep insufflation pressure 10-15 mmHg)
  - High initial insufflation pressure → malpositioned insufflation needle
  - Zero initial insufflation pressure → stopcock is open
- *Are increased*: mean arterial pressure, pulmonary artery pressure, HR, systemic vascular resistance, central venous pressure, mean airway pressure, peak inspiratory pressure, and CO_2
- *Are decreased:* pH, venous return (IVC compression), cardiac output, renal flow secondary to decreased cardiac output
- Hypovolemia lowers pressure necessary to cause compromise
- PEEP worsens effects of pneumoperitoneum
- CO_2 can cause some decrease in myocardial contractility
- Can minimize **respiratory acidosis** from CO_2 pneumoperitoneum by *decreasing* pneumoperitoneum pressure and *increasing* minute ventilation (RR or TV)
- **CO_2 embolus** (see Critical Care chapter)

VENTRAL HERNIA
From previous abdominal incision
- MC type of hernia to recur
- MCC is inadequate fascial closure

Sx's: large abdominal mass after operation
RFs: obesity, smoking, COPD, previous ventral hernia repair
Dx: CT scan - confirms Dx
Laparoscopic repair usually the <u>preferred</u> route *(best option)*
Mesh repair has better long term outcomes compared to primary repair
- Mesh needs to be secured to fascia at least 3-4 cm away from the defect edge
- PTFE (Gortex) commonly used
- <u>No mesh</u> with bowel compromise - just repair enterotomy and close (antibiotics, back in 6 weeks)

0.1% risk of placing veress needle or trocar into bowel / blood vessel
With open repair, just close the skin with sutures or staples
- *Avoid* layered closure of fat (causes fat necrosis) and increased suture material (predisposes to infection)
- *Avoid* drains overlying mesh (predisposes to infection)

MC Cx - **seroma** (bulge or hard mass under skin over mesh)
- Tx - *leave alone* unless very symptomatic
- Usually goes away on its own after 4-6 weeks

Laparoscopic ventral hernia repair compared to open is associated with:
- Lower recurrence
- Fewer overall Cx's
- Lower wound infection rate
- Reduction in ileus
- Shorter hospital stay
- Longer OR time

Recurrence rate for laparoscopic mesh repairs - 5%
- RFs for <u>recurrence</u>: large hernia, long OR time, previous repair, BMI > 40
- MCC for recurrence - **separation of mesh from posterior fascia**

Skin graft over bowel after necrotizing fasciitis, now has ventral hernia→ *leave it alone*
Component separation repair (does <u>not</u> use mesh)
  1) **Rectus sheath** released from **external abdominal obliques** (reduces tension)
  2) External abdominal obliques are separated from internal abdominal obliques
  3) Rectus sheath muscles and attached internal abdominal oblique / transversalis muscles are re-approximated at the midline

Urology

1052. All of the following are true except:
   a. The seminal vesicles are connected to the urethra
   b. Ejaculation failure after proctocolectomy is due to disruption of pelvic sympathetic nerves
   c. Tx for transitional cell CA of the renal pelvis is radical nephroureterectomy
   d. Seizures following TURP are most likely due to hyponatremia

   Answer a. Seminal vesicles are connected to the **vas deferens**. Hyponatemia can occur after TURP due to use of water irrigation instead of saline.

1053. All of the following are true of kidney stones except:
   a. Calcium oxalate stones are MC
   b. Uric acid stones are radiolucent and are likely to appear in patients with gout, ileostomies, or myeloproliferative disorders
   c. Initial Tx of choice for intractable nephrolithiasis is extra-corporeal shock wave lithotripsy (ESWL)
   d. Magnesium ammonium phosphate stones are associated staph aureus

   Answer d. Magnesium ammonium phosphate stones (struvite) are associated **proteus infections** (produce urease)

1054. A 50 yo man presents to the ED with aching scrotal pain. You examine the patient and get an U/S which shows a left sided varicocele. Which of the following tumors is most likely give the presentation:
   a. Testicular seminoma
   b. Lung CA
   c. Pancreatic CA
   d. Renal cell CA

   Answer d. A **new varicocele** on the left side may be a sign of **left sided renal cell CA**.

   The left gonadal vein drains into the left renal vein and the right gonadal vein drains into the IVC. A new left varicocele is worrisome for RCCA compressing the left gonadal vein. A new right sided varicocele is worrisome for an abdominal or pelvic mass causing pressure on the right gonadal vein.

   Varicoceles cause _reduced_ **fertility**
   Hydrocoeles and **spermatoceles** do _not_ affect fertility

1055. A 13 yo boy presents to the ED with an extremely painful testicle after a winter snowball fight. Given the most likely diagnosis, the most appropriate next step is:
   a. Antibiotics only
   b. Inguinal incision
   c. Trans-scrotal incision
   d. Laparotomy

   Answer c. This patient most likely has **testicular torsion**. If the diagnosis is unclear, a duplex U/S can be performed to confirm lack of blood flow to the testicle. Emergent de-torsion through a trans-scrotal incision (not inguinal incision) is indicated.

   Males can have an inherited trait (**bell-clapper deformity**) that allows the testicle to rotate freely in the scrotum. RFs include physical activity and cold climates. Infectious epididymitis is _rare_ in this age group so antibiotics would _not_ be appropriate.

1056. A 1 year old boy is brought to the ED for an enlarged scrotum. You feel a mass-like structure at the internal ring. This is most likely represents:

a. Torsion
b. Epididymitis
c. Hernia
d. Hydrocoele

Answer c. Inguinal hernia. A mass at the internal ring (from intestine or other structure such as bladder or ovary) differentiates a hernia from a hydrocoele.

057. Instead of the above, you do not feel any mass at the internal ring and U/S shows a fluid filled structure in the scrotum. This is most likely due to:
a. Torsion
b. Epididymitis
c. Hernia
d. Persistent processus vaginalis

Answer d. This patient has a communicating **hydrocoele**. This is do to a persistent processus vaginalis. Hydrocoeles (from persistent tunica vaginalis) usually resolve by age 1, if not they are considered communicating (persistent processus vaginalis).

058. A 32 yo man presents with a painful testicular mass. The most appropriate next step is:
a. Orchiectomy through an inguinal incision
b. Orchiectomy through a trans-scrotal incision
c. Transscrotal Bx
d. XRT
e. Chemo

Answer a. Orchiectomy through an inguinal incision (not trans-scrotal incision). This almost certainly represents testicular CA.

059. All of the following are true except:
a. 90% of seminomas have Beta-HCG elevation
b. Seminoma is the MC testicular tumor
c. Seminoma is extremely sensitive to XRT
d. Seminoma is <u>not</u> associated with AFP elevation

Answer a. Only 10% of seminomas have beta-HCG elevation

060. All of the following are true of prostate cancer except:
a. Stage IA disease in an 80 yo man requires no additional treatment
b. A normal PSA is < 4
c. Survival benefit has been established with digital rectal exam (DRE)
d. High Gleason grade confers a worse prognosis

Answer c. DRE has not been shown to improve survival

061. All of the following are true of renal cell carcinoma except:
a. They can synthesize erythropoietin
b. Partial nephrectomy is indicated for tumors < 4cm if creatnine is > 2.5
c. When growing into the IVC, IVC reconstruction is usually needed
d. The classic presentation is pain, abdominal mass, and hematuria

Answer c. Although these tumors have a predilection for IVC invasion, they usually do not attach to the walls and can be plucked out of the IVC at the time of nephrectomy.

Partial nephrectomy is indicated for tumors < 4 cm if creatnine is > 2.5 (avoids permanent dialysis)

062. All of the following are true of bladder cancer except:

a. The MC type is transitional cell carcinoma
b. Schistosomiasis infection is associated with bladder squamous cell CA
c. Transitional cell carcinoma limited to the submucosa can be treated with intra-vesicle BCG or trans-urethral resection
d. Transitional cell carcinoma with invasion of the muscle (T2) is best treated with wedge resection

Answer d. Transitional cell CA with muscle invasion requires total cystectomy and formation of an ileal conduit.

1063. All of the following are true except:
a. Oncocytomas and angiomyolipomas are benign renal tumors
b. Spermatoceles do not affect fertility
c. Preoperative phimosis should be treated with a dorsal slit to open the area
d. Tx for vesicoureteral reflux is ileal conduit
e. The MCC of retroperitoneal abscess is renal in origin

Answer d. Tx for vesicoureteral reflux is re-implantation of the ureter into the bladder.

ANATOMY AND PHYSIOLOGY
- **Gerota's fascia** - fascia that encloses the kidney
- **Anterior to posterior structures** (VAP) - renal vein, renal artery, renal pelvis
  - **Right renal artery** crosses posterior to the IVC
  - **Left renal vein** crosses anterior to the aorta (MC)
- **Ureters** cross _over_ iliac vessels
- **Left renal vein** - can be ligated from IVC
  - Has collaterals (left adrenal vein, left gonadal vein, left ascending lumbar vein)
  - Right renal vein does not have collaterals and cannot be safely ligated
- **Epididymis** - connects to vas deferens
- **Seminal vesicles** - are connected to the vas deferens
- **Erection** - parasympathetic (pelvic splanchnic nerves)
- **Ejaculation** - sympathetic (pudendal nerve)

KIDNEY STONES
- Sx's: severe colicky pain, restlessness
- Dx: **UA** - blood or stones
  - **CT scan** - stones, hydronephrosis; 90% opaque
- Stone Types:
  1) **Calcium oxalate** stones (<u>radio-opaque</u>)
     MC kidney stone (75%)
     ↑ed after **terminal ileum resection** due to **oxalate reabsorption** in colon
  2) **Magnesium ammonium phosphate** stones (<u>radio-opaque</u>)
     Struvite stones
     Associated with **kidney infections** and **urea splitting organisms** such as **Proteus mirabilis** (urease)
     Can cause **staghorn calculi** that fill the renal pelvis
  3) **Uric acid** stones (<u>radio-lucent</u>)
     RFs: gout, **ileostomies**, short gut
     With ileostomy, loss of alkaline fluid from ileostomy lowers urinary pH and volume, leading to uric acid stone formation
  4) **Cysteine** stones (radio-dense to radiolucent)
     Associated with **congenital disorders** of cysteine metabolism
     Prevention - **Tiopronin** (↓s rate of cysteine solidification)
- **ESWL indications** *(best Tx*; extracorporeal shock wave lithotripsy) - intractable pain infection, progressive obstruction, progressive renal damage, solitary kidney, > 6 mm (not likely to pass)

TESTICULAR CANCER

- **#1 cancer killer** in men 25-35
- Sx's: **hard mass** in the substance of testis, may be **painful**
  - Vast majority of testicular masses are **malignant**
- *Testicular mass* - patient needs an **orchiectomy** through an **inguinal incision** (*not a trans-scrotal incision → do not want to disrupt lymphatics*)
  - The testicle and attached mass constitute the Bx specimen
  - Do *not* stick a needle through the scrotum to get Dx
- Dx: U/S (1st test) - helps with diagnosis of testicular CA (vs hernia, hydrocoele)
  - CT scan - to check for retroperitoneal and chest metastases
  - Labs (get *before* orchiectomy so you have levels) - LDH, beta-HCG, and alpha fetoprotein (AFP)
- 90% are **germ cell** - seminoma or non-seminoma
- **Undescended testicles** (cryptorchidism) - increase risk of testicular CA
  - Most likely to get seminoma
- **Seminoma**
  - MC testicular tumor
  - 10% have beta-HCG elevation
  - Should *not* have AFP elevation (if elevated, need to treat like non-seminomatous)
  - *Seminoma is extremely* **sensitive to XRT**
  - Spreads to retroperitoneum
  - Tx: all stages get **orchiectomy and retroperitoneal XRT** (para-aortic and ipsilateral pelvic)
    - Chemo reserved for <u>metastatic disease</u> or <u>bulky retroperitoneal disease</u> (cisplatin, bleomycin, etoposide)
    - Surgical resection of residual disease after above
- **Non-seminomatous testicular CA**
  - **Types** - embryonal, teratoma, choriocarcinoma, yolk sac
  - Spreads to **retroperitoneum** and hematogenously to **lungs**
  - Labs - **AFP** and **beta-HCG** (90% have these markers)
  - *XRT* <u>*never*</u> *used as primary Tx for non-seminomatous*
  - Tx: all stages get **orchiectomy and retroperitoneal node dissection** (prophylactic if Stage I)
    - **Stage II** or greater (beyond testicle) - also get chemo (cisplatin, bleomycin, etoposide)
    - Surgical resection of residual disease after above
- 5-YS (all patients) - **90%**, seminoma better than non-seminoma
- MC location for a <u>primary</u> extra-gonadal germ cell tumor - **mediastinum** (see Thoracic chapter)

PROSTATE CANCER

- MC CA in US for men
- 2nd MC CA death in men (#1 - lung CA)
- Sx's: asymptomatic (MC); obstructive or irritative (eg frequency, dysuria); hematuria; erectile dysfunction
- Screening - survival benefit with screening *not* established (DRE or PSA)
  - PSA - not very specific or sensitive; can be ↑ed with prostatitis, BPH, chronic catheterization; *normal PSA < 4*
- **Alkaline phosphatase** elevation → worrisome for metastases or extracapsular disease
- Dx: **TRUS with Bx** (6-12 Bx's) - histology correlates with prognosis
  - CT scan, PSA, alkaline phosphatase, and bone scan
- MC site - **posterior lobe**
- MC metastatic site - **bone** (osteoblastic - x-ray shows **hyperdense** area)
- Many are **impotent** after resection; can also get incontinence
- **Stage IA** disease found with **TURP** (not palpable, not on imaging) - Tx: <u>nothing</u>
- **Stage I + II** (T1 or T2 - both confined to prostate capsule) get *either*:
  1) **Watchful waiting** (if age > 75 or limited life expectancy) *or*
  2) **XRT** *or*;
  3) **Radical prostatectomy** with pelvic LN dissection (if lifespan > 10 years)

- **Stage III** (extends through the capsule) or **Stage IV** (invades adjacent structures or has metastases) → Tx: **XRT** and **androgen ablation** (leuprolide, flutamide, and/or bilateral orchiectomy)
- **XRT** can help with **bone pain** or **local recurrence**
- Prognosis - high **PSA,** high **Gleason grade,** and **advanced age** are predictors of metastases
- **Androgen deprivation** options:
    1) **Bilateral orchiectomy** *(most effective)*
    2) **GnRH analogues** (leuprolide) - ↓ FSH and ↓ LH
    3) **Anti-androgens** (flutamide) - block androgen receptor

RENAL CELL CARCINOMA (RCC, hypernephroma)
- MC primary tumor of kidney
    - MC kidney tumor - metastases from <u>breast CA</u>
- RFs: **smoking**
- Sx's: **abdominal pain, mass,** and **hematuria** (classic triad)
- Dx: CT scan - tumor disrupts renal contour
    - Can often be fairly certain about RCC based on CT scan but can <u>not</u> exclude RCC with CT scan
    - *Biopsy not useful* - hard to differentiate from oncocytoma; also some risk of bleeding (unfavorable risk-benefit ratio)
    - Essentially all renal masses need some sort of resection unless thought to be a metastasis (then just get CT guided Bx)
    - Cysts are observed unless complex
- Path
    - 90% of primary solid renal masses are RCC (± necrosis, ± calcification)
    - MC subtype - **clear cell** (75%)
    - MC metastatic site - **lung** (30% have metastases at time of Dx)
    - Paraneoplastic syndromes:
        Erythrocytosis from **erythropoietin** secreting tumors *(diagnostic of renal cell CA)*
        HTN from **renin** secreting tumors
        Stauffer syndrome - increased LFTs; improves after resection
- *Wide range of 5-year survival - related to size + degree of spread:*
    Stage I (< 4 cm) > 95% 5-YS
    Stage IV (eg metastases to lungs) 5% 5-YS
- Tx: **radical nephrectomy** with regional nodes
    - Radical nephrectomy takes kidney, <u>adrenal gland</u>, fat, Gerota's fascia, and regional nodes
    - **Partial nephrectomy** should be considered only for patients who would require dialysis after nephrectomy (eg tumor < 4 cm in a patient with a creatinine > 2.5)
    - **Bilateral** small tumors - partial nephrectomies *(avoid dialysis)*
    - RCC has predilection for growth into the **IVC** (even right atrium)
        Pull tumor thrombus out of IVC (± cardiopulmonary bypass)
        They usually *do <u>not</u> attach to the IVC wall* and can be plucked out at the time of nephrectomy
    - Post-op **chemo-XRT** (doxorubicin based), **interferon, IL-2** (all marginal)
- **Isolated lung metastasis** - resection
- **Transitional cell CA of renal pelvis** - Tx: radical nephroureterectomy
- **Oncocytomas** - benign
- **Angiomyolipomas** - hamartomas; tuberous sclerosis; benign
- **Von Hippel-Lindau syndrome** - RCC, CNS tumors, pheochromocytomas

BLADDER CANCER
- MC type - **transitional cell CA** (90%)
- Sx's: **painless hematuria**
- Males; prognosis based on stage and grade
- RFs: smoking, aniline dyes, cyclophosphamide
- Dx: **cystoscopy**

Bladder CA Tx:
- **T1** (*muscle not involved*) - **transurethral resection** _and_ **intra-vesical BCG** (or valrubicin; give for 1 year)
- **T2 or greater** (*muscle involved*)
    - **Cystectomy** (with ileal conduit) + bilateral pelvic node dissection _and_;
        - **Chemo-XRT** (MVAC: methotrexate, vinblastine, Adriamycin, cisplatin)
    - **Men** - include **prostatectomy** in resection
    - **Women** - include **TAH + BSO** and **anterior vaginal wall**
- Metastatic disease - chemotherapy only

Ileal conduit is the standard reconstruction option
- **Reservoirs** or **neobladders** may also be options
- Avoid stasis as this predisposes to infection, stones (calcium resorption), and ureteral reflux

5-YS after <u>cystectomy</u> (all patients) - **60%**
- 5-year survival for T1 tumors - 95%

Squamous cell CA of bladder - schistosomiasis infection

ESTICULAR TORSION
All pre-pubertal and young adult males (age < 25) with testicular pain are considered to have testicular torsion until proven otherwise
Early Dx and Tx are key to helping **avoid testicular loss**
Most accurate sign - **loss of ipsilateral cremasteric reflex**
Can be confused with epididymitis (uncommon prepubertal)
Torsion is usually towards midline (like closing a book)
RFs - inherited trait (bell-clapper deformity), physical activity, cold climates
Dx: **U/S** - can be used to aid in Dx (shows no blood flow to testis)
- If suspicion high → **skip U/S** and **immediate OR detorsion**

Tx: **Trans-scrotal incision** and **de-torse testis** (direction → like opening a book)
- **Bilateral orchiopexy** if testicle viable
- If not, resection and orchiopexy of contralateral testis
- 100% viable if within 6 hours

RETERAL TRAUMA
If going to repair end-to-end →
- Spatulate ends
- Use **absorbable suture** to avoid stone formation
- **Stent the ureter** to avoid stenosis
- **Place drains** to identify and potentially help treat leaks

Avoid stripping the soft tissue on the ureter, as it will compromise blood supply
see Trauma chapter for specific injuries and repairs

ENIGN PROSTATIC HYPERPLASIA (BPH)
Usually arises in **transitional zone**
Sx's: nocturia (wake up at night to urinate), frequency, dysuria, weak stream, urinary retention
Dx: DRE - enlarged prostate; TRUS
Initial Tx:
- **Alpha blocker** - <u>terazosin</u> (Hytrin), relax smooth muscle
- **5-alpha-reductase inhibitors** - <u>finasteride</u> (Proscar), inhibits conversion of testosterone to dihydrotestosterone (inhibits prostate hypertrophy)

Surgery (TURP; trans-urethral resection of prostate)
- **Indications** - recurrent UTIs, gross hematuria, stones, renal insufficiency, failure of medical Tx
- **Post-TURP syndrome** (ie **seizures**) - **hyponatremia** secondary to irrigation with water (as opposed to normal saline); can precipitate **seizures** from cerebral edema; Tx: **Tolvapten** (see Fluid and Electrolytes chapter)

Most patients with TURP have **retrograde ejaculation**

OTHER UROLOGIC DISEASES

- **Varicocele** - abnormal enlargement of veins draining testis (MC on left)
  - Is found in scrotum on the **posterior portion** of the testicle (different from testicular tumor)
  - **New onset left sided** varicocele - worrisome for **renal cell CA** (left gonadal vein inserts into left renal vein, obstruction by renal tumor causes varicocele); Dx - CT scan
  - Can also be from other **intra-abdominal, pelvic,** or **retroperitoneal malignancy** placing pressure on **gonadal veins** (can have right or left sided varicocele)
  - Varicoceles cause **reduced fertility** due to thrombosis, compression, and warmth → **improved fertility** with **high spermatic vein ligation**
- **Spermatocele**
  - *MC cystic structure of scrotum*
  - Fluid filled cystic structure superior and separate from testis along epididymis (different location than varicocele)
  - Tx: surgical removal if symptomatic
  - *Hydrocoeles and Spermatoceles do not affect fertility*
- **Hydrocoele** in adult - if acute, suspect tumor elsewhere (pelvic, abdominal); these are translucent (helps to differentiate from hernia); *hydrocoeles do not affect fertility*
- **Ureteropelvic junction obstruction** (UPJ obstruction; at junction of ureter and renal pelvis) - Tx: pyeloplasty (relieves obstruction)
- **Vesicoureteral reflux** - Tx: ureter re-implantation into bladder with long bladder muscle portion (prevents reflux)
- **Ureteral duplication**
  - **MC urinary tract abnormality**
  - Tx: re-implantation in bladder if obstructed
  - *Not a contra-indication to kidney donation for TXP*
- **Ureterocele**
  - MC at junction of ureter and bladder; MC in females
  - Usually associated with **ureteral duplication**
  - Sx's: UTIs, retention
  - Tx: resect and re-implant ureter in bladder if Sx's
- **Hypospadias** - ventral urethral opening
  - Tx: repair at 6 months with penile skin
- **Epispadias** - dorsal urethral opening Tx: surgery
- **Horseshoe kidney** - usually joined at lower poles
  - Cx's: UTI, urolithiasis, hydronephrosis
  - Tx: may need pyeloplasty for obstruction
- **Persistent urachus** - connection between umbilicus and bladder
  - Causes **wet umbilicus**
  - 10% have bladder outlet obstruction
  - Dx: **voiding cystourethrogram** (looking for an obstruction)
  - Tx: resection of sinus and cyst with closure of bladder; relieve any obstruction
- **Epididymitis** - inflammation or infection of epididymis
  - Sx's: sudden scrotal pain (need to **rule-out testicular torsion** in these patients)
  - MCC of acute scrotal pain in **men** *(not children)*
  - U/S - increased blood flow to epididymis
  - MCC infection - **Chlamydia** (MC); others - Gonorrhea, E coli (Tx: antibiotics)
  - Non-infectious causes - abdominal straining, heavy lifting
- **Pneumaturia** (air in urine)
  - MCC - **diverticulitis** and subsequent colo-vesical fistula (Dx: cystoscopy)
- **Priapism**
  - Tx: aspiration of corpus cavernosum with dilute epinephrine
  - May need to create a communication through glans with scalpel to relieve
  - RFs: sickle cell anemia, hypercoagulable states, trauma, intracorporeal injections for impotence, sildenafil
- **Squamous cell CA of penis** - standard care is penectomy with 2-cm margin
- **IV Indigo carmine** or **methylene blue** - used to check for urine leak
- **Phimosis** found at time of laparotomy - Tx: dorsal slit

- **Neurogenic bladder** (spastic bladder)
    - MC secondary to spinal injury
    - Accidental voiding, often of large amounts of urine
    - Injury above T-12
    - Tx: **surgery to increase bladder resistance**
- **Neurogenic obstructive uropathy** (flaccid bladder)
    - Incomplete emptying of the bladder, can have frequency
    - Injury below T-12; can occur with APR
    - Tx: **intermittent catheterization**
- **Urinary incontinence**
    - **Stress incontinence** (often with cough, sneeze)
        - *MC type of incontinence*
        - MC in **women**
        - Due to **pelvic floor weakness** leading to hypermobile urethra or **loss of sphincter mechanism**
        - RFs: multiparous women, age, obesity, prostatectomy
        - Tx: **Kegel exercises** to strengthen pelvic floor
            - **Alpha-adrenergic agents**
            - Surgery for **urethral suspension** or **pubovaginal sling** *(best Tx)*
    - **Overflow incontinence**
        - Incomplete emptying and enlarged bladder
        - MC in **males**
        - **Obstruction** (eg BPH) leads to distention and leakage
        - Tx: medical Tx of BPH, possible TURP
- **WBC casts** - seen with pyelonephritis and glomerulonephritis
- **RBC casts** - just with glomerulonephritis
- **Retroperitoneal abscess** - MCC is **renal** (usually from pyelonephritis, may involve kidney stones or surgery)
- **Erythropoietin** - ↓ed production with chronic renal failure (**low Hct**)
- **Peyronie's Disease**
    - Thick plaques in tunica albuginea cause penile curvature
    - Tx: **conservative Tx** for up to 1 year (colchicine, Vit E)
    - If that fails to relieve Sx's, need **Nesbit operation** (tissue on opposite side of plaque is shortened to straighten curve – *plaque is __not__ excised*)

Gynecology

1064. A 25 yo old woman presents to the ED with severe abdominal / pelvic pain, abdominal distension, a systolic BP of 60 despite 2 liters of lactated ringers, and a heart rate of 120. The hematocrit comes back at 17. The most appropriate next step is:
   a. Go to OR
   b. FFP and go to the ICU
   c. Send a beta-HCG
   d. Abdominal CT scan

   Answer a. Sometimes you can't wait for a Dx. The most appropriate step here is to go to the OR and figure it out in there. This is highly suspicious for a ruptured ectopic pregnancy.

1065. A 23 yo woman with previous pelvic inflammatory disease presents to the ER with acute abdominal pain. All of the following are true in this patients work-up except:
   a. Unruptured ectopic pregnancy should undergo salpingectomy
   b. A 7 cm tubo-ovarian abscess from pelvic inflammatory disease should undergo percutaneous drainage
   c. Ruptured graafian cysts should be followed
   d. Ovarian torsion requires detorsion and assessment of viability

   Answer a. Unruptured **ectopic pregnancy** should undergo salpingotomy (removal of the ectopic pregnancy), not salpingectomy (which is removal of the fallopian tube). Another option is to abort the pregnancy with methotrexate (MTX).

1066. All of the following are true except:
   a. The fallopian tube (ampullary portion) is MC site of ectopic pregnancy
   b. The round ligament maintains anteversion of the cervix
   c. First trimester bleeding with a closed os and no heartbeat on U/S is consistent with a missed abortion
   d. Seizures are usually the first symptom of magnesium toxicity

   Answer d. Respiratory depression is associated with **magnesium toxicity**

1067. A 21 yo sexually active woman presents with pelvic pain. On pelvic exam and she has cervical motion tenderness and pus discharge. Her Beta-HCG is negative The Tx should be:
   a. Ceftriaxone and doxycycline
   b. Bactrim
   c. Vancomycin
   d. Levofloxacin

   Answer a. This patient most likely has **pelvic inflammatory disease** related to Chlamydia or Gonorrhea. Tx is with ceftriaxone and doxycycline.

1068. A 25 yo woman complains of cyclical rectal bleeding. You perform anoscopy and find a blue mass at 5 cm above the dentate line (3 cm above the levators). Given the likely diagnosis, all of the following are true except:
   a. Sx's of this condition are dysmenorrhea, infertility, and dyspareunia
   b. Ovaries are the MC site
   c. This lesion requires low anterior resection
   d. This lesion can be treated with hormonal manipulation

   Answer c. This patient has **endometriosis** in the rectum, which is usually controlled with OCP's. A blue rectal mass in a young female patient who presents with rectal bleeding should alert you to endometriosis.

1069. All of the following are true of ovarian cancer except:

a. Ovarian CA with peritoneal metastases is usually treated primarily with total abdominal hysterectomy, bilateral oophrectomy, resection of peritoneal metastases, and omentectomy
b. Debulking therapy can be effective
c. Mucinous ovarian tumors can be associated pseudomyxoma peritonei
d. Risk factors for ovarian cancer include oral contraceptive pills (OCPs)

Answer d. Use of OCPs lowers the risk of ovarian CA.

Ovarian CA with peritoneal metastases is treated primarily with **total abdominal hysterectomy, bilateral oophrectomy, resection of peritoneal metastases,** and **omentectomy**. You should try to remove all the carcinomatosis and leave any residual tumor deposits **< 1 cm**. Intra-peritoneal chemotherapy is effective for ovarian CA with peritoneal metastases.

070. A 55 yo post-menopausal woman has a newly discovered ovarian tumor on the right side. All of the following are true except:
a. CA confined to bilateral ovaries is stage I disease
b. An ovarian mass associated with ascites and right hydrothorax is best treated with a peritoneal drain and pleurodesis
c. Serous tumors are the MC ovarian tumor overall
d. The clear cell type of ovarian CA has the worst prognosis

Answer b. Meige's syndrome consists of a pelvic ovarian tumor (classically fibroma) that causes **ascites** and **hydrothorax. Tumor excision** cures the syndrome and relieves the ascites and hydrothorax

CA confined to **bilateral ovaries** is **stage I disease**

071. All of the following are true of ovarian CA except:
a. Intra-peritoneal chemotherapy can be effective for ovarian CA
b. Omentectomy is indicated with surgery for ovarian CA
c. The MC site of initial spread of ovarian CA is the contralateral ovary
d. Ovarian CA is usually diagnosed at an early stage

Answer d. Ovarian CA is usually diagnosed late.

072. At the time of an elective cholecystectomy, a 60 yo woman has an 8 cm cyst attached to her ovary. There appears to be a mass component to the cyst. The most appropriate next step is:
a. Laparoscopic removal of the cyst only
b. Laparoscopic removal of the cyst and ovary
c. Open removal of the cyst
d. Open removal of the cyst and ovary
e. Open TAH and BSO

Answer b Laparoscopic removal of cyst and ovary. A CA diagnosis has not been made, so the morbidity of an open procedure is not indicated (15% CA risk in this patient). Laparoscopic removal of the adnexal cyst and attached ovary (she is not of child-bearing age) is indicated.

073. All of the following are true except:
a. The MC site of endometriosis is the ovaries
b. High grade cervical intra-epithelial neoplasia following conization biopsy requires hysterectomy
c. The MC vaginal CA in young girls is sarcoma botryoides
d. Stage II vulvar CA requires bilateral labial resection and bilateral inguinal and femoral lymph node dissection

Answer b. High grade cervical intra-epithelial neoplasia following **conization biopsy** requires <u>no</u> further therapy.

Stage II vulvar CA requires **modified radical vulvectomy** (entire vulva removed including **bilateral labia majora / minora** and **clitoris**) and **bilateral inguinal/femoral LN dissection**.

NORMAL ANATOMY AND PHYSIOLOGY
- **Fallopian tubes** carry ovum from ovaries to uterus
  - MC site of **ectopic pregnancy - ampullary portion of fallopian tube**
- **Ligaments**
  - **Round ligament** - maintains **anteversion** of uterus (starts at uterus, goes through inguinal canal, eventually attaches to labia majora)
  - **Infundibular ligament** - has **ovarian vessels** (artery, vein) + nerve; a fold of peritoneum that extends from ovary to pelvic wall
  - **Broad ligament** - contains **uterine vessels** (artery, vein); connects the sides of the uterus to the floor and walls of pelvis
  - **Cardinal ligament** - holds cervix and vagina in place at base of broad ligament; contains **uterine artery and vein**

GENERAL
- **U/S** - often study of choice for Dx of disorders in female genital tract
- **Best time for surgery** in pregnancy is early **2nd trimester**
  - Too early risk **spontaneous abortion** (1st trimester; 10-15%)
  - Too late risk **preterm labor** (3rd trimester; 10-15%)
  - 1% risk of fetal demise in 2nd trimester with surgery *(best time)*

ABORTIONS
- **Missed**
  - Dx: 1st trimester bleeding, closed os, U/S - positive sac, no heartbeat
  - Embryo or fetus has died but no miscarriage yet
- **Threatened** - 1st trimester bleeding, positive heartbeat
  - Possibly due to **sub-chorionic hematoma** - Tx: bed-rest
- **Incomplete** - abortion tissue protrudes through os
- **Ectopic** (see below for management)
  - Acute abdominal pain, positive beta-HCG, and negative U/S for sac
  - **Other Sx's** - missed period, vaginal bleeding, hypotension
  - **RFs** - previous tubal manipulation, PID, previous ectopic, smoking
  - **MC location** - ampullary portion of fallopian tubes
  - **Life-threatening hemorrhage** and **shock** can occur

ECTOPIC PREGNANCY
- Sx's:
  - 1) Abdominal / pelvic **pain**
  - 2) **Positive B-HCG**
  - 3) U/S *cannot* find conception
  - 4) **Hypotension**
- The above = **ruptured ectopic pregnancy → go to the OR**
- Other Sx's - missed period, vaginal bleeding
- RFs: previous tubal manipulation, previous pelvic inflammatory disease (PID), previous ectopic pregnancy, smoking
- MC location - ampullary portion of fallopian tubes
- Life-threatening **hemorrhage** and **shock** can occur
- **Laparoscopy** as a 1st step usual
- **Un-ruptured** ectopic pregnancy: Tx - <u>salpingotomy</u>, evacuate hematoma, hemostasis, repair tube; can also try medical Tx (eg methotrexate) to try and terminate pregnancy
- **Ruptured** ectopic pregnancy - Tx: <u>salpingectomy</u> if unstable; otherwise salpingotomy as above

TUBO-OVARIAN ABSCESS
- Sx's: **adnexal pain;** fevers and chills
- RFs: previous PID, intra-uterine device (IUD) use
- Dx: **cervical motion tenderness** and **adnexal mass** on pelvic exam
  - Get **B-HCG** to rule-out ectopic pregnancy
  - **U/S** for Dx (abscess ≥ 6 cm requires percutaneous drainage)
- Tx: **percutaneous drain** (especially if > 6 cm) **+ antibiotics** (doxycycline, ceftriaxone)
  - If you have to operate (can't get drain in or ruptured abscess) → laparoscopy, evacuate abscess, washout, drains *(no oophorectomy)*

MITTELSCHMERZ
- Rupture of **graafian follicle** or follicular swelling
- Pain can be confused with appendicitis
- Occurs 14 days after 1st day of menses
- Negative pelvic exam and negative U/S
- Tx: nothing; if already in OR for RLQ pain and you find this, perform appendectomy and close

ENDOMETRIOSIS
- Sx's: **dysmenorrhea, dyspareunia,** and **infertility** *(classic)*
  - **Rectal involvement** can cause bleeding during menses → rectal endoscopy shows **blue mass**
  - **Catamenial PTX** - endometriosis in lung (causes recurrent PTX)
- **MC site** - ovaries
- Many women with **infertility have endometriosis**
- Tx: OCPs, Danazol, NSAIDs

VAGINAL CANCER
- MC vaginal tumor - *invasion from surrounding structure (eg rectal CA)*
- MC primary type - **squamous cell CA**
- **DES** (diethylstilbestrol) - can cause **clear cell** CA of vagina
- **Botryoides tumor** - rhabdomyosarcoma that occurs in young girls
  - Tx: resection usual
- **XRT** - used for most cancers of vagina

VULVAR CANCER
RFs: elderly, nulliparous, obese; usually unilateral
MC type - **squamous cell CA**; goes to inguinal nodes 1st
Need **2 cm margins** if CA
Tx:
- **Paget's, VIN III** or higher (vulvar intra-epithelial neoplasia), or **carcinoma in situ** - all premalignant (Tx: WLE)
- **Stage I** (< 2 cm) → **WLE** + **ipsilateral** inguinal and **femoral node dissection**
- **Stage II** (> 2 cm) or **Stage III** (beyond vulva or positive nodes) → **modified radical vulvectomy** (entire vulva removed including bilateral labia majora / minora and clitoris) and bilateral inguinal / femoral lymph node dissection
- Post-op **XRT** if close margins
5-YS (all patients) - **75%**

OVARIAN CANCER
Leading cause of gynecologic death
- 2nd MC gynecologic CA (#1 - endometrial CA)
Sx's: abdominal or pelvic pain; change in stool or urinary habits; vaginal bleeding, fullness, dyspareunia (painful sex)
Decreased risk - OCPs, bilateral tubal ligation
Increased risk - nulliparity, late menopause, early menarche, BRCA
Often a **delay in Dx** (60% stage III or IV at Dx)
80% occur in **post-menopausal** patients
Dx: **U/S** and **CA-125**; diagnostic laparoscopy

- **Types** - teratoma, granulosa-theca (estrogen secreting, precocious puberty); Sertoli-Leydig (androgens, masculinization); struma ovarii (thyroid tissues); choriocarcinoma (beta-HCG); mucinous; serous; papillary
- MC type - **serous tumors**
- Worst prognosis - **clear cell** type
- Best prognosis - malignant **germ cell** tumors

Staging of Ovarian Cancer

Stage	Location
I	One or both ovaries only
II	Confined to pelvis
III	Spread throughout abdominal cavity or positive nodes
IV	Distant metastases

- **Bilateral ovary** involvement still **stage I**
- MC initial site of regional spread - **contra-lateral ovary**
- Tx: **total abdominal hysterectomy** and **bilateral oophorectomy** for all stages; *plus*
  - Pelvic and para-aortic LN dissection
  - Omentectomy
  - 4 quadrant washes and Bx's (under right diaphragm, peri-colic recess, pelvic sidewall)
  - Chemo: **cisplatin** and **paclitaxel** (Taxol); **intra-venous** *and* **intra-peritoneal**
  - **XRT** - of some benefit (for residual disease after surgery)
- **Debulking tumor** (cytoreduction of carcinomatosis) - is **effective** (helps intra-peritoneal chemo and XRT; improves prognosis for advanced CA); want residual tumor deposits < 1 cm
- **Peritoneal metastases** - Tx: **resect**
- 5-YS (all patients) - **35%** (late stage at Dx)

- **Krukenberg tumor** - stomach CA that has metastasized to ovary
  - Pathology classically shows **signet ring cells**
  - MC metastasis to ovary - colon CA
- **Meige's syndrome** - pelvic ovarian fibroma that causes **ascites** and **hydrothorax** (MC on the right)
  - Excision of tumor cures syndrome

ENDOMETRIAL CANCER
- *MC gynecologic CA*
- RFs: nulliparity, late 1st pregnancy, obesity, tamoxifen, unopposed estrogen
- Sx's: **vaginal bleeding** (in postmenopausal patients is endometrial CA until proved otherwise)
- Uterine polyps have very low chance of malignancy (0.1%)
- Dx: endometrial curettage or brush Bx; D&C
  - Need routine screening if patient has a RF
- MC type - **endometrioid adenocarcinoma**
- Worst prognosis - **clear cell**
- Need **trans-abdominal approach** (not vaginal) for resection; include para-aortic lymph node dissection
- Tx:
  - **Stage I** (limited to endometrium only) - TAH + BSO
  - **Stage II, III, and IV** or **high grade** tumors →
    1) TAH + BSO + para-aortic / pelvic LN dissection *and:*
    2) post-op XRT
- 5-YS (all patients) - **75%** (early stage at Dx)

CERVICAL CANCER
- Sx's: vaginal bleeding, painful sex, discharge
- PAP smear has greatly decreased incidence of cervical CA
- All associated with **HPV** (MC HPV 16 and 18)
- MC type - **squamous cell CA**; goes to **obturator nodes** 1st

- Dx: **PAP smear** - looks for cervical intraepithelial neoplasia (CIN) or dysplasia; if present, need a Bx (called colposcopy Bx)
  - **Colposcopy Bx** - if high grade CIN (microscopic disease without basement membrane invasion) or more invasive lesion found (eg CIS) → will need conization Bx
  - **Conization Bx** - inner lining of cervix is removed
    - If <u>no</u> basement membrane invasion (eg carcinoma is situ or high grade CIN) → *that is all that is necessary*

Staging of Cervical Cancer

Stage	Location
CIS	Full thickness epithelium; no basement membrane or stromal invasion
I	Cervix only
II	Upper ⅔ of vagina
III	Pelvic side wall, lower ⅓ of vagina; hydronephrosis, or positive nodes
IV	Bladder or rectal invasion (IVA), metastases (IVB)

- Tx:
  - **Microscopic disease** (<u>no</u> basement membrane invasion, eg CIS or CIN) → ***Conization Bx only***
  - **Stages I and II**
    Total abdominal hysterectomy (TAH) and **pelvic LN dissection**
  - **Stages III and IV** - **chemo-XRT** *only* (cisplatin + Taxol); if that fails need <u>pelvic exenteration</u> (TAH-BSO plus vagina, rectum, and bladder)
  - Can **leave ovaries** with cervical CA (unless pelvic exenteration)
- 5-YS (all patients) - **75%** (early stage at Dx due to Pap smear)

OVARIAN CYSTS
- > 95% are benign (follicular, corpus luteum, and thecal cysts)
  - Simple cysts < 10 cm have a < 1% CA risk
- CA usually occurs in **post-menopausal** patients
  - There is a much lower threshold for oophorectomy in post-menopausal patients as they are beyond child-bearing ages and the risk of CA is much higher compared to pre-menopausal patients
- Laparotomy vs laparoscopy
  - In past, removal of a complex cyst was an indication for laparotomy
  - **Laparoscopic** removal using an **endobag** is now *preferred* to avoid over-treating the 90% of patients who end up having a benign lesion
- RFs for **malignancy** in ovarian cyst:
  - Post-menopausal patients
  - Persists beyond 2-3 months
  - Cysts > 10 cm
  - Complex cysts (septated, increased vascular flow on U/S, solid components, papillary projections, thick walls)
  - Elevated CA-125

Post-menopausal
- Complex cysts have a 15% malignancy risk
- If complex, persistent, > 10 cm, or associated with elevated CA-125 → Tx: <u>laparoscopic</u> oophorectomy with attached cyst, intra-op frozen sections, and TAH + contralateral oophorectomy if malignant (convert to laparotomy if malignant; also need staging procedure, see ovarian CA section above)
- If cyst not worrisome for malignancy, follow with U/S
  - If persists or gets larger → laparoscopic oophorectomy with attached cyst and intra-op frozen sections

Pre-menopausal
- Complex cysts have a 1-2% malignancy risk
- A main concern here is avoiding oophorectomy for a benign lesion in a patient who desires future pregnancy
- If thought to be <u>benign</u> and is significantly symptomatic - Tx: <u>laparoscopic</u> removal of cyst only *(leave ovary intact)*

- If thought to be <u>malignant</u> (should be fairly confident about this, eg complex cyst *and* elevated CA-125) - Tx: <u>laparoscopic</u> oophorectomy with attached cyst and intra-op frozen sections
    - Algorithm becomes very complicated after this, weighing how aggressive the CA is (based on histology and stage at operation) compared with whether or not the patient desires future pregnancy
- If cyst not worrisome for malignancy → can follow with U/S; surgery if suspicious findings appear

INCIDENTAL OVARIAN CYST OR TUMOR *(general surgeon perspective)*
- If a cyst, needs to be **complex,** otherwise leave it alone (especially if the patient is pre-menopausal)
    - **Complex cysts** – <u>septated</u>, solid components, <u>papillary projections</u> or <u>increased vascular flow</u> on Duplex U/S
- **Post-menopausal** patients - threshold for oophorectomy is much lower than in pre-menopausal patients
    - If **complex cyst** or highly suspicious **mass** - Tx: <u>laparoscopic</u> oophorectomy with attached cyst / mass and send to pathology
    - If the Dx of CA is made intra-op, all subsequent procedures (including TAH, contralateral oophorectomy, and staging) should be *deferred* to a gynecologic oncologist post-op (2nd procedure)
- **Pre-menopausal** patients - need to be fairly certain this is CA before going with oophorectomy in this scenario as the CA risk is low in this population and oophorectomy will affect future pregnancy
    - If <u>not certain</u> of CA, get Bx of any associated mass, omentum, and any suspicious areas in the peritoneum; 4 quadrant wash for cytology
- Do *not* aspirate the cyst - can spill and upstage the tumor
- Place specimen in an **endobag** before removal to avoid spillage (potentially upstaging the tumor)
- If original procedure **elective** (eg laparoscopic gastric bypass) - may abort procedure depending on findings (eg peritoneal studding)
- If **non-elective** - finish procedure

OTHER GYNECOLOGIC CONDITIONS
- **Ovarian torsion** (adnexal torsion)
    - Sx's: sudden lateralized lower quadrant pain, N/V
    - Dx: U/S
    - Tx: relieve torsion, check for viability; resection if vascular necrosis
- **Ovarian vein thrombosis** - Dx: CT scan with venous phase contrast
    - Tx: heparin
- **Post-partum pelvic thrombophlebitis** - can lead to ovarian vein, IVC, and hepatic vein thrombosis; get liver failure with ascites after pregnancy; Tx: **heparin** and **antibiotics**
- Pregnancy with **acute cholecystitis**
    - Initial Tx: **antibiotics** and **NPO** (>95% treated *without* intervention)
- Pregnancy with **appendicitis**
    - **MC problem requiring surgery with pregnancy**
    - May have *RUQ* pain in 3rd trimester - appendix moves towards RUQ with pregnancy; pain may be exacerbated with patient lying on **right side**
    - Dx: **Get an U/S 1st** (diameter > 7, thickness > 2)
    - Laparoscopic appendectomy if 1st or 2nd trimester; open usual for 3rd
    - If open appendectomy, **mark site of incision over the site of maximal pain** before you put patient to sleep → *appendix is displaced superiorly by uterus*
    - High appendix **rupture, premature labor** (10-15%), and **fetal loss** (5-10%) with appendicitis in pregnancy
- **Pelvic inflammatory disease**
    - Increased risk of **infertility** and **ectopic pregnancy**
    - Sx's: lower abdominal pain, N/V, fever, vaginal discharge
    - MC in **first 1/2 of menstrual cycle**
    - RFs: multiple sexual partners

- Dx: cervical motion tenderness *(best exam finding),* adnexal tenderness, gram stain and cultures (Gonococcus, Chlamydia)
- Tx: **ceftriaxone** and **doxycycline** (admit if severe)

- **Post-menopausal vaginal bleeding**: Dx - endometrial Bx (suspicious for endometrial CA)
- **Uterine Prolapse** (procidentia) - uterus protrudes through vagina
  - RFs: multiparity
  - Tx: weight loss, D/C smoking (↓ cough), pessary, vaginal hysterectomy
- **Polycystic Ovarian Disease**
  - Sx's: amenorrhea, infertility, hirsutism
  - Tx: **clomiphene** citrate
- **Uterine leiomyomas** (eg fibroids)
  - Sx's: under hormonal influence; bleeding (MC Sx), recurrent abortions, infertility
  - Tx: GnRH analogues (eg **leuprolide**)
- **Magnesium toxicity** (for pre-term labor) - can get <u>respiratory depression</u>

Neurosurgery

1074. The most appropriate Tx for a 9 mm cerebral aneurysm (Berry aneurysm) is:
   - a. Craniotomy and clipping
   - b. Endovascular coiling
   - c. Clipping and coiling
   - d. Observation

   Answer d. For **cerebral aneurysms < 10 mm**, the risk of injury trying to exclude it is higher than the rupture risk. These should be **observed**.

1075. All of the following are good indications for sympathectomy except:
   - a. Hyperhidrosis
   - b. Complex regional pain syndrome
   - c. Unresectable pancreatic CA
   - d. Healing of diabetic foot ulcers

   Answer d. Sympathectomy is not been helpful for healing of diabetic foot ulcers

1076. All of the following are true except
   - a. The middle cerebral artery is connected to the posterior cerebral artery by the posterior communicating artery
   - b. Injury with neuropraxia usually recovers
   - c. Epidural hematomas are MC caused by torn bridging veins
   - d. Hemi-transection of the spinal cord is most likely to result in ipsilateral motor and contra-lateral pain and temperature loss

   Answer c. **Epidural hematomas** are most commonly caused by bleeding from the **middle meningeal artery** (see Trauma section).

CIRCLE OF WILLIS
- Circle of arterial circulation in the brain such that if one artery is occluded, the communicating arteries will still allow blood flow
- **Vertebral arteries** - coalesce to form a single **basilar artery**
  - Basilar artery branches into <u>two</u> **posterior cerebral arteries**
- **Posterior communicating arteries** - these connect **middle cerebral arteries** to **posterior cerebral arteries**
- **Anterior cerebral arteries** - branches of **middle cerebral arteries**
  - Connected to each other through <u>one</u> **anterior communicating artery**
- The **internal carotid artery** becomes the **middle cerebral artery**

- **Broca's area** - <u>speech motor</u>, posterior part of anterior lobe
- **Wernicke's area** - <u>speech comprehension</u>, temporal lobe
- **Pituitary adenoma, undergoing XRT, patient now in shock**
  - Dx: pituitary apoplexy Tx: **steroids**
- **Diaphragm innervation** - phrenic nerve (cervical nerve roots 3–5)
- **Microglial cells** - brain macrophages
- **GABA** (Gamma-Amino-Butyric Acid) - chief neuro-inhibitory neurotransmitter in brain; GABA analogues have anti-convulsing, anti-anxiety, relaxing effects

NERVE INJURY
- **Neuropraxia** - mildest form of injury (MC injury)
  - No axon or myelin sheath injury but interruption of **conduction impulse**
  - **Temporary loss of function** (motor >> sensory)
  - Generally all recover
  - **Mildest form** - foot falls asleep while sitting (pressure on sciatic nerve)
  - **Severe** - blunt trauma (make take 6-8 weeks to recover)
- **Axonotmesis**
  - Disruption of **axon** with preservation of myelin sheath
  - Paralysis and loss of sensation
  - MC with **crush injury**

- Wallerian degeneration of nerve occurs (antegrade degeneration towards end plate)
- Nerve has to regenerate for recover (1 mm/day) – can take weeks
- **Neurotmesis**
  - *Worst form of injury* - severe contusion, stretch, complete laceration
  - Disruption of **axon** and **myelin sheath**
  - May not recover or may need surgery for recovery
- Regeneration of **peripheral nerves** occurs at rate of **1 mm/day**
  - *Central nerves do not regenerate*
- **Nodes of Ranvier** - bare sections between myelin sheath cells; allow salutatory propagation of action potentials
- **Sensory function** - 1st to recover after nerve damage

SUBARACHNOID HEMORRHAGE (SAH, non-traumatic causes listed below)
- Sx's: **severe HA** (thunderclap), vomiting, confusion, LOC, seizures
- Etiology - **cerebral aneurysms** (85%, MC at branch points) and **AVMs** (10%)
- Tx: prevent **re-bleeding** (open clips or endovascular coils) and prevent **vasospasm** (calcium channel blocker, volume, phenylephrine to raise BP)
- Asymptomatic cerebral aneurysm **< 10 mm** - *Tx: leave alone (risk of surgery higher than risk of rupture)*

SPINAL CORD INJURY
- **Complete cord transection** - loss of reflexes, flaccidity, anesthesia
  - Autonomic paralysis below level of transection
- **Spinal shock** (neurogenic shock) - **hypotension, normal or slow heart rate,** and **warm extremities** (vasodilated); usually associated with **paraplegia**
  - Occurs with **spinal cord injuries above T5** (loss of sympathetic tone)
  - Tx: fluids initially, may need phenylephrine drip (alpha agonist)
- **Brown-Sequard syndrome** (incomplete cord transection; hemi-section of cord)
  - **MCC** - penetrating injury
  - **Loss of** (occurs below level of injury):
    - *Ipsilateral* motor
    - *Contra-lateral* pain and temperature
  - About 90% recover to ambulation
- **Cauda equina syndrome** - pain and weakness in lower extremities
  - **Loss of bowel or bladder function**
  - Due to compression of lumbar nerve roots
- **Doral nerve roots** (posterior) – generally afferent
  - Carry **sensory** neurons
  - **Spinothalamic tract** - pain and temp
- **Ventral nerve roots** (anterior) - generally efferent
  - Carry **motor** neurons
  - **Corticospinal tract** - motor
  - **Rubrospinal tract** - motor

BRAIN TUMORS
- Sx's: HA, seizures, progressive neuro deficit, persistent vomiting
- **Adults** - 2/3 supra-tentorial
- **Children** - 2/3 infra-tentorial
- **MC primary brain tumor** - gliomas
  - **MC subtype** - glioblastoma multiforme (uniformly fatal)
- **MC metastases to brain** - lung
- **MC brain tumor in children** - medulloblastoma
- **MC metastases to brain in children** - neuroblastoma

SPINE TUMORS
- **MC benign** and **MC overall** - neurofibroma
- **Intra-dural tumors** more likely benign
- **Extra-dural tumors** are more likely malignant
- **Paraganglioma** - can secrete norepinephrine

MYELOMENINGOCELE
- Neural cord defect - herniation of spinal cord and nerve roots through defect in vertebra; looks like big sac off vertebral column
- If sac ruptured - surgery needed to prevent infection of spinal cord
- MC in lumbar region

THORACIC SYMPATHECTOMY
- **Palmar** and **axillary hyperhidrosis** (sweaty palms) - take T2-T4 sympathetic nerves
  - *MC indication for sympathectomy by far*
  - **MC Cx - compensatory sweating** in the lower extremities or abdomen
  - *Avoid taking T1* - can result in **Horner's Syndrome** (ptosis, miosis-small pupil, and anhydrosis; injury to stellate ganglion)
  - **Nerve of Kuntz**
    - Accessory nerve pathway between T1 and T2 that can result in refractory palmar sweating after sympathectomy
    - Need to coagulate on bottom of the 2nd rib to divide the nerve of Kuntz and avoid this complication
- **Complex regional pain syndrome** (Reflex Sympathetic Dystrophy, **causalgia**)
  - Neuron derived pain (neuropathic) - usually after trauma, amputation (phantom pain), frostbite, or previous surgery
  - Continuous pain out of proportion to degree of injury
  - Medical Tx: **gabapentin** and **amitriptyline**; TENS unit
  - *Only use sympathectomy when pain is dramatically relieved by nerve blocks*
  - <u>Not</u> useful for diabetic foot ulcers
  - Location of sympathectomy depends on location of pain:
    - **Unresectable pancreatic CA** causing pain - Tx: lumbar sympathectomy

Orthopaedics

1077. All the following are true of supracondylar humeral fractures in children except:
    a.   Type III will need percutaneous wire fixation
    b.   Type II fractures will likely need wire fixation
    c.   Type I fractures can just be placed in a sling
    d.   Type I fractures need wire fixation

Answer d. Type I supra-condylar humeral fractures can just be treated with a sling.

1078. A 20 yo man falls on an outstretched hand and now complains of tenderness in the "snuff box" of his right hand. You get an x-ray but it is negative. The most appropriate next step is:
    a.   Spica cast up to the elbow, repeat films in 2 weeks
    b.   Exploration
    c.   Nothing
    d.   Tape fingers together

Answer a. Snuff box tenderness is worrisome for a scaphoid bone Fx. These Fx's are hard to see on X-ray. They are at high risk for avascular necrosis. Tx for a patient with snuff box tenderness and a negative x-ray is a cast up to the elbow with follow-up x-ray in 2 weeks.

1079. A 59 yo woman undergoes an abdomino-perineal resection (APR) which takes 12 hours. Post-operatively, you note she has a foot drop on the right. All of the following are true except:
    a.   Proper patient positioning could have likely prevented this problem
    b.   This patient should have a fasciotomy
    c.   This problem is related to the common peroneal nerve
    d.   A foot brace may benefit this patient
    e.   This is not due to tibial nerve injury

Answer b. This patient likely suffered a **common peroneal nerve** injury where the peroneal nerve wraps around the leg at the level of the fibula. This occurred from compression of this area while in the lithotomy position.

The **common peroneal nerve** bifurcates into the **deep peroneal nerve** (dorsiflexion, sensation in 1st toe web-space) and **superficial peroneal nerve** (foot eversion). The **tibial nerve** is found in the deep posterior leg compartment (plantarflexion)

1080. A 24 yo man suffers a supracondylar humeral Fx. Six hours after the event, the patient has his arm reduced and placed in a sling. Shortly afterwards, the patient develops severe forearm swelling and pain. The arm is tense. You have trouble finding distal pulses. The most appropriate next step in management is:
    a.   Emergent open reduction and internal fixation
    b.   Emergency repair of the brachial artery
    c.   Angiogram and stent placement
    d.   Forearm fasciotomies

Answer d. Supracondylar humeral fractures are at high risk for brachial artery injury. **Compartment syndrome (Volkmann's contracture** in this case) can occur after the interruption of blood flow, a delay (4-6 hours), and then restoration of blood flow. This patient needs forearm fasciotomies to the volar and dorsal compartments.

Forearm fasciotomy
    Volar incision - curvilinear (lazy S shape) so that all of the major nerves and arteries are decompressed
    Dorsal incision - longitudinal incision (linear)

The vessel involved in Volkmann's contracture is the **anterior interosseous artery**.

1081. Anterior dislocation of the shoulder is most likely to injure the:
   a.   Subclavian vein
   b.   Subclavian artery
   c.   Axillary nerve
   d.   Thoracic duct

   Answer c. Anterior shoulder dislocation is most likely to injure the **axillary nerve**.

1082. A mid-shaft spiral humeral fracture is most likely to injure the:
   a.   Median nerve
   b.   Radial nerve
   c.   Musculocutaneous nerve
   d.   Ulnar nerve
   e.   Axillary nerve

   Answer b. Radial nerve (weak wrist and finger extension).

1083. Carpal tunnel surgery involves releasing the:
   a.   Superficial radial nerve
   b.   Median nerve
   c.   Ulnar nerve
   d.   Radial nerve

   Answer b. Median nerve using transverse carpal ligament release

1084. A man suffers a minor dog bite and presents 4 days later with pain in a semi-flexed left 2nd digit, tendon sheath tenderness, pain with passive motion, and swelling in the finger. The most appropriate next step is:
   a.   Amputation
   b.   Continued antibiotics
   c.   FNA
   d.   Mid-axial longitudinal incision and drainage

   Answer d. Suppurative flexor tenosynovitis is one of the few orthopedic emergencies. It is caused by an infection in the flexor tendon sheath of the hand. Infection here can rapidly destroy the finger's flexing ability. Tx - **mid-axial longitudinal incision and drainage** (avoid lateral incision along finger - the nerves are there).

1085. A 50 truck-driver presents to the ED with a biceps tendon rupture after rock climbing. The most appropriate next step is:
   a.   Urgent repair
   b.   Discharge with repair within 2 weeks
   c.   Discharge with repair within 1 month
   d.   Discharge with repair within 2 months
   e.   No repair is needed

   Answer b. Flexor tendons generally need repair as they handle a lot of force. For biceps tendon injuries, if the patient is old and frail or perhaps the injury is in their non-dominant arm, repair may not be necessary. The above patient, however, is a truck driver so repair would be indicated.

   Flexor tendon injuries should generally be repaired within 2 weeks to avoid musculo-tendon contraction (at which point a tendon graft becomes necessary). In general, if extensor tendon injuries are going to be repaired they should also be repaired within 2 weeks, although a delay in repair is not quite as problematic as flexor injuries.

1086. Posterior dislocation of the hip is most likely to injure the:
- a. Femoral artery
- b. Femoral vein
- c. Sciatic nerve
- d. Femoral nerve

Answer c. Posterior hip dislocation is most likely to injure the **sciatic nerve**

1087. All of the following are true except:
- a. Tx for an isolated anterior ring Fx (eg pubic rami) with minimal ischial displacement is weight-bearing as tolerated (WBAT)
- b. Salter-Harris III Fx's (crosses the epiphyseal plate) should undergo closed reduction
- c. Humeral spiral Fx's (mid-shaft) are at risk for radial nerve injury
- d. Femur Fx associated with tachypnea is most likely from fat embolus

Answer b. Salter-Harris III Fx's (crosses the epiphyseal plate) should undergo open reduction and internal fixation (ORIF)

1088. All of the following are true except
- a. Acute pain with ankle ecchymosis and a lump behind the knee in a tennis player is most likely a plantaris muscle tendon rupture
- b. Calcaneus Fx is associated with lumbar Fx's in 10% and radius Fx's in 5%
- c. The MC injured nerve with lower extremity fasciotomy is the superficial peroneal nerve
- d. Petechiae, hypoxia, and mental status changes after setting a long bone Fx suggests ETOH intoxication
- e. Ewing's sarcoma often has an onion skin appearance on x-ray

Answer d. Petechiae, hypoxia, and **mental status changes** after setting a long bone Fx suggests **fat embolism.** Risk factors include _delayed_ fixation, young age, multiple Fx's, and conservative Tx of long bone Fx

GENERAL
- **Salter-Harris** fractures III, IV, and V in children - cross the epiphyseal plate and can affect the growth plate (metaphysic) of bone; need **open reduction and internal fixation (ORIF)**
- **Salter-Harris** fractures I and II - **closed reduction**
- Fractures associated with **avascular necrosis (AVN)** - scaphoid, femoral neck, hip dislocation, talus (ankle)
- Fractures associated with **nonunion** - clavicle, 5th metatarsal (Jones' Fx)
- Fractures associated with **compartment syndrome** - supracondylar humerus, tibia, calcaneus
- Biggest risk factor for nonunion - **smoking**
- **Fat embolism**
  - Sx's: **petechiae, hypoxia,** and **mental status changes** (confusion)
  - **Sudan red stain** - fat in sputum and urine
  - MCC - lower extremity Fx's or ortho procedures
  - RFs - delayed fixation, young age, multiple Fx's, conservative Tx of long bone Fx (eg long bone traction)
  - Tx: supportive; may need to intubate
- **Open Fx** - washout, antibiotics, external fixation, soft tissue coverage

BONE SECTIONS
- **Diaphysis** - midsection[shaft
- **Metaphysis** - epiphyseal growth plate (between diaphysis and epiphysis)
- **Epiphysis** - rounded end of long bone

LOWER EXTREMITY NERVES

Obturator nerve	hip adduction
Superior gluteal nerve	hip abduction
Inferior gluteal nerve	hip extension
Femoral nerve	knee extension

HERNIATED LUMBAR DISC

- Sx's: **back pain** aggravated by activity, can **radiate down leg**
  - Herniated disc is **nucleus pulposus**
  - Certain movements increase inter-vertebral pressure at disc (eg attempting to rise out of a chair, bending over at waist)
  - Often have a history of chronic back pain
- **Nerves affected**
  - **L1 to L3 nerves** - weak hip flexion
  - **L4 nerve** (*MC type;* L4–5 disc) - weak knee extension (quadriceps), weak patellar reflex
  - **L5 nerve** (L5–S1 disc) - weak dorsiflexion (foot drop), ↓ sensation in big toe web space
  - **S1 nerve** (S1–S2 disc) - weak plantarflexion, weak Achilles reflex, ↓ sensation in lateral foot
- Dx: **MRI** *(best test)* - needed for patients with neurologic Sx's
- Tx: 90% treated with **NSAIDs** and **pain meds**
  - With time, disc shrinks on its own, decompressing spine
  - Failure of conservative Tx (6 weeks) - consider surgery
  - Surgical decompression removes of part of disc (**discectomy**)
- Consider **emergent decompression** for **severe cord compression** (eg cauda equina syndrome [loss of bowel or bladder function, saddle anesthesia, loss of movement]), progressive muscle weakness, increasing pain, or bone fragments in cord
  - Tx: **dexamethasone**, surgical **decompression**

TERMINAL BRANCHES OF BRACHIAL PLEXUS

- **Ulnar nerve**
  - **Motor** - intrinsic musculature of hand; finger abduction (spreads fingers); **wrist flexion**
  - **Sensory** - all of 5th and ½ 4th fingers; back of hand
  - Injury results in **claw hand**; involved in **<u>cubital</u> tunnel syndrome** at elbow
- **Median nerve**
  - **Motor** - thumb apposition (OK sign); **finger flexors**
  - **Sensory** - most of palm and first 3 and ½ 4th fingers on palmar side
  - Nerve is involved in **<u>carpal</u> tunnel syndrome** at wrist
  - **Injury** - decreased thumb movement, fingers will be extended
- **Radial nerve**
  - **Motor** - wrist extension, finger extension, thumb extension, and triceps
    <u>No</u> intrinsic hand muscles
  - **Sensory** - first 3 and ½ 4th fingers on dorsal side
- **Axillary nerve** - motor to deltoid (abduction)
- **Musculocutaneous nerve** - motor to biceps, brachialis, coracobrachialis

UPPER EXTREMITY

- **Prolonged hand ischemia** (eg laceration of radial and ulnar arteries) - motor function can remain in digits after prolonged ischemia because motor groups are in proximal forearm
- **Clavicle Fx** - usually just treated with sling (risk of vascular impingement)
- **Shoulder dislocation**
  - **Anterior** (90%) risk of **axillary <u>nerve</u> injury**; Tx: closed reduction
  - **Posterior** (seizures, electrocution) risk of **axillary <u>artery</u> injury**; Tx: closed reduction
  - ORIF for either of above if displaced humeral Fx also present
- **Acromioclavicular separation** - Tx: sling (risk of brachial plexus and subclavian vessel injury)
- **Scapula Fx** - sling unless **glenoid fossa** involved, then need internal fixation

- **Proximal humerus: non-displaced** - sling; **displaced** or **comminuted** - ORIF
  - Risk of **axillary nerve damage**
- **Mid-shaft humeral Fx** - Tx: sling (almost all)
  - Surgery only for failed reduction or neurovascular events
  - Risk of **radial nerve damage** (weak wrist + finger extension)
- **Supracondylar humeral Fx**
  - **Adults** → Tx: <u>ORIF</u>
  - **Children**
    - **Non-displaced** → Tx: <u>closed reduction</u>
    - **Displaced** → Tx: <u>closed reduction</u> and internal fixation with <u>Kirschner wire</u>
  - Risk of **brachial artery damage**
  - Risk of **Volkmann's Contracture** (ie compartment syndrome)
- **Monteggia Fx** - proximal ulnar Fx and radial head dislocation
  - Tx: ORIF
- **Colles' Fx** - fall on outstretched hand, distal radius Fx ± distal ulnar dislocation
  - *MC Fx in children*
  - Tx: **closed reduction** for vast majority (adults and children)
- **Nursemaid's elbow** - subluxation of the radius at the elbow caused by a pulling on an extended, pronated arm. Tx: closed reduction
- **Combined radial and ulnar Fx's**
  - **Adults** - ORIF
  - **Children** - closed reduction (preferred)
  - Risk of **ulnar and radial nerve damage** with forearm Fx's
- **Scaphoid Fx** (eg wrist Fx; perilunate wrist Fx)
  - *MC carpal bone Fx (also MC Fx in wrist)*
  - Causes anatomic **snuffbox tenderness** (classic)
  - Can have negative x-ray initially
  - Tx:
    - **Negative X-ray** - *all patients* still get **spica cast to elbow**, follow-up X-ray in 2 weeks to look for Fx healing (occult Fx)
    - **Non-displaced Fx** (scaphoid or lunate) - spica cast to elbow, 6-8 weeks
    - **Displaced Fx** (<u>scaphoid or lunate</u>) - ORIF
  - Risk of **avascular necrosis** with scaphoid Fx (Tx: hip bone graft)
- **Volkmann's contracture**: supracondylar humerus Fx → occluded **anterior interosseous artery** → closed reduction of humerus → artery opens up → reperfusion injury, edema, and **forearm compartment syndrome** (flexor compartment most affected)
  - Sx's: **forearm pain** with passive extension of wrist; weakness; tense forearm
  - **Median nerve** most affected by swelling
  - Tx: **forearm fasciotomies** (both volar and dorsal compartments)
- **Forearm fasciotomy** - need to decompress both compartments
  - **Volar incision** - *curvilinear incision (lazy S shape)* so that all of the major nerves and arteries are decompressed
  - **Dorsal incision** - *longitudinal incision (linear);* need to open both the mobile extensor wad and extensor digitorum communis muscle group compartments
- **Dupuytren's contracture** - associated with diabetes, ETOH
  - Progressive proliferation of **palmar fascia in hand** results in contractures that usually affect the **4th** and **5th digits** (cannot extend fingers)
  - Tx: NSAIDs, steroid injections; excision of involved fascia for significant contraction
- **Carpal tunnel syndrome** - **median nerve** compression by transverse carpal ligament
  - Tx: splint, NSAIDs, and steroid injections; **transverse carpal ligament** release if that fails
- **Trigger finger** - tenosynovitis of the flexor tendon that catches at the MCP joint when trying to extend or flex the finger
  - Tx: tendon sheath steroid injections and splinting (treats majority of cases); if that fails can release the pulley system at the MCP joint

- **Suppurative tenosynovitis**
  - Infection that spreads along flexor tendon sheath (can **destroy tendon**); can occur after minor trauma (eg cat or dog bite)
  - Sx's *(4 classic signs):*
    - 1) tendon sheath **tenderness**
    - 2) **pain** with passive motion
    - 3) **swelling** along sheath
    - 4) **semi-flexed posture** of involved digit
  - Tx: **mid-axial longitudinal incision** and **drainage,** antibiotics *(avoid lateral incision along finger - the nerves are there)*
- **Rotator cuff tears** - supraspinatus, infraspinatus, teres minor, and subscapularis
  - Acutely → sling and conservative Tx
  - Surgical repair if the patient needs to retain a high level of activity or if daily activities affected
- **Flexor tendon injuries** - non-surgical Tx if < 60% laceration
  - If ≥ 60% laceration, repair within 2 weeks to avoid tendon retraction
- **Paronychia** - infection where the skin and nail bed meet
  - Can progress under nail bed (erythema, swelling, pain)
  - Tx: antibiotics; **remove nail** if purulent underneath
- **Felon** - infection in the terminal joint space of the finger
  - Tx: incision over the tip of the finger and along the medial and lateral aspects of the finger tip; prevents necrosis; avoid incision into finger tip pad (key part of finger tip sensation)
- **Prolonged hand ischemia** (eg laceration of radial and ulnar arteries) - motor function can remain in digits after prolonged ischemia because motor groups are in proximal forearm
- **Torus Fx** (greenstick Fx) - buckling of bone cortex in children (eg distal radius); Tx - **cast** (3 weeks)
- **Open fractures** - washout, antibiotics, and external fixation until tissue heals; soft tissue coverage at time of definitive surgery

LOWER EXTREMITY
- **Hip dislocation** (risk of **avascular necrosis** to femoral head)
  - **Posterior** (MC, 90%) - internal rotation, adduction, and shortened leg; risk of **sciatic nerve injury**; Tx: closed reduction
  - **Anterior** - external rotation, abduction, and shortened leg; risk of injury to **femoral artery** or femoral nerve; Tx: closed reduction
  - Reduce in < 24 hours to avoid **avascular necrosis**
- **Pelvic fractures**
  - MC **associated injury - closed head injury**
  - Need to Tx **life threatening hemorrhage** from pelvic Fx 1st
  - Need to assess whether or not the pelvic ring is stable
  - **Isolated anterior ring** with minimal ischial displacement - Tx: weight-bearing as tolerated *(does not need ORIF)*
  - **Bilateral pubic rami Fx's** with minor displacement - Tx: weight-bearing as tolerated *(does not need ORIF)*
  - Generally need ≥ **2 significant Fx's** or **dislocations** for ring to be unstable requiring ORIF
- **Hip Fx** (ie femoral head and acetabulum) - almost all treated surgically (hip replacement)
  - High mortality in **patients aged > 65** (20% mortality in 6 months)
- **Femoral neck Fx** - external rotation, abduction, shortened leg
  - ORIF or partial arthroplasty (hemiarthroplasty)
  - Risk of **avascular necrosis** if open reduction delayed
- **Femoral shaft Fx** - ORIF with intramedullary rod (adults and children > age 6)
  - Children **aged < 6** - spica cast
- **Lateral knee trauma** - can injure the following:
  - Anterior cruciate ligament
  - Posterior cruciate ligament
  - Medial meniscus
  - Medial collateral ligament

- **Anterior cruciate ligament injury** - positive anterior drawer test
  - Present with **knee effusion** and **pain with pivoting action**
  - MRI *(best)* confirms diagnosis
  - Tx: surgery for knee instability (reconstruction with patellar or hamstring tendon); otherwise therapy with leg-strengthening exercise
- **Posterior cruciate ligament injury** - positive posterior drawer test
  - Much less common than ACL injury; present with knee pain and joint effusion
  - Tx: conservative Tx initially; surgery for failure of medical Tx
- **Collateral ligaments**
  - **Medial collateral ligament** injury - lateral blow to knee
  - **Lateral collateral ligament** injury - medial blow to knee
  - Tx: **small tear** - brace; **large tear** - surgery
  - These injuries are associated with injuries to corresponding **meniscus**
- **Meniscus tears** - joint line tenderness; can treat with arthroscopic repair or debridement
- **Posterior knee dislocation** - Tx: closed reduction; all patients need **formal angiogram** to rule out **popliteal artery injury** (25% risk) unless there is a pulse deficit in which case you would just go to the OR
- **Patellar Fx** - Tx: **long leg cast** for most; **ORIF** if comminuted
- **Tibial plateau, tibial shaft,** and **tibia-fibula Fx's** - ORIF fixation unless open Fx, then need external fixator until tissue heals
  - Risk of **compartment syndrome** with tibial plateau Fx
- **Plantaris muscle rupture** - pain and mass below popliteal fossa (contracted plantaris, tennis player) and ankle ecchymosis; *is not repaired (unnecessary for normal function)*
  - These patients are still able to walk unlike Achilles tendon rupture
- **Achilles tendon tear** - re-attachment in OR usual
- **Ankle fracture** - most treated with cast and immobilization; bimalleolar or trimalleolar fractures need ORIF
- **Metatarsal Fx** - cast immobilization or foot brace for 6 weeks
- **Calcaneus Fx** (heel) - cast and immobilization if non-displaced; ORIF for *any* displacement
  - Risk of **compartment syndrome** of foot
  - 5-10% have **lumbar spine** and **distal forearm Fx's** (from fall)
- **Talus fracture** - closed reduction for most; ORIF for severe displacement
- MC injured nerve with lower extremity fasciotomy - **superficial peroneal nerve** (foot eversion)
- **Foot-drop** after prolonged lithotomy position (compression of side of leg while in stirrups), after crossing legs for long periods (temporary), or fibula head fracture - **common peroneal nerve** injury
  - Common peroneal nerve wraps around the neck of the fibula and divides into the deep and superficial peroneal nerves
  - Tx: foot brace for foot drop
- **Infectious arthritis** - swollen erythematous joint; painful
  - MCC - ***staph aureus***
  - Sexually active - ***gonorrhea (diplococci)***
  - Dx: aspiration (arthrocentesis): **> 50,000 WBCs** highly suspicious for infectious arthritis
  - Tx: joint washout to dryness and antibiotics (vancomycin and levofloxacin until cultures back; ceftriaxone if **gonorrhea**)
  - Infected prosthetic joint usually requires removal of the prosthesis

LEG COMPARTMENTS

Anterior - anterior tibial artery, deep peroneal nerve
Lateral - superficial peroneal nerve
Deep posterior - posterior tibial artery, peroneal artery, and tibial nerve
Superficial posterior - sural nerve

COMPARTMENT SYNDROME

Occurs after **restoration of blood flow** following **vascular compromise**
High risk Fx's - supracondylar humeral Fx (Volkmann's contracture), tibial plateau Fx, calcaneus Fx, elbow dislocations; large crush injuries

- Essentially any injury resulting in **interruption** and then **restoration** of blood flow can result in reperfusion injury and compartment syndrome
- MC in **anterior compartment of leg** (get foot-drop) - *most sensitive to area to compartment syndrome*
  - Is a **reperfusion injury** mediated by **PMNs**
  - Can occur in any muscle compartment (pressure in compartment exceeds capillary filling pressure due to swelling of tissues - get **ischemia** and **rhabdomyolysis**)
  - Sx's: Fx or dislocation with loss of blood flow → repair (> 4-6 hours later) → **pain** and **swelling** soon after restoration of blood flow
    - 1st finding - **pain with passive motion**
    - **Swollen** and **tense extremity**
    - Numbness in webspace between the great and 2nd toe (deep peroneal nerve)
    - **Distal pulses** can be present → last thing to go
  - Dx: *based on **clinical suspicion** (if suspected → fasciotomy)*
    - Pressure **> 20 - 25 mmHg** abnormal
  - Tx: **fasciotomy** (for leg - medial incision for superficial posterior + deep posterior compartments and lateral incision for anterior + lateral compartments)
    - With fasciotomy, you are through the fascia when the **muscle bulges**
    - Incise the **total length** of compartment (eg the length of the leg)
    - Remove all **dead tissue** (myoglobinuria if you don't resect)
  - MC injured nerve with lower extremity fasciotomy - **superficial peroneal nerve** (foot eversion)
  - **Rhabdomyolysis** - myoglobin release; also release of K, H, and PO_4^-
    - **Myoglobinemia Tx** - normal saline volume, alkalinize urine (HCO_3^- drip)

FAT EMBOLISM
- Sx's: **petechiae, hypoxia**, and **mental status changes** (confusion) - *classic triad*; other Sx's similar to PE (following long bone Fx)
- **Sudan red stain** - fat in sputum and urine
- **MCC** - lower extremity (hip and femur) Fx's or ortho procedures
- Tx: supportive; may need to intubate

BONE TUMORS
- **MC bone tumor** - metastasis (**MC - breast**, #2 prostate)
  - Tx: ORIF with impending Fx (> 50% cortical involvement); then XRT
  - XRT is good for painful bony metastases
  - **Pathologic fractures** - Tx: ORIF
  - **Colon CA rarely goes to bone**
- MC primary malignant bone tumor - **multiple myeloma**
  - Tx: chemo for systemic disease
- MC bony tumor overall - **osteochondroma**
- MC bony malignant tumor - **osteosarcoma**
- Presence of **pain** with any bone lesion (other than a Fx) is highly suggestive of **malignancy**
- Most important prognostic indicator for bone sarcomas - **tumor grade**
- **Malignant Bony tumors**
  - **Osteosarcoma** (osteogenic sarcoma)
    - *MC primary malignant bony tumor (35%)*
    - MC at **knee** (50%); **young patients** (80% aged < 20 years)
    - Tx: **limb-sparing resection in 90%**; consider **pre-op chemo-XRT** (doxorubicin-based; see Skin and Soft Tissue chapter)
    - Overall 5-YS - **65%**
  - Chondrosarcoma - can arise from **osteochondroma**
  - **Ewing's Sarcoma**
    - MC in adolescents; **painful swelling**; **onion-skin** appearance on X-ray
    - MC location proximal **diaphysis of femur** (long bones)
    - Tx: ***Chemo-XRT is mainstay of Tx***
    - **Chemo** - Doxorubicin based (ifosfamide, etoposide)
    - *All patients get chemo due to high rate of micro-metastases, then XRT resection (can usually spare limb)*

Pediatric Surgery

1089. All of the following are true except:
- a.   Elevated alkaline phosphatase in a child is due to bone growth
- b.   Surfactant is effective for respiratory distress syndrome
- c.   The gallbladder is considered part of the midgut
- d.   Newborns are at increased risk for cutaneous infection due to impaired PMN chemotaxis

Answer c. The gallbladder is part of the foregut (proximal to Ampulla).

1090. The maintenance fluid for a 1 yo 25 kg girl would be:
- a.   45 cc/hr
- b.   65 cc/hr
- c.   85 cc/hr
- d.   105 cc/hr

Answer b. 65 cc/hr (40 cc/hr for 1st 10 kg, 20 cc/hr for 2nd 10 kg, 1 cc/hr for each kg after that).

1091. The safest maintenance fluid for the above child should be:
- a.   LR
- b.   3% NS
- c.   0.45% NS
- d.   0.2% NS

Answer c. Although in the past 0.2% NS was recommended for children, there have been enough significant issues with **hyponatremia** that it is now hard to justify. Either 0.45% NS or NS is the safest resuscitation fluid for a 1 year old.

1092. A neonate has a large hemangioma on his face. All of the following are appropriate in this patient's management except:
- a.   These lesions can usually be observed initially
- b.   These lesions usually regress
- c.   A hemangioma filling the ear canal should be observed
- d.   Persistent large hemangiomas after age 8 will likely need treatment

Answer c. Hemangiomas causing a functional deficit (eg eyelid, ear canal) require Tx. Tx of choice is oral steroids (prednisone) with surgery if that fails.

1093. A 3 yo child has a 0.5 cm hemangioma on her lateral nare that has been present since she was 2 years old. The most appropriate Tx is:
- a.   Multiple pulse dye laser treatments
- b.   Excision and flap closure
- c.   Steroid injection
- d.   Observation

Answer d. Observation is generally indicated for most congenital **hemangiomas** until age 8.

1094. Which of the following is true of teratomas in newborns:
- a.   They are most commonly germ cell type
- b.   The axilla is the MC location in newborns
- c.   Benign vs malignant lesions is most influenced by the 2 month transition mark
- d.   There is always an external component
- e.   Chemo-XRT is the preferred Tx

Answer c. Newborn teratomas are **embryonal** cell type. The MC location in newborns is the **sacrococcygeal** area, some of which can be entirely internal with no exophytic compoenent. The 2-month mark is an important transition (**< 2**

months → usually benign; **> 2 months** → usually malignant). Tx: **coccygectomy** (including the tumor)

1095. Despite 2 weeks of phototherapy, a newborn has persistent jaundice. An attempt at finding a gallbladder on U/S proves difficult. HIDA reveals normal liver uptake but you do not see any radionuclide in the small bowel. The best Tx in this patient would be:
   a. Hepatoportoenterostomy
   b. Hepaticojejunostomy
   c. Choledochojejunostomy
   d. PTC tube
   e. Cyst-enterotomy

   Answer a. Hepatoportoenterostomy (Kasai procedure) is used for **biliary atresia**.

1096. All of the following are true except:
   a. Congenital lobar emphysema is due to failure of bronchial cartilage to develop, resulting in air-trapping
   b. Bronchogenic cysts are abnormal lung tissue outside lung (MC in mediastinum)
   c. CCAM (congenital cystic adenoid malformations) are due to overgrowth of bronchial tissue and are usually connected to the airway
   d. The systemic arterial supply should be addressed last when resecting pulmonary sequestrations

   Answer d. The **systemic arterial supply** should be resected 1st when resecting **pulmonary sequestrations**, otherwise **catastrophic bleeding** can occur.

1097. A newborn is having severe respiratory distress. CXR demonstrates a hyperlucent area in the left upper thorax and opacity of the left lower thorax. The most appropriate next step is:
   a. Left lower lobectomy
   b. Left upper lobectomy
   c. Left sided chest tube
   d. Nasogastric tube
   e. Bronchoscopy

   Answer a. This patient has **congenital lobar emphysema** of the left upper lobe (hyperlucent area) causing collapse of the left lower lobe (opacity) and respiratory distress. Mediastinal shift can also occur causing hypotension. Tx: **emergent left upper lobectomy**. Chest tube should be avoided and could result in catastrophic respiratory compromise.

1098. You are called to the neonatal ICU to see a premature infant with an inguinal bulge and find a mass like structure at the internal ring that is reducible. All of the following are true of this infant's condition except
   a. They are MC on the right
   b. Incarceration risk is higher is premature infants
   c. Repair should be performed before the patient leaves the hospital
   d. Mesh repair should be performed.
   e. It is due to a patent processus vaginalis

   Answer d. High ligation should be performed. Inguinal hernia incarceration risk is higher in premature infants compared to other children. Also, inguinal hernia incarceration risk is higher in children compared to adults.

   Indirect inguinal hernias form from a patent or persistent processus vaginalis. The vast majority (> 99%) of hernias in children age 18 or less are indirect inguinal hernias

1099. A 2 yo boy in the ED has an inguinal hernia. All the following are true except:

4⁹

a. Sedation will help reduce inguinal hernias
b. Inguinal hernias should be fixed 2-3 weeks after reduction
c. To reduce an inguinal hernia manually, the child should be placed in trendelenburg position with knees bent
d. Incarcerated hernias (that are unable to be reduced) should be repaired the same day as discovery to avoid infarction (emergency procedure).

Answer b. Inguinal hernias in children should be fixed 24-48 hours after a reduction (allows inflammation and swelling to subside).

1100. Inguinal hernia repair in a 16 yo boy should consist of:
a. Mesh repair
b. High ligation
c. Pectineal ligament repair
d. Laparoscopic mesh repair

Answer b. High ligation is appropriate until age 16 or so.

1101. A 2 yo is brought in for an umbilical hernia. All of the following are true except:
a. This patient should have surgery at about age 5 if the hernia fails to close
b. This patient is at high risk for incarceration
c. Most of these hernias will close spontaneously
d. These hernias are increased in African-American patients
e. These hernias are increased in premature patients

Answer b. Children with umbilical hernias are at *very low risk for incarceration*. Waiting until age 5 is appropriate as the majority of these close spontaneously. Incarceration risk (and infarction) is higher for adult umbilical hernias. Primary repair (not mesh) should be used for pediatric umbilical hernias.

1102. All of the following are true of cryptorchidism (undescended testicle) except:
a. Complications include infertility, torsion, and testicular CA
b. The MC location of the testicle is the inguinal canal
c. CA risk is reduced if the testicle(s) are brought into the scrotum
d. Division of the spermatic vessels is indicated at re-operation for orchiopexy if inadequate length is still an issue
e. It is associated with Prune Belly syndrome

Answer c. Risk of testicular CA remains the same even if the testicle is brought into scrotum (lifetime surveillance). The blood supply to the **vas deferens** collateralizes to the testicles if the spermatic vessels are ligated.

103. A 15 yo boy develops sudden, severe scrotal pain and a high-riding right testicle. The next appropriate step is:
a. Bilateral exploration of testicles through inguinal incision
b. Unilateral exploration of testicle through inguinal incision
c. Bilateral exploration of testicles through scrotal incision
d. Unilateral exploration of testicle through scrotal incision

Answer c. Tx of choice for testicular torsion is to pexy the involved testicle if still viable (otherwise resection) and to pexy the contra-lateral testicle *(through a **scrotal incision**, inguinal incision for testicular mass).*

104. All of the following are true of neuroblastoma except:
a. N-myc and diploid tumors confers a worse prognosis
b. The MC location is the adrenal gland
c. Catecholamine secretion is common
d. Primary neuroblastomas that cross midline are considered stage II
e. Age > 18 months at diagnosis has a worse prognosis

Answer d. Primary tumors that cross the midline are considered stage III.

1105. All of the following are true of Wilms' Tumor except::
    a.   The most important prognostic indicator is tumor grade (anaplastic worse)
    b.   It is the MC kidney tumor in children
    c.   Lung metastases are initially treated with resection
    d.   Rupture of tumor during resection can *up-stage* the tumor

Answer c. Tx for lung metastases from Wilms' tumors initially is whole lung XRT.

1106. A 2 yo girl presents with painless rectal bleeding. You perform an exam, including DRE, which are normal. Given the most likely cause, which of the following tests will be best to make the diagnosis:
    a.   Abdominal CT
    b.   MRI
    c.   99m-Tc-pertechnate scan
    d.   EGD

Answer c. Meckel's diverticulum is the MCC of painless LGIB in children. It is best diagnosed with a **Meckel scan** (99m-Tc-pertechnate scan).

1107. Treatment for the above patient should be:
    a.   Angioembolization
    b.   Diverticulectomy
    c.   Segmental bowel resection including the Meckel's diverticulum
    d.   Observation

Answer b. Because bleeding is caused by secretion of gastric or pancreatic juices to the **adjacent ileum**, resulting is an **ulcer**, segmental resection of the corresponding ileum along with the Meckel's diverticulum is indicated.

1108. The MC presentation for Meckel's diverticulum in adults is:
    a.   Bleeding
    b.   Obstruction
    c.   Perforation
    d.   Diverticulitis

Answer b. Obstruction, often due to **intussusception**.

1109. A newborn has a gross defect in his abdominal wall. All of the following are true except:
    a.   Gastroschisis is due to rupture of an umbilical vein
    b.   Omphalocele is a failure of embryonal development
    c.   Retention sutures are indicated if having trouble returning the bowel to the abdomen at primary closure
    d.   The most serious complication is sepsis
    e.   The MC associated anomaly with omphalocele is cardiac

Answer c. If having trouble returning the bowel to the abdomen for either **gastroschisis** or **omphalocele**, a silastic silo should be placed (contains the abdominal contents outside the abdomen) which is gradually tightened over time (stretches abdominal wall and makes room for intestines). Primary closure weeks later.

1110. A 2 yo boy in the ED has abdominal distension, pain, vomiting, a mass-like area in the RUQ, and currant jelly stools. Which of the following is true:
    a.   Reduction with barium column height maximum of 2 meters or maximum air pressure of 240 mmHg if using air contrast enema is indicated
    b.   Surgery is indicated if it happens a 2nd time
    c.   The MCC in this age group is Meckel's diverticulum
    d.   Antecedent viral infection is common
    e.   Partial reduction can be observed

Answer d. Antecedent viral infection is common and leads to **enlarged Peyer's patches** (MCC of intussusception). The max column height of barium when trying to reduce an **intussusception** is **1 meter**. The max air pressure if you are using an air contrast enema is **120 mmHg**. If the intussusception does not reduce with those maximums (can keep it there for about an hour), take the patient to the OR and do it manually. You risk **perforation** if you go higher than these values. If the intussusception is not completely relieved despite pneumatic attempt, you need laparotomy for manual reduction.

Surgery is indicated if it recurs a **3rd time**. The MCC of intussusception in _older children_ is usually a pathologic lead point (MC - **Meckel's diverticulum**).

1111. A newborn boy has meconium is his urine. Which of the following is true:
    a.   Emergency colostomy is indicated
    b.   This is considered a low lesion
    c.   The fistula most likely connects to the prostatic urethra
    d.   Associated anomalies are rare
    e.   Males often have cloacal malformations

Answer c. The fistula most commonly connects to the **prostatic urethra** in **males** with **high level imperforate anus** (anorectal malformation). Bowel obstruction is rarely the presenting feature so emergency colostomy is unnecessary, however, colostomy is indicated soon after birth. When the blind rectal pouch is _above_ the levator ani muscles, it is considered a **high lesion**. **Females** can have **cloacal** malformations (fusion of vagina, urethra, and rectum). Associated VACTERL anomalies occur in 60%.

1112. A newborn infant fails to pass meconium in the 1st 24 hours of life and subsequently gets progressive abdominal distension. Plain films which show distended loops of small bowel _without_ air-fluid levels, and have a soap suds appearance. The colon is totally decompressed. The transition point is in the RLQ. On exam, the child has an anus located in the proper position. The most appropriate next test is:
    a.   Upper GI series
    b.   Water soluble contrast enema
    c.   Enteroclysis
    d.   Rectal biopsy

Answer b. The scenario is most consistent with **meconium ileus**. The obstruction occurs in the terminal ileum. No air-fluid levels form because the bowel contents stick to the bowel wall instead of pooling (thick meconium) and give is a soap suds appearance. Water-soluble contrast (gastrografin) enemas can make the Dx as well as relieve the obstruction. N-acetylcysteine enemas can also be used.

113. A 1 week old infant who is otherwise healthy is brought to the ED for vomiting of greenish fluid. He had been taking breast milk normally prior to this and recently passed a well baby check. The most appropriate next test is:
    a.   Upper GI series
    b.   Barium enema
    c.   Enteroclysis
    d.   Rectal suction cup biopsy
    e.   PCR for chloride channel defect

Answer a. Bilious vomiting in any child in the first 2 years of life requires an upper GI series to rule out **malrotation**. This is done _emergently_. Characteristic finding on UGI - _duodenum does not cross midline_

Feeding intolerance _immediately_ after birth could be caused by malrotation, duodenal atresia, annular pancreas, duodenal webs or other conditions. **Upper GI series** would help differentiate.

1114. Upper GI series in the above patient shows the duodenum does not cross the midline and the duodeno-jejunal junction is displaced to the right. Which of the following is appropriate at surgery:
   a. Placement of the duodenum in the left upper quadrant
   b. Placement of the cecum in the right lower quadrant
   c. Placement of the duodenum in the right lower quadrant
   d. Placement of the cecum in the left lower quadrant
   e. Placement of the duodenum in the left lower quadrant

   Answer d. The Ladd's procedure requires placement and fixation of the **cecum** to the **left lower quadrant**.

1115. The bowel in the patient above should be turned:
   a. Clockwise once
   b. Counter-clockwise once
   c. Clockwise until the vascular pedicle is widened
   d. Counter-clockwise until the vascular pedicle is widened

   Answer d. Counter-clockwise until the vascular pedicle is widened

1116. Which of the following is true of duodenal atresia:
   a. Most commonly results in non-bilious vomiting
   b. It is treated with Whipple
   c. It is due to failure of canalization
   d. It is treated with gastro-jejunostomy
   e. It is associated with prenatal U/S finding of oligohydramnios

   Answer c. It is due to failure of canalization of the duodenum. Tx: resection and duodeno-duodenostomy or duodeno-jejunostomy

1117. A 1 month old gets progressive abdominal distension. As a newborn, the infant failed to pass meconium in the 1st 24 hours of life. Your order plain films which show a distended proximal colon with distal decompression near the recto-sigmoid junction. On exam, the child has an anus located in the proper position and on rectal exam there is explosive release of watery stool. The most appropriate next test is:
   a. Upper GI series
   b. Barium enema
   c. Enteroclysis
   d. Rectal biopsy

   Answer d. The scenario is most consistent with **Hirschsprung's Disease**. Dx is made with rectal biopsy, which shows the absence of ganglion cells in the myenteric plexus.

1118. Jejunal atresia is caused by:
   a. A recanalization defect
   b. Placental abruption
   c. Digestive enzyme injury
   d. Meconium
   e. Intra-uterine vascular accident

   Answer e. Intra-uterine vascular accident

1119. A premature infant passes bloody stools and has abdominal distension after the 1st feeding. AXR shows pneumatosis intestinalis. Given the likely diagnosis, which of the following is the most appropriate next step:
   a. Exploration and resection of bowel with re-anastomosis
   b. Exploration and resection of bowel with ostomies
   c. Fluid resuscitation and antibiotics
   d. High frequency ventilation

e.   ECMO

Answer c. This patient most likely has **necrotizing enterocolitis. Fluid resuscitation** and **antibiotics** are the initial step.

1120. All of the following would be indications for laparotomy in the above patient except:
a.   Pneumotosis intestinalis
b.   Persistent metabolic acidosis
c.   Persistent severe thrombocytopenia despite transfusion
d.   Clinical deterioration
e.   Erythema of the abdominal wall

Answer a. Pneumotosis intestinalis is <u>not</u> an indication for exploration by itself in patients with NEC.

1121. A 3 week old infant is brought to the ED for repeated forceful non-bilious vomiting such that it hits the wall opposite the child. On exam, you notice a small protuberance in his RUQ. The vomiting is non-bilious. Which of the following is true of this condition:
a.   Pyloroplasty is indicated
b.   This has a familial link and is more common in females
c.   U/S is not helpful for the diagnosis
d.   Urine pH is usually acidic
e.   Immediate surgery is indicated

Answer b. Projectile vomiting and RUQ "olive" is consistent with **pyloric stenosis**. It has a familial link, is MC in **males,** and the Dx is usually made with U/S.

These patients get **hypochloremic, hypokalemic, metabolic alkalosis** and **paradoxical aciduria.** Fluid resuscitation with **normal saline** <u>before</u> surgery is indicated.

Tx is **pyloromyotomy** in which just the serosa and muscle are divided (the submucosa and mucosa are left intact, unlike pyloroplasty in which they are both divided).

1122. A newborn has severe respiratory distress immediately following birth along with a scaphoid abdomen. CXR shows loops of bowel filling the left chest. All of the following are true except:
a.   Pulmonary hypertension, leading to worsening hypoxia, is common in these patients
b.   The incidence is increased on the left side
c.   Both lungs are dysfunctional
d.   Repair immediately at diagnosis is indicated
e.   These are generally repaired through an abdominal approach

Answer d. The above scenario is most consistent with **congenital diaphragmatic hernia** (99% are Bochdalek hernias for newborns). The scaphoid abdomen is due to displacement of the abdominal contents into the chest. This lesion is associated with a 50% overall survival. These patients should be stabilized <u>before</u> repair (high frequency ventilation, inhaled nitric oxide, possible ECMO).

123. All of the following are true of Morgagni diaphragmatic hernias except:
a.   They are rare
b.   They are MC on the right side
c.   They should be observed
d.   They most commonly present in adulthood

Answer c. Foramen of **Morgagni hernias** (even if asymptomatic) should be repaired due to the risk of bowel incarceration and infarction.

1124. A newborn suffers from severe aspiration and choking with feeds. You try to place an NG tube and cannot get it down. CXR shows the NG tube stops in the mid-esophagus and the stomach is distended. Which of the following is true:
    a.   Pre-op gastrostomy tubes are indicated for the majority of patients
    b.   Barium swallow is required for diagnosis
    c.   Extra-pleural left thoracotomy is indicated, with the lesion generally being found beneath the azygos vein
    d.   The proximal esophagus should be preferentially mobilized at surgery
    e.   The MC associated anomalies are renal

Answer d. The proximal esophagus should be preferentially mobilized as blood supply to the proximal esophagus is generally felt to be superior to the distal esophagus.

Type C is the MC tracheoesophageal fistula (TEF) and involves a proximal esophageal pouch and a distal TEF. You cannot pass an NGT because it gets held up in the pouch. The Dx is almost always made off CXR/AXR and additional studies are not required. Pre-op gastrostomy tubes are indicated only if surgery is to be delayed (eg for 1) prematurity, 2) low birth weight, or 3) sick patients due to pneumonia or cardiac issues). The MC associated anomalies are **cardiac**. Tx of TEF generally involves an extra-pleural **right thoracotomy** with end to end **anastomosis** of the esophagus and closure of the trachea. The fistula is often found beneath the azygos vein which can be divided.

1125. All of the following are true of choledochal cysts except:
    a.   A short common pancreaticobiliary channel is a risk factor
    b.   Congenital choledochal cysts are most likely due to an abnormal pancreaticobiliary junction
    c.   Cyst formation is likely due to the abnormal reflux of pancreatic enzymes
    d.   Inflammation is likely involved
    e.   Caroli's disease involves dilatation of intra-hepatic ducts

Answer a. A _long_ common pancreaticobiliary channel is a risk factor

1126. Treatment for a type I choledochal cyst is:
    a.   Careful follow-up
    b.   Cystogastrostomy
    c.   Cystoduodenostomy
    d.   Cyst resection, hepatic-jejunostomy, and cholecystectomy

Answer d. Choledochal cysts need to be resected because of the risk of forming cancer in the cyst and the risk of cholangitis and pancreatitis. A hepatico-jejunostomy should be performed for Type I cysts. Routine cholecystectomy is performed at the same time.

1127. The MC primary malignant liver tumor is children is:
    a.   Hepatocellular CA
    b.   Fibrolamellar CA
    c.   Angiosarcoma
    d.   Lymphangiosarcoma
    e.   Hepatoblastoma

Answer e. Hepatoblastoma

EMBRYOLOGY AND DEVELOPMENT

- **Foregut** - includes lungs, esophagus, stomach, pancreas, liver, gallbladder, bile duct, duodenum proximal to and including ampulla
    - **Celiac artery** supplies intra-abdominal foregut
- **Midgut** - includes duodenum distal to ampulla, small bowel, large bowel to distal ⅓ of transverse colon
    - **SMA** supplies midgut
- **Hindgut** - includes distal ⅓ of transverse colon to anal canal
    - **IMA** and **internal iliac arteries** supply the hindgut
- Midgut rotates 270 degrees counterclockwise during normal development
- **Umbilical vessels** - **2 umbilical arteries** (from iliac arteries) and **1 umbilical vein** (drains to portal system and IVC)
- ↑ed **alkaline phosphatase** in children compared to adults is from **bone growth**
- **Immunity at birth**
    - **IgA** - from mothers milk
    - **IgG** - only immunoglobulin to crosses placenta
    - **PMNs** have **impaired chemotaxis** *(infants at risk for* **cutaneous** *infections)*
- **Respiratory Distress Syndrome** (RDS; eg hyaline membrane disease)
    - Tx - **surfactant**
- **MCC childhood death** - trauma
    - **Trauma bolus** - 20 cc/kg x 2 (isotonic solution; LR or NS); then blood 10 cc/kg
    - **Hypothermia** occurs more rapidly than in adults
    - **Tachycardia** - best indicator of shock in children

Neonate	>150
Age 0-1 year	>120
Rest	>100

EFFECTIVE FLUID RESUSCITATION

- Initial fluid resuscitation with **dehydration** (eg **pyloric stenosis**) - <u>normal saline</u> 20 cc/kg
- **Neonates** and **infants** - urine output of 2-3 cc/kg/hr
- **Toddlers** and **school age** - urine output of 1 cc/kg/hr
- Children (< 6 months) have only 25% the GFR capacity of adults - poor concentrating ability, be careful with potassium (K) containing fluids
- Children are subject to **hypocalcemia** with massive blood transfusion

MAINTENANCE INTRAVENOUS FLUIDS

- 4 cc/kg/hr for 1st 10 kg
- 2 cc/kg/hr for 2nd 10 kg
- 1 cc/kg/hr for everything after that
- Example - the maintenance fluid for a 25 kg girl would be 65 cc/hr (40 cc/hr for 1st 10 kg, 20 cc/hr for 2nd 10 kg, 1 cc/hr for each kg after that)
- <u>Maintenance</u> solution for <u>all</u> pediatric patients - **½ normal saline** with 5% glucose +/- K (reduces risk of clinically significant **hyponatremia**)
    - *Avoid* 0.2% normal saline *(previously recommended for toddlers)*
    - *Avoid* potassium in neonates
    - *Avoid* potassium in infants and toddlers until making urine
- Children need glucose in maintenance solutions

CONGENITAL DISEASES OF THE LUNG

Congenital lobar emphysema (hyperinflation)
- Sx's: can get **respiratory distress** or **hypotension** due to hyperexpansion of one or more lobes (same mechanism as tension pneumothorax)
- Dx: **CXR** - <u>hyperinflation</u> of a lobe (hyper-lucent area); <u>compression</u> of other structures (eg other lung lobe, mediastinum)
- **Bronchus cartilage** fails to develop - get air trapping with expiration
- Vascular supply is normal
- MC location - LUL
- Tx: **lobectomy**

- **Pulmonary sequestration**
  - Sx's: infection (MC), respiratory distress, hemorrhage
  - Have a **continuous murmur** (DDx: AVM, sequestration, persistent ductus arteriosus)
  - Dx: **CT angio** - shows lung mass with anomalous blood supply
  - MC location - LLL
  - Lung tissue <u>not</u> connected to airway and has <u>systemic</u> **arterial blood supply** (lung tissue can be intra-lobar or extra-lobar)
  - Anomalous arterial supply (*key issue here*)
    - MC off **thoracic aorta**
      - Can also come off **abdominal aorta** (celiac) through **inferior pulmonary ligament**
  - **Intra-lobar** sequestration - pulmonary venous connection usual
  - **Extra-lobar** sequestration - systemic venous drainage usual (MC - **azygos vein**)
  - May have malignant change
  - Tx: *need to ligate systemic arterial supply 1st (can get massive hemorrhage if this isn't performed first)*; then lobectomy (or resection of mass if extra-lobar)
- **Congenital cystic adenoid malformation** (CCAM)
  - Sx's: <u>newborns</u> - respiratory distress, <u>older children</u> - infection
    - **Rapid decompensation** can occur with ventilator - need emergent decompression by removing cyst
  - Usually **intra-pulmonary**; can get **air-trapping**
  - Connected to airway bronchus
  - From **bronchiole tissue overgrowth** (<u>no</u> cartilage; columnar epithelium)
  - MC in **lower lobes**
  - Malignant degeneration reported
  - Tx: lobectomy
- **Bronchogenic cyst**
  - MC cyst of the mediastinum
  - Sx's: can compress airways with **respiratory distress** or become **infected**; newborns can become very ill
  - Are **extra-pulmonary** cysts formed by **abnormal lung tissue** (parenchyma, cartilage); occasionally are intra-pulmonary
  - Are <u>not</u> connected to airway
  - Contain milky liquid; malignant degeneration reported
  - MC location - right side posterior to carina
  - Tx: **cyst resection**

MEDIASTINAL MASSES IN CHILDREN
- **Neurogenic** tumors (neurofibroma, neuroganglionoma, neuroblastoma)
  - *MC mediastinal tumor in children*; usually located posteriorly
- **Respiratory Sx's** and **dysphagia** - common to all mediastinal masses regardless of location
- **Anterior** - T cell lymphoma, **teratoma** (and other germ cell tumors; most common typ of <u>anterior</u> mediastinal mass in children), thyroid CA
- **Middle** - T cell lymphoma, teratoma, cyst (cardiogenic or bronchogenic)
- **Posterior** - T cell lymphoma, neurogenic tumor
- *Thymoma is <u>rare</u> in children*

CHOLEDOCHAL CYST
- Sx's: episodic **abdominal pain, jaundice,** and **RUQ mass** (*classic*, triad in 50%)
  - Other Sx's - pancreatitis, cholangitis
  - **Young females** of **Asian descent** usual
- Mechanism: likely due to an <u>abnormal</u> **pancreaticobiliary junction** that occurs outsi the duodenal wall and formation of a <u>long</u> common channel (> 15 mm). This leads to abnormal **reflux of pancreatic enzymes** during uterine development, inflammation o the biliary system, wall weakness, and cyst formation.
- Dx: **RUQ U/S**; 90% are extra-hepatic
- 5-10% **CA risk** (cholangiocarcinoma)

Types:
- **Type I**: (MC - 85%) saccular or **fusiform dilatation** of the common bile duct (CBD) with normal intrahepatic duct
- **Type II**: isolated **diverticulum** off CBD
- **Type III** or **choledochocele**: arise from dilatation of **duodenal portion of CBD** or where the pancreatic duct joins
- **Type IV**: dilation of both **intra-hepatic / extra-hepatic** biliary system
- **Type V** or **Caroli's disease**: dilatation of **intra hepatic** ducts *only*

Tx:
- **Type I** - cyst excision, **hepatico-jejunostomy** (roux-en-Y) + **cholecystectomy**
- **Type II** - **cyst excised completely** and choledochotomy closed **primarily**
- **Type III** - trans-duodenal approach with **marsupialization** *or cyst excision*; *identify ampulla* → may need sphincterotomy for adequate drainage
- **Type IV** (partially intrahepatic) and **type V** (Caroli's disease, totally intrahepatic) → individualized; may need **partial liver resection** (IV and V), **hepatico-jejunostomy** (IV), or **liver TXP** (IV and V)

YMPHADENOPATHY

Usually acute suppurative adenitis associated with URI or pharyngitis (eg fever, sore throat, cough)

If fluctuant → FNA, culture and sensitivity, and antibiotics; may need incision and drainage if it fails to resolve
- **Chronic causes** - cat scratch fever, atypical mycoplasma

Asymptomatic adenopathy → core needle Bx (*This is **lymphoma** until proved otherwise*)

ONGENITAL DIAPHRAGMATIC HERNIAS

Overall survival 50%

MC on **left side** (85%)

Sx's: **respiratory distress** (severe **hypoxia**, hypercarbia), scaphoid abdomen (abdominal contents are displaced into the chest and compress the lung)

Both lungs are **dysfunctional**
- **Ipsilateral** lung (bowel herniation side) - *severe* **pulmonary hypoplasia**
- **Contralateral** lung - severe **pulmonary hypertension** (pulmonary artery vasoconstriction, leads to worsening **hypoxia**); also *some* pulmonary hypoplasia

80% have associated anomalies (malrotation, cardiac, neural tube defects)

Diagnosis can be made with **prenatal U/S**

CXR - **bowel in chest** (may see NG tube in chest)

Tx: **Intubation** and **NG tube** (decompresses stomach which may be further compressing lungs); may need high-frequency ventilation, inhaled nitric oxide, or ECMO (extracorporeal membrane oxygenation; most devastating ECMO Cx – intracerebral hemorrhage)
- *Stabilize these patients before operating on them*
- Surgery through **abdominal approach** - need to reduce bowel and repair defect usually using mesh
- Look for visceral anomalies (eg **malrotation**)

Bochdalek's hernia *(MC type; MC on the left)* - located posterior-lateral
- Usually do <u>not</u> contain a hernia sac

Morgagni's hernia (rare; *MC on the right*) - located anterior-medial (retrosternal)
- MC in **adults** (pressure creates hernia) - majority asymptomatic
- Usually contain a hernia sac
- **Repair** due to the risk of bowel incarceration (PTFE patch usual)

Eventration - failure of diaphragm to fuse

HEST WALL

Pectus excavatum (sinks in) - sternal osteotomy and strut placement; performed if causing respiratory Sx's or emotional stress
- Nuss procedure places strut without osteotomy
- Possible improvement of pulmonary dynamics

Pectus carinatum (pigeon chest) - strut not necessary; repair for emotional stress
- <u>Not</u> shown to improve pulmonary dynamics

CYSTIC HYGROMA (lymphangioma, benign)
- Classically found in **posterior neck triangle** (posterior and lateral to sternocleidomastoid [SCM] muscle); can also be in axilla or groin
- Fluctuant, multi-loculated area under skin; is a macrocytic **lymphatic malformation**
- Forms **sinuses** and can get **infected** (staph, strep)
- Tx: **resection** (no margins or radical excision needed; preserve all nerves and vessel

BRANCHIAL CLEFT CYST
- Leads to cysts, sinuses, and fistulas; infection can occur
- **1st branchial cleft cyst** - angle of mandible
  - May connect with **external auditory canal**
  - Often associated with **facial nerve**
- **2nd branchial cleft cyst** *(MC location / type)* - anterior border of mid-SCM muscle
  - May go through **carotid bifurcation** into **tonsillar pillar**
- **3rd branchial cleft cyst** - lower neck, **medial** to or through the lower SCM
  - Can have tract to the **piriform sinus**
- Tx for all branchial cysts: **resection**

THYROGLOSSAL DUCT CYST
- Sx's: **midline cervical mass**; usually between hyoid and thyroid isthmus
  - Classically **moves upward** with swallowing
  - May cause dysphagia
- From the descent of the thyroid gland from the **foramen cecum**
- May be only thyroid tissue the patient has
- Risk of **infection**; 1% **malignancy** risk (MC papillary thyroid CA)
- Presents as a **midline** cervical mass
- Goes through the **hyoid bone**
- Tx: excision of **cyst, tract,** and **hyoid bone** (at least the central or mid- portion) through a **lateral neck incision** *(Sistrunk procedure)*

HEMANGIOMA
- MC tumor of childhood and infancy
- Appears at birth or shortly after
- Usually rapid growth within first 12 months of life but then involutes
- MC sites - head and neck
- Tx: *observation initially* - most resolve by **age 6-7** (85%)
- Tx indications (any below):
  - 1) Has **uncontrollable growth**
  - 2) **Impairs function** (airway, eyelid or ear canal)
  - 3) **Persistent** after **age 8**
  - 4) **Ulceration** and recurrent **bleeding**
- Tx if indicated:
  - <u>Oral</u> steroids (*best Tx*; possible lesion injection as adjunct) - **70%** respond we
  - **Pulsed dye laser** (better for more superficial lesions without significant volume eg <u>port-wine stains</u>)
  - Consider resection if steroids not successful
- <u>Rare</u> Cx's of hemangioendothelioma (infants; usually <u>liver</u> hemangiomas)
  - **Kasabach-Merritt syndrome** - consumptive **coagulopathy** (high PT, PTT) ar **thrombocytopenia**; newborns
    - Tx: **embolization** and **steroids** *(best Tx)*; surgery rare
  - CHF (A-V shunt) - Tx: **embolization** and **steroids**; surgery if refractory (rare)
- Congenital capillary malformation (port wine stain); Tx - **pulsed dye laser**

CONGENITAL VASCULAR MALFORMATIONS (AVM's)
- Arterio-venous (MC type to **cause Sx's** and MC **requiring Tx**)
- Surgical indications: hemorrhage, ischemia to affected limb, CHF, functional impairment, limb-length discrepancy (AVM limb longer)
- Tx: **embolization** (may be sufficient) and/or **resection** if Sx's
- **Pulmonary AVM** - continuous murmur; Tx: *embolization only 1st line*
- **Bowel AVM** - endoscopic therapy usual

NEUROBLASTOMA

- *MC solid abdominal malignancy in children*
- *MC malignancy in infancy period*
- MC age ≤ 2 (50%)
  - Children < 1 year have best prognosis
- Sx's: usually presents as **asymptomatic mass**
  - Other Sx's: secretory diarrhea, raccoon eyes (periorbital metastases), HTN, opsomyoclonus syndrome (uncontrolled fast eye movements; unsteady gait), spinal cord compression, limp, skin lesions (metastases - bluish)
- Path: from **neural crest cells** (small round blue cells, **rosette** pattern)
  - MC location - adrenal gland; also occurs on sympathetic chain
  - 90% secrete **catecholamines** (check UA - metanephrines, VMA, HVA)
  - Usually **advanced** at time of diagnosis - 50% have **metastases** (liver and bone)
  - Disease spectrum: ganglioneuroma (benign) → ganglioneuroblastoma (malignant) → neuroblastoma (most malignant)
  - One of the few human malignancies to demonstrate **spontaneous regression** (from a completely undifferentiated state to benign appearance)
  - Neuroblastoma exhibits extreme **heterogeneity** in aggressiveness
- Worse prognosis features (categorized into **low, moderate,** and **high** risk):
  - **Age > 18 months**
  - **Tumor grade** (poor histology, high mitosis index, **diploid** tumors)
  - **Metastases**
  - **N-myc oncogene** amplification (regulates microRNAs)
- Dx: **CT scan** - ± calcifications; compresses renal parenchyma rather than invades (differentiates from Wilms' tumor)
  - **MIBG** - can locate tumors
- Initially unresectable tumors may be resectable after **Doxorubicin**-based chemo
- Tx: **Low Risk** - resection only (**adrenal gland** and **kidney** taken)
  - Moderate or High Risk
    1) **Neoadjuvant chemo** (DECC) - doxorubicin, etoposide, cisplatin and cyclophosphamide *(then* **retinoic acid** if high risk); can downstage tumors
    2) **Resection**
    3) **Post-op XRT** for residual disease or high risk tumors
- 5-YS (all patients) - **40%**
- **Ganglioneuroma** (benign) **Tx** - resection only (need resection to confirm it's benign)

Staging of Neuroblastoma

Stage	Description
I	Localized, complete excision
II	Incomplete excision but does not cross midline
III	Crosses midline +/- regional nodes
IV	Distant metastases (nodes or solid organ)
IV-S	Localized tumor with distant metastases and age < 1

WILMS TUMOR (nephroblastoma; is a kidney tumor)

- *MC kidney tumor in children*
- Sx's: usually presents as **asymptomatic mass**; can have hematuria or HTN; 10% bilateral; associated with aniridia (absence of the iris of the eye) and hemi-hypertrophy (one side of the body is larger than the other)
- MC age > 2 (mean 3 years)
- Most important prognostic indicator - **tumor grade** (anaplastic worst prognosis)
- Frequent metastases to **bone** and **lung**
- Dx: CT scan - replacement of renal parenchyma and not displacement (differentiates from neuroblastoma); no calcifications
- Tx: **nephrectomy** (90% cured)
  - If venous extension occurs into the IVC (through renal vein), the tumor can usually be extracted without IVC resection
  - Need to examine contralateral kidney and look for peritoneal implants
  - Avoid rupture of tumor with resection, which will increase stage
  - **Actinomycin** and **vincristine** based chemo in all unless Stage I and < 500 gm tumor

- Stage V (bilateral kidney involvement) needs nephro-sparing surgery
  - **Pulmonary metastases** - Tx: whole lung XRT
- 5-YS (all patients) - **90%**

Staging of Wilms Tumor

Stage	Description
I	Limited to kidney, completely excised
II	Beyond kidney but completely excised
III	Residual non-hematogenous tumor
IV	Hematogenous metastases
V	Bilateral renal involvement

HEPATOBLASTOMA
- *MC malignant liver tumor in children*; elevated **AFP** in 90%
- Fractures, precocious puberty (from **beta-HCG** release)
- Better prognosis than hepatocellular CA
- Can be pedunculated; vascular invasion common
- Tx: resection optimal; otherwise **doxorubicin**-based chemotherapy → may downstage tumors and make them resectable
- Survival is primarily related to resectability
- **Fetal histology** has best prognosis

MOST COMMONS (in <u>childhood</u> unless otherwise stated)
- MC malignancy overall - **leukemia (ALL)**
- MC solid malignancy class - **CNS tumors**
- MC tumor - **hemangioma**
  - MC tumor in newborn - **sacrococcygeal teratoma**
- MC intra-abdominal malignancy - **neuroblastoma**
  - MC in child < 2 years - **neuroblastoma**
  - MC in child > 2 years - **Wilms' tumor**
- MC kidney tumor - **Wilms' Tumor**
- MC malignant liver tumor - **hepatoblastoma** (benign - hemangioma)
- MC lung tumor - **carcinoid**
- MC malignant <u>intestinal</u> tumor (< 10 years) - **small bowel lymphoma**
- MCC duodenal obstruction - **malrotation**
  - MC in newborns (< 1 week) - **duodenal atresia**
  - MC after newborn period (> 1 week) - **malrotation**
- MCC colon obstruction - **Hirschsprung's disease**
- MCC *painful* <u>lower</u> GI bleeding - **benign anorectal lesions** (fissures, etc)
- MCC *painless* <u>lower</u> GI bleeding - **Meckel's diverticulum**
- MCC <u>upper</u> GI bleeding
  - < 1 year - **gastritis**, esophagitis
  - 1 year to adult - **esophageal varices** (from portal vein thrombosis), esophagitis
- Double bubble sign (gastric + duodenal dilatation on AXR) - **malrotation, duodenal atresia,** or **annular pancreas**

MECKEL'S DIVERTICULUM
- Sx's in <u>children</u> / <u>teenagers</u> - **lower GI bleeding** (*MCC of lower GI bleeding in children and teenagers*)
- MC presentation in <u>adults</u> - **obstruction**
  - Obstruction from **intussusception** or **volvulus** (fibrous band can connect diverticulum to umbilicus, bowel rotates around this)
- Can also get **diverticulitis**
- Rule of 2s
  - 2 feet from ileocecal valve (located in **ileum**)
  - 2 inches in length
  - 2% population
  - 2% symptomatic
  - 2 tissue types: **pancreatic** (MC) and **gastric** (most likely to be <u>symptomatic</u>)
  - Usually present in 1st 2 years of life with **bleeding**
- Found on **anti-mesenteric border** of small bowel

- Embryology - **persistent vitelline duct** (failure of closure of omphalomesenteric duct)
- Is a **true diverticula** (involves all layers of bowel wall)
- Dx: **Meckel's Scan** (technetium-99 pertechnate scintography) - *most accurate diagnostic imaging method for Meckel's Diverticulum* (mucosa lights up)
- Bleeding caused by secretion of **gastric** or **pancreatic juices** to adjacent **ileum**, forming ulcer (not bleeding in the Meckel's diverticulum itself – need segmental ileal resection if bleeding if the Sx)
- Tx:
  - **Incidental** → usually not removed
  - **Diverticulectomy** for: 1) diverticulitis not involving the base, 2)suspicion of gastric mucosa (diverticulum feels thick), or 3) if it has a narrow neck (risk of future obstruction and diverticulitis)
  - **Segmental resection** is needed with any of the following: 1) **bleeding**, 2) diverticulitis involving the base, 3) if the base is >⅓ the size of the bowel (don't want to narrow bowel lumen), 4) if complicated diverticulitis (eg perforation), or 5) compromised bowel (eg strangulation, perforation, or obstruction)

PYLORIC STENOSIS
- MC age: 3 - 6 weeks (1st born white **males**); often **Family history**; RF - **erythromycin**
- Sx's: **projectile vomiting** (non-bilious, *classic*) and **dehydration**
- Can feel **olive mass** in RUQ (the pylorus)
- Have **hypochloremic, hypokalemic, metabolic alkalosis** and paradoxical **aciduria** (see Fluid and Electrolytes chapter)
- Dx: **U/S** *(best test)* – pylorus muscle ≥ 4 mm **thick** or pylorus channel ≥14 mm **length**
- Tx: resuscitate with **normal saline boluses** (20 cc/kg) before OR and until making urine, then switch to D5 ½ normal saline with 10 mEq K maintenance
  - *Avoid* fluid resuscitation with K containing fluids in children with severe dehydration as hyperkalemia can quickly develop
  - *Avoid* non-salt containing solutions in infants as hyponatremia can develop
  - *Infants should always have a maintenance fluid with* **glucose** *because of their limited reserves for gluconeogenesis and vulnerability for hypoglycemia*
- Surgery: **pyloromyotomy** (RUQ incision; divide vein of Mayo, proximal extent should be the circular muscles of stomach; the submucosa and mucosa are not entered)

INTUSSUSCEPTION
- MC age: 3 months to 3 years, **males**
- Sx's: crampy **abdominal pain**, a 'sausage mass' in RUQ, abdominal **distention**; N/V
  - **Currant jelly stools** (bloody; vascular congestion; *not indication for resection*)
  - Often have antecedent **viral infection** leading to enlarged Peyer's patches
- Invagination of one loop of intestine into another (MC - ileum into right colon; **ileocolic**)
- Lead point - hypertrophied **Peyer's patches** (MC overall)
- *Older* children (> 2) more likely to have *pathologic* lead point - **Meckel's diverticulum** (MC) polyps, lymphoma; (older children more likely to require surgery)
- **10% recurrence** after reduction (usually within 1st 24 hours)
  - Surgery if occurs after 2nd time of reduction
- Tx: reduce with **air-contrast enema** → 90% successful; no surgery required if reduced
  - Max pressure with air-contrast enema - **120 mm Hg**
  - Max column height with barium enema - **1 meter** (3 feet)
  - Can keep pressure for about **1 hour**
  - *High* **perforation risk** *beyond above values* → need to proceed to OR if you have reached these values and it is still not reduced
  - Need to go to OR for peritonitis, free air, if unable to reduce after 1 hour, incomplete reduction, or occurs a 3rd time
    - When reducing in OR, do not place traction on proximal limb of bowel; need to apply pressure to the distal limb and milk it out
    - Usually do not require resection in OR unless associated with a lead point (eg Meckel's) or perforation
- **Adults** with intussusception - likely a **malignant lead point** (eg colon CA in cecum) → OR for resection (do not reduce in OR as it is usually malignant – just resect the area unless there is an obvious benign lead point or if taking the bowel would cause short gut syndrome)

INTESTINAL ATRESIAS (jejunal and ileal)
- Develop as a result of **intra-uterine vascular accidents** (ischemia → atresia)
- Sx's: newborn with **bilious emesis** and progressive abdominal distention
  - Most do not pass meconium
- More common in **jejunum**; can be <u>multiple</u>
- RFs: polyhydramnios on prenatal U/S
- Dx: AXR - bowel distension with distal decompression
- Consider rectal biopsy to rule-out Hirschsprung's before surgery
- Tx: NG tube and fluid resuscitation; resection with **primary anastomosis** or bring up **ostomies** if bowel too damaged (look for **multiple lesions**)

DUODENAL ATRESIA
- *MCC of duodenal obstruction in <u>newborns</u> (< 1 week)*
- *MC type of **intestinal atresia***
- MC type - atresia and obstruction **distal** to the ampulla of Vater (80%)
- Sx's: **bilious vomiting**, feeding intolerance immediately after birth, scaphoid abdomen
  - 20% are proximal to the ampulla and have non-bilious vomiting
  - DDx: malrotation, duodenal webs, annular pancreas
- **Etiology** - failure of duodenal **canalization** from its solid state *(<u>not</u> vascular accident)*
- RFs: polyhydramnios on prenatal U/S
- 20% have **Down's syndrome**
  - Also associated with other cardiac, renal, and GI anomalies (eg malrotation)
- Dx: AXR - shows **double-bubble sign** *(classic; proximal duodenum and stomach)*
  - **UGI series** often used to confirm Dx and rule-out other conditions (eg malrotation)
- Tx: resuscitation; **duodenoduodenostomy** or duodenojejunostomy
- **Duodenal webs** can cause persistent obstruction after repair (Tx: resection of web via longitudinal duodenostomy) - look for these at the time of initial repair

MALROTATION
- MCC duodenal obstruction in children (90% occur at age ≤ 1 year) except newborns (duodenal atresia)
- From failure of normal counterclockwise rotation (270 degrees) of intestines
- Sx's: <u>sudden onset</u> of **bilious vomiting** (Ladd's bands cause duodenal obstruction, located in right retroperitoneum; *hallmark Sx*)
  - The patient may have been feeding normally prior to episode
- *Any child (first 2 years of life) with **bilious vomiting** needs an UGI to rule out malrotation - needs to be done **emergently***
- **Ladd's bands** - fibrous stalks of peritoneal tissue that extend from the upper right abdominal sidewall to a displaced cecum (cecum is displaced superiorly and medially; these bands cross and can compress the duodenum, resulting in obstruction (Sx - bilious vomiting)
- **Midgut volvulus** (twisting around the SMA vascular pedicle) can occur in patients with malrotation, causing superior mesenteric artery (SMA) compromise and **intestinal infarction**
  - Volvulus occurs <u>clockwise</u>
  - **Treatment** is therefore **counter-clockwise rotation** of the intestine (may need multiple turns; this untwists and widens the mesenteric vascular pedicle)
- Dx: **UGI** *(best test)* - duodenum does not cross midline; duodenal-jejunal junction is displaced to the right
- Tx: **Ladd's procedure** *(includes **resuscitation**)*
  - **Resect Ladd's bands**
  - **Counterclockwise rotation** of bowel (assess viability if midgut volvulus)
  - *Place and fix **cecum in **LLQ** (cecopexy)*
  - *Place and fix **duodenum in **RUQ***
  - **Appendectomy** (prevents future confounding diagnosis)
- Persistent bowel obstruction after procedure - **duodenal webs** (Tx: resection of web via longitudinal duodenostomy) - look for these at the time of initial repair

MECONIUM ILEUS
- Thick meconium (ie 1st stool) fails to pass; causes **distal ileal obstruction**
- Sx's: failure to pass meconium, abdominal distention, bilious vomiting
- Sweat chloride test or PCR for Cl channel defect - **cystic fibrosis** in 95%
  - Cystic fibrosis transmembrane conductance regulator (CFTR)
  - Thick meconium develops due to deficits in pancreatic enzymes
- AXR: dilated loops of small bowel *without* air-fluid levels (because the meconium is too thick to separate from the bowel wall); can have ground glass or **soap suds** appearance; colon is decompressed
- Can cause ischemia or perforation (meconium pseudocyst or free perforation) → requires laparotomy
- Tx: **fluid resuscitation** important (osmotic load with gastrografin enema will draw fluid, can cause hypotension)
  - Empiric **antibiotics** and **NGT**
  - **Gastrografin** or **N-acetylcysteine enema** *(best test + best Tx)*
    - ***Effectively treats the problem in 80%*** *(done under fluoroscopy)*
    - Can make Dx and Tx's the majority of patients
  - **Surgical indications:**
    - Failure of enema to relieve obstruction
    - Peritonitis (eg perforation or necrosis)
    - Clinical deterioration
  - If surgery required, manually decompress (milk meconium out) through an enterotomy and place a tube enterostomy for N-acetylcysteine antegrade enemas
- Can cause **late strictures** (from ischemia)

TRACHEOESOPHAGEAL FISTULAS (TEF; also includes esophageal atresia)
- Discontinuation of the esophagus and/or presence of a fistula
- Sx's: newborn **spits up feeds**, excessive **drooling**
  - **Respiratory Sx's** with feeding (eg aspiration, choking, coughing)
  - Can't place NG tube in stomach *(classic)*
- RFs: males, diabetic mothers, low birth weight (< 2500 g)
- Prenatal U/S - shows **polyhydramnios**
- Dx **CXR/AXR** (almost always give Dx) - contrast studies / endoscopy *rarely* needed
  - **Proximal atresia** (distal TEF) - distended stomach
  - **Distal atresia** (proximal TEF or none) - gasless abdomen
  - ECHO, renal U/S, spinal and limb X-rays to rule-out VACTERL
- **Type C** - MC type *(85%)*
  - **Proximal esophageal atresia** (blind pouch) and **distal TE fistula**
  - Abdominal x-ray - distended, gas-filled stomach
- **Type A** - 2nd MC type (5%)
  - Esophageal atresia and no fistula
  - Abdominal x-ray - gasless abdomen
- **H-type** (Type E) - TE fistula without atresia; most difficult to Dx
  - MC type to present **later in infancy** (Sx's - aspiration, recurrent pneumonia)
- 70% have associated **anomalies** *(MC - cardiac [20%])*
- **VACTERL Syndrome** - vertebral/spine/sacrum, anorectal malformations (MC - imperforate anus), cardiac (MC - VSD), **TE** fistula, renal/urinary tract, limb anomalies
- **Initial Tx:**
  - Replogle tube (continuous sump drain; goes into proximal esophageal segment)
  - Semi-upright position *(never prone)*
  - If intubation required, place gastrostomy tube (G-tube)
- Tx: **right thoracotomy** (extra-pleural), tie off and divide fistula (or resect atretic segment), tension-free primary esophageal anastomosis (mobilize the **proximal esophagus**, not the distal esophagus), and place G-tube
  - **Azygos vein** often needs to be divided (TE fistula is usually **underneath**)
  - The **proximal esophagus** is considered to be better vascularized (inferior thyroid artery branches) compared to distal esophagus (intercostal arteries)
- **Delayed repair** - infants that are **premature, < 2,500 g**, or **sick** (eg pneumonia, severe cardiac anomaly) → Replogle tube, place G-tube (for decompression or feeding), treat underlying issue, and *delayed* TEF repair

- MC Cx after repair - **GERD**; others - leak, stricture, fistula
- **Survival** related to **birth weight** and associated **anomalies** (**cardiac** most significant)

NECROTIZING ENTEROCOLITIS (NEC)
- Sx's: **bloody stools** and **abdominal distension** after 1st feeding in **premature neonate** *(classic)*
  - Others - feeding intolerance, lethargy, vomiting
- RFs: prematurity, hypoxia, sepsis, neonatal stress
- Mechanism: felt to be bowel ischemia / reperfusion injury
- Abdominal x-ray: may show **pneumatosis intestinalis** (pathognomonic), free air, or portal vein air
- Need serial lateral decubitus films to look for free air (perforation)
- Initial Tx: IV fluid resuscitation, NPO, antibiotics, TPN, orogastric tube decompression, serial exams / abdominal x-rays (Q 6 hours); medical Tx usually for 2 weeks
- *Indications for operation*: 1) free air, 2) diffuse peritonitis, 3) persistent metabolic acidosis, 4) clinical deterioration, 5) persistent severe thrombocytopenia (< 100) despite transfusion, 6) erythema/edema of the abdominal wall (indicates dead bowel beneath), 7) positive paracentesis (fecal material)
  - *Resect dead bowel and bring up ostomies*
  - Extremely ill and can't tolerate laparotomy - *place drain <u>only</u> (in NICU)*
  - Pneumatosis intestinalis by itself is <u>not</u> an indication for drain or laparotomy
- Can get late **stenosis** at previous NEC areas
- Need **barium contrast enema** and **upper GI with SBFT** before taking down ostomies or feeding to rule-out distal obstruction from stenosis
- At risk for **short bowel syndrome** later in life
- Mortality - **10%**

IMPERFORATE ANUS (anorectal malformations)
- Rectum fails to descend through the external sphincter complex
- Rectum ends as a **blind pouch**, usually with a fistulous tract to the **genitourinary system** (eg <u>males</u> - urethra, bladder, scrotum; <u>females</u> - vagina) or **perineal skin**
- Associated with **VACTERL** (60% have an anomaly; see TE Fistula above; MC - urinary tract anomaly)
- Do <u>not</u> typically present with bowel obstruction; low lesions can present with defecation problems
- **Males** often have *high* lesions (> 50%), majority of **females** have *low* lesions (90%)
- *High* lesions (rectum ends <u>above</u> levator ani muscle)
  - **Males** - meconium in **urine** usual (MC - fistula from rectum to **prostatic urethra**)
  - **Females** - meconium in **upper vagina** (may have **cloacal** deformity)
  - Tx: **colostomy** (soon after birth, <u>not</u> an emergency)
  - Later anal reconstruction with **posterior sagittal anoplasty** (places rectum in external anal sphincter complex)
- *Low* lesions (rectum ends <u>below</u> levator ani muscle) - meconium to **perineal skin** (median raphe), **scrotum**, or **lower vagina**
  - Perform **posterior sagittal anoplasty** (pull rectum down into external anal sphincter complex); <u>no</u> colostomy needed
- Need post-op anal dilatation to avoid stricture (patients are prone to constipation)

GASTROSCHISIS
- Congenital **abdominal wall defect**
- Etiology - intrauterine rupture of **umbilical vein**
- RFs - high risk pregnancies, low birth weight
- Only 10% have congenital anomalies *(far less than omphalocele)*
  - MC associated finding - **intestinal atresia**
- To the right of midline, *no* peritoneal sac, stiff bowel from exposure to amniotic fluid
- Tx: initially place saline-soaked gauzes over intestines (to prevent fluid loss), wrap the trunk circumferentially, resuscitate the patient; NPO, prophylactic antibiotics, and TPN; repair when stable
- At operation (when patient is **stable**):
  - Place bowel back in abdomen and close primarily (as long as it is not tight and the bowel is not compromised)

- Often can't get primary repair and have to attach a **silastic silo** to abdominal wall:
  - Contains abdominal contents outside body
  - Progressively tightened over days-weeks to stretch abdominal cavity wall and make room for intestines
  - Primary closure at a later date
- Check for other abnormalities (eg **intestinal atresia**)

MC serious complication - **sepsis**
Mortality - **10%**

OMPHALOCELE

Congenital **abdominal wall defect** (midline defect)
Etiology: **failure of embryonal development**; has **peritoneal sac** with cord attached
Majority (60%) have associated **congenital anomalies** (MC - **cardiac**; others – musculoskeletal, GI, genitourinary; leads to worse prognosis compared to gastroschisis)
- MC associated GI finding - **malrotation**

Sac can contain intra-abdominal structures other than bowel (eg liver, spleen)
Tx: initially place saline-soaked gauzes over intestines (to prevent fluid loss), wrap the trunk circumferentially, resuscitate the patient; NPO, prophylactic antibiotics, and TPN; repair when stable
At operation (when patient is **stable**):
- Place bowel back in abdomen and close primarily (as long as it is not tight and the bowel is not compromised)
- Often can't get primary repair and have to attach a **silastic silo** to abdominal wall:
  - Contains abdominal contents outside body
  - Progressively tightened over days-weeks to stretch abdominal cavity wall and make room for intestines
  - Primary closure at a later date
- Check for other abnormalities (eg **malrotation**)

MC serious complication - **sepsis**
Mortality - **20%** (mostly related to **congenital anomalies**)
- Worse overall prognosis compared to gastroschisis due to congenital anomalies

HIRSCHSPRUNG'S DISEASE

*MCC of **colonic obstruction** in infants*; more common in **males** (4:1)
MC sign → ***infants fail to pass meconium in 1ˢᵗ 24 hours***
- Others Sx's - distension, constipation, vomiting; occasionally get colitis
- Can get explosive release of watery stool with anorectal exam
- Can also present in older patients as chronic constipation (age 2-3)

AXR - **dilated** proximal colon or small bowel (ganglion cells present) with **distal decompression** (no ganglion cells)
Dx: **rectal biopsy** (suction cup biopsy; *best test*)
- Shows *absence* of ganglion cells in Auerbach's myenteric plexus

Due to failure of neural crest ganglion cells to progress in caudad direction
- Disease starts in rectum, moves proximal
- Causes a *functional* colonic obstruction
- In 75% just the rectum is affected
- In 5% the rectum and entire colon is affected

Tx: need to **resect rectum / colon** until proximal to where ganglion cells appear (send margins to path to confirm presence of ganglion cells)
- May need to bring up a colostomy initially (eg Hirschsprung's colitis)
- Eventually connect good residual colon to anus (**Pull-through procedure**; Soave or Duhamel)

Hirschsprung's colitis - may be rapidly progressive
- Sx's: tenderness, foul smelling diarrhea, sepsis, lethargy
- MCC of **death** in Hirschsprung's
- Tx: **rectal irrigation** to try and empty colon; may need **emergency colectomy**

UMBILICAL HERNIA
- Failure of closure of linea alba; most close by age 3, rare incarceration
- RFs: African-Americans, premature infants, males
- Tx: surgery if not closed by **age 5**, **incarceration**, or if patient has **VP shunt**
- Primary repair, not mesh

HYDROCELE
- Most disappear by 1 year
- Formed from persistent **tunica vaginalis**
- Can have connection to peritoneum (**processus vaginalis**, communicating hydrocoele) or not (non-communicating)
  - Non-communicating will resolve
  - Failure to resolve indicates a **persistent processus vaginalis** (communicating hydrocoele)
- Can be in **inguinal canal** or **scrotum**
- Dx: U/S - hydrocoele will <u>transluminate</u> if in scrotum (bowel from hernia will not)
- Surgical indications:
  1) At **age 1 year** if not resolved <u>or</u>;
  2) If though to be **communicating** (size waxes / wanes)
- Tx: **resect hydrocoele** and **ligate processus vaginalis** (inguinal approach)

INGUINAL HERNIA (children)
- In children ≤ 18, almost all are **indirect hernias** from persistent **processus vaginalis**
- MC in **males,** MC on **right**; 10% bilateral if present at birth
- RFs: **prematurity**
- Varying degrees - can go all the way to the scrotum or stop short
- Lump in inguinal canal (eg intestine, cecum) at <u>**internal ring**</u> differentiates **hernia from hydrocoele**
- Can cause **small bowel obstruction** or **incarceration** with bowel strangulation
  Tx:
  - **Incarcerated hernia** *(highest risk age* **< 1 year***)* - tender, firm swelling
    - **Manual reduction** (firm steady pressure) with **sedation**
    - **Trendelenburg** position (head down) with **knees bent**
    - **Emergent operation** if not able to reduce incarceration
    - **If reduced → admit**, repair within **next 24-48 hours**
  - **Incarceration risk**: infants > children > adults
  - **Non-incarcerated → elective repair within 1 week**
  - Inguinal hernia in **premature infant →** repair just <u>*before*</u> discharge
  - Repair - **high ligation** (to age 16 or so); make sure testicle is in scrotum at the end of the procedure
  - Explore **contralateral side** if **left** sided, **female**, or child **< 1 year**

CYSTIC DUPLICATION
- MC in **ileum**; often on mesenteric border
- Tx: resect cyst

BILIARY ATRESIA
- *MCC of neonatal jaundice requiring surgery*
- *MC indication for* **Liver TXP** *in children*
- Progressive jaundice persisting **> 2 weeks** after birth suggests biliary atresia (refractory to phototherapy)
- Dx: liver Bx *(best test)* → bile plugging, periportal fibrosis, eventual cirrhosis
  - U/S (may not see a gallbladder) and **HIDA** (liver lights up but does not go into the intestine) reveal **atretic biliary tree**
  - Labs - elevated **conjugated bilirubin** and **LFTs**
- Get continued jaundice, pruritus, cirrhosis, and eventual hepatic failure
- Tx if **extra-hepatic** ducts *only* (ie **biliary atresia**) → *Kasai procedure* (hepaticoportojejunostomy)
  - Involves resecting the atretic extra-hepatic bile duct segment to the porta hepatis, then sewing an anastomosis between loop of jejunum and porta hepatis

- Need to perform Kasai procedure **before age 3 months**, otherwise get irreversible liver damage
- Majority still go on to **liver TXP** or die from cirrhosis

Tx if **intra-hepatic** ducts involved (ie **ductal hypoplasia**) → liver TXP

ERATOMA (dermoid cyst)

Neonates (have **embryonal** type) - occur along midline (MC - sacrococcygeal)
Adolescents (have **germ cell** type) - ovaries (MC), testicles
MC location - sacrococcygeal teratoma
Can be cystic, solid, or mixed
At risk for **malignant degeneration**
Tx: excision
Elevated AFP or B-HCG suggests **malignant transformation**

Sacrococcygeal teratomas
- MC in **females**; usually presents as a **mass at birth** (can be found on pre-natal U/S - associated <u>hydrops</u> has a very poor prognosis)
- 90% are **benign** at birth
- Most are **exophytic** but can be entirely **internal** (<u>pre-sacral</u>) and diagnosed later in life (can involve the bladder and rectum)
- Great potential for **malignant degeneration** (adenocarcinoma)
- 2-month mark is an important transition - **< 2 months** → usually benign; **> 2 months** → usually malignant
- CT scan to assess abdominal and pelvic extent
- Tx: **coccygectomy** (including tumor) and long-term follow-up
- **AFP** - good marker to follow for recurrence if malignant

NDESCENDED TESTICLES (cryptorchidism)

If undescended bilaterally (30%) - get chromosomal studies
If you cannot feel the testis in the inguinal canal, you need to get an **MRI** to confirm their presence
Path
- MC location - 90% in **inguinal canal**
- Can be anywhere in retroperitoneum, ectopic, or vanished
- **Inguinal hernias** common

Risks of undescended testicle:
- **Testicular CA** (5 x if unilateral, 10 x if bilateral, get **seminoma**)
    - *CA risk stays same even if testicles brought into scrotum*
- **Infertility** - *improves* if testicles are brought down into the scrotum
- **Torsion**

Medical Tx: <u>beta-HCG injections</u> (human chorionic gonadotropin; variable success)
Wait **4-6 months** after birth before surgery to see if they descend on their own
Surgery
- **Orchiopexy** through **inguinal incision** (if testicle in canal); attach testis to scrotum; **high ligation** of processus vaginalis
- If not able to get testicles down (from inadequate length of cord structures; usually associated with intra-abdominal testis) → perform **division of spermatic vessels** (testicular vessels; away from testis, done laparoscopically) to get length, then attach to scrotum (blood supply to **vas deferens** [vas artery] <u>collateralizes</u> to testicles); done as single procedure or staged (after 6-12 months)
- *Want orchiopexy completed by age 2 years*

Adult cryptorchidism - resect testicle (orchiectomy), almost all are non-functional
Prune Belly syndrome - cryptorchidism, absence or hypoplasia of abdominal wall musculature, urinary tract abnormalities, pulmonary hypoplasia, skeletal anomalies

ACHEOMALACIA

Elliptical, fragmented tracheal rings instead of C-shaped; A-P dimension of the trachea collapses; RF - TE fistula or esophageal atresia
Sx's: expiratory wheezing, can have dying spells (usually with feeding); usually gets better after 1-2 years
Dx: narrowing on lateral CXR

- **Awake bronchoscopy** - A-P dimension of trachea collapses (last test to be performed)
■ Usually does <u>not</u> require surgery
■ **Surgical indications** - dying spell (MC indication), failure to wean from ventilator, recurrent infections
■ Surgery - **aortopexy** (aorta sutured to the back of the sternum, opens up trachea)

LARYNGOMALACIA
■ MCC of airway obstruction in infants
■ Sx's: intermittent respiratory distress and stridor; exacerbation in supine position
■ Caused by **immature epiglottis cartilage** with intermittent collapse
■ Most children outgrow this by 12 months
■ Surgical tracheostomy reserved for a very small number of patients

CHOANAL ATRESIA
■ Obstruction of choanal opening (nasal passage) by either bone or mucus membrane; usually unilateral
■ Sx's: intermittent respiratory distress, poor suckling
■ Tx: surgical excision of the obstruction

LARYNGEAL PAPILLOMATOSIS
■ MC tumor of the pediatric larynx
■ Frequently **involutes after puberty**
- Can treat with endoscopic removal or laser but frequently comes back
■ Thought to be caused from HPV in the mother during passage through the birth canal

CEREBRAL PALSY
■ Many develop **GERD**

OTHER
■ **Patent urachus** - connection between umbilicus and bladder (wet umbilicus)
- Tx: resection
■ **Patent omphalomesenteric duct** (vitelline duct)
- Connects ileum and umbilicus; can **drain sucus out umbilicus**
- Tx: resection of the persistent duct
- Meckel's diverticulum forms from this
■ **Persistent omphalomesenteric vessels** (vitelline vessels)
- **Artery** passes from umbilicus to aorta
- **Vein** from umbilicus to portal vein
- MC presents with torsion of bowel with possible strangulation, necrosis
- Can occasionally attach to a Meckel's diverticulum
- Tx: de-torse bowel with resection if necrotic; ligation of persistent vasculature
■ **Omphalitis**
- Infection of **umbilical stump** after birth
- Can lead to **portal vein thrombosis** (elevated LFTs, possible variceal bleeding)
- Tx: **heparin** for acute portal vein thrombosis; **antibiotics** for infection

Skin and Soft Tissue

1128. All of the following are true except:
   a. Stretch marks are due to dermal collagen damage and associated neovascularization
   b. Krause's end-bulbs are involved in cold sensation
   c. Cushing's Syndrome striae are due to loss of collagen and tensile strength
   d. Melanin is formed in keratinocytes

   Answer d. Melanin is formed by **melanocytes** in epidermis basal layer.

1129. A 45 yo woman presents to your office with a lump in her right axilla that she has noticed for 3 months. She denies any Sx's and has had no recent infections. Mammogram is normal. A complete exam reveals no other suspicious lesions. The mass is about 2 cm in diameter, feels hard, and is not painful. There is no surrounding erythema. The most appropriate next step is:
   a. Antibiotics
   b. Core needle biopsy
   c. Close follow-up
   d. Sentinel lymph node biopsy

   Answer b. This mass needs to be biopsied. Antibiotics are not indicated because there has been no antecedent illness and the mass is not inflammatory. Also it would be unusual for an inflammatory mass to last 3 months. Sentinel lymph node biopsy is not indicated. You could resect the mass (excisional biopsy) if the core needle biopsy was indeterminate.

1130. Core needle Bx in the above patient comes back as melanoma. You cannot find any skin lesions on the patient's body. The most appropriate next step is:
   a. Formal axillary lymph node dissection
   b. nothing
   c. Mastectomy
   d. Chemo-XRT only

   Answer a. There are a couple of possibilities with this scenario.
   First is that there is a melanoma primary somewhere and you cannot find it (some melanomas are non-pigmented). Second is that the primary melanoma has regressed spontaneously and the lymph nodes are all that is left of the disease (best scenario). *Error on the side that gives the best chance of survival, which is a **formal axillary lymph node dissection**.*

   Note that axillary dissection for melanoma is different than for breast cancer. For melanoma, you are trying to remove all the disease which means you need to take **level I, II, and III lymph nodes**.

   With breast CA, you only need to take level I and II nodes. You are not trying to remove all the disease with breast CA, but merely staging the patient.

1131. A 65 yo man has a 1 cm diameter dark colored lesion on his arm that looks different according to the patient. You perform a physical exam and find no other lesions. The next appropriate step is:
   a. Resection with 1 cm margin
   b. Punch biopsy
   c. IL-2 therapy
   d. Scrape top layer off and send to cytology

   Answer b. Because you do not know if this is melanoma or not, resection with a margin is <u>not</u> indicated (also, margins are based on depth of lesion, not width). Scraping off the top layer would be inappropriate because you would not be getting the depth of the lesion. The best answer is punch biopsy (although you could also just resect the lesion without margins, and then go back for a re-

resection if it turns out to be cancer). The **punch Bx** should be at the most abnormal looking spot or thickest area.

1132. The punch biopsy in the above patient comes back as melanoma that invades 2.5 mm deep. You perform a physical exam (axillary region) and find no clinically positive nodes. Mets work-up is negative. The most appropriate next step is:
    a.   SLNB and resection of the primary with 2 cm margin
    b.   Axillary lymph node dissection + resection of primary with 2 cm margin
    c.   SLNB and resection of the primary with 1 cm margin
    d.   Axillary lymph node dissection + resection of primary with 1 cm margin

Answer a. Sentinel lymph node biopsy is indicated for lesions > 1 mm deep with clinically negative nodes. A melanoma 2.5 mm (> 2 mm) deep requires a 2 cm margin with resection.

Melanoma in situ (Hutchinson Freckle if on face) - 0.5 cm margin

Melanoma Depth	Surgical Margin
< 1mm (thin)	1 cm
1-2 mm (intermediate)	1-2 cm
> 2 mm (thick)	2 cm

1133. A 45 yo man presents with a suspicious lesion on his temple. Biopsy shows reveals a 2 mm deep melanoma. You do not feel any cervical adenopathy. The most appropriate next step is:
    a.   Resect primary area for margins only
    b.   Resect primary area for margins and superficial parotidectomy
    c.   Resect primary area for margins and SLNB
    d.   Resect primary area for margins, superficial parotidectomy, and SLNB
    e.   Resect primary area for margins, superficial parotidectomy, and MRND

Answer d. Although considerable controversy exists, there is a 20% metastasis rate to the parotid gland for the ear, temple, forehead, and anterior scalp. This is the justification for superficial parotidectomy. Because the lesion is $\geq$ 1 mm deep, a SLNB is indicated.

If there was palpable adenopathy or if the SLNB / parotid gland was positive for tumor, then MRND (+ superficial parotidectomy if not already done) is indicated.

Parotid Basin Melanoma (ear, temple, forehead, anterior scalp) has a 20% metastasis rate to the **parotid gland** (need superficial parotidectomy)
    < 1 mm deep - superficial parotidectomy
    $\geq$ 1 mm deep - SLNB and superficial parotidectomy
    clinically positive nodes - superficial parotidectomy and MRND

1134. All of the following are true of melanoma except:
    a.   Blue is the most ominous color
    b.   Melanoma is the MC metastasis to small bowel
    c.   Ulceration indicates a better prognosis
    d.   Melanoma on the anterior scalp is most likely to metastasize to the parotid gland and anterior cervical chain

Answer c. Ulceration indicates a worse prognosis.

1135. All of the following are true except:
    a.   An appropriate margin for a forearm 2 cm basal cell CA is 0.5 cm
    b.   Morpheaform is the *least* aggressive basal cell CA due to collagenase production
    c.   A 2 cm margin is indicated for Marjolin's Ulcers
    d.   A 2 cm anterior scalp squamous cell CA with clinically negative nodes should undergo primary resection and superficial parotidectomy

Answer b. Morpheaform is the most aggressive **basal cell CA**. Anterior scalp squamous cell CA is at high risk for metastasis to the parotid gland (20%) and parotidectomy is indicated.

1136. A patient has a 5 cm mass in his anterior thigh. All of the following are true except:
   a. MRI is indicated before any biopsy
   b. Core needle biopsy is preferred in most cases
   c. The most important prognostic factor for sarcoma is node status
   d. If open Bx is indicated, the incision should be along the long axis of the extremity

Answer c. Tumor grade is the most important prognostic factor for sarcoma. Sarcomas <u>rarely</u> have nodal involvement.

1137. All of the following are true of sarcomas except:
   a. The MC soft tissue sarcoma is malignant fibrous histiocytoma
   b. The MC mets location is lung
   c. Most extremity soft tissue sarcomas require amputation
   d. Complete resection of a retroperitoneal sarcoma allows the best chance for survival

Answer c. 90% of extremity sarcomas can be treated without amputation. **Complete resection** (with negative margins) of a retroperitoneal sarcoma allows the best chance for survival (take what you have to - eg kidney).

1138. All the following are good prognostic indicators of metastatic sarcoma except:
   a. Disease-free interval < 12 months
   b. < 4 lesions
   c. Primary lesion control
   d. Doubling time > 20 days

Answer a. A disease-free interval > 12 months has a better prognosis.

1139. All of the following are true except:
   a. Alveolar subtype is the worst prognosis rhabdomyosarcoma
   b. The MC location for osteosarcoma is the knee
   c. A painful lesion comprised of blood vessels and nerves near the terminal aspect of the digit is consistent with glomus tumor
   d. Resection is the procedure of choice for Kaposi's Sarcoma (KS)

Answer d. Surgery is not the Tx of choice for KS. These lesions should be palliated (HAART AIDS Tx, systemic interferon alpha, XRT, ect).

140. All of the following are true of Merkel Cell carcinoma except:
   a. It is a locally aggressive neuroendocrine skin CA
   b. Has common mets to bone and LN's
   c. Keratin antibodies show peri-nuclear pattern
   d. Nodes do not need to be assessed

Answer d. These red to purple skin tumors are **very aggressive** with local invasion and metastases to lymph nodes and distant sites (bone MC). Nodes should be assessed.

141. A 35 yo man has several thick and inflamed areas in his axilla with a thick and tough texture. The most likely diagnosis is:
   a. Lymphoma
   b. Sebaceous cyst
   c. Hidradenitis
   d. Lipomas

Answer c. Hidradenitis. These can occur in the axilla, inguinal, and peri-rectal areas.

1142. All of the following are true except:
    a.   Ganglion cysts typically occur over joints and require removal of the check valve if aspiration fails
    b.   Verruca vulgaris (wart) is usually best treated with salicylic acid
    c.   Refractory hyperhidrosis requires ligation of T1-T4 sympathetic ganglia
    d.   Intra-lesional steroid injection after excision if generally the best Tx for keloids

Answer c. Refractory hyperhydrosis requires ligation of T2-T4 sympathetic ganglia; ligation of the T1 ganglia (contributes to stellate ganglion) would result in Horner's syndrome.

1143. All of the following are true of sacral decubitus ulcers except:
    a.   Flaps should not be performed in patients with active infection
    b.   Stage II decubitus ulcers will likely require a flap
    c.   Bone involvement after flap placement requires long term antibiotics
    d.   Stage III ulcers are full thickness down to the subcutaneous fat

Answer b. Stage II decubitus ulcers do not require a flap

1144. Which of the following is true of desmoid tumors:
    a.   They are MC in men
    b.   They frequently metastasize
    c.   Sulindac and tamoxifen are the best therapy for unresectable tumors
    d.   They are composed of myocytes

Answer c. Sulindac and **tamoxifen** are the best Tx for unresectable tumors. Desmoid tumors do <u>not</u> metastasize.

1145. All of the following are true of retroperitoneal fibrosis except:
    a.   Staph infection is commonly involved
    b.   Hydronephrosis is common with the disease
    c.   The ureters are typically deviated medially
    d.   Malignancy should be ruled-out
    e.   Primary therapy is corticosteroids

Answer a. Retroperitoneal fibrosis is generally <u>not</u> related to infection

1146. A 10 yo boy presents with a limp. CT scan shows a retroperitoneal mass compressing lumbar and sacral nerve roots. Core needle biopsy shows malignant fibrous histiocytoma (MFH). Which of the following is true:
    a.   If a pseudocapsule is found, enucleation should be performed
    b.   XRT has been shown to significantly improve survival
    c.   Retroperitoneal lymph node dissection is indicated
    d.   The most important prognostic factor is complete en bloc resection with negative margins
    e.   MFH in this location has a more favorable prognosis

Answer d. The most important prognostic factor for **retroperitoneal sarcoma** is complete en bloc resection with negative margins. These lesions should not be shelled out. XRT improves local control but does not improve survival. Sarcomas almost never have lymph node metastases so lymph node dissection is <u>not</u> indicated. Retroperitoneal sarcomas have a worse prognosis compared other sarcomas.

1147. All of the following are true except:
    a.   Retroperitoneal fibrosis often involves compression of the ureters
    b.   The MC retroperitoneal tumor is lymphoma

c. Hypertrophic scar tissue frequently goes beyond the original injury
d. Peritoneal blood following trauma is absorbed through fenestrated lymphatic channels

Answer c. Hypertrophic scar tissue does not go beyond the original injury. **Keloids** do go beyond the original injury.

SKIN COMPONENTS
- **Epidermis** (top layer) - stratified squamous epithelium (keratinocytes)
  - Melanin is formed by **melanocytes** in epidermis basal layer
- **Dermis** - collagen, elastic fibers, serves as a scaffold for the epidermis
- **Mechano-receptors**
  - **Pacinian corpuscles** - deep pressure
  - **Ruffini's corpuscles** - warmth, skin stretch (slippage of objects)
  - **Krause's end-bulbs** - cold
  - **Meissner's corpuscles** - light pressure and tactile sense
- **Eccrine sweat glands** - aqueous sweat (thermal regulation, is hypotonic)
- **Apocrine sweat glands** - milky type sweat
  - Highest concentration in palms and soles
  - Most sweat released is a result of the sympathetic nervous system via acetylcholine
- **Lipid-soluble drugs** - have increased skin absorption
- Dermis is composed primarily of **Type I collagen** (tensile strength)
- **Tension** - the resistance to stretching (collagen)
- **Elasticity** - the ability to regain shape (branching proteins can stretch out to twice normal length)
- **Cushing's Syndrome striae** - due to **decreased collagen** which results in **loss of tensile strength** and elasticity
- **Stretch marks** - damage to **dermal collagen** with **blood vessel dilatation** and **neovascularization**
- **Tissue expanders** work by local recruitment, thinning of dermis and epidermis, and mitosis (more cells)
- MCC of pedicled or anastomosed free flap necrosis - **venous thrombosis**
- Blood supply to skin for myocutaneous flap - **underlying muscle perforators**

UV RADIATION
Damages DNA (oxygen free radical formation breaks up DNA)
UVB - *most damaging type*
Melanin - single best factor for protecting skin from UV radiation; absorbs UV radiation and dissipates energy as heat

DECUBITUS ULCERS (pressure sores)
Prevention - pressure relieving beds (KinAir beds)
MC - sacrum; others - heel, back of head

Decubitus Ulcers (Pressure Sores)

Stage	Description	Treatment
I	**Erythema**, no skin loss, (confined to epidermis)	Keep pressure off
II	**Partial** skin loss; yellow debris (into the dermis)	Local treatment, keep pressure off (no flap)
III	**Full-thickness** skin loss; subcutaneous fat exposure (completely through the dermis)	Sharp debridement; likely need **myocutaneous flap** (gluteal flap if sacral decubitus ulcer)
IV	Involves **bony cortex, muscle, tendon,** or **adipose tissue**	**Myocutaneous flaps**

Tx (sacral decubitus ulcer):
- **Keep pressure off** the area → **KinAir bed**
- Optimize **nutrition**

- Consider diverting stool with **colostomy** (stage III and IV)
- **Debride wound** in OR; moist dressings
- Bx and send **cultures** with appropriate **antibiotics**
- No flap if the patient has an **active infection**
- When wound looks good, place **gluteal myocutaneous flap** if sacral decubitus ulcer (stage III and IV)

FLAPS
- MCC of pedicled or anastomosed free flap <u>necrosis</u> - **venous thrombosis**
- Blood supply to <u>skin</u> for myocutaneous flap - underlying **muscle perforators**
- <u>No</u> flaps with **active infection**
- **TRAM flaps** (transverse rectus abdominal myocutaneous)
  - Blood supply - **superior epigastric vessels**
  - Most important determinant of TRAM flap viability - **peri-umbilical muscle perforators to skin**
  - Can't use TRAM if previous **CABG with IMA use** - compromises **superior epigastric vessels**
  - Can't use TRAM with previous **transverse laparotomy incision** across upper rectus muscles (eg chevron incision for previous abdominal procedure) – compromises superior epigastric vessels
  - Use contralateral rectus if chest XRT was used for breast CA (internal mammary artery can be compromised)
  - Previous **laparoscopic cholecystectomy** - can still use TRAM flap
  - **Cx's** - necrosis, ventral hernia, bleeding, infection, abdominal wall weakness
  - Some use muscle sparing TRAM or DIEP flap (deep inferior epigastric perforators) to avoid abdominal wall issues

SUSPICIOUS SKIN LESION
- **Punch biopsy** - need to get down to subcutaneous fat
  - <u>No</u> shave Bx *(need to get depth)*
  - **Face, hands,** or **feet** (cosmetic regions or hard to close areas) - always want punch Bx
  - Consider punch Bx for lesions in any location (easy office procedure)
  - Bx at **thickest spot** or **most abnormal looking**
- Can get **excisional Bx** with 1 mm margin for small lesions (< 2 cm) not in a cosmetically sensitive area
  - Make sure you are into the **subcutaneous fat** (need full thickness)
  - Do <u>not</u> try to get surgical margins at this stage, just getting Dx - will go back for surgical margins if it turns out to be CA
- Fix specimen in **formalin**, paraffin embedded permanent section, and H + E stain *(no frozen section)*

MELANOMA
- Represents only 5% of skin CA but accounts for 65% of the deaths
- RFs: fair complexion, easy sun-burning, previous skin CA or XRT
- MC melanoma site on skin - **back** in men, **legs** in women
- **Worse prognosis** - men; ulcerated, ocular, or mucosal lesions; high mitotic rate; increased number of nodes; location on back or posterior arms/ neck/scalp (BANS)
- **Signs of melanoma** (ABCDE)
  - **Asymmetry** (shape of ½ does not match the other)
  - **Borders** that are irregular (ragged, notched)
  - **Color** that is uneven (darkening; **blue** has highest malignant potential)
  - **Diameter** (increase in size or size > 6 mm)
  - **Evolving** over time (few weeks to months)
- MC metastatic site - **lung**
- MC metastasis to <u>small bowel</u> - **melanoma**
- Originates from **melanocytes** (neural crest cells) in epidermis basal layer
- Dx - see suspicious skin lesion above
- **Nevus** with any changes - get punch Bx

- Types:
  - **Melanoma in situ** or **thin lentigo maligna** (ie Hutchinson's Freckle) - just in the **epidermis**, <u>0.5 cm margins</u> are appropriate here
  - **Lentigo maligna melanoma** - least aggressive, minimal invasion, radial growth 1st; presents as an elevated nodule
  - **Superficial spreading** (MC type) - intermediate malignancy; originates from nevus or sun-exposed areas
  - **Acral lentiginous melanoma** - very aggressive; palms / soles of African Americans; **subungal** (below fingernail)
  - **Nodular** - *most aggressive type*; most likely to have metastasized at time of Dx; deepest growth at time of Dx; vertical growth 1st; bluish-black with smooth borders; occurs *anywhere* on the body
  - Melanoma markers: **S-100** protein and **HMB-45**

Staging (metastatic work-up) - CT chest/abdomen/pelvis, LFTs, and LDH for all melanoma ≥ 1 mm; examine all possible draining lymph node sites

Tx for all stages:
  1) resection of primary tumor with appropriate margins *and*;
  2) management of lymph nodes

Melanoma Depth	Surgical Margin
< 1mm (thin)	1 cm
1-2 mm (intermediate)	1-2 cm
> 2 mm (thick)	2 cm

- Need to get down to **muscle fascia** (not through it; elliptical incision with 3:1 ratio length to width)
- Gentle S-shaped incision if over a **joint**
- Do <u>not</u> take a vital structure (eg carotid artery)
- **Head** and **neck** melanomas may require special tailoring; may not be able to get recommended margin
- In-transit metastases → resection
- <u>No</u> Mohs surgery for melanoma

Nodes
- Four general **nodal basins** - inguinal, axillary, cervical, and parotid
- Always need <u>formal lymphadenectomy</u> (eg MRND) if nodes are **clinically positive** or if sentinel lymph node biopsy (SLNB) is **positive** (you are clearing tumor from these areas, not stage, *unlike breast CA*)
- Perform SLNB if nodes are clinically negative and tumor is ≥ 1 mm deep (usually <u>no</u> SLNB if < 1 mm deep)
- **Thin melanoma** (< 1 mm depth) that need **SLNB** (any of the following):
  - Lesion has **ulceration**
  - **Regression** on path (was deeper at one point but regressed)
  - If into **reticular dermis**
  - Has **high mitotic rate**
- **Involved nodes** - usually non-tender, round, hard, 1-2 cm
- **Parotid basin** - **face** and **scalp** anterior to and including **ear** (pinna) and superior to **lip** → 20% have metastases to **parotid gland**
  - *All* need **superficial parotidectomy** *and* **SLNB**
    - If superficial parotid gland is positive, need total parotidectomy and MRND
    - If SLNB is positive, need MRND
    - If clinically positive nodes → need **superficial parotidectomy** and **MRND**

Axillary node melanoma (or any other nodal basin) with <u>no</u> primary →
- Either had regression of primary or is a non-pigmented melanoma
- Tx: <u>complete lymphadenectomy</u> (eg remove Level I, II and III axillary nodes in the axilla - *unlike breast CA*)
- May need to divide **pectoralis minor muscle** to get to Level III nodes in the axilla (lateral pectoral nerve to pectoralis major muscle is here)

Resection of metastases has provided some patients with a long disease-free interval and is the best chance for cure

- Isolated metastases (eg lung, liver) that can be resected with a low risk procedure should undergo resection
- Subungal melanoma
  - Dx: remove nail and get punch Bx
  - Tx by location:
    - **Thumb** - amputate at DIP
    - **Finger** - amputate at PIP
    - **Toe** - amputate at MTP
- **Truncal and extremity melanoma** (below neck):
  - **Line of Sappey** - 2 cm above umbilicus to L2/L3
  - **Above** Line of Sappey → melanoma goes to **axillary nodes** (in general)
  - **Below** Line of Sappey → melanoma goes to **inguinal nodes** (in general)
- **Systemic Tx**
  - **Dacarbazine** *(1st line)* for positive nodes (stage IIIb) or metastases (IV)
  - **IL-2** and **tumor vaccines** can be used for **nodes** or **metastases** (marginal)

BASAL CELL CARCINOMA
- MC CA in U.S. (4x MC than squamous)
- 80% on head and neck; <u>rare</u> nodal disease or metastases
- Pearly appearance, rolled borders, slow and indolent growth
- From epidermis - basal epithelial cells
- Pathology - peripheral palisading of nuclei and stromal retraction
- MC type - **nodular**
- Most aggressive - **morpheaform** (has **collagenase** production)
- Tx: **0.3 - 0.5 cm** margins

SQUAMOUS CELL CARCINOMA
- Overlying erythema; papulonodular with crust and ulceration; red-brown
- May have surrounding induration and satellite nodules
- **Metastases risk**: Melanoma > Squamous cell CA > Basal cell CA
- RFs: actinic keratoses, xeroderma pigmentosum, Bowen's disease, atrophic epidermis, HPV, immunosuppression, sun exposure, fair skin, previous XRT, previous skin CA, old burn scars (Marjolin's ulcer)
- RFs for <u>metastasis</u> - poorly differentiated, greater depth, recurrent lesions, immunosuppression
- Tx: **0.5 - 1.0 cm** margins for most
  - Can treat cosmetic areas with **Mohs surgery** (margin mapping using conservative slices; <u>not</u> used for melanoma) to minimize area of resection (eg lesions on face)
  - Indications for **2 cm margins** - Marjolin's ulcer; penile (penectomy, possibly partial if distal lesion) or vulvar CA
  - Indications for <u>prophylactic</u> lymph node dissection (any below, dissect appropriate lymph node basin):
    1) **> 4 mm** deep
    2) **> 2 cm** in circumference
    3) **parotid basin** lesions (high metastasis rate to parotid gland) – all need **superficial parotidectomy**
  - **Formal regional lymphadenectomy** needed for clinically positive nodes
    Parotid basin lesion with clinically positive nodes → Tx: superficial parotidectomy + MRND
  - **Chemo-XRT** - if nerve, nodal, or vessel invasion or positive margins

SOFT TISSUE SARCOMA
- MC types - #1 **malignant fibrous histiocytoma** (MFH), #2 liposarcoma
- About half arise from extremities; 50% in children
- RFs: **asbestos** (mesothelioma), **PVC** and **arsenic** (angiosarcoma), **chronic lymphedema** (lymphangiosarcoma), **XRT**
- Most sarcomas are large, grow rapidly, and are painless
- Sx's: asymptomatic mass (MC), GI bleed, bowel obstruction, neuro deficit
- Dx: *MRI <u>before</u> biopsy* to rule-out vascular, major nerve, or bone invasion

- Biopsy:
    1) **Core needle Bx** (*best Dx method*; along long axis plane of future incision for en bloc resection; 95% accurate)
    2) If core needle not feasible or insufficient tissue:
        Longitudinal **excisional** Bx if < 4 cm → then go back for margins if sarcoma
        Longitudinal **incisional** Bx if > 4 cm (resect Bx skin site if Bx shows sarcoma when you go back for margins)
        Both of above along **long axis plane of future incision** for en bloc resection (ie incision along **long axis** of extremity)
- **Chest CT** - to check for **lung metastases** (*MC site for metastases*)
- Has **hematogenous spread** (not to lymphatics → node metastases rare)
    - Do not need lymph node dissection
- Most important prognostic factor - **tumor grade** (undifferentiated worst)
    - Staging based on **grade**, not size
- Tx: Want at least **2 - 3 cm margins** (elliptical incision, need margins around previous biopsy site) and at least **1 uninvolved fascial plane** → try to perform limb-sparing operation
    - 90% do not need amputation → *try for perform limb-sparing resection*
    - **Complete resection** best chance for survival
    - **Large tumors** (> 10 cm) may benefit from pre-op chemo-XRT → may allow limb-sparing resection
    - **Place clips** to mark site of likely recurrence → will XRT these later
    - Post-op **chemo-XRT** - for high-grade, close margins, or tumors > 5 cm
        XRT decreases local recurrence; no effect on survival
        Chemo - **doxorubicin** based
    - 5-YS (if complete resection) - **40%**
    - Midline incision favored for pelvic and retroperitoneal sarcomas
    - With resection, try to preserve motor nerves and retain / reconstruct vessels
    - Often have pseudocapsule but do not shell out → leaves residual tumor
    - **Isolated sarcoma metastases** without other systemic disease (eg lung or liver) - Tx: **resect** (best chance for survival; if diffuse metastases - palliate with XRT)
    - **Best prognosis** sarcoma metastases:
        Disease free interval > 12 months
        < 4 metastases
        Doubling time > 20 days
        Primary control
        Complete resection
- **Local recurrence** → re-stage (same as above) resection if resectable
- **Distant recurrence** (eg lung) → re-stage, resection if resectable
- There is a **poor prognosis** for sarcoma overall due to:
    - Delay in Dx
    - Difficulty with total resection and getting negative margins
    - Difficulty getting XRT to pelvic / retroperitoneal tumors (bowel in the way)
- **Head / neck** sarcomas - usually in children (usually rhabdomyosarcoma)
    - Hard to get margins because of proximity to vital structures (eg carotid artery, spinal cord)
    - Post-op XRT for positive or close margins as negative margins may be impossible to obtain
- **Retroperitoneal** sarcomas (MC - **liposarcomas**; others - malignant fibrous histiocytoma, leiomyosarcomas)
    - Almost half of all sarcomas present in the retroperitoneum
    - Generally present as **large tumors** (do not cause Sx's until mass effect occurs)
    - Complete en bloc resection with negative margins is most important prognostic factor - take everything you have to (eg kidney, spleen, colon, portion of liver)
    - Only 25% resectable with negative margins due to proximity to vital organs
    - Best chance for survival is a **negative margin resection**
    - Midline incision for pelvic and retroperitoneal sarcomas
    - **Poor prognosis** for retroperitoneal sarcomas due to:
        Delay in Dx
        Difficulty with total resection and getting negative margins
        Difficulty getting XRT retroperitoneal (bowel in the way)

- Local recurrence 40%
- Worse prognosis compared to sarcomas in other locations
- Often have pseudocapsule but don't shell out *(no enucleation)* → leaves residual tumor
- Need to rule-out **lymphoma** in this area (is the MC tumor in the retroperitoneum; Sx's - night sweats, fevers, chills, adenopathy)

- **Kaposi's Sarcoma** (see Infection chapter)
- **Childhood rhabdomyosarcoma**
  - *MC soft tissue sarcoma in children*
  - Head/neck *(MC site in children)*, genitourinary, extremities, trunk (poorest prognosis)
  - MC subtype - **embryonal**
  - Worst prognosis subtype - **alveolar**
  - **Desmin** - marker for rhabdomyosarcoma
  - Tx: surgery; **doxorubicin** based chemo
  - **Botryoides tumor** - vaginal rhabdomyosarcoma (Sx's - bleeding)
  - *MC malignant aural (ear) tumor of childhood*
- **Genetic syndromes for soft tissue tumors**
  - **Neurofibromatosis** - CNS tumors (acoustic neuroma), peripheral sheath tumors, pheochromocytoma
  - **Li-Fraumeni syndrome** - childhood rhabdomyosarcoma, early onset breast CA, sarcomas, leukemia, brain tumors, many more
  - **Tuberous sclerosis** - angiomyolipoma (benign)
  - **Gardner's syndrome** - familial adenomatous polyposis and intra-abdominal desmoid tumors
- **Neurofibromatosis**
  - Seen in von Recklinghausen's disease; autosomal dominant
  - Affects **neural crest cells** (Schwann cells, endoneurial fibroblasts)
  - Disordered **skin pigmentation** (café au lait spots, axillary freckling)
  - < 10% actually get CA
  - **Type I NF (neurofibromin** mutation)
    - **CNS** tumors (MC - acoustic neuroma)
    - **Peripheral nerve sheath tumors** (MC - neurofibroma, neurolemma)
    - **Pheochromocytoma**
  - **Type II NF (merlin** gene mutation) → *only get **acoustic neuromas***
  - **Schwannomatosis** - multiple schwannomas

MERKEL CELL CARCINOMA
- Neuroendocrine tumor of the skin (80% have Merkel cell virus, polyomavirus)
- Red to purple nodule or indurated plaque
- **Very aggressive** malignant tumor with early regional and systemic spread
  - Spreads through skin and lymph nodes
  - MC metastatic site - **bone**
  - 10% have **metastases** and 25% have **lymph node** spread at Dx
  - Has **neuron-specific enolase, cytokeratin,** and **neurofilament protein** staining (different from other skin CA's)
  - **Keratin antibodies** show **peri-nuclear** pattern
- Tx: resection with **2 - 3 cm margin**
  - All patients get SLNB or formal lymph node dissection
  - Post-op chemo-XRT
- 5-YS (all patients) - **60%**

GLOMUS TUMOR OF SKIN (from glomus body, not glomus cells)
- **Benign** painful tumor comprised of **blood vessels** and **nerves**
- MC location - **terminal aspect of digit** near or under fingernail (can also occur behind eardrum - blanches with pressure)
- Tx: tumor excision
- Is <u>not</u> a paraganglioma

PARAGANGLIOMA (chemodectoma)

- Rarely malignant; neural crest cells
- Part of autonomic nervous system
- From **glomus cells** (chemo-receptors that regulate blood pressure and blood flow to various area of body)
- MC location overall - **abdomen**
- MC ENT location - **carotid body** (ie carotid body tumor)
- MC thoracic location - **aortic arch**
- Can secrete **norepinephrine**; are highly **vascular**
- Tx: tumor excision

RETROPERITONEAL FIBROSIS

- Periaortic and retroperitoneal proliferation of fibrous tissue
- RFs: autoimmune disease, CA, methysergide, previous XRT, hydralazine, beta-blockers
- Sx's: usually related to **trapped ureters** and **hydronephrosis** (flank pain)
- Dx: **CT scan** *(most useful test)* - dense, **confluent mass** encompassing the great vessels and ureters; ureters are pushed **medially**; compression of ureters can occur (elevated BUN, Cr); elevated ESR
  - Need to **rule-out malignancy** (ie get Bx; CA can cause retroperitoneal fibrosis)
  - IVP can show medial deviation of ureters and compression
  - Can get lymphatic obstruction
  - IVC and pelvic vein compression can occur, increasing risk of DVT
- Tx: **corticosteroids** *(mainstay)* and immunosuppression (eg Tamoxifen, Imuran, Infliximab)
- Surgery if **renal function** becomes compromised (**stents** or **ureterolysis** [free up ureters and wrap in omentum]) - rule-out CA while in the abdomen
- Percutaneous **nephrostomy tube** if **pyelonephritis** develops (+ antibiotics), then treat ureters at a later procedure

OTHER CONDITIONS

Lip lacerations - important to line up vermillion border

Xanthoma - yellow, cholesterol-rich, histiocytes; <u>benign</u> tumor; can be associated with familial hypercholesterolemia; Tx - excision

Warts (verruca vulgaris) - HPV origin, contagious, autoinoculable, can be painful; Tx: topical **salicylic acid** *(best)*

Lipomas (MC mesenchymal tumor) - common but rarely malignant; usually on back, neck, or between shoulders

Neuromas - can be associated with neurofibromatosis and von Recklinghausen's disease (Café-au-lait spots, axillary freckling; peripheral nerve, and CNS tumors)

Keratoses
- **Actinic keratosis** - *premalignant*; tan, pink, or red; in sun-damaged areas; need excisional Bx if suspicious; Tx: topical **diclofenac sodium**
- **Seborrheic keratosis** - <u>not</u> premalignant (keratinocytes); trunk, elderly; can be dark (can look like warts)
- **Arsenical keratosis** - associated with squamous cell CA (SCCA)

Keratoacanthoma (from pilo-sebaceous glands)
- Rapid growth, rolled edges, crater filled with **keratin**
- 5% risk of SCCA (low grade)
- May involute spontaneously over months
- Always Bx these to be sure
- Tx: excision usually indicated

Bowen's disease - SCCA in situ; 10% become invasive SCCA; RF - HPV
- Tx: **Imiquimod**, liquid nitrogen cryoablation, topical 5-FU
- *Avoid wide local excision if possible* (high recurrence rate with HPV); get regular Bx's to rule-out invasive SCCA

Desmoid tumors - benign but locally very invasive (fibroblastic spindle cells; collagen)
- RFs: women, pregnancy, trauma, retroperitoneal fibrosis, FAP
- **Anterior abdominal wall** (MC location) - can occur with pregnancy; can also occur after trauma or surgery; usually along fascial plane

- **Intra-abdominal** desmoids are associated with Gardner's syndrome and retroperitoneal fibrosis; often **encases bowel** or mesentery making it hard to get en bloc resection
- High risk of **local recurrence**; no distant spread (do _not_ metastasize)
- Tx: surgery if possible; chemo (**sulindac** and **tamoxifen**) if vital structure involved or too much bowel would be taken (high risk of short bowel syndrome with surgery)
- If significant **small bowel or mesentery would be taken, excision not indicated** due to high recurrence, morbidity, bleeding risk, fistula rate, and risk of short bowel syndrome (give chemo only)

■ Hidradenitis - infection of the **apocrine sweat glands**, usually in **axilla** and **groin** regions; can occur in perianal and genital areas
- **Thick** and **fibrous** soft tissue areas (woody texture) from chronic infections; may have abscesses or sinus tracts; surrounding erythema
- MC organisms - staph / strep
- Medical Tx: antibiotics; avoid antiperspirants; improved hygiene; drain abscesses
- **Chronic refractory axillary hidradenitis** - surgery to remove skin and associated apocrine sweat glands (from fascia to skin) - no surgery with active infection

■ Hyperhidrosis - perfuse sweating, especially noticeable in palms
- Tx: try a variety of antiperspirants over 3 months
- **Sympathectomy** if affecting lifestyle
  - Ligate T2-T4 sympathetic chain (hook cautery)
  - Not above T2 ganglion - will get Horner's Syndrome (injury to T1 and the stellate ganglion)
  - Need to get **crossing nerve of Kuntz** on bottom of **2nd rib**
  - MC Cx - **compensatory sweating** in face, trunks, and legs (15%)

■ Benign cysts
- **Epidermal** inclusion cyst (MC cyst) - have completely mature epidermis with creamy **keratin** material; Tx: resection
- **Trichilemmal** cyst - in scalp, no epidermis (keratin from hair follicles); Tx: resection
- **Ganglion** cyst - over **joints** (MC area - **wrist**); filled with **collagenous synovial fluid**; Tx: aspiration cures 50%, remove check valve if surgery required
- **Dermoid** cyst - intra-abdominal and midline sacral lesions usual; Tx: need resection due to CA risk
- **Pilonidal** cyst - congenital coccygeal sinus with ingrown hair; gets infected and can form abscess; Tx - antibiotics, drainage, and packing if abscess; follow-up surgical resection

■ Keloids - autosomal dominant; dark skinned people higher risk
- **Collagen** (Type I and III) **goes beyond original scar** (main differentiation from hypertrophic scar)
- From **failure of collagen breakdown**
- Tx: **Intra-lesional steroid injection after keloid excision** (best Tx); others - silicone gel sheet or injection (preferably before development of keloids), pressure garments

■ Hypertrophic scar tissue
- Higher risk in dark skinned people
- Often on **flexor surfaces** of upper torso
- **Collagen stays within confines of scar** (differentiates from keloid)
- Often occurs with burns or wounds taking a long time to heal
- Tx: **steroid or silicone injections**; **pressure garments**

Statistics

1148. There were 172,000 new cases of lung CA diagnosed in 2015. This is an example of:
    a.   Prevalence
    b.   Incidence
    c.   Mean
    d.   Mode

Answer b. Incidence is the number of new cases in a certain time frame (usually a year). Prevalence would be the current number of people with the disease (or trait).

1149. In an investigational drug study for breast CA, patients were randomly assigned to either the experimental drug or Tamoxifen. Patients were not aware of which drug they were receiving however the physicians were aware. This would be an example of:
    a.   Cohort study
    b.   Retrospective review
    c.   Double blind randomized control trial
    d.   Single blinded randomized control trial

Answer d. Because the physicians were aware of whether or not the patients were receiving the drug or placebo, it is only a single blinded randomized control trial.

1150. Combining data from several independent trials investigating the same subject is a:
    a.   Cohort study
    b.   Meta-analysis
    c.   Double blind randomized control trial
    d.   Single blinded randomized control trial

Answer b. Meta-analysis combines data from many independent trials

1151. Sensitivity of a test reflects:
    a.   Ability to detect disease
    b.   Ability to say that no disease is present
    c.   Rejecting the null hypothesis when it is true
    d.   Accepting the null hypothesis when it is false

Answer a. Ability to detect disease

1152. Specificity of a test reflects:
    a.   Ability to detect disease
    b.   Ability to say that no disease is present
    c.   Rejecting the null hypothesis when it is true
    d.   Accepting the null hypothesis when it is false

Answer b. Ability to say that no disease is present

1153. Type I error reflects:
    a.   Ability to detect disease
    b.   Ability to say that no disease is present
    c.   Rejecting the null hypothesis when it is true
    d.   Accepting the null hypothesis when it is false

Answer c. Rejecting the null hypothesis when it is true

1154. Type II error reflects:
    a.   Ability to detect disease
    b.   Ability to say that no disease is present
    c.   Rejecting the null hypothesis when it is true
    d.   Accepting the null hypothesis when it is false

Answer d. Accepting the null hypothesis when it is false

1155. Statistical power of a test is:
      a.   = 1- probability of Type I error
      b.   = 1- probability of Type II error
      c.   = 1+ probability of Type I error
      d.   = 1+ probability of Type II error

Answer b. The **power** of a test is the probability of making a right conclusion. A large sample size will increase power (by decreasing the likelihood of a Type II error).

1156. The MC cancer death is from:
      a.   Lung Cancer
      b.   Breast Cancer
      c.   Prostate Cancer
      d.   Pancreatic Cancer

Answer a. Lung cancer accounts for more deaths than any other cancer.

1157. The HPV vaccine given to young women is an example of:
      a.   Screening
      b.   Primary prevention
      c.   Secondary Prevention
      d.   Tertiary Prevention

Answer b. The HPV vaccine is n example of primary prevention.

1158. Given a test with a high positive predictive value:
      a.   A negative result suggests the patient is very likely to have the disease
      b.   Prevalence of the disease in the population has no impact on the test
      c.   The false positives for the test are likely very high
      d.   A positive result suggests the patient is very likely to have the disease

Answer d. A positive result suggests the patient is very likely to have the disease

1159. An epidemiologic study is performed and the odds ratio for smoking and the development of lung cancer are performed. All of the following are true except:
      a.   Odds ratio is the odds of an event occurring in one group compared to the odds of that event occurring in another group.
      b.   An odds ratio of 9 in the above study would indicate smokers are 9 times more like to get lung cancer compared to non-smokers.
      c.   An odds ratio of 1 in a different study would indicate both groups are equally likely to develop the disease
      d.   Odds ratio is equivalent to sensitivity

Answer d. Odds ratio is defined as the odds of an event occurring in one group (group 1) compared to the odds of that event occurring in a separate group (group 2). The higher the odds ratio, the more likely the condition or event is going to occur in the first group.

1160. A retrospective study examined the effect of cytomegalovirus infection on chronic rejection in heart transplant patients. Which of the following is true?
      a.   A students T-test is most appropriate
      b.   An ANOVA test is most appropriate
      c.   A chi-squared test is most appropriate
      d.   There is no good test for this

Answer c. A **chi-squared test** is most appropriate.

BASIC RULES

- **Type I error** - rejects null hypothesis incorrectly (rejecting the null hypothesis when it is true); assumed there was a difference when no difference actually exists
- **Type II error** - accepts null hypothesis incorrectly; falsely assumed there was no difference when an actual difference exists
  - MC due to a **small sample size** (ie a larger sample size would have picked up the difference)
- **Null hypothesis**
  - The hypothesis that no difference exists between groups
  - A **p < 0.05** rejects the null hypothesis
- **p < 0.05** =
  - > 95% likelihood that the difference between populations is true
  - < 5% likelihood that the difference is not true and occurred by chance alone
- **Variance** - the spread of data around a mean value
- **Parameter** - a population
- **Numeric terms** - eg 2, 7, 7, 8, 9, 12, 14
  - **Mode** - the most frequently occurring value = 7
  - **Mean** - the average = 9
    - This is the best measure of **central tendency** when **values are distributed normally** (ie you do not have outliers)
    - There are no outliers in the above set of numbers, so the mean value is a good measure of central tendency
  - **Median** - middle value of a set of data (eg 50th percentile) = 8
    - This is the best measure of **central tendency** when **values are not distributed equally** (ie you have outliers)
    - Take example above, but add 85 and 86 (eg 2, 7, 7, 8, 9, 12, 14, 85, 86)
      - The **mean** would now be = 26 (this is not a good representation of **central tendency** due to the outliers 85 and 86)
      - The **median** would now be = 9 (this is a better representation of central tendency)
  - **Any set of numbers** (eg INR values, weight loss, WBC counts, Hct's, temp's) can be used for the above
- **95% confidence interval**
  - Instead of estimating the parameter by a single value (eg mean), this also includes an interval likely to include the parameter
  - Confidence intervals are used to indicate reliability of an estimate
  - Example:
    Following **lap banding**, mean weight loss for your patients is 125 lb
      95% of your patient have weight loss between 100-150 lb
      The 95% confidence interval for amount of weight loss in your population is (100,150) or there is a 95% probability that following lap banding, your patient will lose somewhere between 100-150 lb
    Written as: mean weight loss 125 lb [100,150]
  - The more narrow the confidence interval, the more accurate the estimate
    Example – for **gastric bypass**, mean weight loss was 130 lb [120,140]; 130 would be a more accurate estimate of weight loss in this population than 125 in the above lap banding population)
- **Prevalence**
  - **Number of people in a population** with the disease (eg number of patients in US with lung CA)
  - Longstanding diseases will ↑ prevalence
- **Incidence**
  - **Number of new cases** diagnosed over a certain time frame (MC annually; eg number of patients in US newly diagnosed with lung CA in 2011)
- **Relative risk** = incidence in exposed population / incidence in unexposed population
- **Odds ratio** - odds of an event occurring in one group (group 1) compared to odds of that event occurring in a separate group (group 2). The higher the odds ratio, the more likely the condition or event is going to occur in the first group.
- **Power of test** (probability of making correct conclusion)
  - = 1 - probability of type II error

- Likelihood that the conclusion of test is true
- **Larger sample size** increases power (by decreasing the likelihood of a type II error)

CLINICAL TRIALS AND STUDIES
- **Randomized controlled trial** (prospective study)
  - Prospective study with random assignment to treatment and non-treatment groups
  - **Avoids treatment bias**
- **Double-blind controlled trial** (prospective study)
  - A prospective study in which _both_ pt and doctor are blind to treatment
  - **Avoids observational bias**
  - Thought to be the best form of trials
- **Cohort study** (_prospective study_)
  - **Cohort** - a group of people who share a common characteristic
  - **Cohort study** - a prospective study comparing the cohort to either the general population of another group that lacks the characteristic
  - Example: prospectively following teenagers who smoke and comparing them to other teenagers who do not smoke in terms of developing lung CA
- **Case-control study** (_retrospective study_)
  - Retrospective study in which those with the disease are compared to a similar population without the disease
  - The frequency of the suspected risk factor is then compared between the two groups
  - _Main limitation for retrospective studies is_ ****selection bias** _(eg control group does not come from the same population as the case group)_
- **Meta-analysis** - combines the data from **different studies** on a specific disease process or treatment (eg combining the data from multiple studies examining the risk of stroke after CABG)

QUANTITATIVE VARIABLES (compares numbers)
- **Student's t test** (unpaired T test)
  - Two independent groups and variable is **quantitative**
  - Compares means (eg mean weight between group A and B)
  - Eg – a new preservation solution is used for lung transplant harvest and pO2 values are measured after transplantation. The average pO2 in the experimenta group is 350 mmHg. The average pO2 in the control group is 250 mmHg. A student's T test is used here to figure out if the 2 groups are significantly different.
- **Paired t tests**
  - Variable is **quantitative** with **before and after studies** (eg mean weight before and after treatment, comparing drug vs placebo)
- **Descriptive Statistics** - quantitatively describes the main features of a collection of data; the aim is to **summarize the data set** rather than use the data to learn about the population (describes the population; eg **age**, proportion of each **sex**, proportion with **co-morbidities**)
- **ANOVA** (analysis of variance)
  - Compares **quantitative** variables (eg means) for more than 2 groups (eg mean weight between groups A, B, C, and D)

QUALITATIVE VARIABLES (compares categories)
- **Non-parametric statistics** - compare **categorical** (qualitative) **variables** (eg diseases, medications, eye color); Non-numerical categories
- **Chi-squared test** - compares two groups based on **categorical** (eg qualitative) **variables** (eg number of obese patients with and without development of hyperlipidemia vs. number of non-obese patients with and without development hyperlipidemia)
- **Kaplan-Meier estimator** - estimates survival

DISEASE DETECTION

	Positive Test	Negative Test
Patients with disease	True-positive (TP)	False-negative (FN)
Patients without disease	False-positive (FP)	True-negative (TN)

Sensitivity
- Ability to detect disease = TP / (TP + FN)
- Indicates number of people who have the disease who test positive
- **With high sensitivity**, a **negative test** result means pt is very unlikely to have disease

Specificity
- Ability to state no disease present = TN / (TN + FP)
- Indicates number of people who do not have the disease who test negative
- **With high specificity**, a **positive test** result means patient is very likely to have disease

Positive Predictive Value - proportion of patients with a positive result who actually have the disease. This value does depend on the prevalence of the disease within a population. Tests with a very high positive predictive value have a low false positive rate and a positive result suggests the patient is very likely to have the disease.

PPV = TP / TP + FP

Negative Predictive value - determines the likelihood of not having the disease given a negative result. A test with a high negative predictive value will have a low false negative rate.

NPV = TN / TN + FN

Accuracy = TP + TN / TP + TN + FP + FN
Predictive value - is dependent on disease prevalence
Sensitivity and specificity - independent of prevalence

PREVENTION

Primary Prevention - avoiding disease altogether (ie vaccinations for HPV)
Secondary Prevention - focuses on early detection of the disease to prevent progression (ie pap smears, stress test, screening colonoscopy, screening mammograms, blood pressure checks)
Tertiary Prevention - decreasing the morbidity related to an established disease (i.e. controlling blood pressure in patients with HTN, screening and treatment of diabetics with eye, foot, and renal problems; HMG-CoA reductase inhibitors in patients with hyperlipidemia)

CPSIA information can be obtained at www.ICGtesting.com
Printed in the USA
BVOW06s1104071115

425672BV00009B/60/P